ESSENTIAL PEDIATRIC GASTROENTEROLOGY, HEPATOLOGY, AND NUTRITION

NOTICE

Medicine is an ever-changing science. As new research and clinical experience broaden our knowledge, changes in treatment and drug therapy are required. The authors and the publisher of this work have checked with sources believed to be reliable in their efforts to provide information that is complete and generally in accord with the standards accepted at the time of publication. However, in view of the possibility of human error or changes in medical sciences, neither the authors nor the publisher nor any other party who has been involved in the preparation or publication of this work warrants that the information contained herein is in every respect accurate or complete, and they disclaim all responsibility for any errors or omissions or for the results obtained from use of the information contained in this work. Readers are encouraged to confirm the information contained herein with other sources. For example and in particular, readers are advised to check the product information sheet included in the package of each drug they plan to administer to be certain that the information contained in this work is accurate and that changes have not been made in the recommended dose or in the contraindications for administration. This recommendation is of particular importance in connection with new or infrequently used drugs.

ESSENTIAL PEDIATRIC GASTROENTEROLOGY, HEPATOLOGY, AND NUTRITION

Stefano Guandalini, MD

Professor of Pediatrics
Chief, Section of Gastroenterology, Hepatology, and Nutrition
Department of Pediatrics
University of Chicago Children's Hospital
Chicago, Illinois

McGraw-Hill
Medical Publishing Division

NEW YORK / CHICAGO / SAN FRANCISCO / LISBON / LONDON
MADRID / MEXICO CITY / MILAN / NEW DELHI / SAN JUAN
SEOUL / SINGAPORE / SYDNEY / TORONTO

The McGraw·Hill Companies

Essential Pediatric Gastroenterology, Hepatology, and Nutrition

2 3 4 5 6 7 8 9 0   DOC/DOC   0 9 8 7 6

ISBN   0-07-141630-7

This book was set in Times Roman by International Typesetting and Composition.
The editor was James F. Shanahan; the editorial assistant was Marta V. Colon.
The production supervisor was Richard Ruzycka.
Project management was provided by International Typesetting and Composition.
The index was prepared by Susan Hunter.
RR Donnelley was printer and binder.

This book was printed on acid-free paper.

Cataloging-in-Publication data for this book is on file at the Library of Congress.

This book is dedicated to my most precious treasure, my family: my father and my mother, who have always encouraged me do my best, resisting however the temptation of taking myself too seriously; my wife, who has constantly and lovingly been my biggest supporter and patiently tolerates my excessive commitments; and my children, the masterpieces of whom I am truly proud.

But ultimately, this book is indeed dedicated to all our patients, from whom we constantly learn, and to whom this effort is caringly directed.

CONTENTS

CONTRIBUTORS

MARC BENNINGA, MD
Division of Pediatric Gastroenterology
Academisch Medisch Centrum
Amsterdam, Netherlands

LYNDA BRADY, MD
Assistant Professor of Pediatrics
Medical Director, Liver Transplantation Team
University of Chicago Children's Hospital
Chicago, Illinois

ROBERTO BERNI CANANI, MD
Department of Pediatrics
University Federico II
Naples, Italy

GRAZIA CAPUANO, MS
University Federico II
Naples, Italy

FRANCESCA CAVATAIO, MD
Children Hospital
"G. Di Cristina"
Palemo, Italy

PIA CIRILLO, MD
Department of Pediatrics
University Federico II
Naples, Italy

RAY E. CLOUSE, MD
Professor of Medicine
Division of Gastroenterology
Washington University School of Medicine
St. Louis, Missouri

NICOLINA DI COSMO, MD
Department of Pediatrics
University Federico II
Naples, Italy

ANGELA DYE, MS, RD, LD
Dietitian
Chicago, Illinois

JOANN KAISER FROEHLKE, MNS, RD, CSP, LD, CNSD
Nutrition Specialist
Pediatric Nutrition Support Service
University of Chicago Hospitals
Chicago, Illinois

RANJANA GOKHALE, MD
Assistant Professor of Pediatrics
Division of Pediatric Gastroenterology
University of Chicago Children's Hospital
Chicago, Illinois

STEFANO GUANDALINI, MD
Professor of Pediatrics
Chief, Section of Gastroenterology, Hepatology, and
  Nutrition
Department of Pediatrics
University of Chicago Children's Hospital
Chicago, Illinois

PUNEET GUPTA, MD
Assistant Professor of Pediatrics
Division of Pediatric Gastroenterology
Georgetown University Medical Center
Washington, DC

ZAHANGIR KHALED, MD
Department of Pediatrics
University of Chicago Children's Hospital
Chicago, Illinois

DONALD LIU, MD
Associate Professor of Surgery and Pediatrics
Surgeon-in-Chief
University of Chicago Children's Hospital
Chicago, Illinois

ERASMO MIELE, MD
Department of Pediatrics
University Federico II
Naples, Italy

JOHN S. MORRICE, MB
Paediatric Gastroenterology
Oxford University
John Radcliffe Infirmary
Oxford, United Kingdom

FERNANDO NAVARRO
Pediatric Gastroenterology
University of Chicago
Chicago, Illinois

GIUSEPPINA ODERDA, MD
Pediatric Clinic
University of Eastern Piedmont
Novara, Italy

LICIA PENSABENE, MD
Fellow in Gastroenterology
Children's Hospital
University of Pittsburgh
Pittsburgh, Pennsylvania

MICHELLE MARIA PIETZAK, MD
Department of Gastroenterology and Nutrition
Children's Hospital of Los Angeles
Los Angeles, California

ALBERTO M. RAVELLI, MD
Department of Pediatrics
University of Brescia
Brescia, Italy

MARIA TERESA ROMANO, MD
Department of Pediatrics
University Federico II
Naples, Italy

JOHN M. RUSSO, MD
Department of Pediatrics
University of Chicago Children's Hospital
Chicago, Illinois

ELIZABETH A. SALHAIMER, MD
Department of Surgery
Massachusetts General Hospital
Boston, Massachusetts

MIGUEL SAPS, MD
Children's Memorial Hospital
Northwestern University
Chicago, Illinois

MELANIE R. SILVERMAN, MD
Department of Pediatrics
University of Chicago Children's Hospital
Chicago, Illinois

ANNAMARIA STAIANO, MD
Department of Pediatrics
University Federico II
Naples, Italy

MINDY B. STATTER, MD
Assistant Professor of Surgery
Director, Pediatric Trauma
University of Chicago Children's Hospital
Chicago, Illinois

PETER B. SULLIVAN, MD, FRCP, FRCPCH
Department of Paediatrics
John Radcliffe Hospital
University of Oxford
Oxford, England

JAN TAMINIAU, MD
Department of Pediatrics
Academic Medisch Centrum
Amsterdam, Netherlands

ANTONINO TEDESCHI, MD
Division of Pediatrics
Reggio Calabria Hospital
Reggio Calabria, Italy

GIANLUCA TERRIN, MD
Department of Pediatrics
University Federico II
Naples, Italy

PIETRO VAJRO, MD
Department of Pediatrics
University Federico II
Naples, Italy

ADAM VOGEL, MD
Children's Hospital
Boston, Massachusetts

STUART ZWANG, MD
Pediatric Surgery
University of Chicago
Chicago, Illinois

PREFACE

The field of pediatric gastroenterology, hepatology, and nutrition has seen an outstanding expansion during the past decade or so. Advances in our understanding of common and complex diseases alike, made possible by new technologies, have made our field increasingly rich and complex.

A pediatric resident presented with a patient with gastroenterologic or liver disorder now faces new and demanding challenges, requiring clear, concise, updated information. While the role of pediatric gastroenterologists as teaching physicians is the cornerstone of an effective learning process, a written reference to adequately support it is necessary.

This book has been created to specifically answer this need.

Authored by a team of national and international experts, it aims to offer a rather comprehensive yet succinct presentation of most of the disorders that the pediatric residents are likely to encounter, with a major emphasis placed on the common ones. The formulary and the wide nutrition chapter are especially likely to be a resident's favorites.

The material included is articulated in convenient sections:

- *Approach to gastrointestinal signs, symptoms, and common tests.* Provides description of common signs and symptoms such as vomiting, diarrhea, constipation, jaundice, and so forth, suggesting an orderly approach to diagnosis and treatment.
- *Gastrointestinal disorders*
- *Liver and pancreatic disorders.* Systematic reviews of gastrointestinal, hepatobiliary, and pancreatic diseases, intend to offer updated and concise pathophysiologic data, followed by relevant clinical information and by correct diagnostic and therapeutic strategies, in line with the principles of evidence-based medicine, whenever possible.
- *Pharmacotherapy and nutrition.* This final section is composed of a formulary covering drugs employed in the treatment of GI and liver diseases, and an extensive chapter on the nutritional support, enriched by exhaustive and updated tables, detailing current data on most of the formulas available and their indications.

It is my hope that pediatric residents will find this manual a friendly and readily available assistant in their practice and a help in the never ending process of learning how to better take care of our patients' needs. Critiques and comments are welcome, as our field constantly evolves, and a new edition will sooner or later be needed!

ACKNOWLEDGMENTS

I am grateful for the enthusiastic support that all the authors gave to this work. They responded adequately to my call to create a unique book, rigorously based on evidence, and yet presenting the material in an accessible way. I wholeheartedly acknowledge their contribution.

ESSENTIAL PEDIATRIC GASTROENTEROLOGY, HEPATOLOGY, AND NUTRITION

I

APPROACH TO GASTROINTESTINAL SIGNS, SYMPTOMS, AND TESTS

C H A P T E R

1

RECURRENT VOMITING

Alberto M. Ravelli

INTRODUCTION

Vomiting is a very common but nonspecific symptom. Occasional and self-limited vomiting does not usually represent a problem, but when vomiting persists and becomes chronic or recurrent, a thorough evaluation and an effective therapeutic intervention are warranted. There are many different causes of chronic or recurrent vomiting, which are not necessarily obvious even after an accurate medical history and clinical examination. Furthermore, some disorders underlying vomiting may have a progressive course and vomiting itself, if not adequately treated, may lead to potentially severe complications. Finally, persistent or recurrent vomiting may impair the quality of life of patients and their families. The physician should therefore have the knowledge and the tools to pursue a rational and balanced approach to diagnosis and treatment of vomiting. Some recent developments—such as diagnostic hypotheses on cyclic vomiting syndrome (CVS), the withdrawal of the prokinetic drug cisapride from the market, and the development of novel antiemetics and potent inhibitors of gastric acid secretion—could have a significant impact on the diagnosis and management of vomiting disorders.

Abbreviations

CNS   Central nervous system
CRF   Corticothropin releasing factor
CT   Computerized tomography
CVS   Cyclic vomiting syndrome
GERD   Gastroesophageal reflux disease
GI   Gastrointestinal
NMRI   Nuclear magnetic resonance imaging

DEFINITION

Vomiting is the expulsion of gastric content through the mouth. The term vomiting is strictly used to identify *emesis*, i.e., the activation of the neural arc known as emetic reflex (see Fig. 1-1). Emesis is characterized by strong contractions of abdominal wall muscles and the forceful expulsion of gastric content through the oral cavity and is typically associated with *nausea*. Activation of the emetic reflex does not necessarily result in vomiting and may be limited to prodromal signs such as nausea, retching, and signs of autonomic arousal. *Regurgitation* differs from vomiting in both quantitative and qualitative terms, since it is the involuntary and effortless expulsion of small amounts or

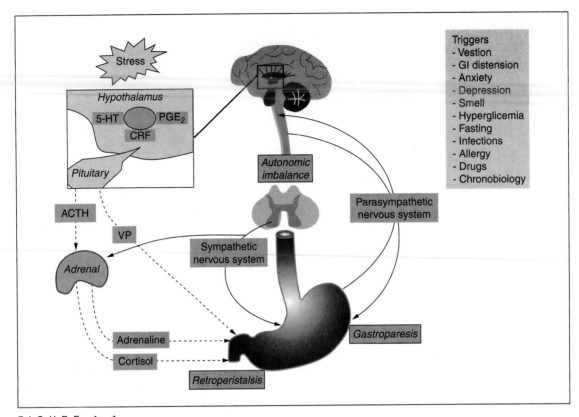

FIGURE 1-1

THE EMETIC REFLEX

"mouthfuls" of gastric contents and is not accompanied by nausea. On the other hand, the pathogenic mechanism underlying regurgitation—i.e., gastroesophageal reflux (see Chap. 13)—often causes the expulsion of large volumes of gastric content. It is important to appreciate, however, that the distinction between the two mechanisms may be difficult to recognize, especially in infants and young children, and the two mechanisms may be operating simultaneously.

According to the appearance of gastric content (which may also change during the day and with the evolution of the disease), four major types of vomiting can be identified:

1. *Alimentary vomiting.* This is made up of undigested or partially digested food, sometimes in abundant amounts. It is the most frequent type of vomiting and may occur immediately or a few hours after a meal. It is more often due to gastroesophageal reflux, either primary or secondary to anatomic malformations of the upper gastrointestinal (GI) tract, or to food intolerance. If it occurs several hours after feedings, it suggests mechanical or functional obstruction (hypertrophic pyloric stenosis, intestinal malrotation, achalasia). Obviously the main complication of alimentary vomiting is malnutrition.

2. *Acid vomiting.* Usually presents with small amounts of whitish, mucousy, and foamy material with pH <5, which may be expelled both during and after meals and sometimes at nighttime. It is often preceded or accompanied by irritability, restlessness, or crying in infants and epigastric pain or heartburn in children. It is

more typical of gastroesophageal reflux disease (GERD) and its main complications are esophagitis and, rarely, peptic stricture.

3. *Bilious vomiting.* It is characterized by the expulsion of thick yellowish-green fluid. In newborns and infants, bilious vomiting is always an ominous sign, suggesting total (atresia) or partial (stenosis) intestinal obstruction distal to the ampulla of Vater in the first place, and requiring immediate diagnostic definition and intensive or subintensive therapeutic support.

In older children, bilious vomiting most often represents the advanced phase of a vomiting attack where it follows the expulsion of food residues, gastric acid, and mucus, and as such is generally related to a persistent activation of the emetic reflex.

4. *Bloody vomiting (hematemesis).* Vomiting of bright red blood or coffee-ground material suggests, respectively, a recent or ongoing bleeding from the upper GI tract (esophagus, stomach, or duodenum). Since hematemesis is a complication rather than an initial manifestation of disease, the infant or child usually has already shown some symptoms or signs that might help identify the cause or site of the bleeding, such as regurgitation, heartburn or epigastric pain (peptic disease), chronic liver disease with portal hypertension (esophageal varices), and purpuric rash (coagulopathy). Intake of nonsteroidal anti-inflammatory drugs (NSAIDs), which may cause GI bleeding in the absence of any other symptom, should always be ruled out. Hematemesis is a potential emergency and the patient should always be evaluated in hospital. If the bleeding is mild and does not result in anemia or hemodynamic changes, the patient can be treated conservatively with antisecretory drugs, keeping in mind that the likelihood of detecting the source of bleeding is considerably reduced when endoscopy is carried out after the first 12–24 h. Hemorrhage from esophageal varices can be massive: this is always an emergency and as such should be immediately directed to a specialized unit for the treatment and support of GI bleeding. Hematemesis does not always

mean bleeding from the GI tract, however. If the patient "spits up" a small amount of blood and complains of a sore throat, hoarseness, or cough, bleeding most likely originates from the tonsils, larynx, or trachea and is generally self-limited. Furthermore, vomiting of dark blood and blood clots often follows a posterior nosebleed, often indicated by a small streak of blood in the oropharynx.

ETIOLOGY AND PATHOGENESIS

There are many different causes of vomiting. Broadly speaking, the major organic causes are digestive (gastrointestinal, hepatobiliary, or pancreatic), neurologic, urologic—which may require medical or surgical treatment—endocrine, and metabolic. Both vomiting and regurgitation can be "functional," i.e., unrelated to known organic causes but rather due to motor and/or sensory dysfunction of the GI tract and its connections with the central nervous system (CNS).

As already mentioned, two major pathogenic mechanisms may underlie the symptom commonly referred to as vomiting: the emetic reflex (*reflex* vomiting) and the incompetence of the antireflux barrier (*reflux* vomiting). The distinction between reflex vomiting and reflux vomiting—or between emesis and regurgitation—is of pathophysiologic value but can also be useful in clinical practice. This distinction is not always easy, however, because of the patient's age (infants and small children cannot report nausea verbally) and because symptoms such as irritability, restlessness, and autonomic arousal (e.g., pallor, sweating, tachycardia, salivation) may be related to activation of the emetic reflex as well as pain induced by acid or esophagitis. Furthermore, in some conditions—e.g., cow's milk allergy, visceral neuropathy or myopathy—both mechanisms can be operating and emesis and regurgitation may coexist.

The major manifestations of the emetic reflex are nausea and vomiting. Nausea is an unpleasant but not painful sensation, referred to the pharynx or the upper abdomen, associated with a desire or feeling of vomiting. Nausea can be brief or persistent, often occurs in "waves," and may precede vomiting or be the only major symptom. Vomiting is the forceful expulsion of gastroduodenal contents through the mouth and is usually, but not always, preceded by retching. Retching does not result in expulsion of gastric contents but involves the same muscle groups. Vomiting may alleviate nausea. As for other neural reflexes, there is a coordinating region, the so-called "vomiting center" in the CNS, where afferent stimuli are processed and integrated. From the vomiting center, coordinated motor outputs are sent to different target organs. The vomiting center is a functional concept rather than a clearly defined anatomic entity. It includes, among others, the reticular formation of the brain stem, the supraoptic and paraventricular nuclei of the hypothalamus, and the area postrema. The main emetic stimuli originate from the cerebral cortex and limbic system (vomiting induced by psychologic stress such as the so-called "anticipatory vomiting"), the vestibular system and the cerebellum (kinetosis or vomiting induced by vection), and abdominal or thoracic viscera (vomiting due to GI or cardiopulmonary disease). These stimuli travel along the afferent sensory fibers of the vagus nerve. The area postrema—previously known as chemoreceptor trigger zone—is a highly vascularized thin strip of gelatinous tissue located in the caudal end of the floor of the IV ventricle, outside the blood-brain barrier. Like carotid chemoreceptors, the area postrema receives inputs from emetic agents in the bloodstream, both endogenous (such as epinephrine, corticothropin-releasing factor [CRF], and cortisol in stressful conditions) and exogenous (such as apomorphine and cancer chemotherapy). Classic experimental studies have shown that ablation of the area postrema abolishes vomiting induced by chemical stimulation ($CuSO_4$) of the gastric mucosa. The stimulation of the vomiting center and area postrema triggers the cascade of events leading to the act of vomiting. Efferent motor outputs coming from the area postrema and vomiting center are both somatic (such as contractions of the diaphragm, anterior abdominal wall, and intercostal muscles) and autonomic. The autonomic output is targeted mainly to the cardiovascular system, respiratory tract, salivary, and sweat glands and results in tachycardia, tachypnea,

pallor, sweating, salivation, and pupillary dilatation. The GI tract is also heavily involved, with three major motor events affecting the foregut: relaxation of the lower esophageal sphincter, relaxation of the gastric fundus, and retrograde peristalsis. The latter two result in a marked impairment of gastric emptying and result from inhibition of the gastric pacemaker and subsequent production of gastric dysrhythmia. At the same time strong contractions of respiratory muscles occur against a closed glottis, resulting in esophageal dilatation. Retching becomes more and more frequent until the esophagus no longer empties its content into the stomach and finally one last violent contraction of abdominal wall muscles causes expulsion of gastric content. Serotoninergic 5-HT_3, dopaminergic D_1/D_2, tachykininergic NK_1, and CRF receptors play a major role in both the central and peripheral mediation of emesis. The neurophysiology of emesis can be used as a framework to explain, at least in part, the mechanisms underlying many cases of persistent or recurrent vomiting, and the chemoreceptor mechanism is indeed the target of most antiemetic drugs.

CONSEQUENCES AND COMPLICATIONS OF VOMITING

Severe vomiting may determine physical, metabolic, and psychologic consequences.

Physical Consequences

A rather common consequence of persistent vomiting is the rupture of capillary vessels in the subcutaneous tissue, presenting as "pinhead" hemorrhages of the face and neck. Severe complications such as esophageal tear (Mallory-Weiss syndrome), which may result in hematemesis and esophageal rupture (Boerhaave's syndrome) are fortunately uncommon in children. Also uncommon are rib fractures and serious abdominal muscle trauma. Herniation of the gastric fundus into the chest may occur in children who suffer from persistent severe retching following an antireflux procedure, especially the Nissen fundoplication. Postoperative vomiting—related to anesthesia and abdominal manipulation—may result in wound dehiscence. Malnutrition and aspiration of gastric content are more typically related to severe gastroesophageal reflux disease, especially in neurologically disabled children.

Metabolic Consequences

Dehydration, alkalosis, hypoglycemia, and ketosis are classic and well-known metabolic consequences of persistent vomiting. *Hypoketotic* hypoglycemia, on the other hand, is typical of certain disorders of amino acid metabolism. In some patients with cyclic vomiting, the syndrome of inappropriate secretion of antidiuretic hormone (SIADH) may occur.

Psychologic Consequences

Nausea is a powerful aversive stimulus. Persistent or recurrent activation of the emetic reflex may induce aversion, conditioning, sensitization, and even cross-reactive sensitization between different stimuli. Typical examples are the persistent aversion to foods which the patient was intolerant to in the past, the anticipatory vomiting in patients undergoing cancer chemotherapy or abdominal surgery, and the nausea and vomiting induced by vection in children with cyclic vomiting syndrome. Both emesis and GERD may induce anorexia, essentially as a consequence of the aversive conditioning determined, respectively, by nausea and heartburn during meals. These observations suggest that the sensitivity of the emetic reflex may be influenced or modulated by higher (cortical) stimuli and previous emetic events, although the neural pathways involved are unknown.

FUNCTIONAL DISORDERS CAUSING VOMITING

Functional Regurgitation of Infancy

This is the physiologic manifestation determined by a transient and relative incompetence of the lower esophageal sphincter leading to gastroesophageal reflux and is treated elsewhere in this book (see Chap. 13).

Rumination Syndrome

This condition is characterized by *voluntary regurgitation into the mouth* of recently ingested food, which is then chewed and swallowed again or, less commonly, spat out. Regurgitation of food is induced by voluntary repetitive contractions of the diaphragm and abdominal muscles, is not associated with nausea or pain, and ceases as the taste of food becomes acidic. The rumination syndrome mainly affects two different groups of patients: (1) infants aged 3–8 months who are neurologically healthy but "disabled" by lack of stimulation and emotional support, in whom malnutrition and developmental delay may develop; (2) patients of any age with psychomotor retardation, in whom rumination seems to be a rewarding and reassuring pastime. Quite often these patients are institutionalized or have emotionally distant or absent mothers. For a correct diagnosis it is essential to observe the patient during a meal without being seen, since the infant stops ruminating immediately if the child spots an observer. Besides malnutrition, signs of environmental, emotional, and affective deprivation may be noticed (including opposition behavior such as avoiding eye contact, hypertonia, and back arching). In these children, rumination may represent a compensatory behavior of rewarding self-stimulation. Occasionally, prolonged contact of the esophageal mucosa with acid may cause typical GERD complications (e.g., esophagitis, reactive airway disease, Barrett's esophagus, and esophageal stricture).

There is no definite therapeutic strategy for rumination syndrome. As in other functional GI disorders, the best results can be obtained with a multidisciplinary approach integrating medical and psychosocial skills ("biopsychosocial approach"). It is essential to reassure and educate the parents on the functional nature of the disorder, whereas pharmacologic therapy (prokinetic and antisecretory drugs) and nutritional rehabilitation should be restricted to those cases complicated by esophagitis and severe malnutrition. The diagnosis of rumination can be confirmed at follow-up, when the improved interaction between patient and caregiver is associated with normalization of feeding behavior and weight gain.

Functional Dyspepsia

Functional (nonulcer) dyspepsia is characterized by a variable combination of symptoms and signs pertaining to the upper GI tract—pain or discomfort, distention, bloating, early satiety, anorexia, nausea, and vomiting—lasting for at least 3 months in children who are obviously able to report such symptoms, i.e., usually school-age children. If these symptoms subside with defecation or are associated with changes in bowel habits, the appropriate diagnosis will be irritable bowel syndrome (IBS). In rare instances, functional dyspepsia and IBS coexist. Depending on the symptom complex, functional dispepsia is classified in subgroups: (a) ulcer-like (if upper abdominal pain prevails), (b) dysmotility-like (if nausea, vomiting, bloating, early satiety, and anorexia prevail), and (c) nonspecific (when the combination of symptoms does not fulfill the criteria for either of the above). Vomiting therefore is not a constant symptom. Dyspepsia symptoms are essentially nonspecific and there are no clinical criteria by which an organic cause can be ruled out with certainty. In these cases a 6–8-week trial with antisecretory drugs (e.g., ranitidine 2.5–5 mg/kg per dose, bid) or prokinetics (e.g., domperidone 0.2–0.4 mg/kg tid or qid) is justified in ulcer-like and dysmotility-like forms, respectively. If treatment fails or symptoms worsen rapidly, the patient should undergo an upper GI endoscopy with biopsy and/or other investigations (full blood count, erythrocyte sedimentation rate [ESR], liver and pancreatic function tests, celiac screen, hemoccult, abdominal ultrasound, lactose breath test). If endoscopy and biopsy show evidence of *Helicobacter pylori* infection, the patient should be prescribed an appropriate eradication therapy and eradication should be confirmed by ^{13}C urea breath test or *H. pylori* stool antigen. It should be remembered, however, that some patients may continue to have dyspeptic symptoms even after *H. pylori* has been eradicated.

Cyclic Vomiting Syndrome

Definition

Cyclic vomiting syndrome is a functional gastrointestinal disorder that can be identified by the occurrence of three or more episodes of intractable nausea and vomiting lasting hours to days separated by symptom-free intervals lasting weeks to months, in the absence of any known metabolic, neurologic, or GI abnormality. The mean frequency of attacks is 12 per year (range 1–70). Other symptoms indicating an autonomic surge such as lethargy, pallor, mild fever, skin blotching, headache, and abdominal pain may occur, and quite often these episodes appear to be triggered by physical or emotional stress.

Etiology and Pathogenesis

Although CVS was first described in the second half of the nineteenth century, its etiology is still unknown. Over the years a number of possible explanations have been proposed: migraine equivalent, abdominal epilepsy, psychodynamic alterations, disorders of gastrointestinal motility (most likely as part of an autonomic neuropathy), hypothalamic dysfunction due to reduced dopaminergic inhibition with secondary adrenal hyperstimulation (Sato's syndrome), fatty acid β-oxidation disorders, mithochondrial DNA mutations resulting in altered energy metabolism (especially disorders of the respiratory chain and fatty acid oxidation), and membrane ion channel disorders ("channelopathies") resulting in periodic depolarization of cell membranes. Indeed, CVS is probably an umbrella term encompassing several disorders of different origin with similar pathogenetic mechanism and clinical picture (Table 1-1). CVS is currently considered by most authors as a dysfunction of the brain-gut axis triggered by physiologic or behavioral reactions. Such a dysfunction may represent an exaggeration of normal defensive mechanisms—first of all the emetic reflex with all its different components—which developed teleologically in order to protect the host from the ingestion of noxious substances. A variety of stresses:

TABLE 1-1

PUTATIVE ETIOLOGIES OF CVS WITH MAJOR SUPORTING DATA

Migraine variant or equivalent

Frequent association of cyclic vomiting with headaches or migraine (including abdominal migraine)

Possible evolution of CVS into migraine

Positive family history of migraine

Similar occurrence (paroxysmal with symptom-free periods)

Several antimigraine drugs successful in CVS

Hypothalamic/adrenal dysfunction (Sato's syndrome)

Lethargy and hypertension common findings during attacks

Several symptoms compatible with adrenal activation

Metoclopramide not effective (and possibly counterproductive)

Possible response to COX-antagonists (e.g., ketorolac)

ADH raised in serum following vection-induced emesis

Effects of stress-induced CRF release on behavior, sympathovagal balance, and GI motility

Autonomic dysfunction

Evidence of autonomic dysfunction in a few patients with CVS

Impaired parasympathetic vagal tone caused by stress-induced CRF release

Increased gastric dysrhythmia and delayed gastric emptying in some patients during attacks

Increased sympathetic modulation and decreased vagal modulation of heart rate

Impaired neuroimmune interactions/food allergy

Functional GI disorders (e.g., IBS)—follows infection or is facilitated by allergic sensitization

Mast cell activation/degranulation in IBS and migraine

Mast cell activation/degranulation partly CRF dependent

Increased production of IL-6 in the stomach of patients with CVS

Attacks prevented in sensitized patients by appropriate exclusion diet

Fatty acid oxidation (FAO) disorder

Attacks triggered and induce ketosis induced by conditions of calorie deprivation

Clinical picture of few known FAO disorders undistinguishable from that of CVS

Normal metabolic profile during periods of well-being for some FAO disorders

Mitochondrial disease

Recurrent vomiting and migraine are common in patients with mitochondrial disease

Mutations of mitochondrial DNA (mtDNA) have been found in CVS patients and their mothers

Ion channelopathy

Similarities with paroxysmal disorder of nerve and muscle due to ion channel defect

Possible therapeutic effect of drugs interfering with ion channel function (Mg, propranolol, and so on)

Gastrointestinal motility disorder

Gastric dysrhythmia and delayed gastric emptying found in some patients during attacks

Possible therapeutic effect of the motilin-agonist erythromycin

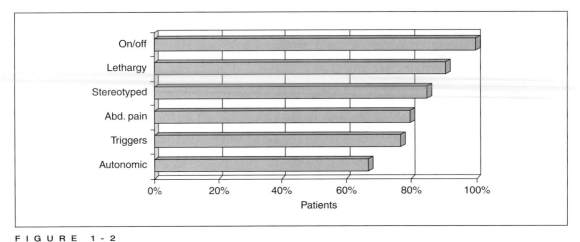

FIGURE 1-2
CYCLIC VOMITING SYNDROME—FEATURES OF ATTACKS

physical, metabolic (e.g., hypoglycemia), immune-allergic, and psychologic (positive or negative) may trigger an attack. As a response to stress, an increased secretion of ACTH releasing hormone (CRF) and vasopressin (ADH) from the hypothalamul-pitutary axis could mediate the activation of the emetic reflex leading to nausea and vomiting.

Clinical Manifestations

To date there are no clinical, biochemical, or instrumental markers of CVS. The diagnostic criteria for CVS are purely clinical and are based on a history of three or more episodes of severe unremitting nausea and vomiting lasting hours to days separated by symptom-free intervals lasting weeks or months, in the absence of any demonstrable gastrointestinal, neurologic, metabolic, or urinary abnormality. In the majority of patients, CVS has its onset in the preschool or school age. A family and/or personal history of migraine, motion sickness, and other functional gastrointestinal disorders (especially IBS) is common, occurring in 40–60% of cases. During the acute attacks the child looks pale, miserable, and usually lethargic. Lethargy can be so severe as to configure a so-called "conscious coma." Functional gastrointestinal symptoms (abdominal pain, diarrhea), migraine-like symptoms (headache, photophobia, phonophobia, intolerance to smell), and manifestations of autonomic arousal (mild

pyrexia, tachycardia, hypertension, skin blotching) often occur. A mild leucocytosis may be present. In the single patient acute attacks tend to be stereotypical with regard to time of onset, periodicity, duration, intensity, and symptoms. A physical or psychologic trigger can be identified in about 80% of cases (Figs. 1-2 and 1-3).

Diagnosis

Several organic disorders can mimic the clinical picture of idiopathic CVS. The differential diagnosis includes mainly brain tumors (particularly brain stem gliomas), obstructive uropathies, recurrent pancreatitis, intermittent intestinal obstruction, chronic intestinal pseudoobstruction, peptic disease, familial dysautonomia or Riley-Day's syndrome, and numerous endocrine and metabolic disorders such as pheochromocytoma, Addison's disease, diabetes mellitus, urea cycle defects, medium chain acyl-coenzyme A dehydrogenase deficiency, propionic acidemia, and acute intermittent porphyria (Table 1-2). Although the clinical history and negative clinical examination may suggest idiopathic CVS, an organic and curable disease should always be ruled out. Since no "minimum" diagnostic criteria exist and the cost/benefit ratio of the various biochemical and instrumental investigations has not been defined, the choice of the tests to be carried out relies on clinical judgment and idiopathic CVS is very

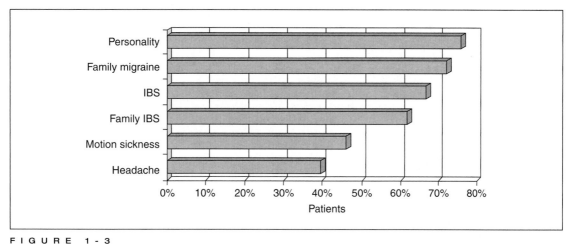

FIGURE 1-3

CYCLIC VOMITING SYNDROME—ACCOMPANYING SYMPTOMS AND FAMILY HISTORY

often a diagnosis of exclusion. A computerized tomography (CT) scan or—even better—nuclear magnetic resonance imaging (NMRI) of the brain and brain stem is recommended to rule out abnormalities of the CNS. A barium meal and follow-through may reveal anatomic abnormalities of the upper gut (e.g., malrotation) whereas abdominal ultrasound can exclude hydronephrosis as well as gallstones. Upper GI endoscopy with biopsy can be helpful to detect mucosal abnormalities such as peptic esophagitis (which is a common complication of CVS), *H. pylori*-related gastritis or ulcer, giardiasis, and allergic gastroenteropathy. Liver, pancreatic, and renal function should be tested and a metabolic screening including blood glucose, electrolytes, lactic and pyruvic acid, ammonia, creatine phosphokinase (CPK), carnitine, and acylcarnitine, as well as urinary amino acids, organic acids, catecholamines, δ-aminolevulinic acid, and porphobilinogen should be carried out. All of these biochemical investigations should be performed during an attack prior to any treatment (infusion of glucose) being given.

Treatment

To date there are no controlled therapeutic trials on CVS, and treatment of CVS remains largely empirical. Whenever possible, triggers should be identified and best avoided. If prodromal symptoms occur,

oral antiemetics (e.g., ondansetron), prokinetics (erythromycin), or cyclooxygenase (COX) inhibitors (ibuprofen, indomethacin, ketorolac) may abort an episode. Patients prone to severe attacks that cannot be controlled at home should be promptly admitted to hospital and treatment should be started as soon as possible. Novel antiemetics such as the 5-HT$_3$ receptor antagonist ondansetron, benzodiazepines such as lorazepam, phenotiazines such as chlorpromazine, and antihistamines such as diphenydramine—alone or in combination—or the antimigraine 5-HT$_{1D}$ receptor agonist sumatriptan may block or shorten an episode. Complications such as dehydration, acidosis, electrolyte imbalance, and peptic esophagitis can be prevented by IV infusion of glucose/saline solutions and H$_2$-antagonists such as ranitidine. The frequency and severity of attacks can be reduced by long-term prophylaxis with antiepileptic drugs (e.g., phenobarbital and carbamazepine), erythromycin (motilin receptor agonist acting as a prokinetic), and several drugs commonly used in the treatment of migraine: cyproheptadine and pizotifen (antihistaminergic and antiserotoninergic), amitriptyline (tricyclic antidepressant with serotoninergic action), propranolol (β-adrenergic receptor antagonist), and sumatriptan. Whenever emotional factors contribute to the disease and situations of conflict exist within the family, a support psychotherapy may be helpful.

TABLE 1-2

DIFFERENTIAL DIAGNOSIS OF CYCLIC VOMITING SYNDROME

Neurologic disease
Brain tumor with raised intracranial pressure
Brain stem glioma
Chiari malformation
Slit ventricle syndrome
Subdural hematoma or effusion
Abdominal epilepsy
Familial dysautonomia (Riley-Day's syndrome)
Anorexia/bulimia nervosa

Gastrointestinal disease
Intermittent gastrointestinal obstruction (e.g., pseudovolvulus, malrotation, and intussusception)
Recurrent pancreatitis
Pancreatic pseudocysts
Cholelitiasis
Chronic intestinal pseudoobstruction
Bochdalek hernia
Recurrent subacute appendicitis
Peptic disease
Intestinal parasites (*Giardia lamblia*)

Urinary tract disease
Obstructive uropathy (acute intermittent hydronephrosis)

Metabolic disease
Medium chain acyl-CoA dehydrogenase (MCAD) deficiency
Short chain acyl-CoA dehydrogenase (SCAD) deficiency
Short chain 3-hydroxy acyl-CoA dehydrogenase (SHCAD) deficiency
Glutaric acidemia type II (late-onset intermittent form)
Propionic acidemia
Isovaleric acidemia (chronic intermittent form)
Partial ornithine-transcarbamylase (OTC) deficiency
Porphyria (acute intermittent form)

Endocrine disease
Pheocromocytoma
Adrenal insufficiency (Addison's disease)
Insulin-dependent diabetes mellitus

Münchausen's syndrome by proxy
Intentional ipecac poisoning

SEVERE INTRACTABLE VOMITING AND DYSPEPSIA

Patients with severe vomiting or dyspepsia—almost always dysmotility-like—unresponsive to conventional medical treatment should be referred to centers specializing in functional and GI motility disorders. Here investigations such as measurement of gastric emptying and intestinal transit, antroduodenal manometry, electrogastrography, and barostat studies can be carried out to identify rare conditions such as intestinal pseudoobstruction (neuropathic or myopathic), gastroparesis, and visceral hyperalgesia. Prior to these specialist investigations, however, a plain abdominal x-ray and a barium meal with follow-through should be carried out, since in most pseudoobstructive disorders air-fluid levels and segmental dilatations of the gut can be seen. In a few cases of unexplained intractable vomiting and dyspepsia gastric electrical activity is severely disturbed ("tachygastria"), leading to electromechanical uncoupling and intractable gastroparesis. In such cases, electrical pacing of the gastric antrum by means of portable devices with electrodes implanted in the gastric serosa may be helpful in relieving symptoms and improving gastric emptying.

DIFFERENTIAL DIAGNOSIS OF CHRONIC AND CYCLIC VOMITING

To correctly address the diagnostic procedure, the possible causes of vomiting should be considered in the light of clinical findings and the personal and family history of the patient. Many patients with CVS, for instance, have a positive family history for migraine, CVS, or IBS. Detailed information should

be obtained regarding symptoms, including age and mode of onset, relation with meals or stressful events (e.g., intercurrent illness, prolonged fasting, and emotional distress), pattern of vomiting (chronic or cyclic, effortless or forceful), and associated signs and symptoms (e.g., nausea and other intestinal or extraintestinal manifestations). This information makes it possible to restrict the range of etiologic possibilities and to better address biochemical and instrumental investigations. A very useful distinction is based on the vomiting pattern (Fig. 1-4). Chronic vomiting is usually not severe but occurs nearly every day with a frequency of <4 emeses per hour and >2 episodes per week, whereas cyclic vomiting is severe but intermittent, with a frequency of ≥4 emeses per hour and <2 episodes per week. "Because the symptom is more severe," children with cyclic vomiting need hospital admission for IV hydration more often than children with chronic vomiting. Neurologic, metabolic, and endocrine causes prevail in children with cyclic vomiting, whereas GI disorders (e.g., GERD) more often underlie chronic vomiting. Furthermore, cyclic vomiting occurs at night much more often than chronic vomiting (Fig. 1-5). Finally, a personal and family history of migraine is much more common in patients with CVS than patients with chronic vomiting.

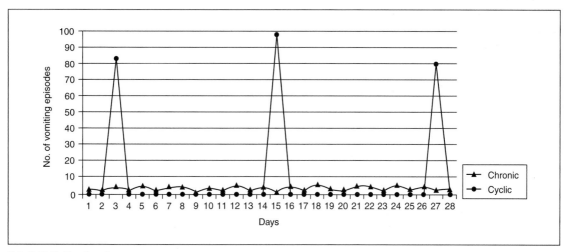

FIGURE 1-4

DIFFERENTIATING RECURRENT VOMITING FROM CYCLIC VOMITING SYNDROME: FREQUENCY OF ATTACKS

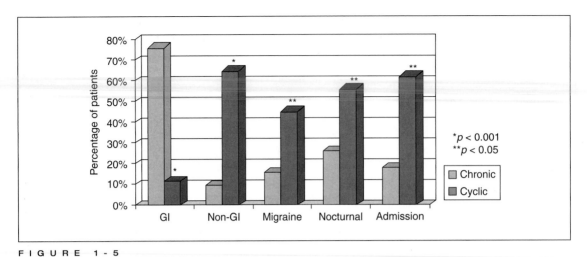

FIGURE 1-5
DIFFERENTIATING RECURRENT VOMITING FROM CYCLIC VOMITING SYNDROME: OTHER FEATURES

Bibliography

Andrews PL, Hawthorn J. The neurophysiology of vomiting. *Baillieres Clin Gastroenterol* 2:141–168, 1988.

Fleisher DR, Feldman EJ. The biopsychosocial model of clinical practice in functional gastrointestinal disorders. In: Hyman PE (ed.), *Pediatric Functional Gastrointestinal Disorders*. New York, NY: Academy Professional Information Services, 1999, pp. 1.1–1.20.

Li BUK, Fleisher DR. Cyclic vomiting syndrome: features to be explained by a pathophysiological model. *Dig Dis Sci* 44(Suppl 8):13S–18S, 1999.

Rasquin-Weber A, Hyman PE, Cucchiara S, Fleisher DR, Hyams JS, Milla PJ, Staiano A. Childhood functional gastrointestinal disorders. *Gut* 45(Suppl):II60–II68, 1999.

Ravelli AM. Cyclic vomiting syndrome: new clues for an old disease. *Gastroenterol Int* 14:65–72, 2001.

2

ACUTE DIARRHEA

Stefano Guandalini

INTRODUCTION

Acute diarrhea is defined as an increased fluid content of the stool above the normal value of approximately 10 mL/kg per day in children and 200 g/24 h in adolescents and adults. For practical purposes, diagnostic criteria in children—except for exclusively breast-fed infants—include a decrease in consistency (loose or liquid) and increase in frequency of bowel movements to ≥3 per 24 h. In acute diarrhea, vomiting is often present too, thus increasing the consequent risk of dehydraton. The familiar term "gastroenteritis" should not be used because: (1) not every instance of acute diarrhea is due to an inflammation of the gastrointestinal (GI) tract as the term implies and (2) even when an infection causes the symptomatology, the involvement of the stomach, as the term would imply, is far from constant.

EPIDEMIOLOGY

Acute diarrhea episodes are for the vast majority due to infections of the gastrointestinal tract and continue to be a major problem for worldwide child health. Even in developed countries, where prevalence of acute diarrhea has drastically declined in the past decades, the attack rate is 1–2 illnesses per individual per year in the general population, and is higher in the first 3 years of life (2.5 episodes per child per year up to 5 in those attending day care centers). In the United States, this leads to more than 200,000 hospital admissions and about 400 deaths per year.[1]

ETIOLOGY

Even though gastrointestinal infections are by far the most common cause for acute diarrhea, the pediatrician should always be aware that acute diarrhea is indeed a symptom that can be caused by many different disorders. Table 2-1 lists these potential *other* causes.

Many pathogens can be responsible for infectious diarrhea. Table 2-2 lists the main microorganisms known to cause acute diarrhea in children of developed countries. The relative incidence of any particular pathogen varies widely between different geographic areas and different age groups. Bacteria are generally more common in the first few months of life and then again in school-age children. *Rotavirus*, the single most pervasive cause of infectious diarrhea worldwide, peaks between the ages of 6 and 24 months. In developed countries, intestinal infections are usually sporadic, but outbreaks of food-borne or water-borne infections are well described and continue to occur.

TABLE 2-1

CAUSES OF ACUTE DIARRHEA NOT RELATED TO INTESTINAL INFECTIONS

Extraintestinal Infections
Urinary tract infections
Upper respiratory tract infections
Otitis media
Meningitis
Surgical Conditions
Acute appendicitis
Intussusception
Drug Induced
Antibiotic associated
Other drugs
Food Allergies
Cow's milk protein allergy
Soy protein allergy
Multiple food allergies
Disorders of Digestive/Absorptive Processes
Sucrase-isomaltase deficiency
Late-onset (or "adult type") hypolactasia
Malrotation
Hirschsprung's disease (enterocolitis variant)
Ileus
Necrotizing enterocolitis
Jejunal and ileal diverticula
Irritable bowel syndrome

TABLE 2-2

MOST COMMON INFECTIOUS CAUSES OF ACUTE DIARRHEA IN CHILDREN IN DEVELOPED COUNTRIES

Viruses
Rotavirus
Calicivirus
Norwalk-like virus
Astrovirus
Enteric-type adenovirus
Bacteria
Campylobacter jejuni
Salmonella
Escherichia coli
Enterotoxigenic (ETEC)
Enteropathogenic (EPC)
Enteroaggregative (EAEC)
Enteroinvasive (EIEC)
Enterohemorragic (EHEC)
Diffusely adherent (DAED)
Shigella
Yersinia enterocolitica
Clostridium difficile
Vibrio parahaemolyticus
Aeromonas hydrophila
Plesiomonas shigelloides
Parasites
Cryptosporidium parvum
Giardia lamblia
Isospora belli

In patients with acquired immunodeficiency syndrome (AIDS), a much wider array of pathogens is seen. Etiologic diagnosis, rarely necessary in sporadic cases occurring in immunocompetent children.

It should be noted that despite a thorough search for the cause of acute diarrhea in children, only in 60–70% of cases is it possible to identify an etiology (usually an intestinal infection). Regardless of the cause, typically acute diarrhea in developed countries runs a mild course and resolves, by definition, in less than 14 days. Currently, it is estimated that the mean duration of acute diarrhea in developed countries is about 5 days, with only 10% of children running a course longer than 7 days.[2] When the course continues beyond 14 days (a rare occurrence), then the clinical definition changes to persistent or prolonged diarrhea, an entity that should be considered and dealt within the realm of chronic diarrhea (see Chap. 3).

In this chapter, the management of acute diarrhea in immunocompetent infants and children will be discussed exclusively.

PATHOGENESIS AND CLINICAL FEATURES

The imbalance between intestinal absorptive and secretory processes that ultimately is responsible for diarrhea in all cases can be the result of many different mechanisms of action. From a practical point of view, it is useful to distinguish between *secretory* (noninflammatory, watery) and *inflammatory* (due to invasive pathogens, dysenteric) diarrhea. Table 2-3[3] reports the prevailing mechanisms for each of the main groups of pathogens according to their location, as well as the corresponding main clinical features.

In secretory diarrhea, the main symptom is profuse, watery, nonbloody diarrhea typically associated with only minor or no vomiting. This pattern is seen when the etiology is from pathogens localizing mostly in the small intestine such as enteric viruses, bacteria that do not invade the intestinal wall or the bloodstream (ETEC, EPEC, DAEC,

EAggEC) and produce enterotoxins, and some parasites (*Giardia*, *Cryptosporidium*). In enterotoxin-induced diarrhea, one or more toxins are released by bacteria adhering to the small intestinal epithelium, that then specifically interact with brush-border bound receptors and then activate a cascade of events leading to the increase of intracellular levels of cyclic AMP, cyclic GMP, or calcium and ultimately resulting in active secretion of chloride and, thus, of water. This occurs in morphologically entirely normal intestine, i.e., without any evidence of inflammation or damage to the intestinal mucosa.

TABLE 2-3

PATHOGENIC MECHANISMS AND CORRESPONDING CLINICAL FEATURES ACCORDING TO LOCALIZATION OF THE MAIN INTESTINAL PATHOGENS

Predominant Pathogenesis[a]	Site of Infection	Agent	Clinical Features
Direct cytopathic effect	Proximal small intestine	Rotavirus Enteric-type adenovirus Calicivirus Norwalk-like virus EPEC *Giardia*	Copious watery diarrhea, vomiting, mild-to-severe dehydration; frequent lactose malabsorption, no hematochezia Course may be severe
Enterotoxigenicity	Small intestine	*Vibrio cholerae* Enterotoxigenic *E. coli* Enteroaggregative *E. coli* *Klebsiella pneunoniae* *Citrobacter freundii* *Cryptosporidium*	Water diarrhea (can be copious in cholera or ETEC), but usually mild course. No hematochezia
Invasiveness	Distal ileum and colon	*Salmonella* *Shigella* *Yersinia* *Campylobacter* Enteroinvasive *E. coli* *Amoeba*	Dysentery: very frequent stools, cramps, pain, fever, and often hematochezia with white blood cells in stools Variable dehydration Course may be protracted
Cytotoxicity	Colon	*Clostridium difficile* Enterohemorrhagic *E. coli* *Shigella*	Dysentery, abdominal cramps, fever, hematochezia EHEC or *Shigella* may be followed by hemolytic uremic syndrome

[a] Elaboration of various types of enterotoxins affecting ion transport has been demonstrated as an additional virulence factor for almost all of the bacterial pathogens.

Inflammatory diarrhea, instead, is characterized by gross (dysentery) or occult blood and/or increased number of fecal leukocytes, and is the result of invasion by bacterial pathogens that can either enter the intestinal wall (*Shigella*, enteroinvasive *E. coli* [EIEC], or *Clostridium difficile*) or potentially even penetrate through it into the bloodstream (*Salmonella*, *Campylobacter*, *Yersinia enterocolitica*, EHEC [O157:H7]).

Some bacterial causes of diarrhea may result in other serious long-term sequelae; EHEC infection may be followed by hemolytic uremic syndrome (HUS) and *Campylobacter jejuni* infection by Guillain-Barré syndrome.

In general, however, diarrhea in developed countries is basically a self-limited condition. If the proper replenishment of water and electrolytes lost with the stools is provided on an ongoing basis, hydration will be maintained, and the condition will fade within a few days. Indeed, presently a vast majority of children presenting for treatment of acute diarrhea in developed countries are either nondehydrated or only mildly dehydrated.

Dehydration remains in any case the most important complication of acute diarrhea, potentially leading to hypovolemic shock in severe cases.

Loss of fluid in the intestine is always accompanied by loss of electrolytes, mostly Na and Cl. In the vast majority of patients the loss is balanced, and so the acute diarrhea results in "isonatremic" dehydration. In developed countries electrolytes derangements are rare, with 1% of admissions having hypernatremia and even rarer findings of hypokalemia or hyponatremia. Hyponatremia is, however, common in children with shigellosis and in severely malnourished children. Signs alarming for hypernatremia include a doughy and velvety skin, dry mucous membrane, muscular signs such as twitching, hyperreflexia, and central nervous system symptoms—especially lethargy, irritability, and seizures. Metabolic acidosis of mild-to-moderate extent is rather common in cases where dehydration is moderate-to-severe.

MANAGEMENT

Assessing Dehydration

Assessment of the degree of dehydration is an essential step in the evaluation of a child presenting with diarrhea, since the degree of dehydration is the main criterion to decide on the type of rehydration (oral vs. intravenous), and thus it also determines the need for hospital admission. Ideally, comparing the actual body weight of a patient with a previous but recent measurement before onset of the disease provides the best estimate of the volume lost. In clinical practice however this is rarely possible; thus, a set of clinical symptoms and signs has been proposed that can be used to estimate the degree of dehydration (see Table 2-4). Dehydration is typically quantified based on the percent of total body weight loss, and categorized as mild (<5%), moderate (5–10%), and severe (>10%).

Managing Dehydration

Rehydration or maintenance of hydration is therefore the cornerstone of treatment. Until the mid-1960s,

TABLE 2-4

ASSESSMENT OF DEHYDRATION IN THE CHILD WITH ACUTE DIARRHEA

Hydration	0–5% Dehydration	5–10% Dehydration	10% or More Dehydration
General	Well	Restless	Lethargic
Eyes	Normal	Sunken	Very sunken
Tears	Present	Absent	Absent
Mouth	Moist	Dry	Very dry
Thirst	Drinks normally	Thirsty	Drinks poorly
Skin	Pinch retracts immediately	Pinch retracts slowly	Pinch stays folded

TABLE 2-5

MANAGEMENT OF DEHYDRATION DUE TO ACUTE DIARRHEA

- Estimate severity of dehydration (see Table 2-4)
- Children not dehydrated or with mild-to-moderate dehydration:

  ORS[a] given to restore hydration over 3–4 h:

      Mild dehydration (<5%): 30–50 mL/kg

      Moderate dehydration (5–10%): 50–100 mL/kg

- After achieving rehydration, prevention of recurring dehydration must be accomplished by supplementing ORS for ongoing losses (10 mL/kg per watery stool)
- Children with severe dehydration (10%) or shock. IV rehydration as follows:

  20 mL/kg of saline in 1 h, followed by:

      Replace 50% of calculate deficit during the first 4 h, 50% during 8 h with 0.45% saline/5% dextrose

      Continue with maintenance fluid therapy, 0.18% saline/5% dextrose. Add KCl 20 mmol/L of fluid after first

        urine is passed

      Switch to ORS as soon as tolerated

      Resume normal diet as soon as possible

[a] In developed countries, hypotonic ORS (Na 60 mmol/L, glucose 74–111 mmol/L) should be used.

this was accomplished almost exclusively via the intravenous route. Subsequently, after it became apparent that enterotoxigenic bacteria such as *Vibrio cholerae* or ETEC leave intact small intestinal mucosal morphology and absorptive functions, and in particular, the glucose-coupled Na influx across the small intestinal epithelial cells, it was realized that the ongoing absorption of Na and glucose during secretion promotes fluid absorption and allows rehydration to take place in spite of the ongoing fluid loss.

These concepts provided the pathophysiologic basis for the *World Health Organization* (WHO)-*United Nations Children's Fund* (UNICEF)-supported and highly successful global program for *oral rehydration therapy* (ORT). Oral rehydration solutions have proved both safe and effective worldwide in hospital settings and also in the home to prevent dehydration. Oral rehydration therapy is grossly underutilized in the United States, where health care providers tend to overuse intravenous hydration. For more than two decades, the WHO has recommended a standard formulation of glucose-based ORS with 90 mmol/L of sodium and 111 mmol/L of glucose, with a total osmolarity of 311 mmol/L. However, many *in vitro* and *in vivo* studies during the 1980s and 1990s had consistently shown that lower concentrations of sodium and glucose enhance solute-

induced water absorption and might therefore be superior to the solution with a higher osmolarity.

Reduced-osmolarity solutions have concentrations of glucose and Na inferior to those in the WHO solution; glucose ranges between 75 and 100 and Na between 60 and 75 mmol/L, so osmolarity is maintained at 225–260 mOsm/L (see Table 2-5). The only two ORS marketed in the United States that have a composition similar to the one described and that have been found safe and effective in maintaining hydration and correcting dehydration in children of developed countries are currently Infalyte (Mead-Johnson) and Pedialyte (Ross). Hypoosmolar ORSs appear to have the additional advantage of allowing a reduced stool output while being just as effective in obtaining and maintaining rehydration and can be safely given throughout the duration of diarrhea, as shown in both developed and developing countries. Indeed, a recent large metaanalysis of all published controlled trials comparing low-osmolarity solutions with standard WHO formulas concluded that "In children admitted to hospital with diarrhea, reduced osmolarity ORS when compared to WHO standard ORS is associated with fewer unscheduled intravenous fluid infusions, lower stool volume post-randomization, and less vomiting. No additional risk of developing hyponatremia when compared with WHO standard ORS was detected."[4]

In a large metaanalysis, ORT was found to provide effective treatment for over 96% of children of developed countries, without any need to resort to intravenous rehydration.

In summary, ORT with a glucose-based ORS must be viewed as being by far the safest, most physiologic, and most effective way to provide rehydration and maintain hydration in children with acute diarrhea and mild-to-moderate dehydration worldwide, as recommended by WHO, *European Society of Pediatric Gastroenterology Hepatology and Nutrition* (ESPGHAN), and the *American Academy of Pediatrics* (AAP).

Intravenous therapy should be used in very few patients with acute diarrhea when the following circumstances are met:

- 10% or more dehydration
- Shock
- Failure of oral rehydration therapy
- Unconscious state

It is safe to assume that a child fulfilling any of these criteria should be admitted to the hospital for proper treatment.

Fluids commonly used instead of proper ORS include tea, cola drinks, fruit juices, and chicken broth. Such beverages contain totally inappropriate electrolyte (low sodium and potassium) and carbohydrate concentrations, are very often hyperosmotic, and are potentially dangerous in a dehydrated child, leading to hypernatremic dehydration.

Table 2-4 provides a scheme of practical recommendations for the management of dehydration in children with acute diarrhea.

Labs to Obtain

Electrolytes

The American Academy of Pediatrics recommends checking serum electrolyte levels in moderately dehydrated children when the history of diarrhea is not obvious, as well as in all severely dehydrated children. Electrolytes should also be measured in children with clinical features suggesting hypernatremic dehydration that can possibly result from ingestion of hypertonic fluids.

Microbiology

Episodes of acute infectious diarrhea resolve for the most part spontaneously without any antimicrobial treatment, which can actually be even contraindicated (as in the case of *Salmonella*, where it may prolong the carrier state or of EHEC, where there is the possibility that treatment enhances release of the cytotoxin responsible for HUS). For this reason, no stool cultures are usually required. In addition, routine stool cultures in acute diarrhea are known to have a very low diagnostic yield (not higher than 5%) and a relatively high cost. When dealing with particular epidemiologic circumstances, such as outbreaks that may carry a public health threat, obviously detection of the responsible pathogen must be sought. Stool cultures should also be obtained in cases where a pathogen potentially treatable is suspected. These circumstances basically coincide with the dysenteric form of diarrhea where, for instance, *Shigella* or *C. difficile* can be found. Finally, a history suggesting food-borne disease should also prompt appropriate stool cultures.

Hospitalized children may acquire intestinal infections leading to diarrhea mostly in the form of either rotavirus (especially during the first 3–4 years of age) or of *C. difficile* (in later ages). These pathogens should therefore be searched in these cases; stool cultures for standard bacterial pathogens are not needed for episodes occurring after third day in hospital, since the yield is very low.

NUTRITIONAL MANAGEMENT

In spite of the time-honored and diffuse practice of withholding feeds during acute diarrhea, many controlled trials have clearly shown the beneficial effect of early feeding. Based on this evidence, ESPGHAN recently recommended, in line with AAP and WHO, that mild to moderately dehydrated children should, after rapid rehydration, be offered a rapid reintroduction of normal feeds. Early feeding has many well-documented positive effects: (1) it reduces the intestinal permeability increased by infection, (2) it minimizes protein and energy deficits, and (3) it maintains growth. All of this is accomplished at no cost in terms of worsening diarrhea, prolonging it, or increasing incidence of emesis.[4]

Breast-feeding

Infants who are exclusively breast-fed should continue breast-feeding at all times. This has long been shown to result in decreased stool output and shorter duration of diarrhea.

Non-Breast-Fed Infants

Lactose-containing formulas have been held responsible for prolongation of diarrhea, and for a long time their use has been discouraged. A number of different formulas—particularly soy-based ones—are being recommended instead. In reality, in the vast majority of children, and especially the well-nourished infants of developed countries, lactose-free formulas do not offer any evident advantages. ESPGHAN[5] recommends that the normal diet should be resumed without restriction of lactose intake. However, if diarrhea does worsen on the reintroduction of milk, stool pH and/or reducing substances should be checked and lactose content reduced if the stool has a pH below 5.5 and contains >0.5% reducing substances. Table 2-6 summarizes recommendations for nutritional management.

TABLE 2-6
NUTRITIONAL MANAGEMENT

> Rapid reintroduction of an age-appropriate normal diet (including solids) should take place after rehydration for 3–4 h with ORS is accomplished
> Routine use of special formula is unjustified
> Routine use of diluted formula is unjustified
> Continuation of breast-feeding at all times is recommended

PHARMACOLOGIC THERAPY

Antibiotics

Acute infectious diarrhea is self-limited and antibacterial drugs are generally unnecessary, even when a bacterial cause is suspected. Routine use of antibacterial agents is recommended only for shigellosis, suspected cases of cholera, symptomatic infection with invasive intestinal *Entamoeba histolytica*, and laboratory-proven symptomatic infection by *Giardia intestinalis*. In addition, antimicrobial therapy is recommended for infections with *Salmonella* in patients who are at increased risk for invasive disease: (1) infants younger than 6 months of age; (2) children with sickle cell disease, malignant neoplasms, HIV infection or other immunosuppressive illness or therapy, chronic gastrointestinal tract disease, or severe colitis. Antibiotic treatment should be preceded by appropriate stool cultures. Table 2-7 reports indications for antimicrobial treatment in acute diarrhea.

Antiemetics

Vomiting is a common symptom in children with acute infectious diarrhea. The common antiemetics metoclopramide, prochlorprezine, and promethazine

TABLE 2-7
ANTIMICROBIAL THERAPY

> Obtain stool cultures
> Antimicrobial therapy is recommended for:
> - Shigellosis
> - Suspected cases of cholera
> - Symptomatic infection by invasive intestinal *Entamoeba histolytica*
> - Documented, symptomatic infection by *Giardia intestinalis*
> - Suspected infection with enteroinvasive bacteria in patients with an increased risk of invasive disease: infants younger than 6 months of age and children with hemoglobinopathies, malignant neoplasms, HIV infection or other immunosuppressive illness or therapy, chronic gastrointestinal tract disease, or severe colitis

hydrochloride all possess however troublesome side effects, including sedation and extrapyramidal reactions, and should be avoided in infants and young children with vomiting associated with acute diarrhea. Ondansetron, a specific serotonin antagonist, decreases vomiting in children with acute diarrhea and may have a valuable role as an antiemetic therapy.

Antimotility Agents

Several agents (e.g., loperamide, diphenoxylate, and codeine) are available that would slow down intestinal motility, thus theoretically improving diarrhea. Although these agents enjoy a wide popularity, they should never be used in cases suspected or proven to be of invasive etiology, for the risk of protracting or worsening the infection. But more in general, no antimotility treatment is needed for acute diarrhea in infants and young children. In fact, these drugs have a very narrow "therapeutic window" and have caused many adverse events. They include lethargy, ileus, respiratory depression, and even death.

New Agents

1. Recently, a new agent that inhibits intestinal enkephalinase has been studied in adults and children with severe diarrhea: racecadotril (acetorphan). The drug, which *in vivo* has been effective in reducing jejunal secretion stimulated by cholera toxin, has been experimented initially in adults with acute-onset diarrhea and later also in children with acute diarrhea of various etiologies, but mostly owing to rotavirus. In both pediatric studies, the drug given at 1.5 mg three times a day significantly reduced the stool output and the duration of diarrhea compared with placebo.[6]

   While these data are certainly promising, the drug will need further studies and analysis of cost-effectiveness before being recommended.

2. One of the most rapidly expanding areas in the treatment and prevention of diarrheal disease has been the use of "probiotics," a term meant to stress the derivation of these bacteria from healthy, live microflora, and their beneficial effect on the host. Among the most thoroughly investigated probiotics, *Lactobacillus rhamnosus* strain GG (ATCC 53103) has been shown to transiently colonize the human gut, unlike the strains employed for the production of commonly marketed yogurts. *Lactobacillus* GG has a number of diverse, potentially beneficial, biological effects, and in several well-conducted clinical trials, it proved effective in the prevention and in the treatment of acute diarrheal disease in children and in adults. The effect is most evident in rotavirus diarrhea, where a shortening of the duration of the illness, prevention of a protracted course, and reduced duration of viral shedding have been documented. Three rigorous metaanalyses have confirmed their safety and effectiveness.[7] This modality of treatment therefore shows exciting promise.

   It must be stressed that the beneficial effects of probiotics in acute diarrhea in children seem to be significant in watery diarrhea and viral gastroenteritis, but not evident in invasive, bacterial-induced diarrhea.

References

1 Herikstad H, Yang S, Van Gilder T, et al. A population-based estimate of the burden of diarrhoeal illness in the United States: FoodNet, 1996-7. *Epidemiol Infect* 129:9–17, 2002.

2 Guandalini S, Pensabene L, Zikri MA, et al. *Lactobacillus* GG administered in oral rehydration solution to children with acute diarrhea: a multicenter European trial. *J Pediatr Gastroenterol Nutr* 30: 54–60, 2000.

3 Guandalini S. Acute diarrhea. In: Walker WA, Goulet, O, Kleinman RE, Sherman PM, Shneider BI, Sanderson IR (eds.), *Textbook of Pediatric Gastrointestinal Diseases*. Hamilton, ON: BC Decker, 2000, pp. 3.1–3.23.

4 Hahn S, Kim S, Garner P. Reduced osmolarity oral rehydration solution for treating dehydration caused by acute diarrhoea in children. *Cochrane Database Syst Rev* CD002847, 2002.

5 Sandhu BK, Isolauri E, Walker-Smith JA, et al. A multicentre study on behalf of the European Society

of Paediatric Gastroenterology and Nutrition Working Group on Acute Diarrhoea. Early feeding in childhood gastroenteritis. *J Pediatr Gastroenterol Nutr* 24:522–527, 1997.

6   Salazar-Lindo E, Santisteban-Ponce J, Chea-Woo E, Gutierrez M. Racecadotril in the treatment of acute watery diarrhea in children. *N Engl J Med* 343: 463–467, 2000.

7   Van Niel CW, Feudtner C, Garrison MM, Christakis DA. Lactobacillus therapy for acute infectious diarrhea in children: a meta-analysis. *Pediatrics* 109: 678–684, 2002.

3

CHRONIC AND INTRACTABLE DIARRHEA

Roberto Berni Canani, Pia Cirillo, and Gianluca Terrin

INTRODUCTION

The intestine is lined with a continuous layer of polarized epithelial cells. The intestinal epithelium has long been recognized as a site for the absorption of nutrients, water, and electrolytes against large gradients. Water freely passes through the intestinal mucosa in response to the osmotic gradient created by Na^+ transport that is accomplished by electrogenic and neutral Na^+ pumps. The presence of mucosal folds, valvulae conniventes, villi, and microvilli in the small intestine produce a 600-fold increase in the absorptive area (approximately 2,000,000 cm^2, or the size of a tennis court, in an average adult). Because the net vector in the healthy intestine is in the absorptive direction, the recognition that the intestinal epithelium is also capable of active secretion of water and ions, even in health, is relatively underestimated. The small intestine secretes fluid and electrolytes under basal conditions and in response to a variety of physiologic stimuli, following food ingestion. Secretion occurs predominantly from the small intestinal crypts. Active secretion, and the fluid secretion that it produces, appears to serve a number of important physiologic functions. For example, the ability of the intestine to secrete water clearly contributes to the fluidity of the intestinal contents. This allows digestive enzymes to reach their targets and, in turn, allows digested nutrients to get the surface of the epithelium, where they are further hydrolyzed and absorbed. The ability of the epithelium to secrete particular ions may also serve specialized roles in specific segments of the intestinal tract. An example of this can be found in the proximal duodenum, where the secretion of bicarbonate by duodenocytes represents an important defensive factor that helps to protect the duodenal epithelium from acid damage. Some authors have also speculated that the ability of the epithelium to rapidly increase the rate of secretory transport may serve as a primitive host-defense mechanism. This would flush the lumen to free it of potentially harmful microorganisms, toxins, and/or antigenic substances, and thus may be a beneficial aspect of the diarrhea that often accompanies enteric infections. Given the physiologic and pathologic importance of secretion by the intestinal epithelium, many investigators have sought to understand its cellular and subcellular basis, as well as the endogenous factors that regulate it (see Table 3-1), and many new insights have been obtained over the last few years with important physiologic and therapeutic implications. In normal conditions, the secretory process is balanced by

TABLE 3-1

MAIN ENDOGENOUS FACTORS INFLUENCING INTESTINAL WATER AND ION TRANSPORT

Absorption	Secretion
Angiotensin II	Acetylcholine
Epinephrine	Atrial natriuretic peptide (ANP)
Enkephalins	Bradykinin
Epidermal growth factor	Cholecystokinin (CCK)
Glucocorticoids	Cytokines (e.g., IL-1β, IL-1α,3,2,8,4)
Growth hormone	Calcitonin gene-related peptide (CGRP), guanylin
Insulin-like growth factor-1 (IGF-1)	Gastrin releasing peptide (GRP)
Cytokines (IL-10)	Glucagon
Mineralcorticoids	Galanin
Norepinephrine	Hystamin
Neuropeptide Y (NPY)	Interferon-γ
Nitric oxide (produced in small quantities	Motilin
by constitutive nitric oxide synthase, cNOS)	Neurotensin
Peptide YY (PYY)	Nitric oxide (produced in large quantities by inducible nitric
Prolactin	oxide synthase, iNOS)
Somatostatin	Prostaglandins
	Serotonin (5-HT)
	Substance P
	Secretin
	Tumor necrosis factor-α (TNF-α)
	Vasoactive intestinal polypeptide

fluid absorption largely by the villous epithelium. Thus, in a normal adult, about 9 L of fluid enter the small intestine—derived from the diet or intestinal secretions, about 1.5 L reach the colon—and only <200 mL is lost daily in the stools.

Diarrhea, a term derived from the Greek "to flow through," is a common manifestation of many gastrointestinal diseases. It consists of a decrease in fecal consistency, and occurs when there is an imbalance between the processes of water and ions intestinal absorption and secretion. This imbalance may be caused by either decreased absorption (osmotic diarrhea) or increased secretion (secretory diarrhea). Both may occur simultaneously (e.g., in celiac disease, inflammatory bowel disease, and giardiasis). Most diarrheal episodes resolve within the first week (acute diarrhea); some, which begin as a typical acute illness,

continue for 2 weeks or longer (persistent diarrhea). Chronic diarrhea refers to the persistence of loose stools (with or without an increase in stool frequency) for at least 4 weeks. Whatever the clinical setting, this definition should include a period long enough to allow most cases of acute diarrhea to run their courses. This is because the causes of acute diarrhea (mostly self-limited infections—the common acute gastroenteritis) and chronic diarrhea (mostly noninfectious etiologies) differ. Chronic diarrhea can have a substantial impact on quality of life and overall health. At its mildest, the condition may be an inconvenience; at its worst, it may be disabling and even life threatening. A wide range of conditions can cause chronic diarrhea, and it is important to identify the underlying cause to ensure that a child receives the most appropriate treatment.

PATHOPHYSIOLOGY

There are two basic pathologic mechanisms for chronic diarrhea: secretory and osmotic, but in some diseases diarrhea may result from a combination of both. Although this kind of classification is dated, it remains an important starting point for the initial diagnostic approach for pediatric patients with chronic diarrhea (see Fig. 3-1).

Secretory Diarrhea

This type of diarrhea is characterized by an up-regulation of the ion transport mechanisms involved in active secretion. The most devastating increase in fluid losses occurs as a result of increased intestinal secretion and particularly that associated with the release of bacterial enterotoxins into the intestinal lumen. The classic enterotoxins produced by *Vibrio cholerae* and enterotoxigenic *Escherichia coli* (ETEC) promote a secretory process in the small intestine without producing significant epithelial cell injury. In cholera, for example, fluid losses can

be massive and approach 24 L in 24 h. A variety of mechanisms can disturb the normal balance between absorption and secretion in the crypt-villous axis. These secretory mechanisms operate through three major effector processes, namely the enterocyte, the endogenous secretagogues, and the enteric nervous system (see Table 3-1). Intestinal fluid secretion results predominantly from the active secretion of Cl^-, and the final common secretory pathway is the Cl^- channel created by a transmembrane protein, the *cystic fibrosis transmembrane regulator* (CFTR). Phosphorylation of the CFTR determines the channel opening, which occurs under the influence of *cyclic adenosine monophosphate* (cAMP), *cyclic guanosine monophosphate* (cGMP), and Ca^{2+}, through the action of specific protein kinases. Three other components of the Cl^- secretion mechanism are located on the basolateral membrane of the enterocyte: (1) the Na^+ pump (which maintains a low intracellular Na^+ concentration relative to the extracellular Na^+ concentration, determining a driving force for the entry of Cl^- by a cotransporter coupled with Na^+); (2) the

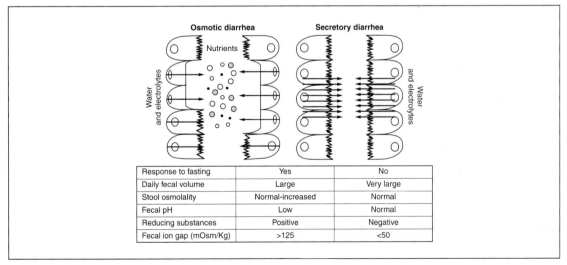

	Osmotic diarrhea	Secretory diarrhea
Response to fasting	Yes	No
Daily fecal volume	Large	Very large
Stool osmolality	Normal-increased	Normal
Fecal pH	Low	Normal
Reducing substances	Positive	Negative
Fecal ion gap (mOsm/Kg)	>125	<50

F I G U R E   3 - 1

THE IMPAIRMENT OF INTESTINAL DIGESTION AND/OR ABSORPTION OF NUTRIENTS AND MACROSCOPIC OR MICROSCOPIC INJURY OF THE INTESTINE ARE THE MAIN FEATURES OF OSMOTIC DIARRHEA (LEFT SIDE)
The unabsorbed nutrients exert an "osmotic force" which is able to drive water and ions into the lumen proportionally to their concentration. Secretory diarrhea is characterized by an active secretion of water and electrolytes, usually without epithelial damage.

Na$^+$-K$^+$-Cl$^-$ cotransporter (an electroneutral mechanism transporting two Cl$^-$ ions for one Na$^+$ and one K$^+$ ion); and (3) the K$^+$selective channels (that enable intracellular K$^+$, entered through the Na$^+$ pump and cotransporter activity, to return to the extracellular fluid). Finally, the secretory process is completed by the paracellular Na$^+$ exit, followed by fluid, which maintains electroneutrality. This complex Cl$^-$ secretory network can be activated directly by enterotoxins, by the liberation of several endogenous secretagogues induced by toxins, by infiltrating inflammatory cells, or by subepithelial neurons that terminate at the basolateral membrane forming the neurosecretory component of the intestinal neuronal reflex. A large number of neurotransmitters have now been identified in the enteric nervous system, many of which are likely to be involved in this network (see Table 3-1), and are therefore potential targets for pharmacotherapy of watery diarrhea. From a clinical standpoint, secretory diarrhea is characterized by large volume of watery stools and by a lack of dependence on oral food ingestion and persistency of the symptom during oral fasting (see Fig. 3-1).

Osmotic Diarrhea

Osmotic diarrhea is caused by an impaired intestinal digestion and/or absorption of nutrients and is generally accompanied by macroscopic or microscopic injury to the intestine. Consequently, these substances exert an "osmotic force" which is able to drive water into the lumen in proportion to their concentration. Whereas secretory diarrhea is predominantly due to dysfunction in the small intestine (however, there are conditions in which the colon is directly involved in the up-regulated secretion), osmotic diarrhea could be related to impaired fluid, electrolyte, and nutrient absorption in the small intestine; or to the appearance of incompletely absorbed nutrients in the colon; or to a direct impairment in the colonic water and ion salvage. Intestinal absorption is dependent not only on intact epithelial processes but also on an adequate time for digestion and contact with the epithelium. Thus, alterations in intestinal transit time, particu-

larly reductions in small-intestinal and whole-gut transit times, may result in impaired intestinal absorption of nutrients, electrolytes, and fluids. Carbohydrate malabsorption is the commonest cause and may result from congenital deficiency of disaccharidases (lactase deficiency) or transport mechanism (glucose-galactose malabsorption), but is more frequently due to muscosal damage. The nonabsorbed sugar may be fermented by colonic microflora to produce lactic and acetic acids, further increasing the osmotic drive of water into the lumen. Fat malabsorption or steatorrhea may result from pancreatic insufficiency, bile salt depletion, or a reduced absorptive surface area. Excessive protein loss occurs in protein-losing enteropathies and may be due to altered gut permeability, inflammation, or lymphatic stasis. The main clinical features of osmotic diarrhea are reported in Fig. 3-1. Stool volume depends on the intake of the unabsorbed nutrients and it is usually not as massive as in secretory diarrhea. In addition, diarrhea regresses with discontinuation of the offending nutrient. The fecal ion gap is >125 because fecal osmolality is not only accounted for by the ions but also by the unabsorbed nutrients and their degradation products.

CAUSES OF CHRONIC DIARRHEA ACCORDING TO THEIR MAIN MECHANISM

Villous Atrophy

Many pathologic conditions, such as celiac disease or cow's milk protein allergy, may determine abnormalities of the small intestinal mucosa. However, the commonest cause of enteropathy is the postenteritis syndrome which induces a mucosal damage less severe than the celiac disease.

Inborn Errors of Electrolyte Transport

Congenital chloride diarrhea (CLD) and *congenital sodium diarrhea* (CSD) are two rare diseases affecting the intestinal electrolyte transport. In CLD, a mutation in the solute carrier family 26 member 3 gene (SLC26A3), located at 7q31, close to cystic fibrosis transmembrane conductance regulator gene, leads to severe intestinal Cl^- malabsorption due the absence or defect of the Cl^-/HCO_3^- exchanger. Massive amounts of Cl^- are lost in the intestinal lumen, and the patients develop a severe watery diarrhea with a prenatal onset (maternal polyhydramnios and distended fluid-filled intestinal loops at ultrasonography). The respective defect in HCO_3^- secretion leads to metabolic alkalosis and intestinal content acidification, which further inhibit Na^+ absorption through the Na^+/H^+ exchanger. Thus, the high intestinal luminal electrolyte content causes a diarrhea with the clinical (massive losses of watery stools) and laboratory (fecal ion gap usually <50) features of secretory diarrhea, but by an osmotic mechanism. Sodium and water losses frequently cause secondary hyperaldosteronism and K^+ wastage leading to both hyponatremia and hypokalemia. In CLD children, supplementation therapy with NaCl/KCl is essential in reducing the risk of severe dehydration. It should be started during the neonatal period and accurately monitored to meet the requirements of increasing body weight. Unfortunately, supplementation therapy is unable to reduce the severity of diarrhea, and many other therapeutic strategies including acetazolamide, colesthyramine, and omeprazole have met with little success.

Patients with CSD show similar clinical features to those affected by CLD. The most important distinguishing features include: (1) the defective Na^+/H^+ exchange mechanism in all parts of the small and large intestine, (2) the presence of much higher Na^+ in the stool (usually >120–145 mmol/L and even in the presence of dehydration >60 mmol/L), and (3) tendency toward acidosis rather than alkalosis. As demonstrated in CLD, absorption of amino acids, glucose, and fatty acids is normal in these patients. The genetic defect of this condition is not known; however, it could be postulated that it is related to a protein involved in the function of the Na^+/H^+ exchanger 3 (NHE3). This molecule is responsible for the exchange at the apical membrane of the enterocyte. The therapeutic approach should include prompt correction of fluid, electrolyte, and acid-base

imbalance in the neonatal period, and life-long replacement with a solution of sodium and potassium citrate.

Carbohydrate Intolerance

It includes lactose intolerance, sucrase-isomaltase deficiency, and congenital glucose-galactose malabsorption. The lactose intolerance, in particular, may come from a congenital lactase deficiency, but this condition is rare, or from an acquired lactase deficiency due to pathologic conditions determining mucosal damage such as celiac or Crohn's diseases or from a progressive loss of lactase activity which affects about 80% of the non-White population.

Inflammatory Bowel Diseases

In these conditions (Crohn's disease, ulcerative colitis, indeterminate colitis, microscopic colitis), the presence of chronic diarrhea could be determined by: (1) malabsorption due to intestinal damage; (2) secretory effect induced by cytokines and other substances, and accelerated transit time; and (3) protein exudates coming from mucosal inflammation, bacterial overgrowth, fistulas-inducing absorptive surface bypass, and blind loops.

Pancreatic Diseases

Pancreatic diseases include conditions associated with a total pancreatic insufficiency, such as cystic fibrosis or Shwachman-Diamond syndrome, or with selective enzyme deficiency, such as congenital lipase deficiency.

Bile Salt Deficiency

Different conditions determine bile salt deficiency through various mechanisms: (1) by reducing their production (cirrhosis), (2) by inducing cholestasis (neonatal hepatitis, biliary atresia), (3) deconjugation (small bowel bacterial overgrowth), or (4) malabsorption (terminal ileum diseases).

Infections

Chronic diarrhea may be associated with intestinal (or extraintestinal, e.g., urinary) infections. In these conditions, it is very important to investigate whether an underlying immune-deficiency may be responsible for the prolonged infectious diarrhea. The commonest causes of an infectious chronic diarrhea are bacterial agents such as *Shigella, Salmonella, Campylobacter jejuni, Aeromonas hydrophila, E. coli, Yersinia*, and *Clostridium difficile*. On the contrary, while viruses typically cause acute diarrhea, they may also result in a prolonged course by inducing a post-enteritis syndrome.

Motility Disorders

The most common cause of chronic diarrhea in infancy not associated with failure to thrive is the Toddler's diarrhea, which is characterized by abnormal intestinal motility and accelerated transit. Other motility disorders may include congenital hyperthyroidism, neurologic disorders, and chronic intestinal pseudoobstruction.

Surgical Causes

Surgical causes include different conditions such as small bowel syndrome, Hirschsprung's disease, necrotizing enterocolitis, and all intestinal abnormalities (stenosis, malrotation, blind loop) leading to small bowel bacterial overgrowth. Chronic diarrhea associated with short bowel syndrome could be explained by the reduced absorptive surface and secondary malabsorption, the higher incidence of bacterial overgrowth, hypergastrinemia, and bile salts deconjugation. Hirschsprung's disease usually determines constipation, but may be associated with diarrhea when enterocolitis or bacterial overgrowth occurs.

APPROACH TO THE PEDIATRIC PATIENT WITH CHRONIC DIARRHEA

A careful history and physical examination are the cornerstones of a successful diagnosis. The most important data obtained from the history are age at the onset of diarrhea and whether it was abrupt or gradual in its appearance. It is important to think in terms of the child's age when establishing a differential diagnosis, as certain conditions first appear only at specific ages (see Table 3-2). If this approach is combined with establishing the diarrhea characteristics (secretory, osmotic, or mixed) and the presence or absence of malabsorption, the diagnostic possibilities are reduced, and tests necessary to establish the diagnosis become more understandable (see Table 3-3). A family history is always crucial in assessing the possibility of inherited conditions or disease. Most infants and children with cow's milk or soy protein allergy come from atopic families, and commonly the parents themselves had vomiting and diarrhea when exposed to milk and soy protein-containing foods. Many infants and children with celiac disease come from families with other affected members or have relatives with dermatitis herpetiformis. The same is often true for children with cystic fibrosis and inflammatory bowel disease (IBD). In infants with microvillous inclusion disease (MID), most of the parents have been consanguineous. In virtually every condition a positive family history is supportive of a specified diagnosis. However, a negative family history does not rule out the possibility that the infant or child has an inherited disease.

As a general rule, the causes of chronic diarrhea are influenced by the socioeconomic status of the population. In developing countries, chronic diarrhea is frequently caused by chronic bacterial, mycobacterial, and parasitic infection, although functional disorders (chronic nonspecific diarrhea or irritable bowel syndrome), malabsorption (such as cow's milk and soy protein intestinal allergy, celiac disease, lactose intolerance), and IBD (Crohn's disease and ulcerative colitis) are also common. In developed countries, such as the United States, the most common causes are functional disorders, malabsorption syndromes, IBD, and chronic infections (particularly in the immunocompromised patient). There are also many other less common causes of chronic diarrhea, and it could be useful to remember that they change markedly with age (see Table 3-2). Another important point in the approach to a child

MAIN CAUSES OF CHRONIC DIARRHEA ACCORDING TO THE AGE OF ONSET

0–30 Days	1–24 Months	2–18 Years
Abetalipoproteinemia	Apple juice and pear nectar	Apple juice or pear nectar
Acrodermatitis enteropathica	Autoimmune enteropathy	Antibiotic-associated
Autoimmune enteropathy	Chronic infection by *C. difficile,*	*C. difficile* colitis
Congenital chloride diarrhea	*G. lamblia*	Chronic infection by
Congenital sodium diarrhea	Chronic nonspecific diarrhea	*C. difficile, G. lamblia*
Congenital short bowel syndrome	Celiac disease	Celiac disease
Congenital lactase deficiency	Cystic fibrosis	Irritable bowel syndrome
Disaccharide intolerance	Food allergy	Inflammatory bowel disease
Food allergy	Postgastroenteritis diarrhea	Lactose intolerance
Glucose-galactose malabsorption		Postgastroenteritis diarrhea
Hirschsprung's disease		
Immunodysregulation, polyendocrinopathy, and enteropathy		
Lysinuric protein intolerance		
Malrotation with partial blockage		
Microvillous inclusion disease		
Neonatal lymphangiectasia		
Primary bile acid malabsorption (PBAM)		
Tufting enteropathy		

with chronic diarrhea is the growth and nutritional assessment. Although there are many ways to perform a nutritional assessment, weight for height is the simplest index of growth failure secondary to malnutrition. Sequential heights and weights, with measurement of head circumference, are critical for determining whether the disease has altered growth and weight gain and whether weight gain was affected before growth, or whether there was no effect on growth. The features can range from normal or excessive growth in overfeeding diarrhea to malnutrition and stunted growth in pathologic conditions such as celiac disease, and delayed growth velocity and puberty in Crohn's disease. Periods of poor weight gain may be due to malabsorption, deficit energy intake, or secondary to changes in metabolic rate, as in hyperthyroidism. A common mistake is a failure to appreciate that because of malabsorption, lack of progress on the growth chart may be due to feeding a dilute hypocaloric formula or clear liquids in an effort to reduce diarrhea. On the contrary, in infants or children who are apparently thriving or overweight while suffering from chronic diarrhea, a careful dietary record should be performed for 1 week to determine whether the youngster is being overfed or is drinking excessive amounts of fruit juices known to induce diarrhea, such as prune juice, apple juice, or pear nectar. The character of the diarrhea (watery, presence of blood and mucus, presence or absence of undigested food particles) may aid in establishing whether its type is secretory, inflammatory, osmotic, malabsorptive, or functional in nature. Frequency and volume estimates may aid in establishing the diarrhea severity. If the patient has been admitted to the hospital and has been electrolyte-depleted and dehydrated on one or more occasions, a more serious diagnosis should be considered. If a child or a teenager has to get up in the night to defecate or becomes incontinent, this suggests an organic basis for diarrhea. These signs together with the presence of blood

TABLE 3-3

QUESTIONS USEFUL IN THE MEDICAL HISTORY OF PEDIATRIC PATIENTS WITH CHRONIC DIARRHEA

Questions	Clinical Implication
Onset	
Congenital	Congenital chloride and sodium diarrhea, microvillous inclusion disease, tufting enteropathy
Abrupt	Infections
Gradual	Everything else
Family history	Congenital absorptive defects, IBD, celiac disease, food allergy
Dietary history	Food allergy, celiac disease
Travel history	Infectious diarrhea
Weight loss	Malabsorption, chronic inflammation, neoplasm, pancreatic exocrine insufficiency
Abdominal pain	Functional disorders, obstruction, celiac disease, IBD, food intolerance, cystic fibrosis, mesenteric vascular insufficiency
Excessive flatus	Carbohydrate malabsorption
Systemic illness symptoms	Diabetes, vasculitis, inflammatory bowel disease, hyperthyroidism, tuberculosis, mastocytosis, Whipple's disease, cystic fibrosis
Immune problems	Primary or acquired immunodeficiencies
Exposure to potentially impure water source	Chronic bacterial infections, giardiasis, cryptosporidiosis
Previous therapeutic interventions: drugs, radiation, surgery	Drug side effects, radiation enteritis, pseudomembranous colitis, postsurgical complications
Secondary gain from illness (Munchausen's syndrome by proxy)	Laxatives
Stool characteristics	
Watery	Secretory diarrhea
Undigested food particles	Malabsorption, functional disorders
Oil	Cystic fibrosis
Blood, mucus	Inflammatory bowel disease, chronic colitis
Nocturnal diarrhea	Organic etiology

and/or mucus in the stools indicate inflammation in the intestine and strongly suggest a diagnosis of IBD. On the contrary, a functional etiology is suggested by protracted smptoms (>12 months), lack of significant weight loss, absence of nocturnal diarrhea, and straining with defecation.

The presence of vomiting indicates a disturbance of intestinal or colonic motility, due to either mucosal or bowel-wall disease or adhesions

from previous surgery. Abdominal distention could be secondary to true obstruction, pseudo-obstruction, malabsorption, or hypersecretion of liquids in the intestine. A review of any systemic or extraintestinal signs and symptoms is useful in the search for other diagnostic clues. The presence of fever is more typically seen in infectious or inflammatory processes. Arthralgia, arthritis, iritis, pyoderma gangrenosum, and hepatic disease are

TABLE 3-4

MAIN INTESTINAL AND EXTRAINTESTINAL MANIFESTATIONS IN PEDIATRIC PATIENTS WITH INFLAMMATORY BOWEL DISEASE

Intestinal	Extraintestinal
Abdominal pain	Recurrent fever
Chronic diarrhea (>6 weeks)	Growth failure
Perianal disease (fissures, skin tags, abscesses, fistulas)	Pubertal delay
Nausea, anorexia, vomiting	Weight loss
Rectal bleeding, hematochezia	Anemia
Tenesmus, urgency, fecal soiling	Arthralgias, arthritis
Recurrent oral ulcers, cheilitis	Erythema nodosum, pyoderma gangrenosum
Malabsorption	Episcleritis, uveitis
	Chronic active hepatitis, steatosis, sclerosing cholangitis, cirrhosis
	Recurrent acute pancreatitis
	Renal calculi, obstructive hydronephrosis, hydroureter

all indications of IBD (see Table 3-4). Recurrent respiratory tract infections could be an indication of cystic fibrosis or congenital and acquired immune deficiency.

If the patient is a neonate with diarrhea in the first days of life, hospitalization is mandatory for an accurate evaluation and therapy. If the stool does not contain occult or gross blood, granulocytes, and eosinophils, an inflammatory or allergic process can be excluded. However, if screening tests (i.e., nutritional indexes) indicate nutrient malabsorption, evaluation must be focused on the assessment of absorption. Diagnosis then depends on determining: (1) whether the patient has sufficient bowel length for digestion and absorption; (2) whether the intestinal villi are intact or congenitally defective, as in microvillous inclusion disease or in tufting enteropathy; or (3) whether there are defects in monosaccharide digestion and absorption or in Cl^- and Na^+ absorption, as occur in congenital chloride diarrhea and congenital sodium diarrhea, respectively. It is important to note that some of these pathologic conditions, starting in neonatal age, are related to genetic defects (see Table 3-5). Thus, molecular analysis could be helpful in the diagnostic approach to these patients, and,

whenever possible in genetic counseling for the family. These patients need upper gastrointestinal small bowel radiology to assess intestinal length and to look for malrotation. Congenital short bowel syndrome may present with malabsorption in the absence of inflammatory changes in the stool. If bowel length appears normal, the patient should have a set of endoscopically obtained small intestinal biopsies to look for characteristic changes seen by light and electron microscopy in primary enterocyte abnormalities. A set of small bowel biopsies should be done in other suspected cases of chronic diarrhea to look for evidence of mucosal injury, such as immune-mediated enteropathy. Finally, during the endoscopic procedure, an aliquot of intestinal fluid may be aspirated for quantitative bacterial cultures, and, if indicated, for pancreatic enzymes.

In infants with chronic diarrhea, a careful feeding history must be obtained. If an infant is or was formula-fed when the diarrhea began, the type of formula and the response to it should be determined. Any change of formula and the respective clinical response should be accurately recorded. If the infant is or was breast-fed when diarrhea began, a careful history of the mother's diet must

TABLE 3-5

GENETICS OF VARIOUS DIARRHEAL DISEASES WITH PRENATAL AND/OR NEONATAL ONSET

Disease	Gene	Location	Function
Specific Transport Defects			
Congenital chloride diarrhea (OMIM 214700)	CLD (OMIM 126650)	7q22-q31.1	Chloride/bicarbonate exchanger
Congenital sodium diarrhea (OMIM 270420)	Unknown		Sodium/hydrogen exchanger
Glucose and galactose malabsorption	SGLT1 (OMIM 182380)	22q13.1	Intestinal sodium/ glucose contransporter
Primary bile acid malabsorption	ISBT (OMIM 601295)	13q33	Ileal sodium/bile salt transporter
Ultrastructural Enterocyte Defects			
Microvillous inclusion disease (OMIM 251850)	Unknown		Unknown
Tufting enteropathy	Unknown		Unknown
Disaccharidase Deficiencies			
Congenital lactase deficiency (OMIM 223000)	Unknown	2q21	Lactase-phlorizin hydrolase activity
Disaccharide intolerance (OMIM 222900)	EC 3.2.1.48	3q25-q26	Isomaltase-sucrase
Multiorgan Transport Defects with Diarrhea			
Abetalipoproteinemia (OMIM 200100)	MTP (OMIM 157147)	4q22-q24	Microsomial triglyceride transfer protein
Acrodermatitis enteropathica (OMIM 201100)	Unknown	8q24.3	Zinc absorption
Immunodysregulation, polyendocrinopathy and enteropathy (OMIM 304790)	FOXP 3 (OMIM 30092)	P11.23-q13.3	Transcription regulator
Lysinuric protein intolerance (OMIM 222700)	y(+)LAT1 (OMIM 603593)	14q11.2	Transport of dibasic amino acids

be determined, especially looking for any response in the infant's symptoms to changes in her diet. The age at which juice or fruit were added should be recorded in these infants; similarly the age at which gluten-containing products were added needs to be established and correlated with symptoms. Onset of diarrhea soon after fruit and juice are added is typical of sucrase-isomaltase deficiency. On the contrary, typical symptoms of celiac disease may not develop for weeks, months, or even years after gluten is added to the diet.

INVESTIGATIONS

Stool Examination

Randomly collected diarrheal stool specimens can be tested for electrolytes, blood, leucocytes, calprotectin, fat, elastase, pH, alpha$_1$-antitrypsin, laxatives, and microbes. If a stool is not passed during the initial part of the visit, a rectal examination can be done to stimulate evacuation and get a specimen.

Fecal electrolyte concentrations are measured in stool water after homogenization of the entire specimen (by manual stirring or in a mechanical blender) and centrifugation of an aliquot to obtain supernatant for analysis. The osmotic gap of fecal fluid is routinely used to estimate the contribution of electrolytes or other substances in determining excessive water content in the intestinal lumen. The osmotic gap is calculated from stool electrolyte concentrations by the following classic formula: stool osmolality (mOsm) $- 2([Na^+] + [K^+])$. In this formula, the sum of the $[Na^+]$ and $[K^+]$ is multiplied by a factor of 2 to account for associated anions. It is important to remember that the stool osmolality within the distal intestine (estimated as 290 mOsm/kg because it equilibrates with plasma osmolality) must be used for this calculation rather than the osmolality measured in fecal fluid, because measured fecal osmolality begins to rise in the collection tube almost immediately, when carbohydrates are converted by bacterial fermentation to osmotically active organic acids. The osmotic gap is large (>125) in pure osmotic diarrhea, in which nonelectrolyte substances (mainly nonabsorbed nutrients) account for most of the osmolality of liquid stool, and small (<50) in pure secretory diarrhea. In mixed osmotic and secretory diarrheas and in cases of modest carbohydrate malabsorption the osmotic gap normally lies between 50 and 125 (see Fig. 3-1). In congenital chloride diarrhea, stool $[Cl^-]$ is >90 mmol/L and exceeds the sum of $[Na^+] + [K^+]$ in the stool. In defective Na^+/H^+ exchanger (congenital sodium diarrhea) stool Na^+ losses are high (>120–145 mmol/L).

If bright red blood is seen or occult blood is found by Hemoccult test, this indicates the presence of an inflammatory, infectious, allergic, or ischemic process in the colon or possibly in the small intestine. At the same time, if white blood cells are found, this indicates an infectious, allergic, or inflammatory process. Eosinophils are typical of intestinal allergies. Recently, a number of leukocyte-derived proteins have been proposed as noninvasive

intestinal inflammation biomarkers, including eosinophilic cationic protein, lysozyme, lactoferrin, and calprotectin. Compared to the other candidates, calprotectin may offer performance advantages based on its biological characteristics. Specifically, this 36.5-kDa nonglycosylated polypeptide accounts for up to 60% of the cytosolic proteins found in neutrophils and macrophages. Additionally, calprotectin is stable in the stools for more than 7 days which may be at least in part due to high Ca^{2+} concentrations in gut lumen that make it resistant to proteolytic degradation, and these are easily measured in the stools by an *enzyme-linked immunosorbent assay* (ELISA). Experiences in IBD children are encouraging and suggest that fecal calprotectin provides reliable information in the diagnostic work-up. A study from our institution showed that calprotectin is actually one of the most sensitive and simple, but not disease-specific, noninvasive marker of inflammation throughout the whole gastrointestinal tract. In fact, high levels of fecal calprotectin have been demonstrated in several common gastrointestinal diseases, such as allergic colitis, celiac disease, polyposis, and gastroesophageal reflux disease (GERD). These considerations open up new prospects for its use in clinical practice to help the diagnosis and follow-up in several gastrointestinal disorders characterized by inflammatory damage, and, as recently demonstrated in adult patients in differential diagnosis with functional bowel disorders. If fat globules are very evident, this strongly suggests pancreatic insufficiency. Microscopic fat could be measured by a semiquantitative method, the steatocrit, that has been validated in pediatric patients in our institution and correlates well with quantitative fat output as measured using the van de Kamer method.

An ELISA test is routinely used to assess elastase 1 as an indirect measure of pancreatic function. This test is more sensitive and specific than fecal chymotrypsin in detecting pancreatic insufficiency, but it does not delineate patients who are pancreatic sufficient. False positives are seen in children with nonpancreatic causes of steatorrhea such as short gut syndrome or small bowel overgrowth. It is possible that these patients may have a secondary pancreatic insufficiency due to an impairment of mucosal release of pancreatic secretagogues. Despite these limitations, the stability of this enzyme allows storage at room temperature for at least 7 days, which could facilitate outpatient postage of fecal samples and the absolute specificity of this test makes it one of the most useful noninvasive pancreatic function tests.

The initial stool specimen should be tested for pH with Litmus paper. Acidic stools (pH <6) usually indicate carbohydrate malabsorption, except in breast-fed infants. If it is ≥6 this indicates the absence of carbohydrate malabsorption. However, if antibiotics are being used concurrently, they may alter the colonic bacterial flora and give a false-negative pH determination. The presence of an amount of reducing substances (detected by Clinitest tablets) more than 0.5% suggests malabsorption of reducing sugars (glucose, galactose, fructose, maltose, and lactose), but a negative result could be obtained with sucrose and other nonreducing sugars (such as lactulose, sorbitol, and mannitol) which need to be hydrolyzed with dilute acid before testing. The most reliable means of detecting carbohydrate malabsorption is stool chromatography. It is essential that the liquid part of the stool is tested. For this, watery diarrhea can be collected by reversing a disposable diaper with the plastic side inward.

A diagnosis of protein-losing enteropathy should be considered when a child has hypoalbuminemia but does not have nephritic syndrome or hepatic dysfunction. Confirmation of enteric protein loss can come from a raised fecal alpha$_1$-antitrypsin in a randomly passed stool. A more accurate diagnosis of protein-losing enteropathy could be obtained through a measurement of fecal clearance of alpha$_1$-antitrypsin. Clearance of this protein from plasma via the intestinal tract is based on the same concept as renal inulin clearance and is calculated in similar fashion. A radioimmunoassay (RIA) kit is used to measure alpha$_1$-antitrypsin concentrations in stools and plasma; total fecal output is calculated from concentration and volume and is divided by plasma concentration.

Measurements of stool electrolytes, osmolality, and magnesium content should be performed in any case of unexplained chronic diarrhea to test for evidence of a Munchausen's syndrome by proxy. Diagnosis of factitious diarrhea requires a high index of suspicion. Low stool electrolytes and osmolality in the presence of diarrhea suggests the addition of water to the stool. If magnesium concentrations in the stool exceed the plasma levels, this indicates a cathartic administration. In all unexplained chronic diarrhea, stools should be tested for phenolphthalein cathartics, emetine, and bisacodyl and its metabolites. Several reports have documented patients with Munchausen's syndrome by proxy using these common over-the-counter cathartics. In these cases spectrophotometric analysis of the stool for these compounds is the more specific test. Because children may ingest laxatives intermittently, negative studies may have to be repeated.

In all pediatric patients with chronic diarrhea, at least three stool specimens should be sent for bacterial culture, toxins, parasites and their ova, and detection of viruses (particularly *Rotavirus* and *Cytomegalovirus*), especially if white blood cells and occult or gross blood are found. A fresh sample is required for parasites. Examination for amebiasis and *C. difficile* must also be considered if stools are positive for blood. Stools should be tested for *Giardia lamblia* by an enzyme-linked immunosorbent assay. In addition, bacterial or parasite species may be identified in duodenal or jejunal biopsies or in duodenal aspirates. Cultures on special media and under specific environmental conditions are required to look for *Aeromonas* or *Plesiomonas* species. The epidemiologic clues raising suspicion for the presence of these organisms include consumption of untreated well water and swimming in fresh water ponds and streams. It is important to remember that in immunocompromised patients (particularly in AIDS patients), but only rarely in the normal child, common infectious causes of acute diarrhea, such as *Campylobacter, Salmonella*, or *Rotavirus*, can cause persistent diarrhea. In this special clinical setting, accurate microbiological studies, including the search for *Cryptosporidium parvum* (evaluated by modified acid-fast stain of the feces and duodenal fluid or by a monoclonal antibody test for direct recognition), *Cytomegalovirus* (CMV) (usually diagnosed

MAIN GASTROINTESTINAL PATHOGENS ISOLATED FROM AIDS-AFFECTED PATIENTS WITH CHRONIC DIARRHEA

Cryptosporidia
Clostridium difficile
Cytomegalovirus
Campylobacter spp.
Entamoeba histolytica
Enteric viruses
Giardia lamblia
Isospora belli
Mycobacterium avium-intracellulare
Microsporidia
Salmonella spp.
Shigella spp.
Strongyloides

MAIN PATHOGENS CAPABLE OF DETERMINING CHRONIC DIARRHEA IN IBD-AFFECTED PEDIATRIC PATIENTS

Bacterial	Viral
Aeromonas	*Adenovirus*
Campylobacter	*Cytomegalovirus*
Clostridium difficile	Rotavirus (group A)
E. coli O157:H7	
Giardia lamblia	
Plesiomonas	
Salmonella	
Shigella	
Yersinia	

from gastrointestinal mucosal biopsy specimens rather than stool samples), *Mycobacterium avium intracellulare* (MAI), *Microsporidia, Isospora belli, Candida albicans*, and other uncommon intestinal pathogens should be performed in any case of chronic diarrhea. A list of potential pathogen causes of chronic diarrhea in AIDS-affected patients are reported in Table 3-6. Unfortunately, a pathogen is found in only about 50–60% of cases, and this could be at least in part due to the multifactorial origin of chronic diarrhea in the HIV-1 infected child, and to the role of the HIV itself in determining modifications in ion transport, mucosal trophism, and nutrient absorption, as recently demonstrated in our laboratory. In addition, it is important to remember that enteric infections may precipitate relapse in children with IBD and should be excluded when the chronic diarrhea is nonresponsive to common IBD treatment. Potential agents capable of determining chronic diarrhea in these patients are reported in Table 3-7. In particular, several aggressive cases of IBD can be due to CMV infection. It is important to detect this organism in IBD-affected patients, because treatment involves rapidly tapering steroids and administering ganciclovir.

Laboratory Tests

Positivity of the acute phase reactants (erythrocyte sedimentation rate and C-reactive protein), together with thrombocytosis, although not specific for IBD, suggests an inflammatory process. A complete blood count should be done in all patients with chronic diarrhea because it may detect abnormalities associated with specific disease entities. Thus, a hypochromic microcytic anemia suggests a chronic disease (such as IBD) or iron deficiency (due to a malabsorption state, such as celiac disease, or blood loss, such as cow's milk allergy or ulcerative colitis). On this matter, it is important to remember that the most reliable confirmation of iron deficiency is a low serum concentration of ferritin. But a normal or high result does not exclude iron deficiency, as ferritin is also an acute phase protein. On the contrary, a macrocytic anemia suggests folate or vitamin B_{12} deficiency (due to Crohn's disease, terminal ileum resection, and stagnant ileal loop). Thrombocytopenia and neutropenia suggest a Shwachman-Diamond syndrome. Finally, lymphopenia can be detected in intestinal lymphangiectasia; and peripheral eosinophilia suggests eosinophilic gastroenteritis, food allergy, or parasitic infestation. If serum albumin and globulins are both abnormally low, this indicates the presence of a protein-losing enteropathy (such as congenital lymphangiectasia) or a liver disease. If plasma albumin is low and globulins are normal, this is more likely to indicate blood loss or malnutrition. On the contrary, if albumin is low and gamma-globulins are elevated this suggests an inflammatory disease (such as IBD). Plasma electrolytes should be monitored in pediatric patients with chronic diarrhea. The presence of either hypokalemia and/or hyponatremia indicates severe fluid and ion losses. If detected in a child with no inflammatory signs, this suggests a secretory process. In this instance, a tumor-driven diarrhea has to be considered, and thyroid function and gastrointestinal hormones should be measured. A plasma *vasoactive intestinal polypeptide* (VIP) is essential for diagnosing patients with VIP-secreting tumors. The measurement of *pancreatic polypeptide* (PP) is also helpful as it is often cosecreted in patients with pancreatic endocrine tumors. It is useful to determine plasmatic gastrin and calcitonin levels in some circumstances. It is useful to determine plasma gastrin and calcitonin levels in some circumstances. Such determinations, however, should only be performed in highly qualified laboratories.

Low serum cholesterol and triglyceride concentrations are seen in abetalipoproteinemia, together with a proportion of acanthocytes of about 50–70% in the peripheral blood film. Vitamin A, C, and E, calcium, phosphate, zinc, magnesium, copper, and selenium should be closely checked, particularly in patients receiving long-term parenteral nutrition, because chronic diarrhea may result in multiple vitamin and trace element deficiencies.

Urine collection may be helpful for laxative identification and for determination of 5-hydroxyindole acetic acid (5-HIAA) (for carcinoid syndrome), vanillylmandelic acid (VMA), metanephrine (for pheochromocytoma), and histamine (for mast cell disease and forgut carcinoids) excretion.

In the case of a suspected cystic fibrosis a sweat test should be performed. It is diagnostic if sweat Cl⁻ is abnormally elevated (>60 meq/L).

To study the small intestine nutrient absorptive capacity a 60-min D-xylose test may be performed by giving PO a standard dose of 5 g. Xylose is a pentose whose absorption takes place in the proximal jejunum and can be considered passive; the sugar is nonmetabolizable, and after appearing in the plasma is excreted intact via the kidneys.

A serum level above 25 mg/dL at 1 h postingestion is considered normal, indicating an intact absorptive capacity of this area of the small intestine. The test is however unspecific, and it may not detect mild-to-moderate injury if the disease is limited to the upper small intestine, and it could give false-negative or false-positive results in over 10% of the cases. Actually, in order to obtain an accurate noninvasive study of small intestine mucosal integrity, the intestinal permeability test (using cellobiose/mannitol permeability ratio) has become more widely used. The permeability ratio represents functional changes in the intestinal mucosa, and it is possible to find abnormal results in any diarrheal disease affecting the integrity of the small intestinal mucosa, such as celiac disease, food allergy, and Crohn's disease. To examine the terminal ileum absorptive function the vitamin B_{12} absorption rate could be studied by the Schilling test. Alternatively, it is possible to detect bile acid malabsorption in two ways. The first method measures the quantity of endogenous bile acids excreted during a quantitative stool collection. The second method involves measurement of the turnover of radio-labeled bile acid. The most common procedure for doing this involves the use of a gamma camera to detect the retained fraction of an orally administered synthetic radio-labelled bile acid (selena-homocholic acid) conjugated with taurine (^{75}Se-HCAT). Alternatively, a measurement of fecal recovery of an oral load of [^{14}C] glycocholate during a 48 or 72-h stool collection and calculation of a retention half-life, or a measurement of serum concentrations of an intermediate product of bile acid synthesis, the 7alfa-hydroxy-4-cholesten-3-one, could be used for evaluating bile acid metabolism. Unfortunately, these tests are not widely available and have been complicated by a lack of standardization of reference values for the pediatric age. In addition, an abnormal test result is not necessarily specific for pathologic bile acid malabsorption but may occur as a result of diarrhea *per se*. Thus, many pediatricians use a therapeutic response to a trial of cholestyramine (a bile acid binding resin) as an indirect test for the possibility that malabsorbed bile acids are the cause of diarrhea.

TABLE 3-8

SEROLOGIC TESTS USEFUL IN THE DIAGNOSTIC APPROACH TO PEDIATRIC PATIENTS PRESENTING CHRONIC DIARRHEA

Test	Clinical Application
Quantitative immunoglobulins/antibodies to HIV	Congenital or acquired immunodeficiencies
IgA-IgG antigliadin (AGA), IgA antiendomysial (EMA), IgA-IgG antitransglutaminase (AntiTGA)	Celiac disease
HLA-DR, DQ typing	Celiac disease
IgG perinuclear staining antineutrophil cytoplasmic antibody (pANCA)	Ulcerative colitis
IgG-IgA antiSaccharomyces cerevisiae antibody (ASCA)	Crohn's disease
Antienterocyte antibody	Autoimmune enteropathy
Antinuclear antibody (ANA)	Vasculitis, microscopic colitis, hypothyroidism, autoimmune enteropathy
Ag p65 for Cytomegalovirus (Ag p65 CMV), CMV DNA	CMV-induced chronic diarrhea

Since immune deficiency may predispose to chronic, recurrent gastrointestinal infections, a comprehensive immunologic work-up (including immunoglobulins, IgG subclasses, T- and B-lymphocytes number and function, phagocyte function, HIV-1 infection tests) is important in frequent or unusual infections, and in *idiopathic intractable diarrhea of infancy* (IDI).

In addition to these "classical" laboratory tests useful for the diagnostic approach to the patient with chronic diarrhea, a continuously growing list of serologic markers is now available. This list is reported in Table 3-8, together with indications for the respective diagnostic application. For a more detailed description of these tests, see specific sections.

Instrumental Diagnostic Procedures

Endoscopy and Mucosal Biopsy

Upper tract endoscopy has become the standard method for obtaining upper small intestine biopsy specimens in patients with suspected malabsorptive disorders. The procedure is performed with a pediatric endoscope that allows specimens to be obtained from the duodenum and proximal jejunum. If bacterial overgrowth is suspected, an aspirate of small intestinal contents can be sent for a quantitative aerobic and anaerobic bacterial culture and for microscopic examination for parasites. Alternatively, pediatric versions of the Crosby or Watson capsules could be used to take biopsies in the small intestine. A characteristic flat mucosa with hyperplastic villous atrophy and crypt hyperplasia is diagnostic of celiac disease (see Fig. 3-2).

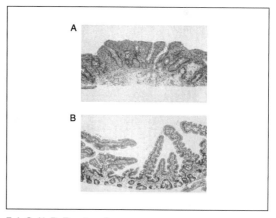

FIGURE 3-2

(A) TYPICAL HISTOGICAL FEATURES OF A SMALL INTESTINE BIOPSY SPECIMEN OF A CHILD WITH CELIAC DISEASE: VILLOUS ATROPHY, CRYPT HYPERPLASIA, AND INFLAMMATION OF LAMINA PROPRIA. (B) THE HISTOLOGY OF A NORMAL INTESTINAL MUCOSA IS REPORTED FOR COMPARISON

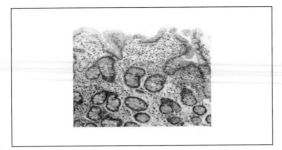

FIGURE 3-3

THE HISTOLOGY OF IMMUNE ENTEROPATHY SHOWS MODERATE VILLOUS ATROPHY WITH CRYPT HYPERPLASIA AND INCREASED CELLULARITY OF THE LAMINA PROPRIA WITH HIGH NUMBER OF INTRAEPITHELIAL LYMPHOCYTES AND EOSINOPHILS

A flat mucosa is also seen in autoimmune enteropathy (see Fig. 3-3). Crypt hypoplastic villous atrophy with an abnormal accumulation of periodic acid Schiff (PAS)-positive material in the upper crypt and villous epithelium with an absence of the usual brush-border staining is typical of microvillous inclusion disease. With electron microscopy, surface epithelial cells show absent or grossly abnormal microvilli as well as numerous vesicular bodies of various size and the characteristic microvillous inclusions (see Fig. 3-4). Other diseases that may be diagnosed by small intestinal biopsy include food allergies, giardiasis, Crohn's

disease, eosinophilic gastroenteritis, Whipple's disease, lymphangiectasia, abetalipoproteinemia, and various bacterial, viral, mycobacterial, fungal, protozoal, and parasitic infections.

Colonoscopy should be performed in all cases of chronic diarrhea in which occult or gross blood is found in the stool. It can enable visualization of the entire colonic mucosa, and in experienced hands, terminal ileal biopsy may be possible. Biopsies should be done from multiple sites even if the colon appears normal, because up to 5% of normal-appearing colonoscopic examinations will yield specimens positive for colitis. Chronic disorders that can be diagnosed by colonoscopy include IBD, pseudomembranous colitis, CMV-induced colitis, amebiasis, and microscopic colitis (lymphocytic and collagenous colitis). A major limitation of current endoscopic procedures is the inability to evaluate small bowel disorders beyond the range of currently available endoscopes. Experience with enteroscopy has been limited in children. This technique requires a large instrument (15 mm), limiting its applicability in the pediatric age group. More recently, swallowable wireless video endoscopy using a small capsule has been proposed to detect obscure Crohn's disease in pediatric patients, but the high costs and the lack of a wide experience in children limit its use (see Fig. 3-5). Finally, 25% of infants with Hirschsprung's disease present with diarrhea. Therefore, any infant with chronic diarrhea,

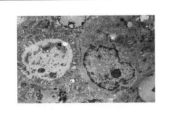

FIGURE 3-4

ELECTRON MICROSCOPY (EM) OF A SMALL BOWEL BIOPSY OF A PATIENT WITH MICROVILLOUS INCLUSION DISEASE SHOWING THE SPECIFIC FINDINGS OF THE DISEASE: MICROVILLUS INCLUSIONS AND INCREASED SECRETORY GRANULES IN THE ENTEROCYTE. THESE TYPICAL EM FINDINGS CAN ALSO BE SEEN IN COLONOCYTES

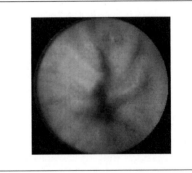

FIGURE 3-5

VIDEO CAPSULE ENDOSCOPY SHOWING A CROHN'S DISEASE-RELATED MUCOSAL DAMAGE IN THE PROXIMAL ILEUM IN A GIRL WITH ABDOMINAL PAIN AND OCCULT BLEEDING

and a history of failure to pass meconium in the first 24 h, should have rectal suction biopsy.

Radiology

A preliminary plain abdominal x-ray is useful for detection of gaseous distention, suggestive of a gastrointestinal obstruction; or intramural or biliary gas, suggestive of necrotizing enterocolitis or intestinal invagination; or calcification, typical of secreting tumors. After this a barium meal and an entire bowel follow-through examination is useful in several ways. Intestinal length may be assessed, as may the presence of any structural abnormalities (such as diverticula, malrotation, stenosis, and pseudoobstruction) that might affect digestion or absorption resulting in chronic diarrhea. Many pediatric patients with mucosal injury from a variety of causes will show characteristic changes in different parts of the intestine, for example: (1) Crohn's disease in the terminal ileum (aphtoid ulcers, cobblestoning, separation of bowel loops, narrowed lumen, skip lesions, hypomotility of intestinal loops or colic segments, and fragmentation of the barium bowel), (2) eosinophilic gastroenteritis in the gastric antrum and duodenum, and (3) excess luminal fluid, dilatation, and irregular mucosal surface in the duodenum and jejunum of celiac disease-affected subjects. A barium enema could be used in the diagnostic work-up of colonic pseudoobstruction and Hirschsprung's disease after the neonatal period. Abdominal ultrasonography should be performed in patients with chronic diarrhea when the results of pancreatic function tests are abnormal. More recently, ultrasonography is also used to evaluate the presence of parietal thickening of last ileal loop (>2.5 mm) or colonic wall thickness (>2 mm), peritoneal effusion, and/or lymphadenopathies in patients with suspected IBD. More recently, *magnetic resonance* (MRN) study of the intestine has been proposed for the diagnostic work-up of patients with suspected IBD. Mesenteric or celiac angiography may be useful in obtaining evidence of intestinal ischemia caused by vasculitis. Computed tomography may be performed if a carcinoid syndrome or a neuroendocrine tumor is highly suspected. In this case, rapid computed tomography scan with thin sections (≤5 mm) through the pancreas following a bolus of intravenous contrast is recommended. When IBD is highly suspected, leukocyte-labeled scintigraphy could provide information on presence, intensity, and extent of the disease.

Breath Tests

The breath hydrogen test, after specific oral loading, can be used for the diagnosis of carbohydrate malabsorption and maldigestion. A high fasting breath hydrogen level points to bacterial overgrowth as the cause of chronic diarrhea, although it is also commonly found in patients with celiac disease. The lactose breath hydrogen test with a long, fast, and careful oral hygiene is an inexpensive and sensitive test for diagnosing lactose intolerance. Recently, a blood test to detect the genetically-induced late-onset lactase deficiency has also become available.

THERAPY

The large number of pathologic conditions presenting chronic diarrhea determines the necessity of a broad spectrum of specific therapeutic interventions.

Drug therapy is only indicated in specific situations including:

- Antibiotics in chronic intestinal infections and in small bowel bacterial overgrowth
- Cholestyramine in bile acid deconjugation and/or malabsorption
- Anti-inflammatory (5-ASA, salazopyrin) and/or immunosuppressor drugs (steroids, azathioprine, cyclosporine, methotrexate, infliximab) in inflammatory bowel diseases and in autoimmune enteropathy
- Growth factors (epidermal growth factor, growth hormone, glucagons-like peptide 2) and antisecretory agents (somatostatin, octreotide, and the enkephalinase inhibitor, racecadotril) in short bowel syndrome, microvillous inclusion disease, and other chronic secretory diarrheal diseases

Empiric or symptomatic therapy (using colesthyramine, octreotide, and other antisecretory agents) is usually adopted in the following clinical conditions: (1) in severe diarrheal diseases as the initial therapeutic approach, before the end of the diagnostic

PEDIATRIC DISORDERS POTENTIALLY TREATABLE BY INTESTINAL TRANSPLANTATION

Short Bowel Syndrome
Congenital malformation
Necrotizing enterocolitis
Trauma
Tumors
Defective Intestinal Motility
Intestinal pseudoobstruction, with or without   concurrent urinary tract pseudoobstruction
Intestinal aganglionosis
Ultrastructural Enterocyte Abnormalities
Microvillous inclusion disease
Tufting enteropathy

work-up; (2) in any case of severe idiopathic diarrhea; and (3) when a diagnosis has been made, but no specific therapy is available or effective.

Surgery may be required to resolve malrotation, stenosis, or blind loops. Various bowel-lengthening procedures have been attempted in short gut syndrome and may be of benefit in selected cases. Finally, intestinal transplantation may be considered in severe chronic diarrheal diseases such as intractable diarrhea of infancy (see Table 3-9).

INTRACTABLE DIARRHEA OF INFANCY

The term intractable diarrhea of infancy indicates a heterogeneous group of diseases with diverse etiology, including immune-mediated enteropathy or ultrastructural abnormalities of the enterocyte. From the first description by Avery et al. in 1968, the original definition (diarrhea of more than 2 weeks of duration, starting within the first 3 months of life, and three or more negative stool cultures for bacterial pathogens) has changed considerably because of a better understanding of intestinal pathology and an improvement in the nutritional and therapeutic approach to these patients. It has recently been suggested that the term intractable diarrhea in infancy must be redefined as severe and protracted diarrhea, with the need for parenteral

nutrition, starts within the first 2 years of life, rapidly becomes life threatening, and leads to dependence on total parenteral nutrition. Histologic analysis seems to be the most important clue for the diagnosis of IDI. Patients present histologically in two clearly different groups. The first is referred to as "immune-enteropathy group" because it has been suggested that the specific histologic findings (villous atrophy, crypt hyperplasia, and cellular infiltration of the lamina propria) are associated with a T-cell activation mechanism. The second group includes severe early onset IDI (usually in the first 2 weeks of life) with villous atrophy without mononuclear cell infiltration of the lamina propria, but with specific epithelial abnormalities. In addition, for a diagnosis of IDI, clinical and histologic data should be taken into account. The main clinical criteria that should be considered are: (1) birth weight, (2) familial history, (3) date of onset and characteristics of diarrhea (watery and/or bloody, persistent despite bowel rest), (4) presence of extraintestinal manifestations, (5) autoantibody (i.e., antibody against the enterocytes), and (6) phenotypic abnormalities. Protracted diarrhea of infectious origin and/or immune deficiency have to be excluded. Microvillous inclusion disease can be excluded by performing periodic acid Schiff staining and electron microscopy. Routine light microscopy of small bowel biopsy specimens allows the detection of all the histologic features. Table 3-10 summarizes the main clinical and histologic features of distinctive disorders included in the IDI group. In conclusion, every classification is probably incomplete, because other forms of IDI with abnormal small bowel mucosa have been described. However, it indicates that there are different pathologic mechanisms operating in the clinical groups and may allow specific treatments to be pursued. In addition, it forms a basis for future research in this exceptionally difficult pediatric clinical condition.

Immune-mediated Intractable Diarrhea of Infancy

The onset of the disease is usually early, during the first 2 years of life (median age 3–5 months).

TABLE 3-10

CLINICAL AND HISTOLOGIC FEATURES OF INTRACTABLE DIARRHEA OF INFANCY

	Ultrastructural Enterocyte Defects		Immune-Mediated Enteropathy	Phenotypic Diarrhea
	Microvillous Inclusion Disease	Tufting Enteropathy	Autoimmune Immune-Mediated	Syndromatic Diarrhea
Date of onset	Neonatal	Neonatal	3–12 months	1–3 months
Type of diarrhea	Watery (100 mL/ kg per day)	Watery (100 mL/ kg per day)	Watery (100–150 mL/ kg per day)	Watery 50–100 mL/ kg per day)
Family history	Frequent	Frequent	Rare	Rare-absent
Commonly associated symptoms	Mucus in the stools	Choanal atresia, keratitis		Low birth weight, facial dismorphism (forehead, broad nose, hypertelorism), tricorrhexis nodosa, immunodeficiency
Villous atrophy	Moderate	Moderate	Moderate to severe	Moderate to severe
T-cell activation	Absent	Absent	↑↑↑	Absent
Intraepithelial lymphocytes	Normal	Normal or ↓	Normal or ↑	Normal
Epithelium	Abnormal PAS	Tufts	Normal to injured	Normal
Crypts	Normal	Hyperplastic, dilated branching	Hyperplastic, necrosis, abscess	Normal
Pathognomonic signs	Abnormal brush-border, secretory granules, membrane inclusions lined by microvilli	Abnormal expression of $\alpha_2\beta_1$ integrin and desmoglein	lamina propria T-cell activation; CD25 + T cells; ↑ HLA-DR	

However, neonatal cases with poor prognosis have also been reported. The stool pattern is characterized by secretory diarrhea, variable in intensity, as well as the presence of blood and mucus discharges. There are usually severe clinical symptoms, protein-losing enteropathy, extensive histologic lesions, and poor prognosis. The vast predominance of males, as well as familial history in several male patients, suggest that some cases may be X-linked. Circulating gut epithelial cell autoantibodies are frequently present. They are primarily IgG and indirect immunofluorescence has shown that they are directed against components of enterocytes brush border or cytoplasm. Immunoglobulins, steroids, and immunosuppressive drugs (including azathioprine, cyclosporine A, cyclophoshamide, and infliximab) have induced durable improvement and even recovery in some patients. Neonatal onset, diarrhea exceeding 150 mL/kg per day, extensive crypt destruction, associated lesions of colon and/or upper digestive tract, severe renal involvement, and high titers of circulating antienterocyte autoantibodies are criteria for a poor prognosis, associated with a poor response to immunosuppressive treatment and a fatal outcome. Successfully compatible bone marrow transplantation in an infant has recently been reported. The most commonly recognized form of immune-mediated IDI is autoimmune enteropathy in which the development of enterocyte autoantibodies occurs in association with a cell-mediated immunopathology characterized by mucosal T-cell activation and a presumed interferon-γ (IFN-γ) mediated up-regulation of crypt epithelial class II MHC (human leukocyte antigen DR) expression. The onset of diarrhea is usually later than other IDI and is often associated with extraintestinal manifestations such as arthritis, diabetes, dermatitis, thrombocytopenia, and renal diseases. Villous atrophy seems to be more pronounced, with severe crypt damage including necrosis and abscess formation. In addition to the typical circulating gut epithelial cell autoantibodies, antigoblet cell IgG may also be detected. Other associated autoantibodies are mainly directed against the nucleus, DNA, smooth muscle, or mitochondria. In some cases of autoimmune enteropathy associated with nephropathy, circulating autoantibodies reactive with the renal tissue have also been reported. The role of gut autoantibodies in the pathogenesis of the disease remains unknown although the partial response to cyclosporin A and the promising use of FK506 further suggest that T cells are involved in the pathogenesis of this disorder. The extraintestinal symptoms may be due to the presence of shared epitopes between tissues producing cross-reacting autoimmunity. It is clear that there is a significant heterogeneity within the autoimmune enteropathy population and that there will not be one single underlying mechanism.

Primary Ultrastructural Enterocyte Abnormalities

Microvillous Inclusion Disease

It is an inherited disorder characterized by loss or absence of the microvilli of the enterocyte brush border, resulting in a reduction of the surface area for nutrient and fluid absorption. There is evidence of a constitutive secretory state, which suggests more central impairment of enterocyte function and polarity, or more secondary inflammation. The typical clinical presentation is characterized by neonatal onset of severe secretory diarrhea.

Histochemical staining with periodic acid Schiff of small intestine biopsy is mandatory for diagnosis. Electron microscopy image shows not only clear abnormalities of microvilli on the brush border but also intracellular abnormalities, with the so-called secretory granules of varying size, unknown composition and function, and membrane-bound inclusions lined by microvilli. The last features suggest an interruption of some pathway transporting microvilli within the enterocyte. Lesions are also present in the large bowel, which may be an easier part of the gut on which to perform biopsy in early infancy. The gene of this likely autosomal recessive disease is not known. The disease requires long-term total parenteral nutrition for survival and the prognosis is poor. Treatment with corticosteroids, colostrums, epidermal growth factor, and octreotide have not been successful. Intestinal transplantation has become the only definitive treatment of this rare intestinal disorder (see Table 3-9 for the main pediatric disorders potentially treatable with intestinal transplantation).

Intestinal Epithelial Dysplasia (Tufting Enteropathy)

This inherited disease is more common than microvillous inclusion disease, particularly within the Middle-East. Histology reveals light to more severe villous atrophy. Abnormalities are mainly localized in the epithelium and include a disorganization of surface enterocytes, with focal crowding resembling tufts. The characteristic tufts of extruding epithelium are seen toward the villous tip and may affect up to 70% of villi. Crypt cell proliferation is dramatically increased, implying secondary T-cell activation, presumably to compensate for the pathologic shedding of enterocytes and increased permeability. The tufting process is not limited to the small intestine, and both gastric desquamation and colonic tufting may be seen. Abnormal lamina, heparan sulfate proteoglycan deposition on the basement membrane and desmoglien distribution have been reported in infants with tufting enteropathy. Basement membrane molecules are involved in epithelial mesenchymal cell interaction and are crucial to intestinal development and differentiation. An alteration of normal distribution of $\alpha_2\beta_1$ integrin adhesion molecules along the crypt-villous axis has been recently reported in patients with tufting enteropathy. The $\alpha_2\beta_1$ integrin is involved in the interaction of epithelium with basement membrane components. Tufts may correspond to groups of nonapoptotic cells that are no longer in contact with the basement. Diagnosis is difficult due to several factors including early onset of diarrhea, failure to demonstrate microvillous inclusion disease, and not very evident tufts of extruding epithelium in several infants. Thus, only repeated duodenal or jejunal biopsies and strict elimination of microvillous inclusion disease allow diagnosis. Another diagnostic difficulty is related to T-cell infiltration in the lamina propria, due to the lack of intestinal permeability, which suggests immune-related enteropathy, particularly when tufts are initially missing or ignored. For these reasons inhibition of T-cell activation by immunosuppressive drugs may significantly improve crypt cell proliferation and enteral absorption, without resolution of the severe diarrhea. A deficiency of intestinal $\alpha_6\beta_4$ integrin has been recently postulated as a cause of tufting enteropathy in a French patient. This integrin is known to be defective in epidermolysis bullosa, in which gross epidermal shedding occurs, although the cutaneous expression of $\alpha_6\beta_4$ integrin appeared normal in the reported French infant. This probably reflects a defect of expression of intestinal integrin isoform or a related and immunohistochemically cross-reactive intestinal integrin deficiency. The clinical features are consistent with the common form of tufting enteropathy.

Several cases of intestinal epithelial dysplasia have been reported as being associated with phenotypic abnormalities (e.g., Dubowitz's syndrome), choanal atresia, rectal atresia, punctiform keratitis, and epidermolysis bullosa. This disease is resistant to all treatment, requires total parenteral nutrition in IDI form, and is an indication to intestinal transplantation. The genetic origin of this disorder is unknown.

Congenital Enterocyte Heparan Deficiency (CEHD)

This extremely rare disorder is characterized by severe enteric protein loss with secretory diarrhea and absorption failure, despite an uninflamed and histologically normal intestine, starting within the first weeks of life. Heparan sulfate is a glycosaminoglycan (GAG) with multiple roles in the intestine including restriction of charged macromolecules, such as albumin, within the vascular lumen. In these patients basement membrane GAGs are almost normal, but there is a virtually complete absence of sulfated GAGs in the enterocyte basolateral membrane in all villi in formalin-fixed small intestinal biopsies. The prognosis is usually poor and some improvement of diarrhea was reported probably not due to a direct effect in GAG synthesis but possibly by increasing water and ion salvage mechanism. Congenital enterocyte heparan deficiency could be an unusual presentation of the carbohydrate deficient glycosylation syndrome type 1. This latter condition in which glycan chain formation is impaired can be detected by aberrant glycosylation of serum transferring.

Syndromic Diarrhea

This disease should be suspected if an infant presents with chronic diarrhea starting in the first 2–6 months of age. Usually the patient is small for gestational age and has an abnormal phenotype (see Table 3-10), defective antibody response, and negative antigen-specific skin tests, despite normal serum immunoglobulins and normal lymphocytic proliferative response *in vitro*, respectively.

Histologically, there are no specific abnormalities, and small bowel biopsy specimens show moderate-to-severe villous atrophy in some cases, with a significant infiltrate of mononuclear cells in the lamina propria. The prognosis is poor since most patients die between the ages of 2 and 5 years. The pathogenesis of diarrhea, and the relationship with low birth weight, dysmorphism, and immunodeficiency in these patients are still largely obscure.

Bibliography

Booth IW, MacNeish AS. Mechanisms of diarrhoea. *Baillieres Clin Gastroenterol* 7:215, 1993.

Donowitz M, Kokke FT, Saidi R. Evaluation of patients with chronic diarrhea. *N Engl J Med* 332:725, 1995.

Fine KD, Schiller LR. AGA technical review on the evaluation and management of chronic diarrhea. *Gastroenterology* 116:1464, 1999.

Goulet OJ, Brousse N, Canioni D, et al. Syndrome of intractable diarrhoea with persistent villous atrophy in early childhood: a clinic-pathological survey of 47 cases. *J Pediatr Gastroenterol Nutr* 26:151, 1998.

Murch SH. The molecular basis of intractable diarrhoea of infancy. *Baillieres Clin Gastroenterol* 11(3):413, 1997.

Russo PA, Brochu P, Seidman EG, et al. Autoimmune enteropathy. *Pediatr Dev Pathol* 2:65, 1999.

Walker-Smith JA. Intractable diarrhea in infancy: a continuing challenge for the pediatric gastroenterologist. *Acta Pediatr Suppl* 83:6, 1994.

CHAPTER

4

FAILURE TO THRIVE/MALNUTRITION

John S. Morrice and Peter B. Sullivan

INTRODUCTION

Considerable diagnostic and therapeutic challenges are presented in the management of the infant or young child (usually less than 2 years old) with *failure to thrive* (FTT). Defining the problem is often the initial difficulty and there has been much debate regarding the meaning and usefulness of the term "failure to thrive." There has been a shift away from the traditional view of FTT being either organic or nonorganic in origin with the recognition that in all cases of FTT the primary insult is that of undernutrition. In addition to this, the historical models which were based on terms such as "maternal deprivation syndrome" have been acknowledged as unhelpful and inaccurate and there is a growing appreciation of the transactional nature of the parent-child relationship. Controversy still exists, however, regarding the treatment of these patients and the impact of failure to thrive in infancy on long-term cognitive function. Regardless of these theoretical arguments, the reality is that numerous clinical consultations bring us face to face with children with FTT and their worried parents.

Occasional reference will be made to children with severe malnutrition, but for a definitive guide to this problem, which is largely confined to children

in the developing world, the reader is referred to the recent *World Health Organization* (WHO) manual on the assessment and management of severe protein-energy malnutrition.[1]

BACKGROUND

Interest in the topic of FTT has grown in the last few years. This is partly because of a realization that the pattern of growth and general health in the early years of life may have an impact on a variety of health parameters in adulthood. There has also been considerable interest in the field of *nonaccidental injury* (NAI), with the diagnosis of neglect being of particular relevance to the topic of FTT.

Progress in the management of FTT has been dogged by a series of incorrect assumptions. The term FTT was first used to describe children in workhouses in the United Kingdom the early 1900s and then during the middle of the last century to describe institutionalized children who were thought to be provided with sufficient calories but did not grow appropriately. The first incorrect assumption was that the reason for this nonorganic failure to thrive was emotional deprivation and much subsequent work tried to establish the physical mechanisms by which a child could consume the appropriate amount of calories and yet fail to grow. It was not until the late 1960s that is was shown that children with FTT in the midst of psychosocial adversity were actually not consuming the requisite amount of calories. For the first time it was acknowledged that undernutrition could be the underlying cause of FTT. The second incorrect assumption was that the lack of nutritional intake leading to FTT was a result of "maternal deprivation." This is now known to be an oversimplification in the majority of cases. What was previously known as maternal deprivation is rare and, with a few exceptions, the mother-infant interaction is not poorer in families of FTT children when compared with controls. Finally, it had been assumed that poverty was eradicated and therefore if a child was not gaining sufficient weight then it could not simply be a result of lack of physical resources. Unfortunately even in the developed world there are those who continue to live in absolute poverty.

Summary

- Even in poor countries the reasons for FTT are complex.
- It was incorrectly assumed in the past that FTT was due to maternal deprivation or neglect.
- It is now known that undernutrition is the unifying cause of FTT.
- Poverty still exists in the "developed" world.

NORMAL GROWTH

Normal growth can be defined as a pattern of progression in weight and height that is consistent with the established standards for age in accordance with the genetic potential of the individual. It is the normal increase in mass and dimensions of the body and is influenced by both genetic and environmental (intra- and extrauterine) factors.

Growth Charts

Growth is monitored by plotting weight and height against standardized reference growth charts. For these charts to be relevant they have to compare like to like, and so the population that they are drawn from has to be comparable to that from which the child comes. Some older reference charts were based on a predominantly White, middle-class population. However, recent versions have reflected with greater precision the more multiethnic and economically diverse communities of the modern developed world. The most recent clinical version of the 2000 *Centers for Disease Control and Prevention* (CDC) growth charts includes a set of curves for infants (birth to 36 months of age) and a set for children and adolescents (2–20 years of age).[2] The charts represent a cross-section of children who live in the United States and breast-fed infants are represented on the basis of their distribution in the U.S. population. They more closely match the national distribution of birth weights than did the 1977 *National Center for Health Statistics* (NCHS) growth charts, and the disjunction between weight-for-length and weight-for-stature or length-for-age and stature-for-age found in the 1977 charts has been corrected. Moreover, the 2000 CDC growth charts can be used to obtain both percentiles and z scores. Finally, body mass index-for-age charts are available for children and adolescents 2–20 years of age. The 2000 CDC growth charts are recommended for use in the United States for routine monitoring of growth in infants, children, and adolescents.

Normal Growth Pattern in First Year of Life

Infants should regain their birth weight by the age of 2 weeks and exhibit steady weight gain (of at least 15–30 g per day) thereafter. However, not all infants will follow the natural growth curves demonstrated in commonly used growth charts. Because birth weight is largely dependent on maternal influences (e.g., maternal weight, parity, smoking, and alcohol consumption) and by 1–2 months of age the true genetic potential for growth is more apparent, the maximum centile achieved between 4 and 8 weeks is a better predictor of the centile at a year than is the centile at birth. Hence "catch up" weight gain is commonly seen in the first few weeks in small-for-date infants. Similarly, "catch down" weight gain can also be entirely normal but is characteristically slower, occurring after 4 months, and ends in normal growth following a lower centile line in a child with normal findings on history and physical examination. The problem can be identifying how much centile shift can be expected in normal infants. From 6 weeks of age there is less variability with only 5% of children crossing through two intercentile lines before their first birthday, and only 1% crossing three intercentile lines. In addition to this it appears that very large and very small babies will regress to the mean so that 5% of children on the 98th centile at birth will fall through three centile spaces.

Dietary Requirements for Normal Growth

The energy needs per kg of infants are three times that of adults. Thus, the *estimated average requirements* (EAR) for energy for infants aged 0–3 months are 115 kcal/kg per day and for children aged 1–3 years 95 kcal/kg per day.

Summary

- Growth is influenced by genetic and environmental factors.
- CDC 2000 growth charts should be used to monitor growth.
- The maximum centile achieved between 4 and 8 weeks reflects genetic potential more accurately than the birth weight.
- A small percentage of normal children will cross centile lines and appear to have FTT.
- The energy requirement per kilogram of body weight of an infant is huge compared to that of an adult.

DEFINITIONS

Failure to Thrive

Failure to thrive is a symptom or a descriptive term rather than a disease or a diagnosis. Therefore, when used to describe a patient the underlying cause or diagnosis should be subsequently identified. The verb "to thrive" means "to do well, to prosper, and to grow strongly and vigorously" and thus implies more than mere physical growth. This notion has been reflected in some definitions of FTT, which have included "evidence of lassitude, loss of energy, and *joie de vivre*." Thus, it is important to assess the psychologic and psychosocial well-being of any child with poor growth as problems in either of these areas can have a huge impact on the child's weight gain and development.

Nevertheless, the current consensus is that any definition of FTT should be primarily weight-based since there are difficulties with the objective assessment of "well-being." FTT implies a failure to achieve a normal rate of growth and so the criterion for diagnosis should involve sustained deviation for a defined period from the expected growth curve (bearing in mind the difficulties in estimating a normal infant's growth pattern as discussed above). A commonly used definition requires a drop in weight below a low centile line, traditionally the third centile. The advantages of this approach were that it was easy to implement and was widely accepted and understood. The disadvantages were that it inevitably included a number of normal but small children and missed those whose weight had dropped from higher centile lines. Therefore, this definition was modified such that children were said to be failing to thrive if their weight fell across two centile lines, although again it is known from normal growth studies that a small number of normal children will be included in this group.

Currently used definitions include the *Social Security Administration* (SSA) guidelines which consider FTT to be present when there is a fall in weight to less than the third centile or to less than 75% of median weight-for-height or weight-for-age in children less than 2 years old.[3] Moreover, there must be no underlying medical disorder, and growth failure should last or be expected to last for at least 12 months. An alternative definition measures the longitudinal ponderal growth trajectory in terms of the discrepancy between a child's predicted and actual weight gain. This has been named the "thrive index" and from this tables have been constructed that calculate the expected and fifth centile weights at 3, 6, 9, 12, and 18 months for children with different 6-week centile positions (see Table 4-1).[4] A third description of FTT requires a weight deviation downward from the true centile (defined as the maximum centile achieved between 4 and 8 weeks of age) crossing two or more centile lines and persisting for more than a month.[5] Although this may pick up a number

T A B L E   4 - 1

THE THRIVE INDEX[a]

6 weeks			Months				
Centile	Weight (kg)		3	6	9	12	18
Boys							
97	5.97	Expected	7.44	9.18	10.21	11.13	12.46
		Lower	6.75	8.07	8.85	9.66	10.79
90	5.56	Expected	6.99	8.73	9.80	10.69	11.99
		Lower	6.36	7.72	8.54	9.32	10.44
75	5.17	Expected	6.57	8.32	9.42	10.27	11.55
		Lower	5.99	7.38	8.25	9.00	10.10
50	4.75	Expected	6.14	7.89	9.03	9.85	11.10
		Lower	5.62	7.04	7.94	8.67	9.75
25	4.36	Expected	5.76	7.51	8.66	9.45	10.68
		Lower	5.28	6.72	7.65	8.37	9.42
10	4.03	Expected	5.44	7.19	8.36	9.13	10.33
		Lower	4.99	6.45	7.41	8.11	9.14
3	3.72	Expected	5.15	6.89	8.08	8.82	10.00
		Lower	4.74	6.21	7.19	7.86	8.89
Girls							
97	5.62	Expected	6.87	8.46	9.46	10.39	11.76
		Lower	6.24	7.44	8.21	9.02	10.19
90	5.23	Expected	6.45	8.04	9.08	9.97	11.32
		Lower	5.87	7.11	7.92	8.70	9.86
75	4.86	Expected	6.07	7.66	8.73	9.59	10.91
		Lower	5.53	6.80	7.64	8.40	9.54
50	4.47	Expected	5.68	7.27	8.36	9.19	10.48
		Lower	5.19	6.48	7.64	8.10	9.21
25	4.10	Expected	5.32	6.91	8.03	8.82	10.09
		Lower	4.87	6.19	7.09	7.81	8.90
10	3.79	Expected	5.02	6.62	7.75	8.52	9.75
		Lower	4.61	5.95	6.87	7.57	8.64
3	3.50	Expected	4.75	6.35	7.49	8.24	9.44
		Lower	4.37	5.72	6.66	7.34	8.39

[a]Predicted attained weight conditional on early centile position: the upper figure is the expected weight (kg) at 3, 6, 9, 12, and 18 months for children with weights on the given centiles at 6 weeks, the lower italicized figure is the weight exceeded by 95% of such children (the fifth centile of the thrive index).

Source: Modified and permission is being sought from reference 4.

of false positives (as many as 22% of the population), it is a reasonable reflection of what many experienced pediatricians would identify as FTT and is simple and easy to remember.

This final point is important as the different definitions are confusing for the average health worker and although recent advances in the development of reference charts are to be welcomed, the danger is that they might compound problems of definition and identification of FTT. A universally recognized definition would potentially enable vulnerable children to be identified earlier and facilitate research and secondary preventative measures.

Classification of Types of FTT

Clearly, growth is not just about weight gain. In order to gain an accurate assessment of a child's nutritional status other anthropometric measurements such as height, head circumference, and *mid-upper arm circumference* (MUAC) should be measured and assessed in the context of age, sex, and parental height. Commonly used indices are weight-for-age, height-for-age, and weight-for-height. A child is *wasted* if there is a deficit in weight-for-height. This is as a result of failure to gain weight or weight loss and usually reflects an acute problem and therefore has the potential to be reversed rapidly. A child is *stunted* if there is a deficit in height-for-age secondary to undernutrition and this signifies a slowing in skeletal growth. This is more likely to be due to a chronic cause and the consequences are subsequently more longstanding.

Summary

- *Normal growth*. A pattern of progression in weight and height that is consistent with the established standards for age in accordance with the genetic potential of the individual.
- *Failure to thrive*. A weight deviation downward from the true centile (defined as the maximum centile achieved between 4 and 8 weeks of age) crossing two or more centile lines and persisting for more than 1 month.

- *Thrive index*. A measure of the discrepancy between a child's predicted and actual growth.
- *Wasted*. A decreased weight-for-age and weight-for-height with a normal height-for-age.
- *Stunted*. A decreased height-for-age and weight-for-age with a normal weight-for-height.
- *Severe malnutrition*. Presence of edema of both feet and/or weight-for-height <70%.[1]

DIFFERENTIAL DIAGNOSIS

A number of conditions are often confused with FTT and these include familial short stature, constitutional growth delay, *intrauterine growth retardation* (IUGR), and the effects of prolonged breast feeding.

Familial Short Stature

This is genetically determined short stature in which the final height is consistent with the mid-parental height. In the early years of life familial short stature may present with a suspicious looking growth curve as children readjust their growth percentile according to their genetic potential. These children grow at constant rates proportional to those of average height with weight appropriate for height and have a normal bone age, and they enter puberty at the expected time. The diagnosis is confirmed as the child maintains a growth channel appropriate for the family without deviation to a lower centile.

Constitutional Growth Delay

A very common diagnosis in children referred for either height or weight gain delay, this condition is actually considered a normal variation of growth. These children usually present with a severe deceleration in growth in the first 2 years of life with a subsequent realignment to a centile line and normal growth increments until adolescence when a growth spurt occurs. It can be very difficult during this period of reduced growth velocity to be confident that such a child is not failing to thrive.

A delayed radiologic bone age and family history of delayed growth and puberty make the diagnosis of constitutional growth delay more likely.

Intrauterine Growth Retardation

Intrauterine growth retardation, defined as a birth weight <10th centile for gestational age, does place children at risk of FTT. Even when infants with IUGR are excluded from the analysis, studies have shown that those infants with FTT have significantly lower birth weights than control groups. Those with symmetrical IUGR (where the length, weight, and head circumference are proportionately reduced) which is associated with intrauterine infections, chromosomal abnormalities, and maternal drug/alcohol ingestion, are particularly vulnerable to ongoing problems with growth. Asymmetrical IUGR, on the other hand, where head circumference (and therefore brain growth) is relatively preserved, has a more favorable prognosis with many infants showing impressive catch-up growth in the first year of life. However, it can be difficult to establish whether the IUGR infant is growing normally without catch-up growth or is, in fact, failing to thrive. Because of the diversity of the etiologic factors and the variability of the time that the fetus has been exposed to the differing environmental, maternal, placental, and fetal factors, the expected growth pattern of an IUGR infant has not been clearly defined. There may be an accelerated growth spurt in the first 3 months of life but significant long-term deficits with regard to height and weight are recognized. Because of their initial small size, a false impression of FTT in an infant with a history of IUGR can easily be made. Thus, it is important to monitor growth of such an infant on appropriate charts. A useful rule of thumb is that if the birth weight is doubled by 4 months and tripled by the first birthday then FTT is unlikely.

Excessively Prolonged Breast Feeding

The effect of prolonged breast feeding on subsequent growth is controversial. There is some evidence to suggest that breast-fed babies have a slower growth velocity. The weight of breast-fed infants drops below the NCHS median value beginning at 6–8 months of age and remains significantly lower than that of formula-fed infants between 6 and 18 months of age. By similar comparison, weight-for-length measurements are also significantly different between 4 and 18 months of age, suggesting that breast-fed infants are leaner than their formula-fed counterparts. Human milk is undoubtedly the ideal and most readily available nutrient for an infant and this is especially true for families in resource-poor settings. How long exclusive breast feeding is adequate and when supplementary food should be introduced has not yet been clarified. A recent study has confirmed that infants who are exclusively breastfed for 6 months do not grow differently to those who are only partially breastfed.[6] Current recommendations from WHO are to exclusively breastfeed for the first 6 months of life.

Summary

- Familial short stature: the final height is consistent with the parental height.
- Constitutional growth delay: is likely if there is a positive family history and if growth continues along a lower centile line.
- IUGR is associated with FTT but such infants can exhibit catch-up growth.
- "Breast is best" but breast feeding beyond 6 months can lead to a relative FTT.

EPIDEMIOLOGY

Although FTT is a common problem, precise epidemiologic data is lacking. FTT accounts for 1–5% of pediatric hospital admissions under 2 years of age. This will be an underestimate of its true incidence, however, as FTT is identified and treated primarily in the community. The population prevalence of FTT has been found to range anywhere between 1.3 and 20.9% depending on the definition of FTT that is used. The imprecision of this data is a reflection of the difficulties in assessing the frequency of the occurrence of FTT in children. Some of these difficulties are discussed below.

Skewed Population

Most early studies have focused on hospital inpatients; this has resulted in a distorted picture of the problem with the higher prevalence of psychosocial dysfunction being a reflection of this selection bias.

Inconsistent Definitions of FTT

If a weight below the third centile is used as the definition then it is of little surprise to find that 3% of the population is failing to thrive. What is clear is that many children, perhaps as many as 50%, with low weight gain are either missed by health professionals or are not followed up or managed appropriately. Weighing children is easy to do but interpreting growth patterns is difficult and it is expensive to train health workers to do this. Considerable anxiety is caused to the parents of those incorrectly identified as FTT. The usefulness of regular weighing of infants is debatable; the current consensus is to be opportunistic and to monitor growth at birth, at 6 weeks, at times of immunization, and at other times where a child presents to health professionals. Assessment of growth and development should be an essential part of the holistic approach to managing any child who presents as an inpatient or in the community.

Preconceptions of Health Workers

Some of the difficulties in compliance with weight surveillance and interpretation of findings are related to a preconception by health workers and researchers that FTT is always linked with poverty. As a consequence of this, most studies of FTT have focused on highly deprived groups and produced skewed and unhelpful results. There is, in fact, little objective evidence to support this putative link with poverty. Indeed recent studies suggest that the majority of patients with FTT come from the larger population of more "average" income backgrounds. In particular it has been noted that because of this assumption that deprivation is a risk factor, children with a weight less than the third centile who are from a low socioeconomic class are more likely to

be labeled as FTT (and hence referred) while similar children from a more affluent background are more likely to be described as "constitutional short stature." Consequently, those children from a higher socioeconomic class are being missed and/or present later than they should. A study from an urban area of the United Kingdom which identified children with FTT using the thrive index, showed: (1) that the majority were not from the most deprived areas of the city, (2) that overt neglect was rare, and (3) that 76% were living in apparently caring homes but were nevertheless undernourished.[7]

Summary

- FTT is common.
- Inconsistent definitions for FTT and preconceptions about FTT being associated with poverty and NAI make assessing true epidemiology difficult.
- Neglect is a rare cause of FTT in children.

ETIOLOGY

Traditional View: Organic or Nonorganic

Traditionally the causes of FTT have been split into two very distinct groups: organic and nonorganic. In organic FTT there is a major illness or organ system dysfunction to account for the poor weight gain while in nonorganic FTT no such cause is found and there has been an assumption that this is the result of psychosocial or psychologic problems, most often centering on the parent-child relationship.

Modern View: Undernutrition in All

In recent years it has been recognized that very few cases, perhaps as few as 5%, of FTT have a pure organic cause. Some have a functional problem that is exacerbated by adverse environmental factors (such as difficulties with feeding) but the vast majority are classified as nonorganic as no physiologic cause is found.

Current thinking on this subject would suggest that the organic/nonorganic split is unhelpful and that insufficient usable nutrition is the underlying

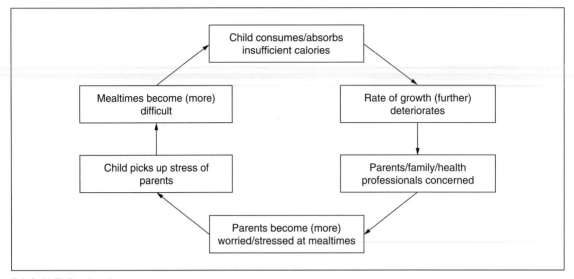

F I G U R E   4 - 1

PROCESS OF FAMILY INTERACTIONS (THE CYCLE OF DESPAIR)

cause in all cases of FTT. The boundaries between the two entities have progressively become blurred with the recognition that many of these children have a mixed etiology. Children with organic FTT can also have nonorganic problems: the child with poor weight gain caused by organic pathology may also exhibit secondary behavioral feeding difficulties and progress into a vicious cycle of undernutrition (Fig. 4-1). Equally, many cases of nonorganic FTT have been found to have organic factors. Stress can cause a neuroendocrine disturbance that can account for a reduction in weight gain. It has also been found that a significant number of children labeled as nonorganic FTT may in fact have oral motor dysfunction and/or poorer cognitive functioning.

There is also a clearer appreciation that the caregiver/child relationship is reciprocal. A mother's desire to nurture her child may be dependent in part on the unique qualities of the child (physical appearance, cry, and response to affection). Therefore, a demanding baby may result in a stressed and anxious mother, equally, a depressed or anxious mother may result in a tense and poorly feeding infant. At the other extreme a slow and quiet baby may be easily ignored and fed less with the subsequent undernutrition making the child even less demanding and more

apathetic. Irrespective of the nature of the initial precipitating trigger of the FTT, there is a danger that the family may be drawn into a vicious cycle of anxiety and distress that further exacerbates the problem (Fig. 4-1). Most parents are upset to learn that their child is not growing satisfactorily and, depending on how the problem is approached, may feel threatened or guilty about the involvement of health professionals. Children are very adept at picking up on this anxiety and thus mealtimes may become even more tense and parents more desperate, even to the extent of force-feeding their child, which inevitably exacerbates the problem.[8]

Precipitating Causes of Failure to Thrive

Undernutrition is consistently found to be the underlying feature of FTT. This may be as a result of several factors in the child or the mother and the consequences of these on their relationship (Fig. 4-2). Most work has focused on the mother-child relationship although it is recognized that there are other relationships (with the father or other family members) which have a significant impact on growth. FTT is known to be associated with a variety of problems such as socioeconomic

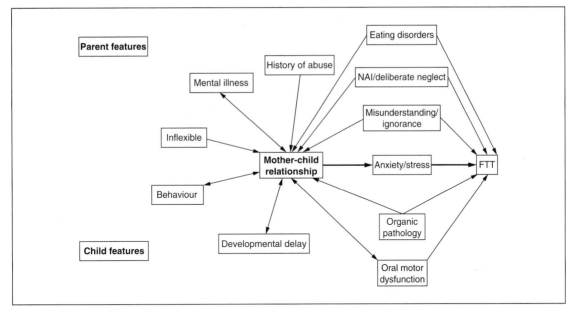

FIGURE 4-2
ETIOLOGY OF FTT

factors (low income, lower maternal education, and impoverished family environment/interactions), neonatal morbidity, acute illness and hospitalization, neurologic and anatomic abnormalities, family dysfunction and abuse/neglect. As Fig. 4-2 demonstrates, these variables stand not in isolation but are interrelated and may precede the FTT and/or be a consequence of it.

Child Factors

Behavior

Infants who fail to communicate their basic needs and/or are unrewarding feeders are at risk of FTT. Some children appear to be less responsive, cry less for feeds, and when fed do not appear as content as other children. These behavioral patterns may reflect the child's personality or indicate either underlying malnutrition or developmental delay. Whatever the cause, they significantly influence the mother-child relationship. Behavioral problems are more common in children with FTT, even in those without a concurrent diagnosis of neurologic or other organic disease.

These children may exhibit increased negative affect and decreased positive affect during feeds but notably no observable differences in behavior from controls in nonfeeding situations.

"Infantile anorexia nervosa" is a term that has been used to describe a group of children characterized by food refusal or extremely fussy eating. This is despite, or possibly because of, parental efforts to increase intake. It commonly occurs between the ages of 6 months and 3 years with a peak at approximately 9 months. It is thought that the behavior stems from the infant's desire for autonomy which leads to a conflict between the caregiver and infant that rages over the dining table—a battle in which the child almost invariably emerges as the victor. Of particular interest in the history is any suggestion of force-feeding in the child's development as this may lead to a significant degree of oral aversive behavior.

Oral-motor Dysfunction

A clear relationship has been demonstrated between feeding difficulties and FTT. These feeding difficulties begin early in life and may be the initial trigger for many of the subsequent mother-child stress responses. It has been found, for instance, that children with FTT take significantly longer to complete a breastfeed. An explanation for this is that these children may have underlying subtle oral-motor dysfunction such that they are slow feeders even at the breast. Such oral-motor dysfunction with perioral hypersensitivity to tactile stimuli may affect up to 25% of FTT infants. This perioral hypersensitivity may be either a secondary phenomenon (e.g., from force-feeding) or a primary problem of subtle neuromuscular incoordination. Whatever the etiology, the oroaversion makes feeding an immensely frustrating experience for the caregivers.

Developmental Delay

Developmental delay has always been closely related to FTT, so much so that it used to be one of the criteria necessary to make the diagnosis. It has been shown that children either hospitalized or being managed in an inner city clinic with FTT have significantly lower than average Bayley Mental Development scores when compared with a control group.

Parental Factors

Misunderstanding/Ignorance

There is often a lack of awareness of the nutritional requirements of the child, particularly in the early months of life when the high energy needs (three times that of adults/kg) may not be appreciated. In an age where there are legitimate concerns regarding obesity and its sequelae there have been reports of children presenting with FTT because of "low fat" diets imposed by well-meaning parents.

Eating Disorders

Mothers with eating disorders have been found to be less facilitating in play and to have children who are less happy at mealtimes and who are consequently lighter than controls. More particularly, children of mothers with anorexia have been found to suffer from food deprivation. Parental eating habits and attitudes are thus significant influences on FTT.

Depression

There are significantly higher levels of depression among women whose children have late onset FTT. It is unclear whether the problems with the child, and particularly with feeding, precipitate the depression or whether the mental health of the mother was an underlying cause of the FTT.

Parenting Skills

All children are different and place particular and unique demands on their parents. Many of these children with "potential" FTT have subtle underlying feeding difficulties and are therefore challenging to feed. Some parents recognize the problem and are able to compensate for these difficulties by adjusting their feeding techniques accordingly. Children of mothers with a lower IQ are known to be at higher risk of FTT and perhaps this is because such mothers are less responsive and fail to compensate for their child's difficult feeding.

History of Abuse

There are few studies looking at this risk factor but those that do suggest that mothers of children with FTT are significantly more likely to have suffered some kind of abuse compared with mothers of normally growing children with as many as 80% of mothers of children with nonorganic FTT in one study stating that they were victims of abuse themselves.

Neglect/Nonaccidental Injury

Abuse and neglect have been associated with FTT ever since it was originally labeled as "maternal deprivation." Although its role has been overstated in the past, recent population studies have found that 5–10% of children with FTT had been registered for abuse or neglect. Furthermore, children with FTT are four times more likely to be abused than controls. Despite this, such families constitute a small proportion of the total number of children with FTT. The experience of most workers is that the parents of the majority of children with FTT are struggling to get calories into their children and have no intention to harm.

Physiologic Causes

There are several ways to approach the etiology of "organic" FTT, none of which are truly comprehensive. One of the most straightforward classifications is to assess intake, absorption, losses, and requirements of nutrients (Table 4-2).

It is important to remember that there can be a primary cause from any of the major systems as shown in Table 4-3.

Infection can be both a cause and a consequence of FTT. Such children are at increased risk of infection as a result of nutrition-related immunocompromise by a variety of known abnormalities including decreased chemotactic response to bacterial endotoxin and phagocytosis of zymogen particles, lower percentages of rosette forming cells (reflecting a reduction in cellular immune function), and reduced Candida killing ability. Evidence of acute or chronic infectious diseases should be sought but in those with *severe* malnutrition there may be few signs and so in these cases it is recommended that antibiotics be routinely given.

Most cases of "organic" FTT can be found to have at least a secondary gastrointestinal abnormality such as dysphagia, malabsorption, or anorexia as a consequence of the underlying pathology.

Examples of Presentations of FTT

Congenital Heart Disease

The child with congenital heart disease may be small because of a primary genetic syndrome of which the cardiac lesion is a component. The child may be hypoxic and breathless leading to *poor food intake*, they may have venous congestion of the gut causing *malabsorption* and/or protein-losing enteropathy, and they may be hypochloremic and alkalotic secondary to diuretic therapy. In addition to this, they may have increased energy consumption (particularly in left-to-right shunts and pulmonary hypertension) so that overall energy intake is insufficient to meet the increased demands. Intake may indeed be appropriate for actual weight but not for expected weight for age.

TABLE 4-2

CAUSES OF FTT

Inadequate Intake	Inadequate Absorption	Excessive Loss	Excessive Requirement
Feeding mismanagement (e.g., errors in formula feed, bizarre/restricted diet, neglect, poverty)	Pancreatic insufficiency (e.g., cystic fibrosis, Schwachman-Diamond)	Vomiting (e.g., CNS abnormality, intestinal obstruction, metabolic abnormality, gastroesophageal reflux)	Chronic illness (e.g., cystic fibrosis, congenital heart disease, inflammatory bowel disease)
Inability to feed optimally (e.g., developmental delay, cleft palate, bulbar palsy)	Small intestine disease (e.g., dissacharidase deficiency, cow's milk protein intolerance, celiac)	Protein-losing enteropathy	Thyrotoxicosis
Anorexia (e.g., chronic illness, "infantile anorexia nervosa")		Chronic diarrhea	Chronic infection (e.g., TB, HIV)
Diencephalic syndrome			Malignancy
			Burns

TABLE 4-3

CAUSES OF FTT BY SYSTEM

Gastrointestinal	*Dysphagia:* neuromuscular incoordination, cleft palate, micrognathia, postoperative esophageal atresia, tracheoesophageal fistula, esophagitis, achalasia
	Anorexia: gastritis, enteric infections, Crohn's disease, celiac disease, motility disorders
	Malabsorption: cystic fibrosis, Schwachman, celiac, cow's milk sensitive enteropathy, short gut, abetalipoprotein anemia, lymphangectasia, bacterial overgrowth, cholestatic liver disease
	Excessive losses: gastroesophageal reflux, pyloric stenosis, incomplete/recurrent obstruction
Renal	Renal tubular acidosis, chronic renal disease, recurrent UTI
Neurologic	Birth injury, asphyxia, chromosomal abnormalities, neurodegenerative diseases, hydrocephalus, intracranial lesions (e.g., diencephalic syndrome, myopathies)
Cardiovascular	Congenital and acquired congestive and cyanotic disease
Endocrine	Hypo- and hyperthyroid, hyperaldosteronism, hypopituitarism, growth hormone deficiency, exogenous hypercortisolism
Respiratory	Chronic hypoxemia, bronchopulmonary dysplasia, cystic fibrosis
Metabolic	Aminoacidopathies, inborn errors of metabolism, idiopathic hypercalcemia
Immunologic	HIV, inflammatory joint disease
Genetic	Fetal alcohol
Chronic infection	TB, recurrent UTI
Hematologic	Fe deficiency, malignancy
Drugs and toxins	Lead

Of note in these infants is the biochemistry of cardiac metabolism. After birth this is normally predominantly fatty acid driven, but in the presence of hypoxia, cardiac metabolism reverts to the fetal glycolytic process and the unmetabolized fatty acids exert a negative effect on carbohydrate metabolism with a subsequent decline in myocardial contractility. It is logical therefore to use carbohydrates and not fats or proteins as a source of extra energy in these infants.

Malignancy

FTT is also a common finding in children being treated for acute lymphoblastic leukemia even when they are provided with aggressive nutritional support. The causes of this, all of which are secondary to the side effects of the intensive chemotherapy used, include toxicity to the intestinal epithelium (leading to *malabsorption*), *anorexia*, and mucositis (causing *dysphagia*). This is particularly true for infants not fully weaned at onset of treatment with subsequent delay in feeding skills and who become increasingly orally aversive with a low solid intake.

Diencephalic Syndrome

Even the very rare causes of FTT, such as diencephalic syndrome, may appear as a gastroenterologic problem as the initial features may only be unexplained poor weight gain. One hypothesis for the pathogenesis for the severe wasting in this unusual low-grade glioma is a disruption of normal appetite control leading to *anorexia*. Typical patients appear at 6–12 months of age with FTT and the features that should prompt the clinician to the diagnosis include an alert appearance, hyperkinesias, vomiting, euphoria, pallor, and nystagmus. Such patients need surgical resection (which is often impossible) and chemotherapy.

Celiac Disease

The child with celiac disease does not fail to thrive only from the primary *malabsorption* but also because of the *anorexia*, vomiting, and abdominal pain associated with the disease (see Chap. 18).

Cystic Fibrosis

Pancreatic insufficiency (and consequent *malabsorption*) is the primary gastroenterologic insult but recurrent chest infections lead to loss of appetite (*anorexia*) and increased energy requirements.

ASSESSMENT OF FTT

As we have seen, the differential diagnosis for FTT is vast but in the majority of cases there are sufficient symptoms and signs to make the correct diagnosis. The assessment of any child with FTT requires a careful history and examination.

Features of the History

Dietary/Feeding History

It is important to obtain a detailed history of feeding from birth. A careful dietetic assessment must be performed, ideally with a 24-h recall of intake and a 3- or 7-day food diary, which should then be evaluated by a dietician for calorie, protein, and micronutrient content. Included in this should be assessment of timing and frequency of meals/feeds, identification of who makes and administers the feeds and how long mealtimes take. Particular attention needs to be paid to the amount of snacking between meals and to fluid intake such as milk, juice, or carbonated drinks. Excessive intake of apparently healthy fruit juices can lead to FTT as they displace more calorie and nutrient dense foods. Evidence of dietary restrictions or exclusions should be sought. Every attempt should be made to observe feeding.

Past Medical History

Perinatal. This should include birth weight, gestational age, birth length, head circumference, and any need for medical intervention. Perinatal factors exert a significant influence on postnatal growth. Many babies born with IUGR continue to be relatively small and can easily be misdiagnosed as having FTT. Prematurity also puts infants at increased risk of a range of respiratory, neurologic, and gastrointestinal pathologies as well as behavioral and cognitive dysfunction that also may lead to postnatal undernutrition.

Postnatal. Growth disturbance can occur secondary to almost all severe and chronic childhood illnesses.

Systemic Enquiry

A thorough systemic enquiry is essential to rule out organic pathology. In the context of gastrointestinal disease in particular a clear idea of whether the child is vomiting, has abdominal pain, or an abnormal bowel habit is important.

Family History

Heights, weights, developmental delay, constitutional short stature, and chronic illnesses in first degree relatives are all potentially crucial clues in assessing the potential etiology of FTT.

Developmental History

It is sensible as part of a holistic approach to the care of children with FTT for them to undergo in their initial assessment a standardized developmental assessment (such as the Bayley scale of infant development for those <30 months and the McCarthy scales for older children). At the very least the basic developmental milestones should be documented.

In the older child, an attempt should also be made to ascertain their educational achievement and ability. Many of these children, because of the FTT and its associated psychosocial and physical problems, are less likely to do well at school and will require additional support in this setting.

Psychosocial History

Parental health beliefs. Parental misconceptions regarding what constitutes an appropriate diet for a child or infant may also lead to FTT and so an assessment should be made of their own feeding habits and diet. Mothers with eating disorders such as anorexia nervosa can be restricting their child's intake and particularly foods that they consider unhealthy or fattening. Children of parents who hold to a strictly vegan diet may be at risk of poor growth because of a bulky diet that restricts energy intake as well as iron deficiency anemia, vitamin B_{12} deficiency, and rickets.

Poverty. Poverty is associated with childhood malnutrition. It is essential, therefore, to establish the economic status of the family concerned: the parents' employment, their housing circumstances, and whether they have sufficient funds to buy adequate food and the means by which to prepare it appropriately.

Parental coping ability. Chronically ill children may overwhelm the caregiver abilities of perfectly able, adequate, and loving parents. Moreover, children may appear to thrive as hospital inpatients, where many trained staff share the burden of care, but fail to thrive at home when looked after by a struggling parent. Caring for a chronically ill child can lead to huge additional stresses on a family leading to marital discord, depression, abuse of alcohol and drugs, and isolation from the extended family and wider community.

Summary

- Dietary: what is the child eating and how successfully?
- Perinatal: identify risk factors such as prematurity and IUGR.
- Systemic enquiry: make a thorough exploration for clues of cause of FTT.
- Developmental: identify underlying delay contributing to FTT and/or feeding problems.
- Psychosocial: explore issues such as parental beliefs and attitudes to food and feeding, economic status, education, and general parenting skills.

Features of the Physical Examination

General Examination

A thorough general and systematic examination is required. In particular any evidence of chronic illness or dysmorphic or dwarfing syndromes should be sought. The possibility of NAI should be borne in mind and telltale physical signs such as suspicious bruising, burns, or abrasions for which there is no adequate explanation given should be noted. Evidence of acute or chronic infectious diseases should be looked for but there may be few signs, particularly in those with severe malnutrition.

Signs of underlying gastroenterologic disorders such as finger clubbing, perianal skin tags, mouth ulcers, and anal fissures or fistulae are easily missed if not specifically looked for.

Anthropometry

Weight, height, head circumference, and ideally also skin fold thicknesses (e.g., triceps, subscapular, suprailiac) and mid-upper arm circumference should be measured.

Weight. The child's naked weight should be measured on an electronic scale.

Length/height. Length and height are more difficult to measure accurately. Length in those under two years of age is measured lying horizontally on a measuring board and requires an assistant to hold the legs straight and feet as flat as possible against the footboard with the head held straight against the sliding headboard which incorporates a measuring scale (see Fig. 4-3). In the older child, height is measured with a wall mounted stadiometer with particular attention paid to keeping the head upright with eyes and ears level by gentle traction applied to the mastoid processes, knees should be straight and feet flat on the ground with heels touching the back of the board (see Fig. 4-4).

From these measurements the body mass index can be calculated (weight in kg/height in m^2).

Weight and height should be plotted against a comparable population such as the 2000 CDC

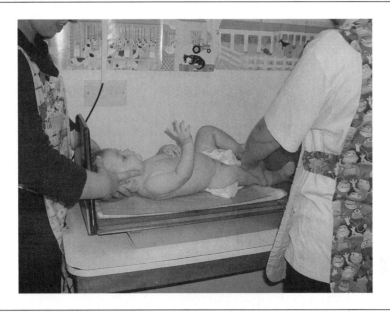

FIGURE 4-3

MEASUREMENT OF INFANT'S LENGTH

growth charts.[2] Growth parameters should be corrected for gestational age (head circumference until 18 months, weight until 24 months, and height/length until 40 months chronologic age).

Skin fold thickness/MUAC. Accurate measurement of skin fold thickness requires training and is performed using calipers usually in the triceps and subscapular regions. These measurements can be used to provide an assessment of subcutaneous fat stores. MUAC is measured using a narrow nonstretching tape applied midway between the acromion and olecranon processes (see Fig. 4-5).

Behavior

Observing feeding. This is crucial in understanding the pathogenesis of a child's FTT. Ideally it should be conducted in the family home where the child's positioning for feeds, presence of inappropriate distractions (e.g., television), interruptions of feeding, and multiple and/or inconsistent feeders can be observed. A video recording taken by the parents can also be instructive and may be more practical to arrange.

Nutritional deficiencies. Some nutritional deficiencies such as zinc and iron can cause alterations in behavior with iron deficiency in particular being associated with anorexia, irritability, apathy, and delayed psychomotor development.

Summary

- Accurately assess weight, length/height, and head circumference (+/− MUAC and skin fold thickness).
- Look specifically for evidence of dysmorphic syndromes, NAI, and infection.
- Exclude underlying "organic" pathology.
- Assess degree of malnutrition and in cases of severe malnutrition examine for central hypothermia, pallor, dehydration or shock, decreased level of consciousness, decreased peripheral perfusion, localizing infection (particularly secondary skin infection), eye signs secondary to vitamin A deficiency, and skin changes secondary to kwashiorkor and bilateral pitting edema.[1]
- Observe a feed, ideally in the home situation.

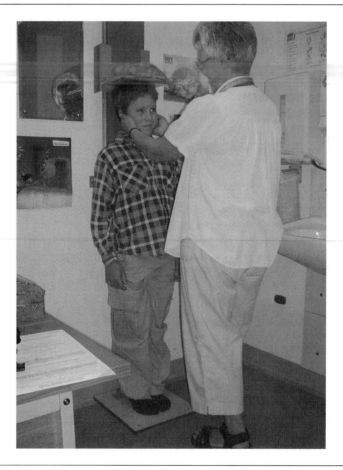

FIGURE 4-4

MEASUREMENT OF HEIGHT

Laboratory Investigations

The list of possible laboratory investigations is extensive (Fig. 4-6). However, necessary investigations are indicated by the clinical findings and will be undertaken to either: (1) identify or exclude an underlying cause, or (2) assess the impact of the nutritional insult.

Routine Screening to Identify/Exclude Cause

Screening for causes of organic FTT is rarely of help. In one study by Sills in Buffalo in 1978, 185 children with FTT underwent 2607 investigations of which only 36 (1.4%) were of positive diagnostic assistance. Therefore, the investigations listed in Fig. 4-3, even those in the first line, should strictly be considered in the light of the findings in the history and examination.

Assessing Impact of Nutritional Insult

Biochemistry. Investigations for evaluation of nutritional status may be of some use. Proteins such as albumin and transferrin have been used as nutritional markers but their long half-life limits their usefulness. Other protein markers that have been studied include prealbumin (also increased with infection

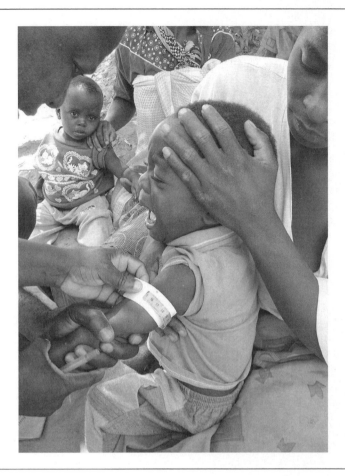

FIGURE 4-5

MEASUREMENT OF MUAC

and inflammation), retinal binding protein (which seems more affected by energy than protein deficiency), fibronectin, insulin-like growth factor (IGF)-1 (low levels of which would also be consistent with constitutional short stature), and erythrocyte Na-K-ATPase (ENKA). ENKA is an enzyme involved with the active transport of sugars and amino acids and with cellular thermogenesis and accounts for approximately one-third of all basal energy requirements. A fall in energy intake leads to a lower basal energy requirement and a reduction in ENKA activity.[9]

Nutritional deficiencies of iron and calcium may enhance the absorption of lead and toxic metals and children with FTT have been found to

have significantly higher lead levels than matched controls with 16% having blood levels high enough to warrant chelation therapy.

Immunology and hematology. Immune dysfunction is a common feature and resolves with a return to normal nutritional status. Many patients with a severe degree of malnutrition have a depressed lymphocyte count ($<1.5 \times 10^9$/L) and energy, which can therefore be a useful indicator as to the severity of malnutrition. The possibility of HIV infection should be considered in areas of the world where there is a high prevalence. In such contexts FTT is often a presenting sign of underlying

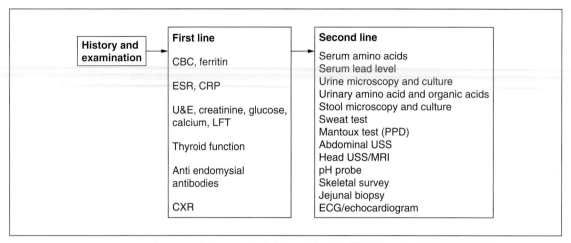

INVESTIGATIONS TO CONSIDER IN A CHILD WITH FTT

infection. Indeed, in many African countries a breast-fed child presenting with FTT in the first year of life would be presumed to have HIV infection, particularly if the child or either parent has had a chronic illness and/or other siblings had died or were failing to thrive.

Specific Gastroenterologic Investigations

There are particular investigations that may be relevant in a gastroenterologic setting. If there are concerns regarding possible malabsorption as either a primary or secondary component of the FTT then serum albumin and ferritin (as general markers for malabsorption) as well as stool for fecal elastase and chymotrypsin (to assess pancreatic exocrine function) could be indicated. Antiendomysial antibodies and/or IgA tissue transglutaminase may be requested to exclude celiac disease. Evidence of malabsorption and FTT may necessitate a small bowel biopsy.

Crohn's disease is another condition that can present with FTT but usually in the older child with poor weight gain/weight loss, and in these children there may be few other clinical clues as to the underlying diagnosis. A radiologic small intestinal lesion is present in at least 80% of young adults with Crohn's disease and so contrast studies (a barium meal and follow through or ideally a small bowel enema) as well as endoscopy (upper and lower) should be considered.

TREATMENT

General Management

Assessment

The treatment of these children is based on the foundation of a comprehensive clinical assessment, which will have identified the particular problems that the child or the family have and indicate the ways in which these problems can be addressed.

Collaboration

There have been remarkably few studies looking at the impact that the diagnosis of FTT has from a parent's point of view. The few that do exist have been damning with many parents reporting that they felt dismissed and/or were given false reassurance and/or were doubted. Most importantly parents often report that they feel threatened and undermined. The very term FTT might be seen by parents to imply a failure on their part and there are calls for the term to be dropped. Therefore, it is imperative that once the diagnosis has been made that feelings of inadequacy and guilt, which will feed into the spiral of undernutrition (Fig. 4-1), are addressed and that the relevant healthcare workers work in collaboration with the parents. Parents are to be empowered by working in partnership with the members of the multidisciplinary team.

Who? Personnel Involved in Intervention

Multidisciplinary team

A multidisciplinary team approach is essential to the effective management of FTT. The etiology of the problem can be complex and multifactorial and accordingly the remedy may be complicated and multifaceted. Few studies have specifically evaluated the superiority of a multidisciplinary team and in different centers such a team will consist of a variety of health professionals including general pediatricians, pediatric gastroenterologists, community pediatricians, dieticians, social workers, pediatric nurses, developmental specialists, behavioral therapists, occupational therapists, health visitors, speech and language therapists, psychologists, psychiatrists, and nursery nurses. The core membership of a hospital-based team should include a pediatrician, a specialist health visitor/community health worker, and a dietician.

A potential pitfall in such an approach is that of poor communication between the different professionals involved and one of the key roles of the pediatrician can be to take a lead role in coordinating the care provided.

Where? Location of Intervention

Inpatient

In the past many children with FTT would be admitted to hospital, the goal being to ensure adequate dietary intake, to assess feeding, to observe the behavior of the child and family and family-child interactions, and to see whether the child would gain weight while an inpatient. Such admissions are no longer routine and the only absolute indications for an inpatient stay would be refractory cases or when there are concerns regarding the possibility of NAI and the presence of severe malnutrition.

Outpatient

It has been long recognized that hospitalization is not ideal for most of these children; the real debate is whether they should be managed in the outpatient clinic or at home. An advantage of the clinic approach is that it is more cost-effective. It is a relatively expensive option to have health workers regularly on home visits when the patient and family can come to a central clinic. One-stop clinics where the family can be seen by a number of professionals during a single visit are preferable and they reduce the risk of conflicting advice from different health care workers.

Community

As part of the assessment process already described the importance of observing the child feeding at home was stressed. Similarly, it would make sense for any intervention to place emphasis on the home setting. Few studies, however, have been able to prove that home interventions are any more successful than those undertaken from the outpatient setting. Work from Baltimore in 1997 concluded that the additional provision of home intervention in the form of lay visitors supported by a community nurse led to an improvement in the receptive language and home environment for the younger children and on longer-term follow-up an improvement in motor development for all children. It is likely that parents feel less intimidated and more involved in an active partnership in the intervention if it is happening in their home.[8]

What? Methods of Intervention

Nutrition

Calorie intake. Inability to achieve an adequate calorie intake is the fundamental problem with FTT and so nutritional management is the cornerstone of treatment. The ultimate goal is to promote "catch-up" growth and thus to restore deficits in weight and height. For a child of about 6 months of age, for example, a weight gain of 45 g per day can be considered to be catch-up growth. To achieve catch-up growth the child will need to receive nutrients in excess of the EAR. A common mistake is for energy requirements to be based on the child's current weight and not the expected weight for age. Formulas are available that account for this problem such as

$$\text{kcal/kg} = 120 \times \frac{\text{median weight for current height (kg)}}{\text{current weight (kg)}}$$

Using this formula will provide 1.5–2 times the expected calorie intake for age, and protein intake must be increased at a similar proportion to achieve maximum growth. A minimum of 9% energy from protein is necessary in order to achieve maximum nitrogen retention in malnourished children.

The child is unlikely to be able to increase the volume of oral intake sufficiently and so fortification of the diet is necessary to provide a more calorie-dense feed. In a young breast-fed infant the maternal diet should be assessed and improved if necessary. If maternal dietary supplementation does not lead to an improvement in the infant's growth, then supplementation of breast feeds may be required, while in the meantime not suppressing breast milk production, if possible. For the non-breast-fed child many strategies can be employed to encourage increased energy intake (Table 4-4). A potential disadvantage of the use of calorie supplements is that this can "medicalize" the problem of (nonorganic) FTT and lead to parents feel-

ing disempowered. Nevertheless, if the child does not show "catch-up" growth then they are not getting enough calories, and further, energy enhancement is required under dietetic supervision.

Micronutrient intake. Micronutrient deficiencies also need to be addressed. A multivitamin preparation that includes iron and zinc is recommended for all undernourished children. Iron deficiency is seen in as many as 50% of children with FTT, while vitamin D deficiency and rickets have also been described. Zinc deficiency has been implicated in impaired linear growth. Such vitamin and mineral deficiencies may only become apparent once the child begins to gain weight.

Methods of feeding. Nasogastric tube feeding is sometimes required in some cases of severe malnutrition or if there is failure to gain weight or there are oral-motor problems. In the majority of cases this is a short-term measure while oral feeding is established. However, in those children with severe neurodisability for whom there are concerns about the safety of swallow and/or with inordinately prolonged feeding times (>3 h per day) such that it adversely affects the quality of life of the caregivers, then the insertion of a gastrostomy feeding tube should be considered.

Psychosocial

The psychosocial factors influencing the ability of a child to thrive are many and complex and may require considerable time and several interviews and/or home visits to be fully addressed. There may be a role in this setting for the health professional to act as an advocate if it is thought that poverty is a significant contributing factor and where intervention from government or private agencies may alleviate this. The family may, however, simply require help in accessing the services that are already available to them. If there are issues with regard to a significant breakdown in the caregiver-child relationship (a minority of cases) then the child may benefit from a brief placement in foster care, or preferably with other members of the extended family, with frequent visits from the natural parents. These are invariably difficult situations and the

TABLE 4-4

STRATEGIES FOR INCREASING CALORIE INTAKE

Dietary
Three meals and two snacks per day
Increase number and variety of foods offered
Increase "high energy" food/drinks offered (e.g., add cheese, butter, cream)
Decrease "low energy" food/drinks offered (e.g., fruit juices, water)
Behavioral
Offer meals at regular times
Positive reinforcement when food is eaten
Gently encourage children to eat, avoid conflict
Never force-feed

common sense of a wise social worker in the multi-disciplinary team can be absolutely invaluable.

In the older child with an organic cause for poor weight gain (e.g., Crohn's disease), some of the issues regarding physical growth and maturation need to be approached with great sensitivity. Time must be taken with the patient and family to explain the treatment options and the patient dealt with in a manner that reflects his or her age and not their physical size.

How? The Nonconfrontational Approach

It is best to offer the least specialist (and therefore potentially least stigmatizing) service first (from a well trained and supported community worker) unless there are additional concerns about the severity of the FTT, possible organic causes, or NAI. Simple advice concerning feeding practices may be all that is required. If this is unsuccessful then it is important that the community worker has access to the multidisciplinary team described above. A pediatrician is often required to clinically assess the child at this stage and, in the minority where an organic cause is identified, there may be a need for further clinical follow-up. However, in the majority of cases once any investigations are completed the child should be managed primarily in the community for continuation of nutritional care and with support from other specialists as required.[10]

Summary

- A thorough assessment guides subsequent management choices.
- Always work in collaboration with the parents.
- Involve a multidisciplinary team, which includes a dietician.
- Center management in the community and in the home.
- Calorie supplementation is essential.
- Address underlying psychosocial problems.

PROGNOSIS

As always, long-term prognosis is dependent on the final diagnosis. If there is underlying organic pathol-ogy then the outcome will be influenced by the course of this illness. For all those with FTT continued follow-up is required and this should ideally be carried out in the community with monitoring of growth and development. Few long-term systematic studies of FTT exist—these report ongoing problems with growth, cognition, and behavior.[3]

Behavior

Children with FTT are known to have more behavioral problems than their peers with increased negative affect and decreased positive affect, particularly during feeds and these problems may contribute to their failure to gain weight. At the time of diagnosis of FTT they are also more likely to have evidence of insecure attachment and problems with communication and mood. Follow-up of children with FTT reveals that these children have significantly more family problems, worse psychologic development, and more behavioral deficits than do control groups.

Growth

Although the majority of children with FTT seem to improve during the first 5 years of life, many are left with a lasting short fall in growth. Studies from the developed world show a significant association between FTT and suboptimal weight-for-height and weight-for-age and this persists despite evidence that the interventions instigated at the time of diagnosis had improved nutritional intake. Similarly, in developing countries children with FTT have poorer growth in terms of weight, height, and head circumference and again this is long-standing despite interventions. Although earlier intervention does seem to have an impact on long-term outcome, these findings raise the possibility of early "programming" of growth in the face of nutrient deficiency at an early age and emphasize the need for early and intensive interventions.

Development/Cognition

The impact of FTT on head growth is reflected in the consequences that undernutrition has on cognition and development. The brain appears particularly vulnerable to nutritional insults from midgestation through to the early preschool years.[11] The growing brain accounts for 60% of the body's glucose usage despite accounting for only 3% of body weight. Germinal stem cell populations divide to form neurons but will cease to do so after the first 3 years of life. Cerebellar neurons continue to replicate after birth and can be affected by early undernutrition resulting in persistent fine and gross motor dysfunction. Not only are neurons affected but also glial cells which are needed in the myelinization of nerve cells essential for nerve conduction. Although these cells are constantly replaced, it is thought that early undernutrition can result in a large enough deficit that they are never fully restored. The effects of undernutrition on the brain will depend on the timing and the severity of the insult with the areas that are most active in their maturation at the time of the deficit most likely to be affected. It is no surprise to find, therefore, that the prognosis is poorest if a child is exposed to undernutrition during the first 6 months of life.

Despite the apparent critical nature of the brain's development there have been suggestions recently that the cognitive impact may not be as great as was feared.[10] Studies in the 1980s, however, suggested that children with FTT manifested significant intellectual delays at 3-year follow-up and delays in language development, reading age, and verbal intelligence 13 years later. Four more recent studies have addressed this question. One found that children with a history of FTT had a clinically and statistically significant cognitive deficit; the other three found that FTT was associated with decreased cognitive, motor, or neurologic measures compared to controls.[3] The impact of FTT is dependent on its severity and timing with early onset at less than 6 months being potentially devastating with regard to long-term outcome. Therefore, the priority must be early identification and appropriate and effective management.

Summary

- Underlying physiologic causes of FTT must be investigated.
- Children with FTT are often left with a long-term suboptimal growth.

- The impact on cognition is dependent on the timing and severity of the FTT with the first 6 months being of particular importance.
- Early identification and effective intervention is required.

References

1 *Management of the Child with a Serious Infection or Severe Malnutrition: Guidelines for Care at the First-referral Level in Developing Countries.* Geneva: World Health Organisation, 2000. Available at: http://www.who.int/child-adolescent-health/publications/referral_care/homepage.htm

2 Ogden CL, Kuczmarski RJ, Flegal KM, et al. Centers for Disease Control and Prevention 2000 growth charts for the United States: improvements to the 1977 National Center for Health Statistics version. *Pediatrics* 109(1):45–60, 2002.

3 Perrin EC, Cole CH, Frank DA, et al. Criteria for determining disability in infants and children: failure to thrive. *Evidence Report/Technology Assessment* 72. Boston, MA: Tufts-New England Medical Centre, 2003.

4 Wright CM, Matthews JNS, Waterston A, et al. What is the normal rate of weight gain in infancy? *Acta Paediatr* 83:351–356, 1994.

5 Edwards AG, Halse PC, Parkin JM, et al. Recognising failure to thrive in early childhood. *Arch Dis Child* 65(11):1263–1265, 1990.

6 Aarts C, Kylberg E, Hofvander Y, et al. Growth under privileged conditions of healthy Swedish infants exclusively breastfed from birth to 4-6 months: a longitudinal prospective study based on daily records of feeding. *Acta Paediatr* 92(2):145–151, 2003.

7 Wright CM. A population approach to weight monitoring and failure to thrive. In: David TG (ed.), *Recent Advances in Paediatrics.* Edinburgh: Churchill Livingstone, 1995, pp. 73–87.

8 Batchelor JA. Failure to thrive in young children, research and practice evaluated. London: The Children's Society, 1999.

9 Maggioni A, Lifshitz F. Nutritional management of failure to thrive. *Pediatr Clin North Am* 42(4): 791–809, 1995.

10 Wright CM. Identification and management of failure to thrive: a community perspective. *Arch Dis Child* 82(1):5–9, 2000.

11 Frank DA, Zeisel SH. Failure to thrive. *Pediatr Clin North Am* 35(6):1187–1206, 1988.

5

CONSTIPATION

Alberto M. Ravelli

INTRODUCTION

Constipation is one of the most common gastrointestinal (GI) problems affecting infants and children. Approximately 3% of all pediatric visits and 25% of pediatric gastroenterologist consultations are motivated by a suspected disorder of defecation, more often constipation. In the vast majority of cases constipation is a functional disorder, meaning that there is no recognizable underlying organic disorder. Organic disorders such as anatomic malformations of the anorectum and Hirschsprung's disease are usually diagnosed in the neonatal period and require surgery. It is possible, however, that in a few cases of "functional" constipation a mild intestinal myopathy or neuropathy exists, leading to chronic constipation poorly responsive to conventional therapies and progressing into adulthood. There are a number of misconceptions regarding constipation in children—such as its being "psychologic" or "psychosomatic" in nature—that often result in underestimation or misdiagnosis of the disorder and inadequate or incorrect therapeutic approaches. Although there are defecation disorders which are clearly related to psychosocial problems (see "Functional nonretentive fecal soiling"), voluntary fecal retention is usually a consequence rather than the cause of constipation. Since constipation essentially begins as a difficulty in passing the stools, an infant or child may accumulate large masses of hard feces in the rectum leading to an increasingly difficult and often painful defecation that the child will understandably try to avoid or delay as much as possible, thereby worsening the problem.

Abbreviations

CNS	Central nervous system
EAS	External anal sphincter
GI	Gastrointestinal
IAS	Internal anal sphincter
IBS	Irritable bowel syndrome

PHYSIOLOGY OF COLONIC TRANSIT AND DEFECATION

Colonic Motility

The colonic musculature must alternatively mix food without propulsion (for water reabsorption), act as a storage site, move its content aborally, and finally expel feces. To accomplish these different functions, the colon must not have a restricted dominant pattern of motor activity and indeed, unlike the smooth muscle of gastric antrum and small intestine, the colonic smooth muscle does not exhibit a typical omnipresent pacemaker activity. The colon may display electric quiescence as well as electric activity at a wide variety of frequencies. As a consequence, the colon exhibits different patterns of motor activity. In the cecum and proximal colon, circular smooth muscle produces a slow nonpropulsive segmental mixing rhythm and only occasional propulsive contractions. In the distal colon, the combined action of circular and longitudinal smooth muscle (teniae coli) produces both segmental mixing and slow propulsion, and occasional powerful mass movements propel fecal material toward the rectum.

Anorectal Motility and Defecation

The descending fecal bolus distends the empty rectum, stimulating sensory receptors in the bowel wall and pelvic floor. Ascending sensory fibers allow conscious awareness of rectal distention. There is a transient contraction of the voluntary striated muscle external anal sphincter (EAS) and the puborectalis sling, the so-called inflation reflex. Transmission of the nerve impulse distally by the myenteric plexus of the lower rectal wall produces a reflex inhibition of the involuntary internal anal sphincter (IAS), the rectosphincteric relaxation reflex, followed by the inhibition of the EAS involving reflex pathways as well as facilitatory cortical pathways. Relaxation of the puborectalis muscle allows widening of the anorectal angle (from resting 60°–105° to 140°), resulting in an unobstructed anal canal. The increased abdominal pressure and rectal peristalsis result in expulsion of feces and emptying of the entire rectum. Prior to the acquisition of voluntary control, rectal distention results in EAS loss of electrical activity and tone (inhibition reflex). By 24–30 months of age, the maturation of myenteric ganglion cells is associated with persistence of EAS tonic activity mediated by a spinal reflex and augmented by supraspinal cortical centers, allowing the normal inflation reflex and conscious control of defecation.

DISORDERS OF DEFECATION

In children and adults, constipation is generally regarded as a reduction in the number of bowel movements. In healthy newborns and infants, however, bowel movements are quite variable and may be influenced by feeding. Breast-fed babies may open their bowels up to 10 times a day, whereas in formula-fed infants defecation is usually less frequent. Therefore, for an appropriate definition of constipation other parameters should also be taken into account, such as the passage, consistency, and volume of stools. Furthermore, constipation is not the only disorder of defecation and other conditions exist where newborns, infants, and children may present with decreased and/or difficult bowel movements. Functional defecation disorders have recently been defined by an international expert panel and their diagnostic criteria are the basis for a positive diagnosis.

Infant Dischezia

An otherwise healthy infant strains, gets red in the face, and cries for at least 10 min before evacuating soft normal-looking stools, and similar episodes can occur several times a day. This is due to abdomino-pelvic dyssynergia, i.e., a poor coordination between intraabdominal pressure and relaxation of the pelvic floor, and crying corresponds to a Valsalva maneuver. The clinical examination should include a careful inspection of the anorectum to rule out anorectal abnormalities. Since symptoms subside spontaneously in a few weeks no pharmacologic therapy is needed. Parents should be reassured, however, as they may get quite anxious about the problem.

Functional Constipation

Functional constipation is the most common defecation disorder in pediatric patients. It typically affects infants and children between 6 months and preschool age and is defined by a ≥2-week history of ≤2 bowel movements per week with hard, large, or pellety stools in most evacuations, in the absence of structural, endocrine, or metabolic abnormalities.

The transition from breast to formula feeding is often associated with the development of functional constipation, though recent studies suggest that intolerance to cow's milk protein may be responsible for a significant proportion of cases of "functional" constipation (see "cow's milk protein intolerence" and see also Chap. 14).

Functional Fecal Retention

Functional fecal retention is the most common cause of constipation associated with fecal soiling from early infancy to adolescence. Patients have a ≥3-month history of difficult or painful passage of large stools with a frequency of ≤2 per week. The previous experience of painful defecation leads these children to avoid opening their bowels by strongly contracting the pelvic floor muscles and assuming the typical retentive posture. As a consequence of the fecal overload and rectal distention (secondary megarectum), other symptoms may develop such as encopresis (overflow soiling), irritability, abdominal pain, and early satiety with reduced food intake. While looking absent and uninterested, the child is actually worried and feels lonely and isolated. All these symptoms typically subside following a complete evacuation of the rectum.

Functional Nonretentive Fecal Soiling

Functional nonretentive fecal soiling is an altogether different matter. It is a manifestation of an emotional disorder usually affecting school-age children and is characterized by a ≥3-month history of defecation occurring in places and situations inappropriate to the social context, in the absence of fecal retention and without any structural or biochemical abnormalities. These patients are not actually constipated, as they open their bowels daily and often evacuate completely in their underwear, without any other GI signs or symptoms.

Irritable Bowel Syndrome

The presence of recurrent abdominal pain/discomfort related to bowel movements in a child with consti-pation or irregular bowel habits should raise the suspicion of irritable bowel syndrome (IBS), the diagnostic and therapeutic criteria of which are dealt with in detail elsewhere (see Chap. 6).

Cow's Milk Protein Intolerance

Recent studies show that more than 60% of infants and preschool children with constipation refractory to conventional medical therapy may respond to withdrawal of cow's milk protein from the diet. Many such patients have a personal and/or family history of atopic disease, but serum IgE and skin prick test to cow's milk protein may be negative. In these patients, rectal biopsies consistently show an eosinophilic inflammatory infiltrate in the lamina propria ("allergic proctitis") (Fig. 5-1). Colonic transit studies often demonstrate a rectal "hold-up" of indigestible pellets (Fig. 5-2) and barium enema shows irregular narrowing of the rectum and a transition zone reminiscent of Hirschsprung's disease. It is conceivable that allergic inflammation may impair neuromuscular function of the sigmoid and rectum in these patients.

Defecation Disorders in Children with Neurologic and Neuromuscular Disease

Children with disorders of the central nervous system (CNS) and especially spastic cerebral palsy, as well as children with severe muscular dystrophy, often suffer from severe constipation. Although usually regarded as functional, constipation in these patients is multifarious; lack of physical activity, insufficient fluid and fiber intake, and spasticity or reduced tone of abdominal muscles may impair defecation and promote fecal retention. The involvement of the enteric nervous system is possible and may impair gut motility and reduce visceral sensitivity, contributing to fecal overload and anorectal incoordination. In some patients with Duchenne's muscular dystrophy, GI smooth muscle can also be affected leading to gastroparesis and intestinal pseudoobstruction. Furthermore, these unfortunate children often suffer from other GI problems such as gastrosophageal reflux disease and feeding difficulties due to

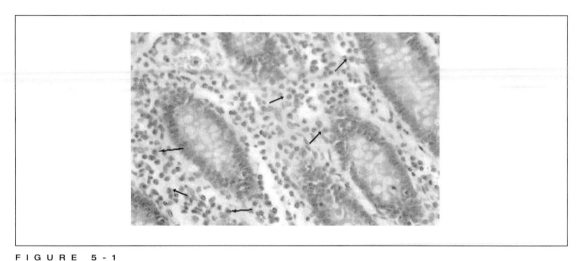

FIGURE 5-1

A PROMINENT EOSINOPHILIC INFILTRATE IS EVIDENT IN THIS RECTAL BIOPSY

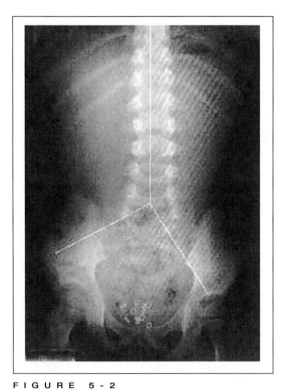

FIGURE 5-2

RADIOLOGIC IMAGE OF THE ABDOMEN SHOWING PELLETS IN THE PELVIC AREA, AS THEY ARE RETAINED IN THE SIGMOID AND RECTUM IN A CASE OF SECONDARY MEGARECTUM

defective swallowing. Although therapeutic measures are essentially the same as in neurologically normal children, constipation in these patients can be very difficult to treat and requires a great deal of patience, understanding, and dedication. In particularly severe cases, recurrent bowel obstruction due to fecal impaction can be prevented by periodic anterograde colonic enema (ACE), which is made possible by the endoscopic placement of a colostomy tube through which the left colon can be flushed periodically.

DIAGNOSIS

A detailed personal history and a careful clinical examination are often all that is needed to make a correct diagnosis of a functional defecation disorder. The above-mentioned criteria are in fact particularly useful for a positive diagnosis and should be applied to reduce laboratory and invasive investigations to a minimum. A delayed meconium passage in the neonatal period suggests the possibility of Hirschsprung's disease. If growth and developmental retardation or signs of malnutrition are present, organic disorders should be considered such as enteric neuropathy or myopathy (again including Hirschsprung's disease), endocrine or metabolic disease (e.g., hypothyroidism), cystic fibrosis, and possibly celiac disease (gluten-sensitive enteropathy), although this is more commonly associated with diarrhea. A distended abdomen also suggests conditions such as intestinal dysganglionosis or malabsorption syndrome. A personal or family history of atopic disease may suggest the possibility of constipation secondary to cow's milk allergy.

A thorough clinical examination should include: (1) abdominal palpation to establish the presence, site, and extension of fecal masses; (2) inspection of the lumbar and sacral area to detect signs of occult spina bifida such as local pigmentation, hypertricosis, lipoma, or skin pit at the level of spinal lesion; (3) sensory stimulation of the perianal area (in cooperative patients) and stimulation of the external anal sphincter reflex in order to assess the integrity of sensory-motor pudendal nerve fibers, which may be altered in the presence of occult spina bifida; (4) anal inspection to detect venous congestion, fissures, or other skin lesions and to exclude malformations of the anorectum; and (5) careful rectal examination to assess the anal sphincter tone and the presence or absence of feces in the ampulla (with the latter again suggesting Hirschsprung's disease). Rectal examination is controversial in children with fecal retention; some believe it should be postponed to the second visit, once a good and trustful relation with the patient has been established. Rectal examination should be carried out maintaining eye contact and a friendly attitude and using a well-lubricated index or little finger—depending on the patient's age and size—with the child lying on a side or on his or her back. Anal sphincter tone and abdomino-pelvic coordination can be assessed in cooperative patients asking them to squeeze and push.

CLINICAL INVESTIGATION

If the major features of functional constipation are present (Table 5-1), there is usually no need for specific investigations to confirm the diagnosis. Some well-targeted laboratory investigations, however, may be useful in patients with a known underlying disease, an uncertain personal history, and/or equivocal clinical findings such as abdominal distention, growth impairment, and neurodevelopmental delay (Table 5-2). A sigmoidoscopy with biopsies may be useful to confirm the suspicion of constipation related to cow's milk allergy, which is characterized by a prominent eosinophilic infiltrate of the rectal and sigmoid mucosa (Fig. 5-1). If a child is suspected of having a colonic motility disorder, a colonic pellet transit study can be carried out, where a plain abdominal x-ray is taken at day 1 and 5 after ingestion of 20–30 indigestible radiopaque pellets to visualize the number and site of retained

TABLE 5-1

FEATURES SUGGESTING FUNCTIONAL CONSTIPATION

- Normal meconium passage
- Onset during transition periods (breast to bottle feeding, diaper withdrawal, beginning of nursery school) or intercurrent febrile illness
- Absence of vomiting, diarrhea, severe food refusal
- No overtly distended abdomen
- No retentive posturing during avacuation
- Normal growth
- Mild congestion of perianal veins, perianal erythema, occasional anal fissures
- Overflow soiling
- Stools in ampulla at rectal examination
- Satisfactory response to medical therapy

TABLE 5-2

LABORATORY INVESTIGATION TO DETECT UNDERLYING CAUSES OF CONSTIPATION

Test	Disorder
Celiac disease screening (total serum IgA, htTG)	Celiac disease
Serum electrolytes	Electrolyte imbalance
Thyroid function screening (FT3, FT4, TSH)	Hypothyroidism
Fecal elastase or chymotrypsin, Sweat test	Cystic fibrosis
PRIST, RAST, and/or skin prick test to cow's milk protein[a]	Cow's milk allergy
Serum and urine lead	Lead poisoning

[a]Cow's milk-related constipation possible if positive, but not excluded if negative.

pellets. In children with colonic inertia the pellets are usually scattered throughout the colon, whereas in children with functional outlet obstruction or secondary megarectum pellets are usually retained in the sigmoid and/or rectum and therefore are located radiologically in the pelvic area (Fig. 5-2).

TREATMENT

In functional constipation, the primary goal of therapy is to empty the rectal ampulla thereby producing painless bowel movements with a frequency >3 per week. Rectal washout can be achieved with evening enemas for at least 2–3 consecutive days. This should be followed by a maintenance treatment for a minimum of 4–5 months with nonabsorbable osmotically active sugars such as lactulose or lactitol at an initial daily dose of 1 g/kg. Subsequently the dose can be adapted to the clinical response, but the treatment period should be prolonged until the bowel frequency becomes normal (ideally one bowel movement per day, or at least ≥4 per week). The pharmacologic therapy should be associated with a toilet training and an adequate intake of fluids and natural fiber (approximately 1 g/kg daily). Complete resolution of the problem can be achieved in 50% of patients at 12 months and 48–65% after 4–5 years follow-up.

In children with fecal retention, mineral oil should be given daily to gradually remove from the rectum the fecal mass around which liquid feces may flow and produce soiling. Controversy exists regarding enema, which some consider counterproductive as it may frighten the patient, while others regard as extremely useful in that it gives immediate relief thereby calming down the patient. Phosphate enemas should be avoided, however, as they may result in hypocalcemia. In extreme cases manual disimpaction may be necessary, and this should be carried out under general anesthesia. As with functional constipation, a long maintenance therapy with stool softeners is necessary to ensure prolonged periods of painless defecation, until the condition subsides.

Oral electrolyte-free polyethylene glycol (PEG) solutions can be used as an alternative to enemas to remove fecal impaction at a dose of approximately 1–1.5 g/kg daily for 3 days. PEG 0.8 g/kg can subsequently be given daily as a maintenance treatment instead of nonabsorbable sugars. The treatment of fecal impaction and the maintenance therapy of functional constipation are summarized in Table 5-3.

The therapeutic approach to functional nonretentive fecal soiling is difficult. Oral laxatives and biofeedback have given conflicting results. A therapy aimed at increasing the attention level and the responsibility of the young patient by means of toilet training techniques seems more useful. Once parents have been reassured about the absence of an underlying organic disease, a psychosocial support for emotional problems is advisable.

TABLE 5-3

MEDICAL TREATMENT OF FECAL IMPACTION AND FUNCTIONAL CONSTIPATION

Laxative	Dose	Side Effects and Precautions
Lubricants		
Mineral oil	15–30 mL for each year of age (max. 250 mL), single dose or 2 divided doses. Maintenance: 1–3 mL/kg daily, in single dose or 2 divided doses	Not recommended in children <1 year; more likeable if cooled. Lipoid pneumonia if aspirated (caution in children with swallowing problems, dysphagia, or gastroesophageal reflux disease)
Lavage		
PEG solution	1–1.5 g/kg orally for 3 days; 25 mL/kg per hour (max. 1000 mL/h) or 20 mL/kg per hour for 4 h daily	Bad taste, may require hospital admission for NG tube placement. Nausea, vomiting, bloating, abdominal cramping
PEG 3350 (Miralax) (electrolyte-free)	1–1.5 g/kg daily, for 3 days. Maintenance: 0.8 g/kg (8.5–34 g) daily	Flatulence, diarrhea; expensive but easy to take because it is tasteless
Osmotic		
Magnesium hydroxide	1–3 mL/kg daily of 400 g/5 mL solution, in 2 divided doses. Maintenance: modulate dose as to obtain one bowel movement daily for 1–2 months	Overdose may lead to hypermagnesemia, hyperphosphatemia, secondary hypocalcemia; caution in small children and children with renal insufficiency
Magnesium citrate	>6 years: 1–3 mL/kg daily; 6–12 years: 100–150 mL daily; >12 years: 150–300 mL daily; in single dose or 2 divided doses	As for magnesium hydroxide
Lactulose	1–3 mL/kg daily, in 2 divided doses. Maintenance: modulate dose as to obtain one bowel movement daily for 1–2 months	Flatulence, abdominal cramping; well tolerated in the long term
Sorbitol	1–3 mL/kg daily, in 2 divided doses. Maintenance: modulate dose as to obtain one bowel movement daily for 1–2 months	Flatulence, abdominal cramping; less expensive than lactulose
Stimulant		
Senna	2–6 years: 2.5–7.5 mL daily, in single dose; 6–12 years: 5–15 mL daily, in single dose (same for fecal disimpaction and maintenance therapy)	Hepatitis (idiosyncratic), melanosis coli, hypertrophic osteoartropathy, iatrogenic renal damage (analgesics)
Bisacodyl	≥2 years: 0.5–1 g suppository or 1–3 tablets, in single dose (same for fecal disimpaction and maintenance therapy)	Abdominal pain, diarrhea, hypokalemia, anomalies of rectal mucosa

Bibliography

Fleisher DR, Feldman EJ. The biopsychosocial model of clinical practice in functional gastrointestinal disorders. In: Hyman PE (ed.), *Pediatric Functional Gastrointestinal Disorders*. New York, NY: Academy Professional Information Services, 1999, pp. 1.1–1.20.

Iacono G, Cavataio F, Montalto G, Florena A, Tumminello M, Soresi M, Notarbartolo A, Carroccio A. Intolerance of cow's milk and chronic constipation in children. *N Engl J Med* 339:1100–1104, 1998.

Rasquin-Weber A, Hyman PE, Cucchiara S, Fleisher DR, Hyams JS, Milla PJ, Staiano A. Childhood functional gastrointestinal disorders. *Gut* 45(Suppl):II60–II68, 1999.

6

RECURRENT ABDOMINAL PAIN AND IRRITABLE BOWEL SYNDROME

Licia Pensabene, Miguel Saps, and Stefano Guandalini

INTRODUCTION

The past several decades have witnessed numerous studies on the subject of *recurrent abdominal pain* (RAP) of childhood. RAP is in fact one of the most common pediatric complaints, yet it remains one of the most frequently misunderstood pediatric disorders.

The classic definition of recurrent abdominal pain derives from the description by Apley and Naish, who, in their landmark article on abdominal pain,[1] defined RAP as three or more bouts of pain, severe enough to limit activities, over a period of at least 3 months.

It is crucial for the clinician to recognize that the term "recurrent abdominal pain" implies a description, not a diagnosis. Not a single, homogeneous entity, RAP can actually be a manifestation of multiple disorders. Although a number of organic as well as functional conditions can cause RAP, the term RAP has historically implied that no organic disease is present. Indeed, in clinical practice most children and adolescents presenting with this symptom have a *functional* disorder (a condition defined as a variable combination of chronic or persistent symptoms occurring in the absence of biochemical or structural abnormalities, tissue damage, or inflammation). Because the exact etiology and pathogenesis of functional pain are unknown, functional abdominal pain has largely been a diagnosis of exclusion. However, *positive* diagnostic criteria for *functional gastrointestinal disorders* (FGIDs) have been defined recently by an International Working Team, the pediatric Rome Committee. The work of these experts has resulted in the so-called "Rome Criteria," a set of diagnostic criteria that have evolved into well-respected clinical tools in the field of gastroenterology. The original criteria were recently revised and expanded to produce the *Rome II Criteria*, a symptom-based classification system that provides a framework for a *positive diagnosis* of FGIDs.[2] Based on them, functional gastrointestinal disorders that are associated with abdominal pain are classified into five subtypes:

- Irritable bowel syndrome (IBS)
- Functional dyspepsia

- Functional abdominal pain syndrome (FAPS)
- Abdominal migraine
- Aerophagia

The emphasis of most of this chapter will be on "functional" abdominal pain, in particular on IBS, one of the most common functional bowel disorders, with only a brief description of the organic diseases causing abdominal pain in the section dedicated to the differential diagnosis.

EPIDEMIOLOGY

Recurrent abdominal pain in children is a common disorder that affects 10–25% of school-age children and adolescents and accounts for a significant number (2–4%) of office visits to primary care physicians. The prevalence of RAP and IBS increases with age into adolescence.[1,3] Age and gender interact, with an equal gender ratio in early childhood but predominant female symptom reporting in late childhood and adolescence.[1] Hyams and colleagues studied 507 adolescents in a suburban town in the United States and they found that abdominal pain occurred at least weekly in 13–17% of adolescents, but that only half of these individuals had sought medical attention within the preceding year; they also found that up to 6% of middle-school students and 14% of high-school students observe symptoms consistent with IBS.[3]

Recurrent abdominal pain has also been associated with significant functional impairment, particularly school absenteeism, and with greater risk for potentially dangerous and unnecessary medical investigations and procedures. Recent estimates of the direct and indirect medical expenses associated with IBS were up to $30 billion a year. In addition, IBS can have a serious impact on a patient's daily activities and quality of life.

PATHOPHYSIOLOGY

In this section, the functions of the patients most likely involved in generating functional recurrent abdominal pain will be reviewed.

Brain-Gut Interaction

The Enteric Nervous System

Embedded within the wall of the *gastrointestinal* (GI) tract are two networks of neurons, the myenteric plexus (Auerbach's plexus), situated between the external longitudinal and internal circular muscle layers, and the submucosal plexus (Meissner's plexus), lying between the circular muscle layer and the mucosa. The myenteric plexus is larger and contains the neurons controlling motility; the submucosal plexus is smaller and includes more sensory cells and the neurons that control gland secretion. Between the nerve terminals and the smooth cells there are the *interstitial cells of Cajal* (ICC) that have properties of both muscle and nerve cells. The ICC are believed to act as the gut *pacemaker*, controlling the frequency and propagation of intestinal contractions. These complex layers of microcircuitry are connected by interneurons and constitute the *enteric nervous system* (ENS). Structurally and functionally, the ENS can be considered analogous to the *central nervous system* (CNS). This highly integrated system has been called the "*little brain*" or "*gut brain*." Although the ENS receives input from the central and autonomic nervous systems, it can function independently: the ENS has the unique characteristic of performing most of its functions in the absence of CNS control. Despite this ability, the ENS is under the constant influence of the CNS. It is common even for healthy individuals to experience gastrointestinal symptoms under stressful circumstances. Classic examples include accelerated colonic transit leading to diarrhea or delayed gastric emptying resulting in vomiting when worried about important events.

In summary, there is a constant bidirectional dialogue between brain and gut and functional abdominal pain may develop when this communication is altered, as a result of increased sensory and/or motor activity in the gastrointestinal tract.

The Gut as a Sensory Organ

Symptoms may also occur in response to amplification or aberrant processing of the information received at the central (brain) level. Studies with advanced imaging techniques have suggested abnormal cerebral processing of visceral stimuli in patients with FGIDs, revealing an increased activity in the areas involved in the affective and emotional component of the symptom in patients with IBS compared to asymptomatic individuals.[4]

The autonomic nerves contain afferent (sensory) fibers that carry information from the viscera to the CNS and efferent fibers that transmit information from the CNS to the viscera. Under physiologic conditions, most of these processes do not reach the level of conscious perception. There are visceral sensations, such as abdominal pain or the urge to vomit, which inform the individual about potentially noxious events (e.g., inflammation of the mucosa or serosa and distention of the organ are stimuli to the viscera that are perceived as painful). In the majority of patients with functional bowel disorders, the stimulus associated with visceral pain is intestinal distention.

An alteration in afferent thresholds may have significant effects on gastrointestinal functions. Chronic functional abdominal pain seems to be associated with an increased activity of sympathetic nerves or with a decreased vagal activity.

The ENS and the brain use multiple neurotransmitters for chemical signaling and exchanging information, including excitatory neurotransmitters, such as acetylcholine and gut inhibitory neurotransmitters, such as nitric oxide, norepinephrine, epinephrine, and others. Serotonin (5-hydroxytryptamine; 5-HT) has recently emerged as an important enteric neurotransmitter. Serotonin has been implicated in the pathogenesis of IBS and higher levels of plasma serotonin are found postprandially in patients with diarrhea-predominant IBS. The use of different selective serotonin receptor antagonists and agonists is emerging as one of the most promising therapies for functional bowel disorders (see related section).

Visceral Hyperalgesia

The visceral hyperalgesia hypothesis proposes that greater sensitivity of visceral afferent pathways or central amplification of visceral input lead to an enhanced perception of visceral stimuli. Different experiences may alter visceral perception and lead to development of visceral hyperalgesia. For example, in children with chronic intestinal pseudoobstruction, repeated surgery and painful diagnostic procedures as well as pain from inflammatory conditions may alter sensation peripherally or centrally. Like the skin on a scar site that may remain very sensitive to touch for years, internal tissues damaged by surgery may be left more sensitive to a variety of stimuli. Release of inflammatory mediators may also sensitize nerve endings causing pain to persist once the inflammation has resolved, very much like the skin may be left hypersensitive after a burn.

Controlled studies show that compared to healthy individuals most IBS patients experience rectal discomfort at lower volumes or pressures of intraluminal distention and have diminished tolerance to intestinal gas loads. Di Lorenzo et al. found that children with functional abdominal pain exhibited generalized visceral hyperalgesia, with less severity in the rectum, whereas IBS patients had rectal hyperalgesia without gastric hypersensitivity.[5] Most of the patients had their symptoms reproduced by the distention only at the site of predominant hyperalgesia, providing a physiologic explanation of different symptoms in children who have distinct functional GI disorders.

Motor Abnormalities in FGIDS

For many years it was believed that abnormal motility was the cause of most functional bowel disorders (i.e., excessive contractile activity may cause abdominal pain). The term "spastic colon" is still used to describe IBS.

In addition to a greater sensory response, patients with FGIDs may indeed display abnormal motility. Though the pathophysiology of IBS is commonly attributed to dysfunction of the large intestine, evidence exists to incriminate the small bowel as well. Typical abdominal colic episodes have been associated with the passage of high-amplitude contractions through the ileocecal region.

Antroduodenal manometric studies have demonstrated similar abnormality (postprandial antral hypomotility) in a proportion of children and adults with functional dyspepsia. Bloating has been explained by an abnormal transit and pooling of gas in conjunction with gut hypersensitivity. It has been suggested that rather than having a persistent motility abnormality, patients with FGIDs may exhibit an abnormal motor response (that is neither specific nor predictable) to a variety of physiologic stimuli.

Inflammation

"My son was doing well until the entire family developed a gastroenteritis; everybody recovered except him. Since that time he has had belly pain." Pediatricians commonly hear such a story. There is evidence that IBS can occur following a gastrointestinal infection resulting in transient inflammation; the term "postinfectious IBS" has been used to describe these conditions. It has been reported that 20–25% of patients admitted to the hospital for bacterial gastroenteritis developed symptoms consistent with IBS in the first 3 months. Mild mucosal inflammation may perturb neuromuscular function not only locally but at distal noninflamed sites. Inflammatory stimuli may provoke a hyperalgesic state and alter the motor function in patients with IBS. This gut dysfunction may persist even after resolution of the mucosal inflammation.

Immunity

Several recent studies seem to indicate that immunity plays a role affecting the brain-gut axis. The enteric mast cells seem to be involved in stress-induced gut hypersensitivity and seem to be an essential component in the psychoimmunologic response of the gut.

Stressors

Stressful events have been long believed to be important in the development of symptoms in FGIDs. Some studies have shown that children with RAP had greater exposure to stressful life events. There is evidence that both psychiatric disorders and sexual and physical abuse are associated with IBS.

Dysregulation of the hypothalamic-hypopituitary-adrenal axis is likely to mediate the effects of stress on gastrointestinal function. *Corticotrophin-releasing hormone* (CRH), presumably released from the hypothalamus, seems to be the hormonal mediator of the stress response. Use of CRH antagonists abolishes the increased gut sensitivity to stress in animals. Studies in humans have suggested that IBS patients have a hyperreactive gut that overreacts to emotional or stressful stimuli. Patients with IBS can develop dysmotility of the small intestine and colonic hypermotility in response to stress. These alterations may presumably cause diarrhea, constipation, or abdominal distention depending on the predominant abnormality.

Genetics

Heredity has been suggested to explain the finding that IBS tends to run in families. Twin studies have shown a 17% concordance for IBS in monozygotic patients with only 8% concordance in dizygotic twins. Although these data suggest a specific role of heredity in the development of IBS, it has been reported that having a parent with IBS accounts for more variance than having a twin with IBS, suggesting that social learning (parental reinforcement and modeling) has an equal or greater influence.

Biopsychosocial Model

The biopsychosocial model of medical care is an alternative to the conventional medical model. In the medical model, a patient presenting with a symptom is assumed to have a disease, with objectively demonstrable tissue damage and malfunction. In contrast, the biopsychosocial model is concerned not only with *disease*, involving abnormality of the structure and/or function of organs and tissues (physical component) but also with *illness*, a patient's subjective sense of feeling unwell, suffering, or disability (psychologic component).[6] Both genetics (previously discussed) and *early life experiences* influence an individual's susceptibility to functional bowel disorders. The developing brain and nervous system are modulated by early life

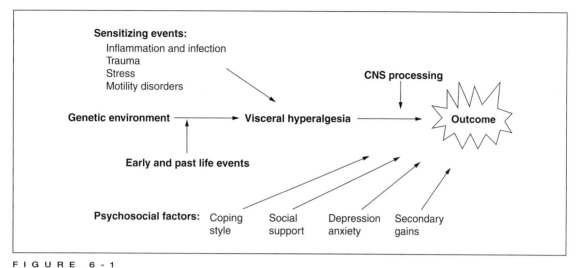

FIGURE 6-1

PATHOPHYSIOLOGIC MODEL OF FUNCTIONAL BOWEL DISORDERS

experiences. Early life experiences modify thinking, behavior, and coping style. When a child complains of abdominal pains, there is the potential for a wide range of responses from parents, teachers, and peers. The responses may reinforce or discourage future pain-related and health care-seeking behaviors. This particular background is also affected by physical and environmental exposures such as infection, food intolerance, and social exposures that influence the patient's attitude toward illness. The biopsychosocial model expands the role of the physician for accurate diagnosis and for therapeutic interventions; it enables the clinician to address illness rather than being confined to the diagnosis and treatment of physical disease which the patient with a functional symptom does not have.

A Unifying Pathophysiologic Model

An attractive pathophysiologic model that has been proposed to explain the development of functional bowel disorders in adults is one that views gut visceral hypersensitivity as the final common pathway for different sensitizing events such as infections, inflammatory insult to the bowel, traumas, motility abnormalities, or other physical or psychologic stressors. These factors may act on a susceptible individual to produce increased bowel sensitivity in response to noxious (hyperalgesia) and non-noxious (allodynia) stimuli. Early or past life events and an appropriate genetic environment may be facilitating factors in the onset of visceral hyperalgesia. This model has been confirmed by multiple studies in adults and is beginning to find confirmatory evidence in children as well (Fig. 6-1). This brain-gut connection seems to be a mechanism that links the psychoemotional state with gastrointestinal dysfunction. As we develop a better understanding of this brain-gut interaction in FGIDs, our emphasis of treatment is moving beyond the biomechanical toward a biopsychosocial model.

CLINICAL SIGNS/SYMPTOMS

Despite their limited validation, the most widely accepted criteria for definition of all functional bowel disorders are the *Rome II Criteria*, a symptom-based classification system. The Rome II Com-mittee identified five functional bowel disorders associated with abdominal pain or discomfort: (1) IBS, (2) functional dyspepsia, (3) abdominal migraine, (4) aerophagia, and (5) FAPS.

Irritable Bowel Syndrome

IBS is the most common functional disorder of the gastrointestinal tract. It is characterized by alterations in bowel function accompanied by pain and discomfort.

The *Rome II Criteria* for irritable bowel syndrome are as follows:

In children old enough to provide an accurate pain history, in at least 12 weeks, which need not be consecutive, in the preceding 12 months, of

I. Abdominal discomfort or pain that has two out of three features:
   a. Relieved with defecation
   b. Onset associated with a change in frequency of stool
   c. Onset associated with a change in form (appearance) of stool
II. There are no structural or metabolic abnormalities to explain the symptoms. The following symptoms also support a diagnosis of IBS:
   a. Abnormal stool frequency defined as greater than three bowel movements per day or less than three bowel movements per week
   b. Abnormal stool form (lumpy/hard or loose/watery)
   c. Abnormal stool passage (straining, urgency, or feeling of incomplete evacuation)
   d. Passage of mucus with stool
   e. Bloating or feeling of abdominal distention

A history that meets these criteria, in the presence of a normal physical examination and growth, with the aid of negative results of a limited diagnostic evaluation, is consistent with a diagnosis of childhood IBS. Regarding the "limited diagnostic evaluation" it should be emphasized that in the absence of evidence suggesting disease, a positive diagnosis of IBS can be made and no further testing is warranted; however, in practice the clinician may want to perform some laboratory studies to reassure the patient and the family (discussed in the section of diagnostic testing).

It is also possible to distinguish, among the patients with IBS, those who tend to have constipation, those with a predominance of diarrhea, and those whose symptoms alternate from diarrhea to constipation. However, there are several additional historical features that the clinician should elucidate. In those patients with constipation, an assessment of the adequacy of dietary fiber and fluid intake should be made. In those with diarrhea and bloating, an inquiry should be made about the ingestion of poorly absorbable carbohydrates such as sorbitol (sugar free gums, candies, fruits) and fructose (fruits, soft drinks, juices). IBS symptoms are frequently observed following viral illnesses that cause acute gastrointestinal symptoms (postinfectious IBS). A careful psychosocial history is also part of initial and follow-up visits.

Functional Dyspepsia

Dyspepsia is defined as recurrent or persistent pain or discomfort centered in the upper abdomen.

The *Rome II Criteria* for functional dyspepsia are as follows:

In children mature enough to provide an accurate pain history, in at least 12 weeks, which need not be consecutive, within the preceding 12 months, of

1. Persistent or recurrent pain or discomfort centered in the upper abdomen (above the umbilicus)
2. No evidence (including upper endoscopy) that organic disease is likely to explain the symptoms
3. No evidence that dyspepsia is exclusively relieved by defecation or associated with the onset of a change in stool frequency or stool form

Although not rigorously defined or proven, there appear to be subtypes of patients with dyspepsia. These include the following

Ulcer-like dyspepsia. Pain centered in the upper abdomen is the predominant (most bothersome) symptom.
Dysmotility-like dyspepsia. An unpleasant or troublesome nonpainful sensation (discomfort) centered in the upper abdomen is the predominant

symptom; this sensation may be characterized by or associated with upper abdominal fullness, early satiety, bloating, or nausea.

Nonspecific dyspepsia. Symptomatic patients whose symptoms do not fulfill the criteria for either ulcer-like or dysmotility-like dyspepsia.

The diagnosis is based on symptoms as no specific tests exist to confirm it, although it does require exclusion of organic disease that could explain the symptoms (including a negative esophagogastroduodenoscopy).[7]

Abdominal Migraine

Abdominal migraine is a paroxysmal disorder affecting about 2% of school-age children. It is most prevalent in children around 10 years of age, declining rapidly thereafter, although occasionally it may persist into adulthood. It is characterized by paroxysmal occurrence of severe midline abdominal pain that lasts for hours and is often accompanied by pallor and anorexia. It may be associated with a personal and/or family history of migraine headaches (present less than half of the time). Most importantly, these children are well in between episodes of pain, and the attacks come on acutely, usually following a stereotyped pattern in each individual patient. Diagnosis is clinical and there is no laboratory test to confirm it.

The *Rome II Criteria* for abdominal migraine are as follows:

I. In the preceding 12 months, three or more paroxysmal episodes of intense, acute midline, abdominal pain lasting 2 h to several days, with intervening symptoms-free intervals lasting weeks to months
II. Evidence of absence of metabolic, gastrointestinal, and central nervous system structural or biochemical diseases is absent
III. Two of the following features:
   a. Headache during episodes
   b. Photophobia during episodes
   c. Family history of migraines
   d. Headache confined to one side only

e. An aura or warning period consisting of either visual disturbances (e.g., blurred or restricted vision), sensory symptoms (e.g., numbness or tingling), or motor abnormalities (e.g., slurred speech, inability to speak, paralysis).

Aerophagia

Aerophagia is defined as a disorder of excessive air swallowing. It is associated with abdominal distention and discomfort that characteristically worsen over the course of the day and resolve during sleep. Abdominal discomfort is often such that children limit their food intake.

The *Rome II Criteria* for aerophagia are as follows:

At least 12 weeks, which need not be consecutive, in the preceding 12 months of two or more of the following signs and symptoms:

1. Air swallowing
2. Abdominal distention due to intraluminal air
3. Repetitive belching and/or increased flatus

Functional Abdominal Pain Syndrome

There are many children and adolescents with functional abdominal pain who do not fulfill criteria for IBS, functional dyspepsia, abdominal migraine, or aerophagia. The pain is usually located in the periumbilical region and does not relate to defecation, eating, or other specific events. It may be continuous or recurrent, frequently affects daily activity, and makes it difficult for the child to fall asleep. This group of patients is considered to have the "functional abdominal pain syndrome" that the Rome II Committee members defined as one of the categories of abdominal pain, being an entity by itself.

The Rome II Criteria for functional abdominal pain syndrome are as follows:

At least 12 weeks of

1. Continuous or nearly continuous abdominal pain in a school-aged child or adolescent
2. No or only occasional relation of pain with physiologic events (e.g., eating, menses, or defecation)

3. Some loss of daily functioning
4. Pain not feigned (e.g., malingering)
5. Insufficient criteria for other functional gastrointestinal disorders that would explain the abdominal pain

Affected children frequently have headache, dizziness, light-headedness, nausea, and vomiting. Often there is a great dissociation between dramatic subjective complaints (marked pain severity/impairment in performing age-appropriate activities such as school, play) and lack of objective findings. Specific inquiries should seek to identify psychosocial factors that may be contributing to symptoms. As with other forms of pain of functional origin the diagnosis is clinical.

In reality, most children present with symptoms that overlap one or more of those five subtypes of functional bowel disorders associated with abdominal pain or discomfort. There is also evidence that symptom profiles may shift over time and patient with predominant dyspepsia or IBS can flux between the two conditions. This can be explained by the fact that there may be overlap among different functional bowel disorders or by the hypothesis that patients cycle in and out a continuum of functional disorders.

DIFFERENTIAL DIAGNOSIS

The diagnostic evaluation of a child with abdominal pain begins with a history to distinguish chronic from acute pain, to subcategorize the clinical presentation, and to address alarm signals that affect differential diagnosis. The presence of a number of clinical features ("red flags") has been classically associated with a greater likelihood of an organic condition; while some of those symptoms can occasionally be found in children with FGIDs (e.g., weight loss), their presence should heighten suspicion of disease and prompt further evaluation. Moreover, the presence of an isolated symptom (such as isolated abdominal pain) is usually thought to be consistent with a functional disorder, while multiple symptoms (such as abdominal pain with

weight loss, vomiting, or diarrhea) are more likely to be due to an organic condition (Table 6-1). There are multiple causes of chronic abdominal pain in children, including functional (Table 6-2) and organic causes (Table 6-3). A diagram outlining uncommon surgical entities based on the location in the abdomen of the presenting complaint is provided in Fig. 6-2.

Among the functional causes of abdominal pain, besides the five subtypes of FGIDs already described, chronic constipation should be considered. This condition is specifically treated in a separate chapter. The following paragraphs will outline the more common of the multiple organic causes of chronic abdominal pain in children.

Carbohydrate Intolerance

Lactose intolerance or malabsorption of other carbohydrates such as sorbitol should be considered as potential primary etiology of chronic abdominal pain, in particular in the presence of increased flatulence, bloating, and diarrhea. The breath hydrogen test following a lactose or fructose load will confirm the diagnosis. Exclusion of the offending agents may improve the symptoms. On the other hand, as a result of the high independent prevalence of both conditions in the general population, the presence of chronic abdominal pain and lactose intolerance in one patient may be merely coincidental. Hamm et al. found lactose malabsorption in 21–25% IBS American patients,[8] a prevalence considered comparable to that in the general U.S. population. Moreover, lactose-free elimination diet resolved symptoms in a similar percentage of patients in the lactose absorber and in the lactose malabsorbers. Thus, an exclusion diet may be helpful in the resolution of symptoms only in a limited number of patients.

Esophagitis/Gastritis/Duodenitis/Peptic Disease

A study evaluating findings on endoscopic examinations in 62 Indonesian children with recurrent abdominal pain revealed pathologic abnormalities

TABLE 6-1

DIFFERENTIATING FUNCTIONAL FROM ORGANIC ABDOMINAL PAIN

Diagnostic Criteria Suggesting a Functional Etiology

Chronic history, greater than 3 months (which need not be consecutive)

Compatible age range (5–14 years)

Characteristic features of abdominal pain (as described by Rome II Criteria)

Presence of an isolated symptom (such as isolated abdominal pain)

Evidence of physical or psychologic stressful stimuli

Environmental reinforcement of pain behavior

Normal physical examination (including rectal examination and stool occult blood)

Normal laboratory evaluation (CBC with differential, ESR, urinalysis, stool O&P)

Signs and Symptoms ("Red Flags") Suggesting an Organic Etiology

Presence of more than one symptom (e.g., pain and fever; pain and diarrhea)

Pain further away from the umbilicus

Pain awakening the child at night

Persistent vomiting

Hematemesis

Involuntary weight loss

Growth deceleration

Blood in stools (gross or guaiac-positive)

Changes in bowel function

Perianal disease

Dysuria, hematuria

Joint involvement (arthritis)

Fever

Elevated erythrocyte sedimentation rate

Elevated white count

Anemia

Hypoalbuminemia

Family history of inflammatory bowel disease, peptic ulcer disease

TABLE 6-2

FUNCTIONAL CAUSES OF CHRONIC ABDOMINAL PAIN

Irritable bowel syndrome

Functional abdominal pain syndrome

Dyspepsia

Abdominal migraine

Aerophagia

Chronic constipation

including erosions, esophagitis, and duodenitis in 50% of the patients. In the absence of peptic ulcers, it is unclear how much these pathologic findings contribute to the patients' symptoms. Multiple conditions (e.g., infection, allergy, Crohn's disease) can cause esophagitis, gastritis, and duodenitis in childhood and need to be considered in the differential diagnosis of RAP; in the following section we will briefly discuss some of them.

Gastroesophageal reflux disease (GERD) should be suspected when heartburn (defined as a

TABLE 6-3

ORGANIC CAUSES OF CHRONIC ABDOMINAL PAIN

Gastrointestinal	**Psychiatric**
Esophagitis	Conversion reaction
Gastritis	**Hepatobiliary**
Duodenitis	Chronic hepatitis
Peptic ulcer	Cholelithiasis
Eosinophilic gastroenteritis	Cholecystitis
Malrotation	Choledochal cyst
Cysts (duplication or	Sphincter of Oddi
mesenteric)	Dysfunction
Carbohydrate intolerance	
Celiac disease	**Pancreatic**
Polyps	Pancreatitis
Parasites	Pseudocyst
Hernias	**Gynecologic**
Tumor	Hematocolpos
Foreign body	Endometriosis
Intussusception	Mittelschmertz
Inflammatory bowel disease	Tumor
Respiratory	**Metabolic**
Infection, tumor or	Porphyria
inflammation in vicinity of	Diabetes
diaphragm	Lead poisoning
Urinary	**Musculoskeletal**
Ureteropelvic junction	Trauma
obstruction	Inflammation
Recurrent pyelonephritis	Infection
Recurrent cystitis	Tumor
Hydronephrosis	
Nephrolithiasis	
Hematologic	
Angioedema	
Collagen vascular disease	
Sickle cell disease	

retrosternal burning discomfort that radiates toward the head) or oral regurgitation of sour or bitter gastric contents, is a prominent part of the history. A study investigating the presence of GERD in children with recurrent abdominal pain concluded that pathologic gastroesophageal reflux is a frequent finding in children with recurrent abdominal pain. Treatment of gastroesophageal reflux in this group

of patients resulted in resolution or improvement of abdominal pain in 71% of cases.

Abdominal pain is by far the most frequent presenting symptom of *chronic peptic ulcer disease* in children. The pain is usually epigastric in location, nonradiating, but may also be generalized or periumbilical; it is a food-related pain (frequently children experience exacerbation rather than relief with meals), and it is not uncommon for ulcer pain to awaken the patient at night. The most common associated symptoms are nausea, vomiting, or heartburn. Evidence of GI bleeding is not uncommon, manifested by positive stool guaiac testing and iron deficiency anemia. However, the clinical presentation of peptic ulcer disease may have symptoms that overlap with functional dyspepsia. The presence of the "red flag" findings noted in Table 6-1 and a favorable response to antacids or H2 blockers may orient toward a suspicion of peptic disease; but there is evidence that antisecretory therapy may also be effective in functional dyspepsia. Therefore, as symptoms and therapeutic response may be indistinguishable, the definitive diagnosis of peptic disease requires esophagogastroduodenoscopy.[2]

In the absence of worrisome features, the child or adolescent with dyspepsia can be treated without prior evaluation (see also Chap. 17). Short-term (6–8 weeks) empirical medical therapy with an H2 blocker or proton-pump inhibitor is an acceptable diagnostic test of self-limiting upper GI inflammation in patients with symptoms less than 3 months. If predominantly painful dyspeptic symptoms do not improve with a short-term antisecretory empiric therapy, or quickly return after cessation of treatment, and in untreated patients with symptoms beyond 3 months, upper gastrointestinal endoscopy should be performed to look for evidence of disease. The findings of disease (e.g., *H. pylori* infection, Crohn's disease, discussed later) will prompt specific therapy. The absence of mucosal disease supports a diagnosis of functional dyspepsia.

Together with *H. pylori, nonsteroidal antiinflammatory drugs* (NSAIDs) are the most important exogenous factors associated with peptic ulcer. In any patient being evaluated for recurrent abdominal pain with dyspepsia, a careful history is required to ensure that possible NSAIDs consumption is

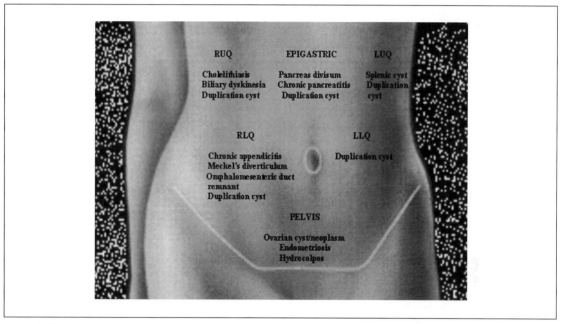

RUQ

Cholelithiasis
Biliary dyskinesia
Duplication cyst

EPIGASTRIC

Pancreas divisum
Chronic pancreatitis
Duplication cyst

LUQ

Splenic cyst
Duplication
cyst

RLQ

Chronic appendicitis
Meckel's diverticulum
Onphalomesenteric duct
remnant
Duplication cyst

LLQ

Duplication cyst

PELVIS

Ovarian cyst/neoplasm
Endometriosis
Hydrocolpos

FIGURE 6-2

LOCALIZING SURGICALLY TREATABLE CAUSES OF RECURRENT PAIN BY ABDOMINAL REGION

detected and NSAIDs should be stopped if they are frequently used.

Pancreatitis

Chronic pancreatitis has been defined as a continuing inflammatory disease of the pancreas characterized by irreversible morphologic changes that typically cause recurrent or persisting abdominal pain and/or permanent loss of exocrine and endocrine function in certain individuals. Recurring, severe pain is the primary clinical manifestation of chronic pancreatitis. The pain is most commonly located in the epigastrium, radiating to the sides or back; other frequent symptoms include anorexia, nausea, and persisting vomiting. Eating is a common aggravating factor of pain and vomiting. Severe abdominal tenderness in the epigastric area and decreased bowel sounds are characteristic. The major entities associated with the development of chronic pancreatitis in childhood include metabolic causes (e.g., hypercalcemia, hyperlipidemia), idiopathic, hereditary pancreatitis, cystic fibrosis, autoimmune pancreatitis, sclerosing

cholangitis, and obstructive chronic pancreatitis (e.g., pancreas divisum, choledochal cyst, sphincter of Oddi dysfunction).

Biliary Tract Disease

Biliary tract disease is uncommon in the pediatric age group. Chronic cholecystitis related to cholelithiasis is more common in the pediatric population than in acute gallbladder pathology. Pigment gallstones are seen with higher frequency in pediatric patients with hemolytic anemia, sepsis, long-term parenteral nutrition; cholesterol or "mixed type" stones, seen commonly in adults in the United States, are less commonly identified in the pediatric population. However, in older children, obesity, ileal disease (resulting in reduced bile salt absorption), and a family history of childhood gallstones have been associated with cholesterol or mixed type stones. Children with gallstones may have colicky or nonspecific pain or remain asymptomatic. The pain is mostly located in the right upper quadrant or in the epigastrium and may radiate to the back or right shoulder; usually the pain persists for hours and occurs episodically. Nausea and vomiting are very common associated symptoms.

Chronic gallbladder pain may also be present in the absence of stones. Chronic acalculous cholecystitis and biliary dyskinesia (a dysfunction of gallbladder contraction resulting in a reduced ejection fraction) are rare causes of biliary-type pain in the absence of cholelithiasis.

Other biliary tree pathologies such as choledochal cyst may present with abdominal pain. Classically, presenting symptoms include jaundice, prevailing in children, and abdominal pain, more common in adults; moreover, an abdominal mass is palpable in about 24% of patients.

Infections

Parasitic infections, particularly *Giardia lamblia*, *Dientamoeba fragilis*, *Cryptosporidium*, and *Blastocystis hominis* are the most common infections associated with chronic abdominal pain and altered bowel pattern, often accompanied by anorexia, abdominal distention, and diarrhea. In contrast, positive fecal ova and parasite tests were found in only 2% of adult patients with IBS.[8]

Chronic *Clostridium difficile* diarrhea may be seen in children, associated with crampy abdominal pain (and history of antibiotic ingestion).

Microscopic Colitis

"Microscopic colitis" is an umbrella term covering cases of colitis in which there is histologic but no macroscopic, colonoscopic, or barium abnormality. Three specific subclassifications should be considered: (1) a *form frust* of chronic idiopathic inflammatory bowel disease, in which intraepithelial lymphocytes and chronic inflammation of the lamina propria are associated with gland distortion, (2) lymphocytic colitis, in which the lamina propria contains an inflammatory infiltrate of plasma cells and neutrophils, and the epithelium is invaded by lymphocytes and occasional neutrophils, and (3) collagenous colitis, which is histologically similar to lymphocytic colitis with the addition of subepithelial collagen table thickening. Microscopic colitis presents with chronic watery diarrhea, commonly

associated with crampy abdominal pain. The large volume of diarrhea (400–1200 g per day) distinguishes patients with lymphocytic or collagenous colitis from those with IBS, where stool weight in excess of 300 g per day is rare.

For other gastrointestinal disorders that may present with recurrent abdominal pain such as inflammatory bowel disease, small intestinal bacterial overgrowth, and celiac disease, see the specific chapters.

Gynecologic Disorders

In adolescent girls, a history of midlower abdominal pain was found to have low sensitivity but high specificity for gynecologic diseases. Gynecologic disorders such as endometriosis, ovarian neoplasms, congenital abnormalities, or adhesions following pelvic inflammatory disease should also be considered in the differential diagnosis of abdominal pain. Endometriosis (defined as the presence of benign endometrial tissue outside the uterus) can be the cause of chronic abdominal pain in postmenarchal adolescents. Clinically, it may manifest with cyclic abdominal pain (thought to be secondary to swelling before and during menstruation), nausea, vomiting, constipation, or diarrhea. Ovarian neoplasms are uncommon in children and fortunately, the majority of the lesions are benign. Chronic abdominal pain may be the only manifestation of these lesions; physical examination may reveal a palpable mass. However, some of the acute causes of gynecologic pain may also lead to chronic pain (including ovarian cysts that represent the majority of ovarian masses in children). Hydrometrocolpos due to imperforate hymen or vaginal and cervical stenosis or atresia may present with periodic lower abdominal pain. Physical examination is characterized by a lower midline abdominal mass in postmenarchal girls.

Urinary Disorders

While in infants with urinary tract infection or pyelonephritis, fever, vomiting, and diarrhea are frequent presenting symptoms, in older children, fever accompanied by diffuse abdominal/flank pain may be the presenting symptoms of pyelonephritis. Obstructive conditions such as ureteral or pelviureteric junction obstruction are also known to present with recurrent episodes of periumbilical and crampy pain, usually associated with vomiting. Hematuria can be present in the setting of urinary tract infections, abuse, trauma, Henoch-Schönlein's purpura, or renal stones. Dysuria associated with abdominal pain can represent a sign of pyelonephritis, abuse, trauma, or a sexually transmitted disease.

Congenital Anomalies

Symptomatic intestinal malrotation usually presents early in life with 85% of all cases of midgut volvulus occurring in the first year of life. In neonates symptoms are usually dramatic with sudden onset of bilious vomiting and a visibly seriously ill patient. Older infants may present with episodes of colicky abdominal pain. In one series, 20% of cases of malrotation in patients over 1 year of age presented with chronic abdominal pain. These patients often have vague, long-standing abdominal complaints with or without emesis. The pain is often postprandial and may be accompanied by bilious emesis and diarrhea or evidence of malabsorption or protein-losing enteropathy associated with bacterial overgrowth.

Duplications of the alimentary tract are uncommon congenital abnormalities. Duplications are cystic, spherical, or tubular structures lying within the wall of the alimentary tract or in the mesentery. The clinical presentations may be vague and diverse depending on the location of the duplication. Presenting signs and symptoms include abdominal mass, vomiting, decreased oral intake, gastrointestinal bleeding, periumbilical tenderness, and abdominal distention.

Musculoskeletal Pain

A musculoskeletal diagnosis can usually be confirmed by clinical examination alone, the key to which is reproducing the patient's pain by either a movement or more specifically a palpation over the structure that is the source of the pain.

Pain related to trauma is usually well localized and sharp in nature and may be exacerbated by movement. Costochondritis pain originates in the anterior chest wall, from where it may radiate into the chest, back, or abdomen; pain is reproducible by palpating the affected costal cartilage.

Familial Mediterranean Fever

Familial Mediterranean fever (FMF) is an autosomal recessive disorder that primarily affects Jewish, Armenian, Turkish, and Arab populations; FMF is characterized by recurrent and self-limited attacks of fever of unknown origin usually accompanied by polyserositis (peritonitis, pleuritis, and/or synovitis). Amyloidosis is the most severe complication of FMF. Fever, abdominal pain, chest pain, and arthritis/arthralgia are the leading symptoms. Severe abdominal pain similar to acute peritonitis is present in 95% of patients. A typical attack usually lasts from 1 to 4 days. The frequency of the attacks varies from weekly to one every 3–4 months or less. During attacks, acute-phase reactants may be elevated; between attacks, FMF patients are asymptomatic and appear healthy.

DIAGNOSTIC TESTING

As previously discussed, functional abdominal pain is too often perceived as a diagnosis of exclusion. In patients with no alarm symptoms, the Rome Criteria provide a framework for a *positive diagnosis* of FGIDs, having a positive predictive value of approximately 98%. A history that meets these criteria, in the presence of a normal physical examination and growth, is consistent with a diagnosis of FGIDs. The physician should avoid performing exhaustive investigations in attempts to "rule out" an organic disease at all cost. Performing multiple tests may provide results that often are unrelated to the presenting symptom or have no clinical relevance (such as a mildly elevated sedimentation rate). The physician should reassure the patient that no test is necessary at this point but if further symptoms present or the current symptoms worsen, the physician will not hesitate to proceed with further workup.

However, in clinical practice, the physician may want to perform some laboratory studies to reassure the patient and the family; inexpensive and easily available diagnostic tests are as follows:

- Complete blood cell (CBC) count
- Erythrocyte sedimentation rate (ESR)
- Chemistry panel
- Liver function tests (LFTs)
- Thyroid function tests
- Urine analysis
- Stool examination for blood, ova, and parasites
- Breath hydrogen testing for lactose malabsorption

It should be stressed, however, that screening tests are known to yield a low incidence of thyroid dysfunction, ova and parasite infestation, and colonic pathology in patients fulfilling at presentation the diagnosis of IBS. Finally, even though the lactose hydrogen breath test is often used to diagnose lactose intolerance in patients with FGIDs, the cause-effect relationship between lactose intolerance and symptoms is equivocal at best.

The need for *other* diagnostic tests should be based on history and physical examination: the presence of "red flag" warning signals raises the possibility of other disorders and additional evaluation, such as endoscopy, radiography, and/or celiac antibodies should be performed. Also, the diagnosis of functional dyspepsia does require the exclusion of an organic disease to explain the symptoms (including a negative esophagogastroduodenoscopy); this is the only type of functional abdominal pain syndrome in which endoscopic study is necessary for a firm diagnosis.

The diagnostic yield of a sonographic examination of the abdomen in children presenting with FGIDs seems to be extremely low; abnormalities were found in only 10 of 644 ultrasound studies performed in children with the diagnosis of recurrent abdominal pain, suggesting that only children who have abdominal pain with atypical clinical features should receive sonographic screening.

TREATMENT

There is no uniformly successful treatment for FGIDs. The pathophysiologic model of dysregulation of the brain-gut interaction provides several targets for possible medical and nonmedical interventions for patients who seem to defy the traditional biomedical model. Patient-physician interaction, education, reassurance, cognitive treatments, decrease sensory input, viscero-somatic convergence (acupuncture, massage), reduction in luminal stimuli (dietary changes, anticholinergics), and visceral analgesics (serotonin receptor agonists and antagonists, tricyclic antidepressants) are all possible treatment options in FGIDs. The treatment strategy is thus best based on the nature and severity of the symptoms.

General Treatment Approach

Education and Reassurance

Initial treatment of functional pain is based on reassurance, emphasizing the usually benign nature of this condition and the absence of an organic disease. An effective physician-patient-family relationship is the cornerstone of effective treatment. It is essential to assure the family and the patient that the physician believes the symptoms are "real," despite the benign aspects of the history, physical examination, and laboratory tests.[8] It is of great importance to give an extensive explanation of the nature of the disorder discussing the problem as a common diagnosis and not just an exclusion of an organic disease. Comparisons with other common and benign entities such as headaches or muscle cramps may help.

The main goal of the therapy is to reestablish a normal daily life for the patient and the family. The family should be discouraged from reinforcing the symptoms by allowing the child to miss school and sport activities. The parents' attitude toward the pain experience should be balanced, showing support and understanding, but being aware that excessive attention to the painful experience and missing activities may allow some patients (especially the ones with low self-worth) to develop a sick role, perpetuating the symptoms.

Due to the high index of symptomatic success with reassurance, medications are not necessary for every patient with functional abdominal pain. Drug therapy should only be recommended for patients with symptoms interfering with satisfactory quality of life.

Dietary Modification

Food-induced symptoms are commonly reported among IBS patients, with 20–65% attributing their symptoms to adverse food reactions. Patients are, however, more likely to experience symptoms as a generalized effect of eating, and at times may even become conditioned to reduce eating to avoid post-prandial discomfort.[8] However, certain dietary substances (fatty foods, gas-producing foods, caffeine, lactose in lactase-deficient individuals, excess fiber) may aggravate symptoms in some individuals. The avoidance of gas-forming foods such as legumes, complex carbohydrates, lactose, and a limited fat intake (fats potently activate motor reflexes) may provide symptomatic relief in some patients.

Although high-fiber diets have been long used in adult IBS patients, the data in children are still preliminary, and a substantial increase in fiber consumption may be difficult for pediatric patients to achieve. Nevertheless, the addition of fiber each day seems to be a simple and inexpensive intervention that might benefit some children with RAP.

Pharmachotherapy Targeted at Specific Symptoms

Laxatives

See the chapter 5.

Anticholinergic and Antidiarrheal Medications

Some patients with diarrhea seem to benefit from an antidiarrheal preparation such as loperamide (1–2 mg once or twice a day) that decreases stool frequency and urgency while improving stool consistency.

For pain and bloating, antispasmodic (anticholinergic) medication, particularly when symptoms are exacerbated by meals, should be considered, even if this therapy has not yet been proved to be useful in children with RAP. Metaanalyses of adult studies and anecdotal experience seem to demonstrate that some of these agents may be effective.[8] Smooth muscle relaxants

such as hyoscyamine and dicyclomine seem to retain efficacy when used on an as-needed basis up to three times per day, whenever the symptoms are present (much like analgesics are used for headaches), but become less effective with chronic use.

Tricyclic Antidepressants

Tricyclic antidepressants (TCAs), such as amitriptyline and imipramine, are commonly prescribed for treatment of a variety of chronic pain conditions and functional disorders, including IBS, in smaller doses (0.2–0.4 mg/kg per day, 5–50 mg per day) than needed for treatment of major depression. These agents are especially effective in diarrhea-predominant patients. It should be stressed with the patients' families (often concerned at the idea of beginning an antidepressive drug) that the analgesic effects of TCAs are independent of its effects on depression. Family and patients need to understand that they are not being treated for a psychiatric problem. Minimization of side effects (predominantly sedation) can be achieved by giving the medication at bed time. Moreover, the possibility of cardiac arrhythmias demands caution when prescribing these drugs (ECG monitoring should be performed before starting treatment). It is recommended that the medication be started at low doses, increasing the dose progressively as needed to achieve a full dose in weeks.

Selective Serotonin Reuptake Inhibitors

Selective serotonin reuptake inhibitors, such as paroxetine, fluoxetine, or sertraline also seem to be effective in relieving symptoms in adult patients with FGIDs. Among the antidepressant medications, *selective serotonin reuptake inhibitors* (SSRIs) are often prescribed because of their lower side-effect profile, but there are only a few controlled studies of their efficacy in managing chronic pain syndromes. Furthermore, physiologic studies suggest that SSRIs increase motility in the small intestine, while the TCAs slow intestinal transit. Thus, a patient in whom the main symptom is constipation may benefit most from an initial trial of an SSRI, whereas TCAs are especially effective in diarrhea-predominant patients.

Serotonin Receptor Antagonists and Agonists

Serotonin (5-HT) has recently emerged as an important enteric neurotransmitter with diverse sensory and motor functions in the GI tract. Serotonin has been implicated in the pathogenesis of IBS and higher levels of plasma serotonin are found postprandially in patients with diarrhea-predominant IBS.

A number of *selective 5-HT₃ antagonists* have been developed including ondansetron, granisetron, tropisetron renzapride, and zacopride. Ondansetron demonstrated some benefits in diarrhea-predominant IBS, but no improvement in abdominal pain. Similarly, no reduction in pain was seen with granisetron administration. Alosetron, a newer 5-HT₃ receptor antagonist, has greater potency than ondansetron, and good bioavailability. Treatment with alosetron leads to significant relief of abdominal pain and discomfort in women with diarrhea-predominant IBS. Constipation is the most common adverse event reported, but its use has also been associated with ischemic colitis, resulting in significant restriction of its licensed indications by the *Food and Drug Administration* (FDA).

Selective 5-HT₄ receptor agonists such as tegaserod and prucalopride have been developed for patients with IBS and constipation. Tegaserod has repeatedly proven effective in the relief of abdominal pain and discomfort in adult women with constipation-predominant IBS, by accelerating orocecal and colonic transit without altering gastric emptying. The most significant adverse events are transient diarrhea and headache.

Alternative and Complementary Therapy

Several reports have documented the greater use of alternative therapies such as diet supplements, probiotics, and Chinese medicine in patients with FGIDs, especially those who failed the previously discussed therapies. Efficacy of alternative therapies has been difficult to ascertain, in view of the lack of controlled trials. However, placebo-controlled studies have shown an overall improvement in IBS patients who used *peppermint oil* (*Mentha piperita*); this spasmolytic agent that relaxes gastrointestinal smooth muscle, relieving pain, is commonly found in many over-the-counter preparations for IBS. Moreover, a randomized controlled trial in Chinese medicine demonstrated that *Chinese herbal therapy* is effective in the management of symptoms related to IBS. Natural and herbal medications are not without adverse effects, and patients should not take these products without provider supervision. Another alternative therapy for FGIDs in Chinese medicine is *acupuncture*. There are no high quality studies of acupuncture for IBS in adults and no studies for this condition in children. However, several recent studies have shown that contrary to expectations a pediatric population accepts acupuncture treatment well and there is preliminary data suggesting the effectiveness of acupuncture in treatment of pediatric chronic pain.

Effective psychologic treatments include cognitive-behavioral interventions, psychotherapy, and stress management. Techniques of cognitive behavioral therapy can be used in the pediatric clinic to identify obstacles to school attendance and to design interventions that help children with functional abdominal pain return to school and other activities. A systematic review of the literature concludes that the efficacy of psychologic treatment for IBS could not be established yet, because of methodologic inadequacy in all the studies.

Probiotics are live microbial food supplements that benefit the host animal by improving intestinal microbial balance. Despite alterations of enteric flora that may play a role in irritable bowel syndrome, the role of probiotics in IBS has not been clearly defined. Some studies have shown improvements in pain and flatulence in response to probiotic administration, whereas others have shown no symptomatic improvement. Although probiotics hold great promise and appear to be useful in some settings, more clinical study is needed to firmly establish the relevance of probiotic therapy. It is possible that the future role of probiotics in IBS will lie in prevention, rather than cure.

In chronic cases of refractory pain, referral to specialized treatment centers for an interdisciplinary pain management approach may be the most efficient method of treating disability. It is likely that a referral for counseling would be more acceptable if it were presented as a referral for relaxation training, pain management, or other specific aspects of counseling that the parents value.

NATURAL HISTORY

Functional abdominal pain is not always a benign condition with a satisfactory outcome. Long-term psychiatric disorders have been identified in patients suffering from functional abdominal pain in childhood.[9] Young adults with a childhood history of RAP are significantly more likely to endorse anxiety symptoms and disorders, hypochondriacal beliefs, greater perceived susceptibility to physical impairment, poorer social functioning, antidepressant treatment and a family history of generalized anxiety disorder, with over 80% meeting criteria for a lifetime psychiatric diagnosis.[9] Children with abdominal pain do not necessarily continue to experience physical symptoms in adulthood, but may have an increased risk of adult psychiatric disorders. A large population-based cohort study showed that childhood RAP is significantly associated with an increased risk of internalizing psychiatric disorder in adulthood, but with no somatic distress if one controls for psychiatric disorder. Childhood RAP likely predicts IBS later in life, as well as migraine.[9] Follow-up studies have shown an evolution of children with abdominal migraine into adults with migraine headaches and these episodes of abdominal pain have been considered a prodrome of migraine headaches. Consequently, interventions during childhood may have the potential to prevent or reduce the incidence and/or severity of functional bowel and other disorders in adults.

CONCLUSION

The initial evaluation of the child with recurrent abdominal pain should be performed by the primary care physician. It is crucial for the clinician to

CASE STUDY 6-1

A girl aged 16 years presents with a 10-year history of worsening recurrent abdominal pain. She describes her pain as intermittent, occurring once a day, lasting from 5 min to several hours, relieved with defecation and located in the lower left quadrant. At times, she also complains of epigastric, cramping pain after eating, increased gassiness, and bloating. Stools are usually normal without any blood or mucus; occasionally they are loose and at times she has to strain to pass pellet-like stools. She remains active and denies weight loss, joint pain, or mouth ulcers. Treatment with neither hyoscyamine nor lactulose was helpful. She has had worsening of symptoms since an attempt was made to wean her off ranitidine that seemed to give some relief of the epigastric pain in the past. Physical examination does not reveal any abnormality; she is between the 25th and 50th percentile for both weight and height.

A screening blood workup (including CBC, ESR, thyroid function, celiac antibodies, LFTs, amylase, lipase), urinalysis, and stool studies (O&P) is negative; she thus undergoes upper endoscopy with biopsies (symptom recurrence on stopping medication should prompt further investigation), which reveals no pathologic diagnosis on duodenal, antral, and esophageal biopsies. An abdominal x-ray shows a significant amount of stool scattered throughout the right and left colon.

In summary, given the significant workup that she has had and the lack of organic signs or symptoms, she has likely mixed features of different functional disorders: irritable bowel syndrome with constipation and dyspepsia. She would benefit from a trial of treatment with amitriptyline, polyethylene glycol, and continued ranitidine.

recognize that the term "recurrent abdominal pain" is a description, and not a diagnosis, and both organic and functional pain should be considered. A careful history and physical examination with limited laboratory evaluation is sufficient to suggest a diagnosis of an FGID in most cases and to start the treatment. Red flag signals of disease should always lead to further evaluation, but in the absence of obvious disease, children fulfilling symptom-based criteria for FGIDs can be treated for their problems without initially extensive diagnostic studies.

Since these disorders tend to be chronic and do not respond to initial therapy in most cases, the specialist is frequently consulted; he/she is thus charged with making sure an organic condition has not been missed, confirming or refuting a diagnosis of an FGID, and addressing the correct treatment.

References

1   Apley J, Naish N. Recurrent abdominal pain: a field survey of 1000 school children. *Arch Dis Child* 33:165–170, 1958.

2   Rasquin-Weber A, Hyman PE, Cucchiara S, et al. Childhood functional gastrointestinal disorders. *Gut* 45(Suppl II):II60–II68, 1999.

3   Hyams JS, Burke G, Davis PM, et al. Abdominal pain and irritable bowel syndrome in adolescents: a community-based study. *J Pediatr* 129:220–226, 1996.

4   Drossman DA, Ringel Y, Vogt BA, et al. Alterations of brain activity associated with resolution of emotional distress and pain in a case of severe irritable bowel syndrome. *Gastroenterology* 124(3):754–761, 2003.

5   Di Lorenzo C, Sigurdsson L, Griffiths J, et al. Rectal and gastric hyperalgesia in children with recurrent abdominal pain. *Gastroenterology* 114: A743, 1998.

6   Hyams JS, Hyman PE. Recurrent abdominal pain and the biopsychosocial model of medical practice. *J Pediatr* 133:473–478, 1998.

7   Hyams J, Colletti R, Faure C. Functional gastrointestinal disorders: Working Group Report of the First World Congress of Pediatric Gastroenterology, Hepatology, and Nutrition. *J Pediatr Gastroenterol Nutr* 35:S110–S117, 2002.

8   Drossman DA, Camilleri M, Mayer EA, et al. AGA technical review on irritable bowel syndrome. *Gastroenterology* 123(6):2108–2131, 2002.

9   Campo JV, Di Lorenzo C, Chiappetta L, et al. Adult outcomes of pediatric recurrent abdominal pain: do they just grow out of it? *Pediatrics* 108:E1, 2001.

7

INTESTINAL OBSTRUCTION

Mindy B. Statter and Elizabeth A. Sailhamer

INTRODUCTION

Intestinal obstruction represents an important and common cause of surgical emergencies in children. The classic presentation of vomiting and abdominal pain should alert the clinician that obstruction is a possibility, but the differential diagnosis for intestinal obstruction is broad, and must be pursued with further history, physical, and selective diagnostic studies. The etiology and presentation of bowel obstruction can vary dramatically in infants and children within certain age groups. The optimal imaging approach can be determined by the child's age and findings on the abdominal radiograph. Although most cases of bowel obstruction require surgical intervention, the surgical approach and urgency of the interventions differ, and some can be managed nonoperatively. Therefore, prompt preoperative diagnosis is imperative.[1]

ETIOLOGY

Pediatric intestinal obstruction is generally caused by one of the following: (1) atresia or stenosis, (2) extrinsic compression including incarcerated hernia, (3) intussusception, (4) anomalies of rotation, (5) inspissation of bowel contents, (6) peristaltic dysfunction, (7) intrinsic masses, or (8) inflammatory lesions, e.g., perforated appendicitis.[2]

Extrinsic Compression

- Incarcerated hernia
- Malrotation (Ladd's bands), midgut volvulus
- Meckel's diverticulum with omphalomesenteric duct remnants
- Superior mesenteric artery (SMA) syndrome
- Postoperative adhesions
- Seatbelt syndrome
- Perforated appendicitis

Intrinsic Obstruction

- Inspissation of bowel contents
- Peristaltic dysfunction
  a. Hirschsprung's disease
  b. Intestinal pseudoobstruction
  c. Intestinal neuronal dysplasia (IND)
- Intussusception
- Intestinal stenosis and atresia
- Intrinsic mass or polyp
- Pyloric stenosis

PATHOGENESIS

Intestinal obstruction in children can be either partial or complete, and may be due to intrinsic lesions or extrinsic compression of the lumen. When the intestinal lumen becomes obstructed, the bowel proximal to the obstruction becomes dilated and begins to secrete fluid into the lumen. As the intestine proximal to the obstruction becomes distended, blood flow to the dilated bowel wall is compromised. This can result in loss of mucosal integrity, which can lead to bacterial translocation with resultant bacteremia or sepsis. With progressive bowel wall distention, venous drainage becomes impaired resulting in bowel wall edema. The increased transmural pressure compromises arterial inflow leading to ischemia and intestinal necrosis.

Clinical Signs and Symptoms

Abdominal distention, bilious vomiting, and failure to pass meconium are the cardinal signs and symptoms of mechanical obstruction in the newborn. The diagnosis is often suspected antenatally because of maternal polyhydramnios. Likewise with a child of any age, the cardinal symptom of intestinal obstruction is vomiting. The association of abdominal distention with vomiting should prompt thorough evaluation for a possible intestinal obstruction with ileus being a diagnosis of exclusion.

Nausea and Vomiting

Vomiting is the hallmark of intestinal obstruction. The quality of emesis may change as the obstructive process evolves. The emesis may be initially nonbilious and progress to feculent over the ensuing 24–36 hours indicating a complete obstruction. Nonbi-lious vomiting is present in intestinal obstructions proximal to the ampulla of Vater (such as pyloric stenosis), whereas bilious vomiting is present in obstructions that are distal to the ampulla of Vater (such as malrotation). Feculent emesis may be observed with distal small bowel obstruction and results from stasis of small bowel contents and overgrowth of bacteria in the succus entericus. Blood-tinged emesis signifies an irritative or inflammatory process in the *upper gastrointestinal* (UGI) tract.[3]

Abdominal Pain

Pain is one of the most common complaints among children who present to the emergency department. Children may be able to describe the pain, or if

unable to verbalize, they may present with persistent crying, irritability, inconsolability, poor feeding, failure to thrive, or sleeplessness. The location (localized vs. diffuse), timing (acute vs. gradual onset), and quality of the pain (sharp vs. dull; intermittent colicky vs. constant) are important to characterize when possible. Periumbilical, crampy abdominal pain (colicky pain) is classic for intestinal obstruction, because it results from distention of the loops of bowel proximal to the obstruction, which wax and wane with the timing of peristalsis. Peritoneal signs (rebound tenderness, rigidity, or guarding), along with fever and tachycardia, may suggest an ischemic or perforated bowel.[4]

Abdominal Distention

As with any cause of complete intestinal obstruction in a child, the degree of abdominal distention is directly related to the anatomic site of obstruction. Distal obstruction (jejunal or ileal) is characterized by abdominal distention; however, with proximal obstruction (gastric or duodenal) the abdomen may appear scaphoid. In distal obstruction, the proximal bowel loops become air- or fluid-filled; the abdominal wall is firm and may be tympanitic to percussion if the bowel loops remain air-filled.

Change in Bowel Habits

Constipation and obstipation are signs of bowel obstruction anywhere in the GI tract. Diarrhea, especially bloody diarrhea, can often be a late finding in obstruction, signifying ischemia to the intestinal wall, resulting in necrosis and mucosal sloughing. Bloody diarrhea may be seen with malrotation with midgut volvulus and intussusception ("currant jelly stool"—stool composed of mucous and blood). If frank blood is absent, digital rectal examination and stool guaiac should be performed to assess for occult blood, and for the presence or absence of stool in the vault.

Bowel Sounds

Bowel sounds are an unreliable finding; in the neonate, bowel sounds may be audible with ischemic intestine and conversely, may be absent in a non-pathologic state.

Nonspecific Complaints

Children may also present with anorexia, lethargy, and fever, among other nonspecific complaints. They are often dehydrated from vomiting, and may present with dry mucous membranes, sunken fontanelles, tachycardia, oliguria, and hypotension. Any abdominal scars suggesting past abdominal surgeries should be noted. In addition, the inspection of the external genitalia is imperative; the presence of an irreducible inguinal bulge suggests an incarcerated hernia. The male patient with abdominal pain and a nonpalpable undescended testis may have intraabdominal testicular torsion.

Medications such as nonsteroidals or herbal family remedies should be elicited from the history.

DIFFERENTIAL DIAGNOSIS

In distinguishing between the various etiologies for mechanical obstruction in children, it is most helpful to classify children by age. The etiology and presentation varies significantly with age.

Neonates

- Often congenital etiologies
- Intestinal atresia or stenosis (duodenal, jejunal, or ileal)
- Malrotation (with or without midgut volvulus)
- Pyloric stenosis (highest incidence between 2 and 6 weeks of age)
- Inspissation of bowel contents (meconium ileus)
- Peristaltic dysfunction (Hirschsprung's disease)
- Incarcerated hernia

Infants

- Malrotation with midgut volvulus
- 75 percent become symptomatic in the first month of life
- 90 percent become symptomatic in the first year of life
- Intussusception (incidence between 3 months and 3 years)
- Incarcerated hernia

Preschool Children (Less Than 5 Years)

- Intussusception
- Incarcerated hernia
- Perforated appendicitis

School-Aged Children (Older Than 5 Years)

- Acquired intestinal stenosis secondary to ischemia (posttraumatic, e.g., "seatbelt syndrome")
- Inflammatory lesions such as Crohn's disease or perforated appendicitis
- Extrinsic compression such as incarcerated hernia, perforated appendicitis, or postoperative adhesions
- Intrinsic lesions such as masses, polyps
- Meckel's diverticulum

It is important to remember that malrotation, with midgut volvulus, may present at any age, and must be included in the differential diagnosis any time a child presents with bilious vomiting (Table 7-1).

DIAGNOSTIC MODALITIES

Making the diagnosis of intestinal obstruction is relatively straightforward using a combination of plain radiographs, contrast enema, and upper gastrointestinal contrast study. However, the actual etiology of the obstruction, e.g., atresia, congenital adhesive band, and internal hernia may not be determined until exploratory laparotomy.

The plain abdominal radiograph (AXR, commonly referred to as "KUB") is the initial diagnostic study for children with intestinal obstruction, but should never be used as an isolated study to "rule in or rule out" any pathology. The "obstructive series" includes a supine and lateral decubitus, or upright

TABLE 7-1

DIFFERENTIAL DIAGNOSIS OF INTESTINAL OBSTRUCTION[a]

Etiology	Age	Classic Presentation	Diagnosis
Malrotation with/without midgut volvulus	Any age 50–75% <1 month 90% <1 year	Bilious emesis, minimal abdominal distention, with a late finding of blood in stool	UGI: ligament of Treitz not located to left of midline; "bird's beak/"corkscrew" appearance
Duodenal atresia or stenosis	First week of life	Bilious emesis. Epigastric distention only Down's syndrome	UGI: blunt end termination of contrast
Jejunoileal atresia or stenosis	First week of life	Bilious emesis and progressive abdominal distention. The more distal the obstruction, the later the onset of emesis and abdominal distention	Contrast enema to distinguish small from large bowel obstruction. Presence of microcolon indicates unused colon due to proximal obstruction
Meconium ileus	1–2 days	Absent or delayed passage of meconium. Bilious emesis, abdominal distention	Barium enema for diagnostic and therapeutic purposes. Sweat test for cystic fibrosis
Hirschsprung's disease	Any age	Delay or failure to pass meconium, sepsis, abdominal distention, bilious emesis	Barium enema, rectal biopsy
Pyloric stenosis	2–6 weeks	Projectile, nonbilious vomiting. Olive-shaped mass	US UGI
Intussusception	5–9 months (range: 3 months to 3 years)	Colicky abdominal pain with periods of lethargy, bilious vomiting, currant jelly stool. Sausage-shaped mass	US Barium enema (or air inflation) for diagnosis and therapeutic reduction.
Incarcerated hernia	Any age	Inguinal mass	Physical examination Ultrasound
Postoperative adhesions	Any age	Postoperative	Barium enema or UGI
Lap belt complex	Any age	Posttrauma	Barium enema or UGI
Perforated appendicitis	Any age	Anorexia, vomiting, abdominal pain	US
Meckel's diverticulum			Radionuclide scan

[a]UGI: upper GI barium study; US: abdominal ultrasound; AXR: abdominal x-ray.

abdominal films, in addition to an upright *chest x-ray* (CXR). Typical findings are distended air-filled bowel loops, the presence of air-fluid levels, and the absence of distal air in the colon and rectum (Fig. 7-1). A paucity of bowel gas may be apparent due to the replacement of air by fluid in the dilated bowel. The presence of free intraperitoneal air (pneumoperitoneum) should be noted, especially on the upright CXR. There are no pathognomonic findings on plain films for malrotation. The information

operator dependent in terms of the quality and interpretation of the study.[5]

When malrotation and midgut volvulus are included in the differential diagnosis, the imaging evaluation must be considered an emergency and executed until malrotation is eliminated from the different diagnosis. Upper gastrointestinal contrast studies are the definitive diagnostic modality for malrotation. The UGI demonstrates that the duodenojejunal junction is normally located to the left of the midline and differentiates obstruction related to rotational anomalies (malrotation) from intrinsic duodenal obstruction (duodenal atresia).

It should be noted that in the neonate, it is difficult to differentiate small intestine from large intestine radiographically. The contrast enema is helpful in that the colon will be delineated; if a "microcolon" is demonstrated, as well as a collapsed terminal ileum, the diagnosis of distal small bowel obstruction is made.

Computerized tomography (CT) is of limited use in the emergent evaluation of intestinal obstruction. Diagnostic evaluation requires complete opacification of the intestinal tract with enteral contrast which can contribute a significant delay in diagnosis.

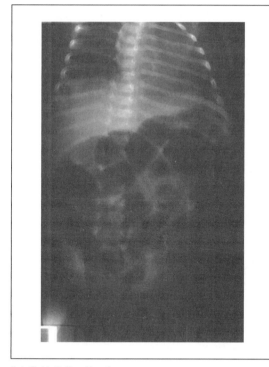

FIGURE 7-1

PLAIN ABDOMINAL X-RAY DEMONSTRATING MARKEDLY DILATED BOWEL LOOPS CONSISTENT WITH INTESTINAL OBSTRUCTION

obtained with each study determines the next step in the evaluation. In the neonate, it is difficult to tell whether the dilated bowel loops are small or large intestine. The contrast enema is therefore used to confirm the diagnosis of small bowel obstruction demonstrating a microcolon. Barium enema is also used to exclude meconium ileus and intussusception, which are both conditions that often respond to nonoperative management.

Ultrasound (US) is becoming recognized as a useful noninvasive imaging modality, with good sensitivity and specificity in certain disease processes. It is the diagnostic modality of choice for pyloric stenosis. It is also a useful alternative to invasive contrast radiography, and can be used as a screening tool in intussusception. The advantages of US include no radiation exposure, discomfort, or contrast medium. The disadvantages are that it is

TREATMENT

Initial management of any child who presents with mechanical bowel obstruction should include fluid resuscitation and monitoring. Children often present with intravascular depletion secondary to decreased oral intake, emesis, and increased secretory losses into the dilated intestine. Therefore, stabilization of the patient with fluid resuscitation (nonglucose-containing isotonic solution, e.g., lactated Ringers or normal saline) and electrolyte replacement are crucial, with bladder catheterization to monitor the urine output and assess the adequacy of the resuscitation. In any vomiting child, a *nasogastric tube* (NGT) should be placed for decompression, and the patient *should not have any oral intake* (NPO). Consideration should be given to starting broad-spectrum antibiotics in neonates and infants or if ischemia and bowel compromise is suspected. Early surgical consultation is imperative. After appropriate resuscitation and workup, the necessity for operative intervention is determined. Indications for emergent exploratory laparotomy include: (1) malrotation with or without midgut volvulus, (2) pneumoperitoneum, (3) an irreducible intussusception, and (4) peritonitis.

SPECIFIC ETIOLOGIES

Malrotation and Midgut Volvulus

Although generally thought of as neonatal pathology, malrotation is encountered throughout childhood, adolescence, and even adulthood. Malrotation with acute midgut volvulus represents the most dreaded cause of bilious vomiting in a child because it can result in ischemia and necrosis of the entire small bowel in a matter of several hours, leading to short gut syndrome.

Incidence

Malrotation is estimated to occur in one in 6000 live births. Acute midgut volvulus eventually develops in about two-thirds of patients with malrotation, and is present in 50% of patients who come to surgery for rotational abnormalities. Most patients with midgut volvulus (50–75%) present in the first month of life, and 90% present within the first year. The remaining 10% can present at any time during childhood or adulthood. There is an 8–12% incidence of duodenal (intraluminal) webs in patients undergoing operation for malrotation.[6]

Pathogenesis

The midgut normally herniates out of the peritoneal cavity and into the umbilical cord at the fifth week of gestation and returns to the abdominal cavity at 10 weeks. Normal intestinal rotation and fixation is complete by 12 weeks of gestation. The respective duodenojejunal and cecocolic limbs undergo a 270 degree counterclockwise rotation. The duodenojejunal limb makes the rotation around the superior mesenteric artery and the cecum descends into the *right lower quadrant*

(RLQ). Peritoneal bands form to anchor the ascending and descending colon, respectively, in the right and left paracolic gutters. If the cecum and ascending colon do not fully rotate and descend, peritoneal bands, Ladd's bands, secure the cecum in the RUQ and cause extrinsic compression of the duodenum. Normally, there is a broad-based attachment of the intestinal mesentery, from the ligament of Treitz in the left lower quadrant (LUQ) to the cecum in the RLQ. This broad-based attachment prevents axial rotation of the mesentery and intestine. In malrotation, the duodenojejunal junction is to the right of midline (instead of in the LUQ) resulting in a narrow point of fixation and the mesenteric pedicle containing the superior mesenteric artery and *superior mesenteric vein* (SMV) can undergo volvulus. Obstruction is usually the result of external compression of the duodenum by the congenital peritoneal bands (Ladd's bands) or by acute midgut volvulus.[2]

Ladd's bands. These are aberrant peritoneal bands fixating a malpositioned cecum to the posterior abdominal wall. These bands extend across the duodenum, resulting in extrinsic compression and obstruction of the lumen without volvulus. This may manifest as chronic, partial obstruction with intermittent colicky abdominal pain, occasional bilious vomiting, and failure to thrive, even without volvulus.

Acute midgut volvulus. The superior mesenteric artery perfuses the midgut, which includes the small intestine from the ligament of Treitz to the midtransverse colon. Without normal fixation by a broad-based mesentery the narrow mesenteric pedicle is prone to volvulus. This results in acute bowel obstruction and acute vascular compromise of the SMA, leading to ischemia and necrosis of the midgut in a matter of hours, if not detected early.

Intrinsic duodenal obstruction. Malrotation is associated with other congenital anomalies in children, and obstruction can be due to duodenal stenosis, webs, or atresia in 8–12% of children with malrotation.

Chronic midgut volvulus. Older children (>2 years old) with malrotation may present with symptoms of recurrent abdominal pain resulting from intermittent episodes of partial midgut volvulus. The partial volvulus results in lymphatic and venous obstruction (instead of arterial occlusion), resulting in intermittent episodes of abdominal pain and bilious vomiting or hematemesis, bloody diarrhea, constipation, weight loss, and failure to thrive.

Internal hernia. The lack of fixation of the bowel provides potential spaces for internal hernias, which can result in bowel obstruction and strangulation.

Symptoms and Signs

Unexplained bilious vomiting in an infant is malrotation with midgut volvulus until proven otherwise. Bilious emesis is the cardinal manifestation of intestinal obstruction, and is almost uniformly present. On physical examination, there are few early findings. The abdomen is usually not distended, because the obstruction is very proximal. Guaiac positive stool or hematochezia resulting from mucosal injury is a relatively common early finding with volvulus. If transmural necrosis ensues, in addition to peritonitis, other evidence of an intraabdominal catastrophe may be present, such as hypotension, acidosis, respiratory failure, and thrombocytopenia.

Diagnosis

Any newborn with bilious emesis should undergo emergent imaging evaluation initially consisting of plain films. There are no pathognomonic findings for malrotation or midgut volvulus on plain abdominal radiograph. The AXR in malrotation with volvulus may demonstrate a paucity of air due to resorption of intraluminal air and the accumulation of fluid within bowel loops. The definitive imaging study is the UGI when the diagnosis of malrotation is suspected. This study identifies the normal location of the duodenojejunal junction (ligament of Treitz) to the left of the midline, rising

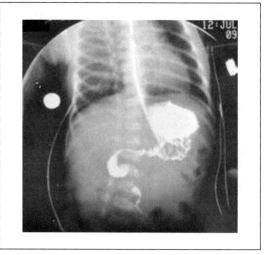

FIGURE 7-2

UGI DEMONSTRATING MALROTATION WITHOUT MIDGUT VOLVULUS
The ligament of Treitz is not observed to the left of the midline; the duodenum and proximal jejunum descend to the right of the spine.

posteriorly to the level of the pylorus. The diagnostic findings of malrotation include the absence of a normally positioned ligament of Treitz with the duodenum and proximal jejunum descending on the right (Fig. 7-2). Additionally, if volvulus is present, the contrast may abruptly taper into a "bird's beak" or "corkscrew" appearance at the level of the second portion of the duodenum.

Treatment

For the symptomatic patient, evaluation, resuscitation, and preoperative preparation should be conducted at the same time so that the diagnosis can be immediately followed by emergent laparotomy. This urgency is related to the fact that a delay in diagnosis of a few hours may determine whether ischemic intestine remains viable and salvageable at laparotomy. Initial management includes intravenous fluid resuscitation, nasogastric decompression, bladder catheterization, and intravenous broad-spectrum antibiotics. The operative procedure includes assessment of the bowel viability by complete evisceration of the intestine and mesentery.

If present, midgut volvulus is relieved by rotating the intestine counterclockwise. Correction of the malrotation includes division of Ladd's bands to release the compression on the duodenum, and broadening of the mesentery to prevent future volvulus. If necessary, infarcted intestine is resected. At the conclusion of the procedure, the intestine is replaced into the abdomen without mesenteric torsion; generally the small intestine on the right and the cecum and colon on the left. Appendectomy is considered standard because future diagnosis of acute appendicitis may be difficult being that the cecum is positioned on the left side of the abdomen.

Prognosis

Results after surgical correction of malrotation are generally excellent. Mortality rate for operative correction of malrotation ranges from 3% to 9% overall. Recurrent volvulus after correction is rare. Morbidity and mortality of malrotation is related to the extent of intestinal necrosis and short gut syndrome.

Incarcerated Inguinal Hernia

Inguinal hernia repair is the most common procedure performed in childhood. It is also one of the most common causes of small bowel obstruction in children.

Incidence

One to two percent of all children have inguinal hernias, with greater prevalence in premature males. Approximately, 10% of inguinal hernias become incarcerated, with 70% occurring in the first year, and most of those occurring in the first 6 months.[2]

Pathogenesis

Inguinal hernias in children are most commonly indirect hernias, in which a loop of bowel (or ovary in females) herniates through the inguinal canal via a congenitally patent processus vaginalis. Initially, a hernia is often reducible and only appears as an inguinal "bulge" on a Valsalva maneuver; however, if a loop of bowel becomes incarcerated (or nonreducible) this can lead to SBO—and possibly a strangulated hernia in which the herniated loop is ischemic or even necrotic.

Symptoms and Signs

Children are often brought to see a physician because swelling or a "bulge" was noticed by the parents during crying or any Valsalva maneuver. It is important to note if the mass can be reduced. Incarcerated hernias are irreducible, and can be erythematous and tender. Children will often present with symptoms of SBO, including nausea and vomiting, obstipation, abdominal distension, and poor feeding. The differential diagnosis also includes testicular torsion or testicular tumor; examination of the external genitalia and confirmation that both testes reside in the scrotum is imperative.

Diagnosis

The diagnosis of incarcerated inguinal hernia is made primarily by physical examination. AXR can show an obstructive pattern, with bowel gas in the scrotum. After a difficult or inconclusive examination, US of the inguinal canal and scrotum can identify bowel in the herniated sac.[1]

Treatment

Incarcerated hernia without evidence of strangulation can be reduced nonoperatively in 80% of cases. It is highly unlikely that bowel with significant vascular compromise or necrosis can be reduced without operation. If irreducible, the patient should be taken to the operating room for urgent surgery. If reducible, the patient may be scheduled for elective inguinal hernia repair in the near future. Often, patients are admitted and undergo inguinal hernia repair the next day. The advantages of reduction include allowing time for fluid resuscitation and resolution of edema, making subsequent hernia repair technically less difficult.

Postoperative Adhesions

The possibility of adhesive obstruction should be considered in any patient with a history of previous abdominal surgery who presents with obstructive symptoms.[2]

Incidence

Adhesive obstruction probably occurs more frequently in children than in adults following abdominal surgery, with a reported incidence of 2% in one series.

Pathogenesis

Obstruction due to adhesions can occur anywhere from the immediate postoperative period to many years after an abdominal surgery. In the early postoperative period, it is difficult to distinguish paralytic ileus from mechanical causes of postoperative obstruction, such as adhesions, postoperative intussusception, volvulus, or internal hernia.

Symptoms and Signs

The patient typically experiences sudden onset of crampy abdominal pain followed by anorexia, nausea and vomiting, and abdominal distension, relative to the location of the obstruction. The patient may initially have a few small bowel movements that represent evacuation of the intestine distal to the obstruction, but thereafter no stools are passed. Physical findings vary with the stage of the condition at the time of presentation. The abdomen may be initially soft and nondistended. Bowel sounds generally are hyperactive, occurring in rushes. With time, the overdistended intestine becomes aperistaltic. Hiccups may occur due to irritation of the diaphragm by the distended bowel loops. Significant fever, leukocytosis, and signs of peritonitis indicate compromised intestine.

Diagnosis

It is difficult to diagnose acute intestinal obstruction that occurs in the early postoperative period. An "obstructive series" is the initial diagnostic study. An upright CXR can rule out pneumonia as a cause of paralytic ileus and evaluate for the presence of free intraperitoneal air. AXR reveals an obstructive pattern, but is also used to evaluate for air in the colon, which would suggest either ileus or partial obstruction (Fig. 7-3). Uniform distribution of air in moderate-sized loops of small and large intestine on a plain film is suggestive of ileus. However, any of these findings, in association with crampy abdominal pain and auscultation of periodic rushes suggests mechanical obstruction. Contrast enema is most helpful when the obstruction is likely to be in the distal GI tract. UGI studies are helpful when a proximal obstruction is suspected.

Treatment

Initial management of postoperative adhesive obstruction includes intravenous fluid hydration, nasogastric decompression to reduce distention and bowel wall edema, and broad-spectrum antibiotics to suppress bacterial translocation. The character of the gastric aspirate may be informative because bile-stained aspirate and feculent intestinal contents are signs of high-grade or complete obstruction. When signs, symptoms, and radiographs suggest incomplete obstruction, a trial of decompression is warranted. The goal of therapy is to alleviate obstruction prior to the development of ischemic intestine.

Perforated Appendicitis

Incidence

Appendicitis with perforation is more common in children than adults. Approximately 1% of all children <15 years of age develop appendicitis, with a peak incidence between 10 and 12 years of age. The incidence of perforation is 20–50%. This may be a consequence not only of the inability to communicate effectively with the toddler or pre-school-age child, but the tendency for parents and physicians to attribute all childhood fevers and gastrointestinal symptoms to viral illnesses contributing to a delay in presentation and diagnosis.[7]

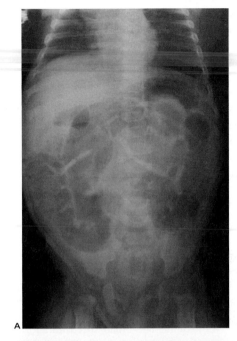

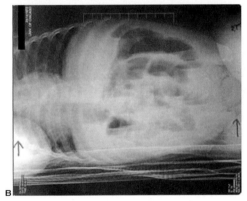

FIGURE 7 - 3

SIX-MONTH-OLD MALE WITH PAST SURGICAL HISTORY SIGNIFICANT FOR REPAIR OF A JEJUNOILEAL ATRESIA PRESENTS WITH BILIOUS EMESIS
(A) The supine plain film demonstrates dilated bowel loops. (B) The left lateral decubitus film demonstrates significant air-fluid levels. His small intestinal obstruction was secondary to postoperative adhesions.

Pathogenesis

The pathogenesis of appendicitis begins with luminal obstruction; intraluminally due to a fecalith in 30–50% of patients or extrinisically by lymphoid hyperplasia. With luminal obstruction, the mucosa continues to secrete mucous resulting in distention, increases transmural pressure, impaired venous drainage and edema, and subsequent impaired arterial inflow with local tissue ischemia. Appendiceal mucosal ulceration allows bacteria to invade the appendiceal wall. The combination of bacterial infection and tissue ischemia leads to gangrene and rupture.

Signs and Symptoms

The goal of management is to diagnose acute appendicitis before perforation. The risk of perforation within 24 h of onset of symptoms is <30%. Conversely, after 48 h of onset of symptoms the probability of perforation is >70%.

The symptoms of perforated appendicitis include anorexia with vomiting, severe, generalized abdominal pain, fever (>38°C), and diarrhea. Nonverbal children may present with right hip pain mimicking a septic hip. Children <5 years of age, with their sparse omentum, are less capable of "walling off" the perforation and often present with generalized peritonitis.

Diagnosis

Radiographic studies are reserved for children with atypical, equivocal, or confusing findings. A calcified fecalith is apparent in 10% of patients. With the finding of small bowel obstruction on abdominal plain film in young children, the differential diagnosis must include perforated appendicitis (Fig. 7-4). Ultrasound may show matted bowel loops in an inflammatory mass without abscess formation in the right lower quadrant, without visualization of the appendix. CT scans may be useful in patients with perforated appendicitis to distinguish phlegmon from abscess and to plan therapeutic interventions such as percutaneous, transrectal, or transvaginal abscess drainage.

Treatment

Preoperative resuscitation includes intravenous fluid hydration, nasogastric decompression, and for suspected perforation, broad-spectrum antibiotic

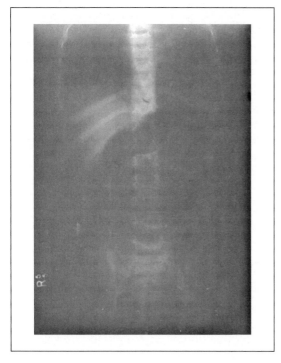

FIGURE 7-4

THREE-YEAR-OLD FEMALE PRESENTS WITH HISTORY OF DECREASED APPETITE, NONBILIOUS EMESIS, ABDOMINAL DISTENTION, AND LETHARGY WITH THIS PLAIN FILM DEMONSTRATING DILATED BOWEL LOOPS (SEE CASE STUDY 7-2).

coverage (gram negative) and anaerobic coverage is indicated. Standard therapy includes ampicillin, gentamicin, and clindamycin or metronidazole. Exploratory laparotomy and appendectomy are indicated for perforated appendicitis without phlegmon or abscess formation, as may occur in the pre-school-age child. Postoperatively, antibiotics are continued until fever and leukocytosis have resolved. The standard approach to perforated appendicitis has been limited laparotomy, with drainage of an abscess if present and appendectomy. It has been argued that with this approach, due to the inflammation involving the cecum and surrounding bowel, the procedure can be complicated by greater blood loss, increased risk of bowel injury, and subsequent development of postoperative abdominal and/or pelvic abscesses by entering an established abscess.

Alternative approaches depend on whether the mass is a phlegmon or an abscess, as determined by ultrasound or CT. If the mass is determined to be a phlegmon, intravenous antibiotics and volume resuscitation without immediate laparotomy are a safe and effective treatment provided the patient demonstrates clinical improvement, e.g., resolution of fever, leukocytosis, and the abdominal pain. Elective interval appendectomy can be planned 6 weeks later, generally with postoperative hospital stay of 1 day. Laparotomy is indicated if clinical improvement does not occur after 24 h of nonoperative management. If an abscess is identified, after volume resuscitation and intravenous antibiotics, drainage by percutaneous, tranvaginal, or transrectal routes may be performed. With clinical improvement, antibiotic therapy is continued until the patient is afebrile and the leukocytosis and abdominal tenderness have resolved. Elective interval appendectomy can be planned for 6 weeks later, generally with postoperative hospital stay of 1 day.[8]

Superior Mesenteric Artery Syndrome

Superior mesenteric artery syndrome is a condition in which the third portion of the duodenum is compressed by the SMA[9] (Fig. 7-5). Predisposing factors include weight loss with loss of the fat from the mesentery surrounding the SMA, rapid structural growth, prolonged supine positioning, immobilization in spinal orthosis, and spastic quadriparesis.[10]

Symptoms and Signs

Weight loss is followed by early satiety, postprandial nausea, bilious vomiting, upper abdominal distention, and abdominal pain. There is relief of obstruction when child lies prone or in the left lateral decubitus position after feeding, allowing the SMA to fall off the duodenum.

Diagnosis

Diagnosis is made by UGI study demonstrating dilatation of the first and second portions of the duodenum, and abrupt obstruction of contrast flow at the site where the SMA crosses the third part of the duodenum (Fig. 7-6).

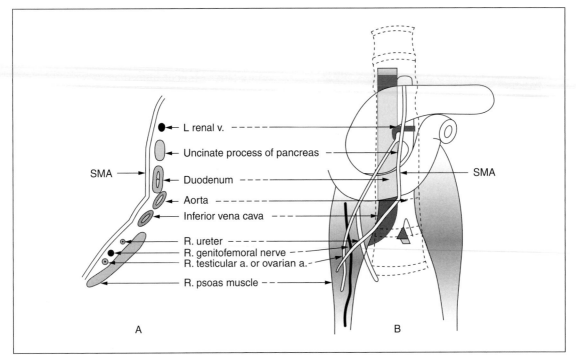

FIGURE 7-5

(A) DIAGRAM IN SAGITTAL SECTION OF THE ANGLE FORMED BY THE SUPERIOR MESENTERIC ARTERY
AND AORTA CONTAINING THE THIRD PORTION OF THE DUODENUM. (B) DIAGRAM OF THE ANTERIOR VIEW
OF THE SUPERIOR MESENTERIC ARTERY CROSSING THE THIRD PORTION OF THE DUODENUM.
Source: Adapted from Skandalakis et al. 1983, reprinted with permission.

Treatment

Conservative management includes nutritional support, repositioning the child (left lateral decubitus) during feeding to facilitate gastroduodenal emptying, or placement of a feeding tube into the jejunum, bypassing the obstruction. Surgical options include division of the suspensory muscle (ligament of Treitz) or duodenojejunostomy. Both of these procedures may be performed from either an open or a minimally invasive laparoscopic approach.

Lap Belt Complex

The "seatbelt syndrome" first described by Garrett and Braunstein in 1962 and renamed "lap belt complex" by Newman in 1990 refers to the spectrum of injuries associated with lap belt restraints. These injuries include intestinal tears, perforations, and transactions; mesenteric disruptions; and lumbar fractures, distractions, and dislocations (chance fractures). Compared to adults, the intraabdominal organs of young children are less protected by the bony thorax and pelvis. With rapid deceleration, "jack-knifing" or hyperflexion over the lap belt may occur with compression and injury of abdominal viscera.[11]

Pathogenesis

The intraabdominal injuries sustained in the lap belt complex include crush injuries, as the intestine is compressed against the spinal column, and ischemic injuries from mesenteric avulsion. At laparotomy, the injuries are identified and treated; but if intestinal injury remains undetected, it may scar, creating a stricture, adhere to adjacent intestinal loops resulting in kinking of the intestinal loops, or create a point of

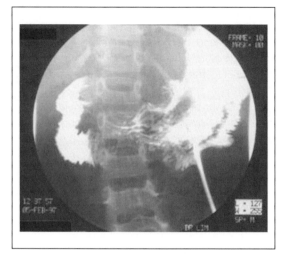

FIGURE 7-6

UGI DEMONSTRATING ABRUPT OBSTRUCTION OF
CONTRAST FLOW AT THE SITE WHERE THE SUPE-
RIOR MESENTERIC ARTERY (SMA) CROSSES THE
THIRD PART OF THE DUODENUM.

fixation and potential volvulus, presenting as
delayed intestinal obstruction. Intestinal injuries
generally occur at or near points of intestinal fixation, e.g., ligament of Treitz or cecum.

Symptoms and Signs

The hallmark indicator of the lap belt complex is
abdominal or flank ecchymosis—"lap belt sign."
Peritoneal signs may be present at the time but may
be difficult to discern from the discomfort associated with rectus muscle hematomas associated with
the lap belt sign. A delayed presentation of traumatic
intestinal stricture may present as bilious vomiting
and abdominal distension, with a remote history of
a motor vehicle collision.

Diagnosis

Plain films may demonstrate air-fluid levels or a
paucity of bowel gas as air becomes resorbed and
bowel loops become fluid filled.

Treatment

Initial management, as with other causes of intestinal obstruction includes intravenous fluid hydration, nasogastric decompression to reduce distention
and bowel wall edema, and broad-spectrum antibiotics to suppress bacterial translocation. Contrast
studies provide a "road-map" delineating the point
of obstruction. Emergent laparotomy is planned
after adequate resuscitation.

CASE STUDY 7-1

A 4-Week-Old with Abdominal Distention

A 4-week-old male infant presented, after transfer from an outside hospital, with a diagnosis of possible
bowel obstruction. The pediatric surgical team was informed of the transfer and was involved from the time
of the patient's arrival. There was a 2-day history of slight irritability and poor feeding and several episodes
of nonbilious emesis. Plain films and a contrast enema were sent with the patient. The plain films revealed
diffusely dilated bowel loops, and the contrast enema completely filled the colon. Physical examination
revealed a crying, 3.5 kg infant, with good color and capillary refill <2 s. The abdomen was diffusely distended with no abdominal wall discoloration or edema. The abdomen was firm and nontender.

There were no inguinal hernias and both testes were palpated in the scrotum. Digital rectal examination
revealed no stool in the rectum and the mucous was hemoccult negative. IVF resuscitation was initiated
and a nasogastric tube was placed; there was no return of bilious effluent. An emergent UGI was performed to rule out malrotation; the ligament of Treitz was in a normal location. With the findings of a normal
contrast enema, and a normal UGI, the diagnoses of intussusception (based on this patient's age, intussusception would be relatively unlikely) and malrotation were eliminated from the differential diagnosis.
Based on the 2-day history of poor feeding and the degree of abdominal distention, the patient was taken

emergently to the operating room with a diagnosis of small bowel obstruction of unknown etiology for exploratory laparotomy. Preoperatively, the patient received broad-spectrum antibiotics. The patient was explored through a right lower quadrant transverse incision. At exploration, an inflammatory band was noted in the right lower quadrant completely obstructing the distal ileum with marked thinning of the bowel wall at the point of compression with no evidence of perforation. After releasing the band, the thinned segment of ileum was resected and an anastomosis was performed. An appendectomy was also performed because this patient would subsequently have a right lower quadrant incision that could prove confusing at the time of evaluation for abdominal pain in the future. Postoperatively, the patient received antibiotics for 48 h and had gradual resolution of his ileus and was discharged to home on postoperative day 7 once he was tolerating oral feeds.

CASE STUDY 7-2

A 3-Year-Old with Abdominal Distention

A 3-year-old female presented to the emergency room with a 3-day history of decreased appetite, nonbilious emesis, abdominal distention, and lethargy. The patient was evaluated by the pediatric emergency medicine team, IVF resuscitation was initiated, and a plain supine abdominal film was obtained. The film demonstrated dilated small bowel loops. Laboratory values were significant for a leukocytosis. Pediatric surgical consultation was requested. Physical examination revealed a febrile (39.2°C), listless child with clear lung fields and a marked distended abdomen. There was diffuse tenderness to palpation without localization and no evidence of tenderness to percussion (no peritoneal signs). A complete obstructive series was obtained and the possibility of pneumonia masquerading as an abdominal process was ruled out on the CXR. The abdominal films demonstrated an ominous stacked pattern with air-filled bowel loops in the right lower quadrant and an UGI was initiated that showed no evidence of malrotation. While waiting for the contrast to flow through the normal-appearing proximal jejunal loops, an ultrasound of the right lower quadrant was obtained that showed an inflammatory mass. The combination of findings eliminated intussusception and malrotation from the differential diagnosis, and supported a diagnosis of perforated appendicitis. The patient received broad-spectrum antibiotics and was emergently taken to the operating room for exploratory laparotomy. Exploration revealed perforated appendicitis with purulent fluid in the abdomen and pelvis. Appendectomy was performed. The patient received approximately 4 days of broad-spectrum antibiotics and had rapid resolution of her fever, ileus, and leukocytosis and was discharged to home on postoperative day 5.

References

1   John SD. Imaging of acute abdominal emergencies in infants and children. *Curr Probl Diagn Radiol* 29:141, 2000.

2   O'Neill JA, Rowe MI, Grosfeld JL, et al. *Pediatric Surgery*, 5th ed. St. Louis, MO: Mosby, 1998.

3   Davenport M. ABC of general surgery in children. Surgically correctable causes of vomiting in infancy. *Br Med J* 312:236, 1996.

4   D'Agostino J. Common abdominal emergencies in children. *Emerg Med Clin North* Am 20:139, 2002.

5   Schwartz MZ, Bulas D. Laboratory evaluation and imaging. *Semin Pediatr Surg* 6:65, 1997.

6 Ashcraft KW, Murphy JP, Sharp RJ, et al. *Pediatric Surgery*, 3rd ed. Philadelphia, PA: WB Saunders, 2000.

7 Oldham KT, Colombani PM, Foglia RP. *Surgery of Infants and Children: Scientific Principles and Practice*. Philadelphia, PA: Lippincott-Raven, 1997.

8 Weiner DJ, Katz A, Hirschl RB, et al. Interval appendectomy in perforated appendicitis. *Pediatr Surg Int* 10:82, 1995.

9 Skandalakis JE, Gray SW, Rowe JS. *Anatomical Complications in General Surgery*. New York, NY: McGraw-Hill, 1983.

10 Delgadillo X, Belpaire-Dethiou MCB, Chantrain C, et al. Arteriomesenteric syndrome as a cause of duodenal obstruction in children with cerebral palsy. *J Pediatr Surg* 32:1721, 1997.

11 Newman KD, Bowman LM, Eichelberger MR, et al. The lap belt complex: intestinal and lumbar spine injury in children. *J Trauma* 30:1133, 1990.

8

JAUNDICE IN THE NEWBORN AND YOUNG INFANT

Lynda Brady

INTRODUCTION

Jaundice or icterus refers to the yellow discoloration secondary to bilirubin deposit. Jaundice indicates that there is hyperbilirubinemia. The degree of yellow discoloration correlates with the level of bilirubin. There are two types of bilirubin: (1) conjugated (direct, or "post-hepatic") and (2) unconjugated (indirect, or "pre-hepatic").

Neonatal jaundice is a common condition; 30–50% of children are jaundiced in the newborn period. The vast majority of those children have unconjugated hyperbilirubinemia, associated with physiologic jaundice. This hyperbilirubinemia peaks at day of life 3–5 and resolves within the first 3 weeks of life. Any child still jaundiced beyond 3 weeks of age must have a conjugated bilirubin level evaluation, as conjugated hyperbilirubinemia indicates liver disease. In the newborn period, this may be secondary to *biliary atresia* (BA), a condition that makes a timely diagnosis imperative to initiate appropriate therapy. Conjugated hyperbilirubinemia always warrants referral to a pediatric gastroenterologist.

UNCONJUGATED HYPERBILIRUBINEMIA

Unconjugated hyperbilirubinemia refers to an elevation in unconjugated bilirubin. Unconjugated bilirubin is normally bound to albumin and the free level is low. Free unconjugated bilirubin can cross the blood-brain barrier and cause kernicterus, the most serious complication of this condition.

Increased levels of free unconjugated bilirubin may be secondary to

- Increased production of unconjugated bilirubin
- Decreased albumin levels
- Increased competitors for albumin binding such as drugs or free fatty acids from intralipids

See Table 8-1 for a list of causes of elevated unconjugated bilirubin, which are discussed below.

Physiologic Jaundice

Physiologic jaundice is secondary to decreased bilirubin glucuronsyltransferase activity. The jaundice

CAUSES OF INCREASED PRODUCTION OF UNCONJUGATED BILIRUBIN

Physiologic jaundice

Breast-feeding jaundice

Systemic disease

   Hemolysis

      Maternal-fetal blood group incompatibility

      Extravascular blood in tissues

      Red cell abnormality

   Sepsis

   Hypothyroidism

Inherited disorders

   Crigler-Najjar type I and II

   Rotors

   Dubin-Johnson

begins after the first 24 h of life and is associated with moderate elevations in bilirubin. The jaundice peaks in 3–5 days and then resolves. A healthy newborn, with a normal physical examination whose jaundice begins after 24 h of life and with a total bilirubin under 12 mg/dL does not need further investigation (see Fig. 8-1). On the other hand, jaundice which occurs before 24 h of life, or is associated with bilirubin greater than 12 mg/dL should be investigated.

Breast-Feeding Jaundice

The pathogenesis of breast-feeding jaundice is unclear. Breast-feeding jaundice begins after 5–7 days of age. The jaundice usually peaks in the second week but can last for months. Diagnosis can be made according to Table 1. The diagnosis is supported when breast feeding is stopped and the total bilirubin drops by 50%.

Hemolysis

The most common reason for early severe neonatal jaundice is maternal-fetal blood group incompatibility. Maternal immunization occurs when fetal cells cross into maternal circulation (maternal sensitization). Maternal IgG antibodies cross into the fetal circulation causing destruction of fetal red blood cells (RBC). This incompatibility can be due to ABO or minor antigens. Rh incompatibility is rare and secondary to the use of anti-D γ-globulin in Rh negative mothers.

Hemolysis can also be due to abnormalities in red blood cell morphology from glucose-6-phosphate dehydrogenase deficiency, spherocytosis, or hemoglobinopathy.

Metabolic Diseases

Crigler-Najjar disease is an autosomal recessive, congenital deficiency of bilirubin *uridine diphosphate* (UDP) glucuronosyltransferase. This leads to an inability to conjugate and excrete bilirubin. Patients have severe persistent jaundice. Bilirubin levels may rise to 25–35 mg/dL (1 mg/dL = 17 μmol) without treatment. There are two types of Crigler-Najjar disease.

Type I is a complete lack of the enzyme. These children have severe unconjugated hyperbilirubinemia. There is no evidence of liver disease. Treatment is with prolonged phototherapy for up to 15 h a day. There is no response to phenobarbital treatment. Neonates with this syndrome are at great risk for kernicterus, especially if there are confounding factors such as sepsis or dehydration. Although the greatest risk for kernicterus is during the neonatal period, sudden late neurologic decompensation has been reported.

Type II Crigler-Najjar is due to a partial defect in UDP glucuronosyltransferase. These patients have lower bilirubin levels and will have significant decrease in the bilirubin level in response to phenobarbital treatment (10–15 mg/kg per day).

Gilbert's syndrome is characterized by recurrent mild unconjugated hyperbilirubinemia with normal liver function. There is a decrease in the level of bilirubin UDP glucuronosyltransferase. In Northern Europe, North America, and Africa this is due to mutations in the promoter region of the UDP glucuronosyltransferase gene. In Asia other mutations have been described. Gilbert's is rarely clinically apparent before puberty. There have been

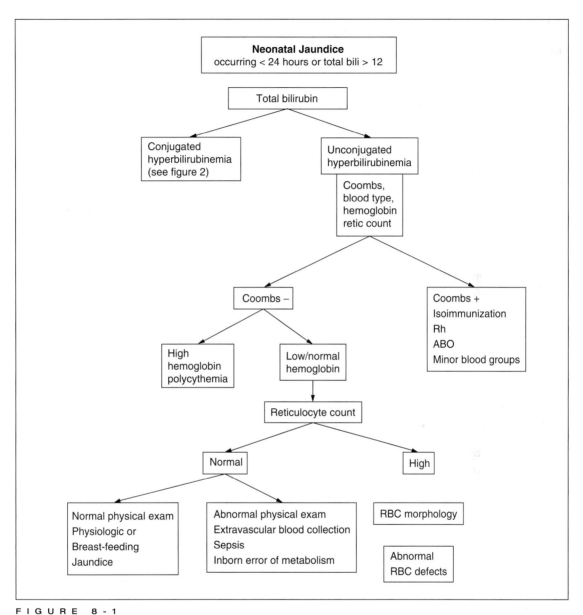

FIGURE 8-1

WORK-UP OF UNCONJUGATED HYPERBILIRUBINEMIA

some studies which demonstrate predisposition to hyberbilirubinemia in infants with Gilbert's. Although the clinical course is benign in the majority of patients, the decreased ability of glucuronidation may lead to decreased ability to metabolize certain drugs. No specific treatment is necessary.

Rotors syndrome is a familial disorder with mild elevation in both conjugated and unconjugated bilirubin. There are normal liver enzymes and histology. The syndrome is due to lack of intrahepatic intracellular binders. The hepatocytes are unable to bind the bilirubin and it "leaks" back into the serum. In addition, patients have abnormal urinary excretion of coproporphyrins. The total level is elevated and the coproporphyrin isomer I makes up less than 80% of the total. No treatment is necessary for this entity.

Dubin-Johnson syndrome is associated with elevations in conjugated and unconjugated bilirubin. The syndrome is due to a defect in the ability of the multidrug-resistant associated protein 2 (MRP2) to transport anions across the hepatocytes cannicular membrane. This leads to increased intracellular bilirubin levels that "leak" back into the serum. Severe cholestasis has been reported in the newborn period. Diagnosis is made in a patient with mild elevation in both conjugated and unconjugated bilirubin and abnormal excretion of urinary coproporphyrins. In this syndrome the type I isomer makes up more than 80% of the total coproporphyrins excreted. No treatment is necessary.

Toxicity

Kernicterus is the most serious complication of severe unconjugated hyperbilirubinemia. This develops secondary to bilirubin binding to specific areas of the brain, particularly the basal ganglion, hippocampus, cerebellum, and floor of the fourth ventricle.

Clinical findings include

- Sluggish Moro reflex
- Opisthotonus
- Hypotonia
- Hyperpyrexia
- Seizures

The exact bilirubin level when kernicterus occurs is unknown. Kernicterus is likely to occur with unconjugated bilirubin levels greater than 30 mg/dL and unlikely to occur with levels below 20 mg/dL. Premature infants will develop kernicterus at much lower levels and treatment should be individualized for infants <37 weeks gestation.

TREATMENT

Hyperbilirubinemia is a frequent reason for neonatal hospital admission. Treatment may vary depending on the etiology of the hyperbilirubinemia, so determination of the cause is important. The mainstay of treatment is phototherapy. In severe cases exchange transfusion may be necessary. Recommendations depend on the age of the child, the bilirubin level, and the cause of the bilirubin elevation; specific recommendations can be seen in Table 8-2.

Dehydration and decreased number of stools have been associated with increased bilirubin levels. Children should be fed frequently and kept well-hydrated. Breast-feeding should be optimized with frequent feeding. Interruption in breast-feeding will decrease bilirubin in children who have

TABLE 8-2

MANAGEMENT OF HYPERBILIRUBINEMIA IN THE HEALTHY TERM NEWBORN

Age (hours)	TSB Level, mg/dL (pmol/L)			
	Consider Phototherapy	Phototherapy	Exchange Transfusion If Intensive Photo Therapy Fails	Exchange Transfusion and Intensive Phototherapy
≤24	Work-up according to flow chart			
25–48	≥12 (210)	≥15 (260)	≥20 (340)	≥25 (430)
49–72	≥15 (260)	≥18 (310)	≥25 (430)	≥30 (510)
>72	≥17 (290)	≥20 (340)	≥25 (430)	≥30 (510)

breast-feeding jaundice, but interruption in nursing is not necessary.

Other treatments have included

- Bilirubin binders (cholestyramine)
- Inducers of UDP glucuronosyltransferase (phenobarbital)
- Inhibitors of heme oxygenase (tin mesoprotoporphyrin)

Although tin mesoprotoporphyrin has been shown to eliminate the need for phototherapy in breast-fed babies it is not widely used. Phenobarbital is the mainstay of treatment for children with Crigler-Najjar type II. Crigler-Najjar type I is treated with life-long phototherapy. This is a cumbersome treatment for the patient and there has been neurologic deterioration reported despite aggressive phototherapy. There have been reports over the past 15 years of children treated with liver transplants, auxillary liver transplants, and hepatocyte transplants. All of these therapies have eliminated the need for phototherapy but carry the risks associated with these procedures. Recently, gene therapy has been successful in animal models and is a hope for the future for these patients.

CONJUGATED HYPERBILIRUBINEMIA

Conjugated hyperbilirubinemia almost always indicates liver disease. There is a large list of diseases that can cause a child to be jaundiced. A few of them are responsible for the vast majority of cases, and this chapter will focus on that. The differential diagnosis of cholestasis depends on the age and clinical presentation of the patient; newborns who are ill-appearing with cholestatic liver disease are likely to have a viral illness or a metabolic disease, while a 1-month-old, well-appearing infant is more likely to have one of the entities outlined in Table 8-3.

Cholestatic Newborns

Newborns within the first week or two of life are likely to be cholestatic from

TABLE 8-3

DIFFERENTIAL DIAGNOSIS OF CHOLESTATIC INFANT

Ductular
Biliary atresia
Neonatal hepatitis
Choledochal cyst
Ductal paucity
Alagille's syndrome
Progressive familial intrahepatic cholestasis
Hepatocellular
Metabolic disease
α_1 antitrypsin deficiency
Galactosemia
Hereditary fructose intolerance
Cystic fibrosis
Disorders of bile acid synthesis
Tyrosinemia
Infection
Urinary tract infection
Hepatitis A, B
Endocrine
Hypopituitarism
Hypothyroidism
Toxic
Total parenteral nutrition
Drugs (unusual)

1. Infections
   a TORCH
   b Syphilis
   c Enteric viruses
   d HHV 6
   e Parvovirus B19
   f Bacterial infection outside the liver
2. Metabolic causes
   a Neonatal hemochromatosis (NH)
   b Galactosemia

Infections

TORCH is the acronym for viral infections which occur in the mother and affects the fetus (toxoplasmosis, rubella, CMV, herpes). Most of the TORCH infections cause mild maternal morbidity, but have serious fetal consequences.

Toxoplasmosis infection is acquired when an infected cat sheds the oocytes in feces. Infected newborns may have microcephaly, chorioretinitis, intracranial calcifications, and purpuric rash. Most children with congenital toxoplasmosis have hepatomegaly but the jaundice is variable. Liver biopsy shows hepatitis with necrosis. The organism can be demonstrated with the use of fluorescent antibody staining. Diagnosis is made by detection of IgM/IgA antibody in the infant. Polymerase chain reaction can demonstrate infection in the newborn's blood or prenatally in amniotic fluid or the placenta. Mothers with known infections can be treated with sulfadiazine and pyrimethamine in an attempt to prevent congenital infection. Infants with documented infections may be treated with these drugs but they will not affect preexisting damage.

Congenital rubella is extremely rare because of immunization programs.

Cytomegalovirus (CMV) is the most common congenital infection. The majority of children are asymptomatic. Infants who are symptomatic are low birth weight, thrombocytopenic, microcephalic, and have purpuric rash, periventricular calcifications, and progressive deafness. Hepatosplenomegaly and cholestasis are common. Liver biopsy demonstrates giant cell hepatitis and viral inclusions. Diagnosis is by culturing CMV from the infant or by detection of CMV DNA. Treatment with gancyclovir has been shown to decrease deafness. There are no studies demonstrating efficacy of treatment in isolated liver disease. Children with mild hepatitis will have complete remission. There have been reports of progressive liver disease but neurologic sequelae and progressive deafness are more common.

Congenital herpes infections can be life-threatening to a newborn. The infection comes from mothers infected with HSV II or postnatally from contact with persons infected with HSV I. There is an increased risk of infection when there is prolonged rupture of membranes or invasive monitoring is used during labor and the risk is decreased by Cesarean section delivery. The liver disease is severe with jaundice, hepatomegaly, and coagulopathy. It is often associated with encephalitis but can occur in isolation. Treatment must be initiated early to avoid morbidity and mortality. The liver histology will demonstrate large areas of necrosis and intranuclear inclusion bodies. Immunohistochemical staining can demonstrate herpes virus within the liver tissue. Antiviral therapy with acyclovir is the treatment. There have been reports of successful liver transplantation when antiviral therapy fails.

Despite routine maternal screening, congenital syphilis remains a cause of neonatal liver disease. Patients may present at birth or symptoms develop over the first few weeks of life. Mild cases have characteristic rash on palms and soles, hepatosplenomegaly, poor weight gain, and purulent nasal discharge (snuffles). More severe cases have significant anemia, thrombocytopenia, hydrops fetalis, jaundice, periostitis, skin rash, and lymphadenopathy. Liver histology may demonstrate a nonspecific hepatitis but silver stain will show the spirochete. Diagnosis is made through serologic testing including the *Venereal Disease Research Laboratory* (VDRL) and confirmed with specific anitspirochete antibodies. Treatment is with parenteral penicillin.

Enteroviruses are a rare cause of massive liver necrosis in the newborn period. Patients present with lethargy, poor feeding, and jaundice. There will be severe coagulopathy. Diagnosis is made through viral culture of the nasopharynx or rectum. Treatment is supportive, although new antivirals such as pleconaril have been used to treat these infants. There have been reports of Parvovirus B19 and HHV 6 associated with liver disease in the newborn period.

Bacterial infections outside the liver can cause conjugated hyperbilirubinemia. There is absence of hepatosplenomegaly and elevated transaminases. Blood as well as urine cultures should be obtained in infants with new onset hyperbilirubinemia.

Metabolic Diseases

Although there are a host of metabolic diseases which can affect newborns, most do not present with hyperbilirubinemia and liver disease.

Galactosemia is one of the metabolic diseases that can present with cholestasis in the newborn period. Most cases of galactosemia are diagnosed through newborn screening. The clinical presentation of galactosemia can vary; newborns can present after the first ingestion of milk with abdominal distention, vomiting, and hypoglycemia. Infants who do not have this striking presentation in the nursery will present in the first weeks of life with failure to thrive, vomiting, or diarrhea. Conjugated hyperbilirubinemia and hepatomegaly develop over the first week of life. Infants with galactosemia will develop cataracts shortly after birth and mental retardation will occur with continued exposure to galactose. Galactosemia is an autosomal recessive disorder due to the lack of enzymes in the degradation pathway of galactose to glucose. Most patients have galactose-1-phosphate uridyltransferase deficiency. Galactokinase and uridine diphosphate galactose-4-epimerase are the other two enzymes which can be deficient. Diagnosis is made by demonstrating decreased enzyme activity. All patients with galactosemia exposed to galactose will have reducing substances in their urine; therefore, all patients with cholestasis in the newborn period should have reducing substances analyzed. Treatment is restriction of galactose in the diet. Treatment will reverse the liver damage and the child will have normal growth. Despite restriction of galactose, children may develop learning disabilities and other neurologic deficits.

Neonatal hemochromatosis is the other metabolic liver disease likely to present in the newborn nursery. NH is a rare disorder secondary to iron overload *in utero*. Patients present with liver failure characterized by coagulopathy, thrombocytopenia, hypoglycemia, and hypoalbuminemia but there are normal to slightly elevated transaminases due to the decreased hepatic mass. There is an extremely elevated ferritin level. Jaundice develops over the first days of life. On physical examination there will be splenomegaly but a small, firm liver. NH is difficult to distinguish from sepsis but should be suspected in children with the clinical presentation and negative cultures. The pathogenesis of NH has not been elucidated but there is some evidence it may have to do with iron transport between mother and fetus. Familial occurrence of the disease is well recognized. The disease is extremely rare in first

pregnancies. Subsequent pregnancies after the birth of a child with NH carry a high risk of recurrence suggesting a maternal factor. Diagnosis is made by demonstrating the iron overload. Although the iron deposition in NH is most notable in the liver, it also is present in the heart, pancreas, exocrine and endocrine organs, intestines, and gastric and salivary glands. MRI of the pancreas or a buccal biopsy will demonstrate iron overload. Liver histology demonstrates nodular cirrhosis with severe cholestasis. NH is universally fatal. There have been anecdotal reports of using an "antioxidant cocktail" with desferrioxamine, *N*-acetylcysteine, selenium, and vitamin E. Liver transplantation in these patients has been successful.

Cholestatic Infants

Infants between 1 and 12 months of age develop cholestasis from diseases which affect hepatocytes or the biliary duct system, as outlined in Table 8-3.

Biliary atresia is the most important entity in the differential diagnosis of an infant with cholestasis. Biliary atresia is the end result of a destructive inflammatory process, which affects the intra- and extrahepatic bile ducts. It occurs in 1:8000–1:10,000 live births. It is the leading cause for liver transplantation in pediatrics. There is extensive research being done to discover the etiology and pathophysiology of the disease. Viral infections, defects in the morphogenesis of the biliary system, and immune-mediated injury are thought to play a role in the development of the disease.

There are two clinical forms of biliary atresia: *fetal* and *postnatal*.

The *fetal form* occurs in approximately 10% of cases. These infants have similar laboratory findings as the postnatal form, but are jaundiced from birth and are likely to have associated malformations:

1. Splenic anomalies
   a. Polysplenia
   b. Asplenia
2. Portal vein anomalies
   a. Preduodenal
   b. Absence
   c. Cavernous transformation

3. Situs inversus
4. Malrotation/gut atresia
5. Cardiac anomalies

The *postnatal* biliary atresia has a consistent clinical presentation. The patient is a full-term baby, normal size who is gaining weight, and is jaundiced past the age of 2 weeks. On physical examination there may be hepatomegaly. There may be dark urine and acholic stools. If no intervention is performed, the liver disease will progress and by 3–4 months of age failure to thrive will ensue. Later, as cirrhosis develops, the child will have muscle wasting, ascites, hepatosplenomegaly, and bleeding. Laboratory evaluation will demonstrate:

- Conjugated hyperbilirubinemia
- Elevated alkaline phosphatase
- Elevated gamma-glutamyltranspeptidase
- Mildly elevated transaminases

Ultrasound should be done to rule out other causes of cholestasis. If there is no gallbladder found after a 4-h fast, the test is consistent with BA. Other findings on ultrasound have been used to support the diagnosis of BA, and they include: (1) triangular cord sign, (2) the shape of the gallbladder and (3) the shape and thickness of the gallbladder wall. Liver histology is very specific and demonstrates bile duct proliferation, bile plugs, and portal tract edema. The diagnosis is confirmed with an intraoperative cholangiogram.

It is imperative to intervene early with a Kasai procedure. The Kasai procedure is a total resection of the extrahepatic biliary tree to the porta hepatis (within the liver). Biliary drainage is reestablished by using a Roux loop, which is anastomosed to the porta hepatis. Drainage is established in 80% of cases done prior to 8 weeks of age. Recent studies have shown children undergoing Kasai prior to 5 weeks of age may have better long-term success. After 12 weeks of age the success drops to 20%. Kasai procedures are probably not warranted in children over 14 weeks of age. The Kasai procedure is palliative and the vast majority of patients will undergo liver transplantation. The combination of Kasai and liver transplantation allow for long-term survival in a disease that was universally fatal 40 years ago.

TABLE 8-4

CLASSIFICATION OF CHOLEDOCHAL CYSTS

Type I	Cystic dilatation of the common bile duct
Type II	Diverticulum of the common bile duct and/or the gallbladder
Type III	Choledochocoele
Type IV	Multiple intra- or extrahepatic cysts
Type V	Fusiform intrahepatic dilatation

Neonatal hepatitis occurs in up to 25% of infants with cholestasis. The etiology of this entity is unknown but it can recur in a family. Patients tend to be small but otherwise have no distinguishing physical features. The laboratory examinations are similar to that of biliary atresia. The two diseases can be distinguished with a liver biopsy. In neonatal hepatitis the liver histology demonstrates giant cell transformation and although most have normal ducts, bile ductular proliferation can be a feature. The prognosis is good with only 10% of patients developing progressive liver disease. Treatment is supportive.

Choledochal cysts are cystic dilation with the biliary tree. There is a female predominance (female:male 5:1). There are five types (see Table 8-4) according to the location with the biliary tree. Type I is the most common in the United States and United Kingdom. Conjugated hyperbilirubinemia is the clinical presentation in infants. In older children, choledochal cysts present with the triad of jaundice, fever, and abdominal mass. Diagnosis is made by ultrasound. Treatment is by surgical resection of the cyst, and surgery should be done immediately in infants with cholestasis. In asymptomatic children, surgery can be scheduled within the first 2 months of life. There is a significant risk of carcinoma in cyst tissue. The dismal prognosis once cholangiocarcinoma occurs warrants complete excision of the cysts even in asymptomatic children.

Alagille's syndrome is characterized by

- Cholestasis with pruritus and fat malabsorption
- Characteristic facies with broad forehead, deep set eyes, small pointed chin; the facies may not be evident in infants

- Cardiac anomalies including peripheral pulmonic stenosis, severe hypoplasia of the pulmonary, and multiple other anomalies
- Eye findings—posterior embryotoxins
- Butterfly vertebrae
- Failure to thrive

The less prominent associated symptoms include renal disease, mental retardation, xanthomas, and vascular abnormalities. Alagille's syndrome is an autosomal dominant disorder with variable penetrance. It is due to defect on chromosome 20 for the JAG1 protein. Diagnosis is made by clinical presentation. Laboratory investigations demonstrate conjugated hyperbilirubinemia, elevated alkaline phosphatase, elevated GGTP, mildly elevated transaminases, and very high cholesterol. Liver histology demonstrates paucity of bile ducts and cholestasis. Treatment is supportive. Death can occur because of heart disease and progressive liver failure. Liver transplantation should be reserved for those patients with liver failure and severe pruritus unresponsive to medical therapy. Growth failure does not resolve after liver transplantation.

Progressive familial intrahepatic cholestasis (PFIC) was previously known as Byler's syndrome. The disease is characterized by cholestasis beginning in early childhood, pruritis, and growth failure with low GGTP levels. PFIC is three separate entities. PFIC 1 and PFIC 2 are due to two genetic defects but they are very similar clinically. PFIC 1 is due to a mutation in the familial intrahepatic cholestasis (FIC1) locus at 18q21-22. PFIC 2 is due to a mutation in the bile salt export pump (BSEP) gene at 2q24. PFIC 3 has been identified in cholestatic children with elevation in GGTP. It is due to mutation in the *multidrug resistant* (MDR) 3 gene. Liver histology demonstrates ductal paucity, hepatocellular cholestasis with pseudoacinar transformation. Without intervention PFIC is a progressive disorder which leads to cirrhosis. First line medical treatment is to address cholestasis and pruritus. Surgical treatment with partial cutaneous biliary diversion has been shown to relieve pruritus, growth failure, and arrest the progression of liver disease. Liver transplantation is often necessary in patients who do not respond to medical therapy.

There are several metabolic liver diseases that present in this age group. The most important and second leading cause for pediatric liver transplantation is α_1 **antitrypsin deficiency**. The incidence is 1:1600–1:2000 live births. The protease inhibitor (PI), α_1 antitrypsin, is mainly produced in the liver. Only 15% of individuals with α_1 antitrypsin deficiency develop liver disease but it is the leading cause of emphysema in young adults. The deficiency is due to a mutation in PI locus on chromosome 14. The most common deficiency is due to a single amino acid replacement (lysine for glutamic acid at position 342). The protease inhibitor is characterized by electrophoresis. The normal PI type is MM and the disease state is ZZ, but there are 75 structural variants described. The liver disease is caused by accumulation of the abnormal protein in the hepatocyte (PAS positive granules on histology). The disease is characterized by cholestasis in infancy, hepatomegaly, and laboratory investigation similar to biliary atresia. Homozygotes will have low levels of α_1 antitrypsin in their serum. Liver histology demonstrates PAS positive, diastase negative granules after 6–8 weeks of life. There can be ductular proliferation and giant cell transformation. Treatment is supportive. The prognosis is varied. Approximately half of the patients with liver disease do well although there may be mild elevation in transaminases. The other half does poorly and will eventually require a liver transplant.

Bile acid synthesis defects are uncommon disorders that cause progressive cholestatic liver disease in infancy or early childhood. Children present like those with neonatal cholestasis but have normal or slightly elevated GGTP. No primary bile acids can be measured in the serum as opposed to other cholestatic diseases where the serum bile acids would be elevated. Diagnosis is based on demonstration of abnormal bile acids through mass spectrometry of urine and serum. Pathogenesis of liver injury is related to reduction in levels of normal bile acids and accumulation of abnormal, hepatotoxic, bile acids. Bile acid replacement therapy is usually effective. Regression of liver damage has been documented during treatment of patients who were diagnosed early in life.

Patients with **galactosemia** may present in this age group and the characteristics are the same as those outlined above.

Hereditary fructose intolerance can present in this age group in infants who have been exposed to fructose. This is a common exposure even before introduction of fruits because pediatric medications are made with sorbitol (which converts to fructose in humans). Hereditary fructose intolerance is an autosomal recessive disease with an incidence of 1:20,000. The disease is due to a lack of fructose-1-phosphate aldolase. Presentation of the disease can vary with the age of the patient. In infancy the patient presents with vomiting, poor feeding, hepatomegaly, and jaundice. Laboratory investigation will demonstrate elevated transaminases, coagulopathy, conjugated hyperbilirubinemia, and metabolic abnormalities:

- Hypoglycemia
- Hypphosphatemia
- Hypomagnesemia
- Lactic acidosis
- Hyperuricemia

Since the presentation can mimic other entities, a careful diet history is critical. Urine reducing substances will be positive. The diagnosis can be confirmed by measuring the fructose-1-phosphate aldolase in the liver. Treatment is restriction of fructose, sucrose, and sorbitol. Long-term survival is normal in those who abide with these restrictions.

One-third of patients with **cystic fibrosis** have abnormal liver function tests and/or abnormal histology. There can be a wide variety of histologic pictures and cystic fibrosis should be considered in the differential diagnosis of a cholestatic neonate, especially if there is associated failure to thrive, edema, or pulmonary disease. Treatment of the liver disease is supportive.

Outside of the neonatal period, **infections** are a rare cause of hepatic dysfunction in the first year of life. Hepatotrophic viruses do not cause jaundice except in the rare cases of fulminant failure in this age group. Infants exposed to hepatitis B and C are more likely to become chronic carriers. Bacterial infections outside the liver are still a cause of cholestasis and urine cultures should be done on all infants with new onset cholestasis.

Endocrine disorders such as hypopituitarism and hypothyroidism can cause cholestatic liver disease. Liver biopsy findings in children with hypopituitarism demonstrate intracellular bile pigment accumulation and variable giant cell formation which can help to distinguish it from neonatal hepatitis (see Fig. 8-2).

Complications and Treatment of Cholestasis

Cholestasis is the lack of normal bile flow. Complications arise from decreased delivery of bile acids to the small bowel (fat malabsorption), regurgitation of constituents of bile into the systemic circulation (pruritis, hypercholesterolemia), and retention of substances normally excreted in bile within the liver leading to hepatotoxicity.

Treatment is aimed at preventing complications of cholestasis until the underlying disease is treated or resolved.

Ursodeoxycholic acid (UDCA), the major bile acid in black bears, is useful in the treatment of cholestatic liver disease in humans for several reasons. UDCA replaces hydrophobic bile acids which accumulate during liver disease and prevents the hepatotoxicity caused by those hydrophobic bile acids. It has a hypercholeretic effect (increased bile flow). UDCA is an immune modulator, reducing the immune-mediated damage in some cholestatic liver disease. Since UDCA combats all of the complications of cholestasis it should be the first line treatment. The dose of UDCA is 5–10 mg/kg per dose three times per day.

If a patient is cholestatic, they are unable to absorb fats or fat soluble vitamins effectively. Formulas containing medium-chain triglycerides, which do not require bile acids for absorption, are easier to absorb than most formulas which contain long-chain triglycerides. Complications of vitamin deficiency will develop if vitamin A, D, E, and K are not supplemented. Cholestasis causes a deficiency of essential phospholipid fatty acids (linoleic acid and arachidonic acid) which improve with supplementation and treatment with UDCA.

Pruritus can also be a complication of cholestatic liver disease. UDCA relieves pruritus in a small percentage of patients. In patients who do not

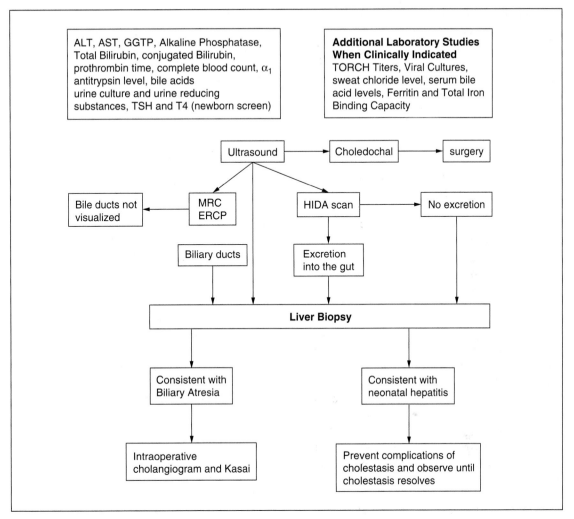

ALT, AST, GGTP, Alkaline Phosphatase,
Total Bilirubin, conjugated Bilirubin,
prothrombin time, complete blood count, α_1
antitrypsin level, bile acids
urine culture and urine reducing
substances, TSH and T4 (newborn screen)

**Additional Laboratory Studies
When Clinically Indicated**
TORCH Titers, Viral Cultures,
sweat chloride level, serum bile
acid levels, Ferritin and Total Iron
Binding Capacity

Ultrasound → Choledochal → surgery

Bile ducts not visualized ← MRC ERCP

HIDA scan → No excretion

Biliary ducts

Excretion into the gut

Liver Biopsy

Consistent with Biliary Atresia

Consistent with neonatal hepatitis

Intraoperative cholangiogram and Kasai

Prevent complications of cholestasis and observe until cholestasis resolves

F I G U R E   8 - 2

LABORATORY WORK-UP FOR CHOLESTATIC INFANTS

respond to UDCA, diphenhydramine and local skin care, rifampin is the next treatment of choice. Rifampin is effective in more than 50% of patients with pruritus. Long-acting opiate antagonist can be used in patients who do not respond to rifampin.

As liver disease progresses, nutritional assessment and support are critical. Patients with end-stage liver disease and steatorrhea have high energy expenditure. These patients may require many more calories than normal infants. Hepatosplenomegaly, ascites, and fatigue may make feeding difficult. Nutritional supplementation with high calorie for-

mula and nasogastric feeds should be considered to maintain normal growth.

Bibliography

Chardot C, Carton M, Spire-Benedelac N, et al. Prognosis of biliary atresia in the era of liver transplantation: the French National Study 1986–1996. *Hep* 30(3): 606–611, 1999.

Clayton PT. Inborn errors of metabolism presenting as liver dysfunction. *Semin Neonatol* 7(1):49–63, 2002.

Durand P, Debray D, Mandel R, et al. Acute liver failure in infancy: a 14 year experience at a pediatric transplant center. *J Pediatr* 139(6):871–876, 2001.

Emerick KM, Whitingtom PF. Molecular basis for neonatal cholestasis. *Pediatr Clin North Am* 49(1):221–235, 2002.

Feranchak AP, Ramirez RO, Sokol RJ. Medical management of cholestasis. In: Suchy F, et al. (eds.), *Liver Diseases in Children.* Philadelphia, PA: Lippincott Willaims & Wilkins, 2001, pp. 195–238.

http://aappolicy.aappublications.org AAP practice guidelines for the treatment of hyperbilirubinemia in the newborn.

McKiernan PJ. Neonatal cholestasis. *Semin Neonatol* 7(2):153–165, 2002.

Murray KF, Kowdley KV. Neonatal hemochromatosis. *Pediatrics* 108(4):960–964, 2001.

Roberts EA. The jaundice baby. In: Kelly DA (ed.), *Diseases of the Liver and Biliary System in Children.* London: Blackwell Science, 1999, pp. 11–46.

9

PORTAL HYPERTENSION AND ASCITES

Lynda Brady

INTRODUCTION

Portal hypertension is defined as an elevation in portal pressure above 10 mmHg. This is a result of increased portal blood flow and an increase in resistance to flow; and is a complication of a wide variety of pediatric liver diseases. Portal hypertension is a major cause of morbidity and morality in children with liver disease. Systemic investigations of the pathophysiology and treatment of portal hypertension have been almost exclusively limited to adults, with only anecdotal reports in the pediatric literature. Portal hypertension in pediatric patients may be different from that in adults and caution should be used when extrapolating adult data to children.

ETIOLOGY AND PATHOPHYSIOLOGY

Understanding portal hypertension requires knowledge of the anatomy of the portal system (see Fig. 9-1). Portal capillaries originate in the mesentery of the intestine and the spleen and end in the hepatic sinusoids. Capillaries of the mesentery and the spleen supply nutrient and hormone-rich blood to the portal vein. The portal vein enters the liver and branches into smaller vessels eventually

ending in the hepatic sinusoids. The partially oxygenated blood from the portal vein combines with oxygenated blood from the hepatic artery to give the liver unique protection against hypoxia. These two blood sources combine in the hepatic sinusoids, a unique well-fenestrated capillary system. The blood exits the liver via the hepatic veins. Portal hypertension (P) is the result of a combination of increased portal flow (F) and increased resistance (R) to flow ($P = F \times R$).

The etiologies are numerous (see Table 9-1). They are divided according to the location of the lesion causing the portal hypertension. Causes of portal hypertension are classified as extrahepatic or intrahepatic or they are classified as pre- and postsinusoidal. Table 9-1 uses both classifications. The most common extrahepatic cause of portal hypertension in pediatrics is portal vein clot with cavernous transformation. The majority of cases are of unknown etiology. One-third is due to umbilical catheterization, trauma, or hypercoagulable states. Obviously, a clot in the vessel would lead to increased resistance to flow.

Intrahepatic causes are further divided into biliary tract disease and hepatocellular disease. When portal hypertension is due to intrahepatic causes, there is portal inflammation and scarring secondary

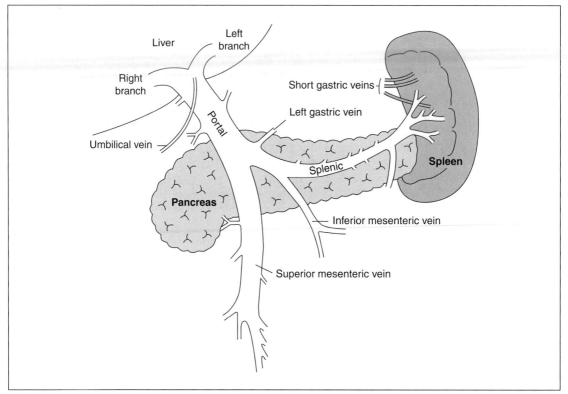

FIGURE 9-1

ANATOMY OF THE PORTAL SYSTEM

to the underlying etiology; this leads to impingement of the intrahepatic portal venules and decreased sinusoidal space resulting in increased resistance. In addition to the scarring there is release of vasoactive substances within the liver. Endothelin-1, one such vasoactive substance, is increased in patients with cirrhosis. In one pediatric study, endothelin-1 levels were elevated in cirrhotics versus controls and increased in those with ascites versus those without.

Increased resistance may be the primary event leading to portal hypertension but a variety of hemodynamic changes contributes to increased portal blood flow. Patients with portal hypertension have increased cardiac output, decreased splanchnic arterial tone, and decreased responsiveness to vasoconstrictors. The increase in cardiac output is due to increase in return to the heart (preload) and a decrease in the vascular resistance (afterload), the latter being the first event. Studies in animals indicate that a number of humoral mediators are involved including glucagons, prostaglandins, and nitric oxide (NO). Nitric oxide levels are in fact increased in pediatric patients with portal hypertension, and inhibitors of NO have been found to reverse the decreased vascular resistance and the decreased responsiveness to vasoconstrictors in studies in adults.

The vasodilatation results in a decreased effective plasma volume; in turn, this activates the rennin-aldosterone system resulting in sodium retention accompanied by fluid retention. The final change is alterations in the serotonergic and sympathetic tone in the splanchnic vasculature.

The signs and symptoms are secondary to decompression of venous pressure via portosystemic collaterals and can be best understood by

TABLE 9-1

CAUSES OF PORTAL HYPERTENSION

Presinusoidal

Extrahepatic
  Portal vein obstruction
  Splenic vein obstruction

Intrahepatic
  Biliary tract diseases
    Biliary atresia
    Sclerosing cholangitis
    Intrahepatic cholestasis syndromes
      Alagille's syndrome
      Persistent familial intrahepatic cholestasis/
        Byler's syndrome
      Congenital hepatic fibrosis
      Caroli's disease
  Hepatocellular diseases
    Hepatitis (B, C, autoimmune)
    Wilson's disease
    α_1 antitrypsin disease
    Toxins
  Miscellaneous
    Schistosomiasis
    Hepatoportal sclerosis
    Idiopathic portal hypertension

Postsinusoidal

Extrahepatic
  Budd-Chiari syndrome
  Constrictive pericarditis
  Congestive heart failure

TABLE 9-2

SIGNS AND SYMPTOMS OF PORTAL HYPERTENSION

Variceal bleeding
Portal hypertensive gastropathy
Splenomegaly
Rectal hemorrhoids
Visible abdominal wall veins
  (caput medusa)
Ascites
Hepatic encephalopathy

the retroperitoneal/paravertebral system (RPPV). Blood flows from the portal vein to the pancreatico-duodenal veins and into the RPPV system. This phenomenon can be seen on ultrasound but does not cause clinical symptoms.

The shunting of blood away from the liver leads to symptoms of portal hypertension (see Table 9-2). Intravascular homeostasis is controlled by hydro-static pressure in the capillaries and plasma colloid osmotic pressure. In a patient with portal hypertension there is an increase in the capillary hydrostatic pressure. In addition, children with chronic liver disease produce less albumin leading to decreased osmotic pressure. These factors plus the increased sodium and fluid retention contribute to accumulation of intraperitoneal fluid which is ascites.

Hepatic encephalopathy is due to shunting of blood away from the liver, interaction of gut metabolites with the central nervous system, hepatocellular dysfunction, and altered neurotransmitter function. Although encephalopathy more often occurs in children with liver disease, it is not necessarily linked to liver disease. In fact, it can also be seen in patients with portal hypertension from other reasons who have a large intake of protein. Ammonia is usually elevated in children with encephalopathy, but the degree to which the ammonia is elevated does not correlate with the degree of encephalopathy. Other symptoms such as hepatopulmonary and hepatorenal syndromes present in patients with significant liver disease associated with their portal hypertension. Mechanisms and treatment are discussed in Chap. 28.

examining the anatomy of the vessels (see Fig. 9-1). The most common symptoms come from esophageal varices, one of several portosystemic collaterals. Gastroesophageal varices result from increased flow through the coronary vein, left gastric vein, and the short gastric vein. The second most common symptom is splenomegaly that results from increased flow into the splenic vein. Rectal hemorrhoids are a result of increased flow in the inferior mesenteric vein. Increased flow through the umbilical vein will produce the visible abdominal wall vessels, caput medusa. The final engorged system is

CLINICAL PRESENTATION

The clinical presentation of portal hypertension can be quite dramatic. The most common presentation is gastrointestinal (GI) bleeding. Patients can have hematemesis or melena, as a result of bleeding from gastroesophageal varices or from portal hypertensive gastropathy. Bleeding from other sites in the gastrointestinal tract is rare in pediatrics. In children with known chronic liver disease the signs and symptoms may be expected. In children with silent liver disease or extrahepatic causes of portal hypertension, the GI bleeding may be the initial presentation of a previously undetected disease. Splenomegaly or hypersplenism with thrombocytopenia or leukopenia may be the presenting sign of portal hypertension.

Portal hypertension is less likely to present with ascites or encephalopathy initially, but clinicians must definitely keep monitoring for them. Ascites should be suspected in any patient with liver disease who has an increase in abdominal girth or large weight gain. Spontaneous bacterial peritonitis presents with acute abdominal pain in patients with ascites or portal hypertension. Hepatic encephalopathy may be difficult to recognize in children, particularly infants. Early signs are subtle and include irritability, developmental delay, school difficulty, lethargy, and sleep problems. Untreated encephalopathy can progress to decreased consciousness or coma.

DIAGNOSTIC WORK-UP

Portal hypertension should be suspected in any child presenting with a significant GI bleed, particularly if splenomegaly is noted. Physical examination should be directed to look for signs of chronic liver disease: growth failure, muscle wasting, cutaneous finding (telangiectasia, caput medusa), jaundice, ascites, or encephalopathy. Laboratory examination should include a complete blood and platelet count, hepatic indices (ALT, AST, alkaline phosphatase GGTP, and bilirubin), and markers of hepatic function prothrombin time, albumin, and ammonia. Although many studies have been done in adults to determine the most accurate radiologic examination to determine the etiology of portal hypertension, few studies have been done in pediatric patients. An ultrasound to look at portal circulation in combination with an endoscopy can determine if there is portal hypertension or varices. In the majority of patients, this combination of procedures is sufficient to make the diagnosis.

All patients with GI bleeding from suspected portal hypertension must undergo endoscopy. More invasive radiologic procedures, such as angiography, should be reserved to clearly delineate the vasculature or measure portal pressures.

Once the diagnosis of portal hypertension is made, the underlying etiology should be determined. Portal vein clot or hepatic vein obstructions are usually seen on ultrasound. More invasive radiologic procedures may be needed to confirm the diagnosis. A diagnosis of portal vein clot or Budd-Chiari syndrome requires the physician to look for an underlying coagulation defect (hypercoagulable state). If physical examination or laboratory findings indicate there is underlying liver disease the cause must be sought (see Table 9-3).

TABLE 9-3

WORK-UP FOR PATIENTS WITH PORTAL HYPERTENSION

Laboratory Evaluation

Portal Vein Clot
  Antilupus anticoagulant
  Anticardiolipn antibody
  Protein S, C antithrombin III levels
  Factor V Leyden mutations

Suspected Liver Disease
  Hepatitis B and C antibody
  Cerruloplasm (Wilson's disease)
  α_1 antitrypsin level (α_1 antitrypsin disease)
  Antismooth muscle antibody, antinuclear antibody,
    antiliver kidney microsomal antibody
    (auto-immune hepatitis)
  Liver biopsy to confirm diagnosis

COMPLICATIONS AND TREATMENT

The treatment of portal hypertension is directed at management of the symptoms. The most important manifestation is variceal bleeding. The management of varices can be divided into prophylaxis of initial or recurrent bleeds and emergent treatment of variceal hemorrhage. Most of the data concerning the management of varices comes from controlled trials in adults; pediatric literature is descriptive and anecdotal.

Treatment of Esophageal Varices

Bleeding esophageal varices in children is a life-threatening emergency (see Fig. 9-2) and they should be taken to the closest hospital. Once the patient is hemodynamically stable and has secure intravenous access they should be transferred to a tertiary care center with an experienced endoscopist. In patients with chronic liver disease there may be coagulopathy and thrombocytopenia. In addition to the crystalloid and packed red blood cells these patients should be given fresh frozen plasma, platelets, and vitamin K. Significant bleeding and hypotension impairs hepatic blood flow. This may cause further damage to an already diseased liver causing increase in ascites, coagulopathy, and encephalopathy. The blood within the GI tract is a large protein load and can precipitate encephalopathy.

The initial management of variceal bleeding should include pharmacologic agents which constrict the splanchnic vasculature. The most studied drug is vasopressin. In a study of 215 children, 184 had cessation of bleeding with conservative management and vasopressin. The occurrence of significant side effects has limited the use of the drug. Somatostatin or its analogue octreotide are as effective as vasopressin with very few side effects.

Despite fluids, blood, correction of coagulopathy, and splanchnic vasoconstriction, 15% of pediatric patients continue to bleed and need emergent endoscopy to control bleeding. The two endoscopic methods to control bleeding are band ligation and sclerotherapy. In adult studies, band ligation is equally as effective as sclerotherapy with fewer adverse events.

If bleeding persists after endoscopic intervention, a transjugular intrahepatic portosystemic shunt (TIPS, see Fig. 9-3) should be considered in patients with decompensated liver disease and an open portal vein. This is considered a bridge to liver transplant. If a patient has decompensated liver disease and a clotted portal vein, TIPS is not an option and emergent liver transplant is needed. In patients with a portal vein clot or a surgically correctable lesion, surgical intervention should be considered. In a patient with decompensated liver disease the mortality of surgical shunt is as high as 50%. In those patients TIPS is the treatment of choice because they will require transplant in the near future.

The next problem is what to do after a patient has had a first variceal bleed. There is a 50% chance of rebleeding after the initial variceal bleed. There are three choices: pharmacologic, endoscopic, or portosystemic shunt.

The only pharmacologic agent is the β_2 blocker propranolol. There are several adult studies demonstrating the efficacy of propranolol prophylaxis. The aim of the therapy is to decrease resting heart rate by 25% or decrease the hepatic venous pressure gradient to below 12 mmHg. The mechanism is β blockade in the splanchnic bed and unchecked α adrenergic stimulation leading to decreased splanchnic and portal flow. In addition, the decreased heart rate decreases the cardiac output which is contributing to the portal hypertension.

The second type of prophylaxis is endoscopic. There are two types of endoscopic intervention: chemical sclerotherapy or band ligation. Sclerotherapy has many more complications than band ligation, and band ligation has become the choice for prophylaxis. Endoscopic prophylaxis is the therapy of choice in patients with extrahepatic portal vein clot and no liver disease. The success of this procedure has decreased the need for surgical portosystemic shunts.

The final type of prophylaxis is portosystemic shunts. They are reserved for patients who have bleeding despite pharmacologic and endoscopic intervention or are not candidates for those therapies. There are four types of surgical shunts. The first three (portacaval, mesocaval, and splenorenal)

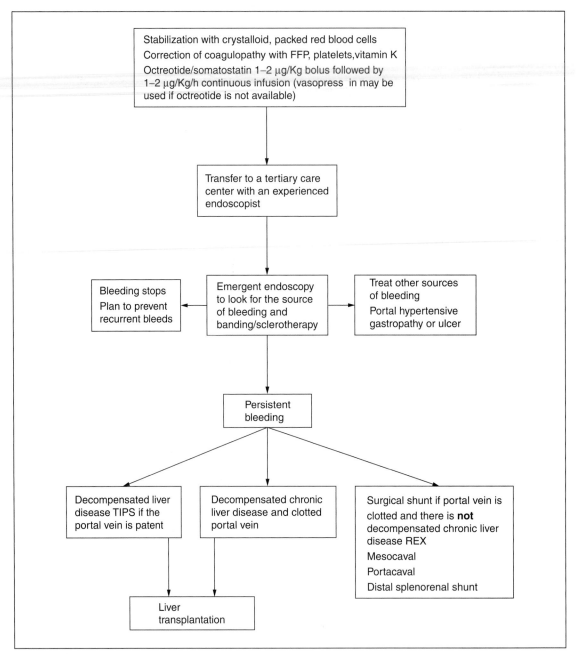

FIGURE 9-2

TREATMENT OF ACUTE VARICEAL HEMORRHAGE

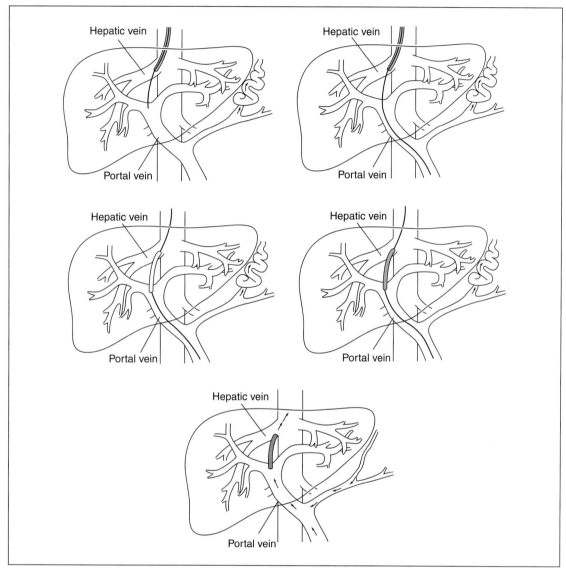

FIGURE 9-3

THE TRANSJUGULAR INTRAHEPATIC PORTOSYSTEMIC SHUNT ("TIPS")

divert blood away from the liver. Shunting blood from the liver can cause encephalopathy. A newer shunt for patients with extrahepatic portal vein clot is a meso-REX shunt where blood is shunted from the mesentery into the left intrahepatic portal vein via the umbilical vein. The major advantage is this shunt returns normal hepatic flow avoiding the risk

of encephalopathy. Prior to the extensive use of endoscopic intervention, surgical portosystemic shunts were used in large number of children with good results. The good results from shunts were seen in patients with extrahepatic portal hypertension. In contrast, those patients with decompensated liver disease had a 50% mortality rate. A better choice in those patients is a transjugular intrahepatic portosystemic shunt (see Fig. 9-3). This is a radiology procedure where the hepatic vein is accessed through the jugular and a shunt between the portal vein and the hepatic vein is established. This shunt is safer and has fewer complications in patients with end-stage liver disease than surgical shunts. These shunts are more likely to clot and are viewed as temporary bridges to transplant.

The question of whether to do TIPS or surgical shunt in a patient with no evidence of decreased synthetic function of the liver (compensated liver disease) is currently under debate. There are some data to suggest surgical shunts could be a choice for patients with compensated liver disease. In adult studies with patients who had stable chronic liver disease, surgical shunts were more cost-effective and lasted longer than TIPS. That decision would have to be made with a transplant team and experienced surgeon.

If the patient's portal hypertension is diagnosed prior to an esophageal bleed there needs to be a decision whether to use primary prophylaxis. Should you treat someone who has not had an initial variceal bleed? The answer is not clear. In pediatric patients who are close to medical attention primary prophylaxis is probably not necessary. In a patient who does not have close easy access to medical care primary prophylaxis should be considered.

Treatment of Ascites

The second most common problem in patients with portal hypertension is ascites. The management of ascites involves several steps:

- Salt and fluid restriction
- Diuretics
  a. Loop
  b. Antialdosterone
  c. Thiazide
- Paracentesis
- TIPS

Any patient with new onset of ascites or sudden increase in the amount of ascites should undergo paracentesis. This is to determine the fluid is a transudate and not infected. Sodium restriction decreases the sodium and fluid retention and is the initial step in the management of ascites in adult patients. Caution must be used when restricting the diet of a child, especially a patient awaiting liver transplantation. Growth is important and restricting a patient's diet may contribute to growth failure. Those patients who do not respond to salt restriction or are not candidates for salt restriction should be placed on diuretics. Loop diuretics (furosemide), aldosterone antagonist (spironolactone), and thiazide diuretics are the most common diuretics used. Loop diuretics are rapid acting and cause sodium loss. These may be used in the initial treatment of ascites. Spironolactone (starting dose 1–2 mg/kg per day) is a good long-term choice because the antialdosterone works against the increased rennin-aldosterone state in portal hypertension. Thiazide diuretics may be added to those patients who do not respond to a single diuretic. In adults, a patient with resistant ascites undergoes frequent taps where large amounts of fluid are removed. Albumin infusions are given during the removal of fluid to avoid decrease in intravascular volume. Children rarely develop resistant ascites but if there is respiratory compromise large volume paracentesis should be done. Finally, patients who do not respond or cannot tolerate large volume paracentesis, TIPS may be used to treat their ascites while awaiting transplant.

Encephalopathy is rarely seen in patients without underlying liver disease. Mild encephalopathy may develop after a GI bleed because of the increased protein load. Management of mild hepatic encephalopathy is aimed at decreasing ammonia production. Details about pathogenesis and treatment of encephalopathy can be found in Chap. 28.

LONG-TERM PROGNOSIS

The long-term prognosis of portal hypertension depends on the underlying cause. Studies looking at patients with extrahepatic portal vein clot have found patients have variable time to presentation and variable chance of having GI bleeding. More importantly, children with recurrent bleeding from varices tended to "outgrow" their problem in adolescence. This is thought to be due to recanalization of the portal vein or development of a natural portosystemic shunt. For these reasons, portal vein clots may be considered a benign condition and should be treated conservatively. Surgery should be reserved for those who do not respond to medical management.

Unfortunately, the same cannot be said for patients with underlying liver disease. A majority of those patients will develop progressive liver disease. Patients with signs of poor synthetic function in native livers when they present with their portal hypertension are candidates for liver transplantation. Their portal hypertension will be managed for a "short" time until they are transplanted.

Patients who fall somewhere in the middle of this spectrum are those patients with chronic liver disease but no evidence of decreased synthetic function. The classic example in pediatrics is a patient with biliary atresia. Patients with biliary atresia and functioning Kasai procedures can live a long period of time with their native livers. They are no longer cholestatic but develop cirrhosis and portal hypertension. The difficult choice is long-term treatment for portal hypertension when synthetic function is still normal. Band ligation or β_2 blocker are the treatments of choice for prophylaxis against recurrent variceal bleeding but will not treat other symptoms of portal hypertension. Surgical shunts to treat recurrent esophageal bleeds and ascites resistant to medical therapy have been shown safe and effective in adults but may increase encephalopathy especially in patients with liver disease. The ultimate treatment for biliary atresia is liver transplantation. Survival after liver transplantation is 85–90% at 1 year. This is an appropriate treatment for persistent portal hypertension in patients with underlying liver disease. The decision of how to treat portal hypertension in a patient with stable underlying liver disease must be made by the family with an experienced surgeon and a transplant team.

Bibliography

Herman HB, LeBerge JM. Role of TIPS in the treatment of portal hypertension in children. *J Pediatr Gastroenterol Nutr* 29:240–249, 1999.

McKiernan PJ. Treatment of variceal bleeding. *Gastroenterol Endosc Cilin North Am* 11:789–812, 2001.

Rykman FC, Alonso MH. Causes and management of portal hypertension in pediatric population. *Clin Liver Dis* 5:789–788, 2001.

Sabri M, Saps M, Peters JM. Pathophysiology and management of pediatric ascites. *Curr Gastroenterol Rep* 5:240–246, 2003.

Schneider BL. Portal hypertension. In: Suchy F, et al. (eds.). Philadelphia, PA: Lippincott Willaims & Wilkins, 2001, pp. 129–154.

Sheppard R. Complications and management of chronic liver disease. In: Kelly DA (ed.), *Diseases of the Liver and Biliary System in Children*. London: Blackwell Science, 1999, pp. 189–212.

10

INTERPRETATION OF SOME COMMON GI TESTS AND PROCEDURES

Puneet Gupta

INTRODUCTION

This chapter describes some common tests and procedures used in diagnosis and management of common gastrointestinal (GI) disorders. It is only meant to provide a quick reference to guide the resident in the understanding of the indications and limitations of the test, and should not be intended as an exhaustive or in-depth review of all available investigations. The tests and procedures are presented—grouped according to their main clinical indications—and then manometric and endoscopic procedures are briefly illustrated.

MALABSORPTION

Malabsorptive syndromes present with similar signs and symptoms: abdominal distention; pale, foul-smelling, bulky stools; muscle wasting; poor weight gain or weight loss; and growth retardation. Laboratory tests are often required to confirm the diagnosis and find the etiology of malabsorption syndrome. Tests can be divided into stool tests and blood tests.

Stool Testing

Fecal Fat

A useful screening test for malabsorption is a microscopic examination of stool for fat. This test can be performed by mixing a small amount of stool with Sudan red stain. The presence of more than six to eight droplets per low-power field is abnormal and suggests presence of triglycerides and neutral fat. The addition of acetic acid protonates ionized fatty acids and identifies free fatty acids as orange droplets with Sudan stain. In disorders with pancreatic insufficiency (cystic fibrosis or Shwachman's syndrome), the fat droplets number in the hundreds to thousands.

Quantitative Fecal Fat

A more definitive test for fat malabsorption is the 72-h stool collection for fat analysis. Excretion of excessive fat (see the following formula, according to age) demonstrates fat malabsorption. A dietary record during this period is used to calculate the fat intake. Patient should be on normal diet (<35% fat). Amount of calories and fat ingested is recorded for

3 days during the test. Stool samples are collected and frozen during this time. Coefficient of fat (CA) absorption is calculated as

$$CA = \frac{\text{fat ingested (g)} - \text{fat excreted (g)}}{\text{fat ingested (g)}} \times 100$$

where infants CA is >85–90% and >3-year-old CA is >95%.

Although the test is highly reliable to show fat malabsorption, it is however cumbersome, and is currently only rarely performed.

Fecal pH

Stool pH lower than 5.5 is suggestive of carbohydrate malabsorption. This is the result of the transformation by colonic bacterial flora of unabsorbed carbohydrates that generates lactic acid and other organic acids. Clearly, however, the test is nonspecific: acidic stool pH may in fact be also the result of other conditions, including congenital chloridorrhea.

Stool Reducing Substances

Measurement of carbohydrates in the stool using the Clinitest reagent for reducing substances is easily performed by combining 10 drops of water with 5 drops of stool and then adding a Clinitest tablet. The color change can be quantified as trace to 4+ using a color sheet provided by the manufacturer; >0.5% or 2+ reducing substance suggests carbohydrate malabsorption.

It should be noticed that sucrose is *not* a reducing substance and stool needs to be boiled with 1 mmol/L HCl for 30 s before testing. This treatment in fact releases glucose and fructose allowing the former sugar—which is reducing—to react with Clinitest.

Stool Osmotic Gap

Malabsorptive disorders are often associated with osmotic diarrhea. Stool osmotic gap is calculated as follows: stool osmolality (mOsm) − 2([Na$^+$] + [K$^+$]). In this formula the sum of [Na$^+$] and [K$^+$] is multiplied by a factor of 2 to account for associated unmeasured anions. It is important to remember that the stool osmolality within the distal intestine (estimated as 290 mOsm/kg because it equilibrates with plasma osmolality) can and should be used for this calculation. The osmotic gap is large (>125) in purely osmotic diarrhea, in which nonabsorbed nutrients and their metabolites account for most of the osmolality of liquid stool; the osmotic gap is small (<50) in purely secretory diarrhea. In mixed osmotic and secretory diarrheas and in cases of modest carbohydrate malabsorption the osmotic gap normally lies between 50 and 125.

Fecal Elastase

Fecal elastase 1 is a human pancreas-specific endoprotease that remains viable up to 1 week at room temperature. Its excretion and fecal concentration is not altered by pancreatic enzyme supplementation. An enzyme-linked immunosorbent assay (ELISA) is used to measure fecal elastase 1 as an indirect measure of pancreatic function and is more sensitive than measuring fecal chymotrypsin.

Stool Alpha$_1$ Antitrypsin

Measurement of spot stool alpha$_1$ antitrypsin levels is helpful in establishing a diagnosis of protein-losing enteropathy. This serum protein is of similar molecular weight as albumin and is resistant to digestion and therefore, in contrast to albumin, it can be measured in stool. Meconium normally contains high level of alpha$_1$ antitrypsin, so levels are difficult to interpret in infants less than 1 week of age. Patients with protein-loosing enteropathy have fecal alpha$_1$ antitrypsin level >2.6 mg/g of stool (NL 0.98 ± 0.17 mg/g).

Blood Tests

Various nutrients can be measured in blood to assess adequate absorption. Useful tests include serum iron, transferrin, folic acid, calcium, magnesium, zinc, 25-(OH)-vitamin D, vitamin A, vitamin E, and vitamin B$_{12}$ levels. Vitamin K stores can be assessed by measuring prothrombin time. Serum albumin and prealbumin levels can be useful in assessing protein malabsorption.

Breath Hydrogen Test

The breath hydrogen test can be used to evaluate carbohydrate malabsorption like sucrose or lactose malabsorption. Malabsorbed carbohydrate passes into the colon, where it is metabolized by bacteria with release of a number of metabolites, including the gas hydrogen (H_2). To test for malabsorption of a specific carbohydrate, hydrogen gas in expired air is measured after oral load of the carbohydrate.

After fasting for 6 h, the child is given a 2 g/kg (maximum 50 g) of desired sugar as a 10–20% solution. End expiratory air is collected before sugar load and every 30 min for 2 h thereafter to measure H_2 gas. A rise in H_2 gas >20 ppm above the baseline suggests the malabsorption of the tested carbohydrate. A rise in H_2 within 30 min of ingestion suggests small bowel bacterial overgrowth or rapid transit due to short gut or gastric dumping syndrome.

The patient should not receive antibiotics within 1 week before performing this test because they alter the colon flora and suppress hydrogen gas production. The major problem with the breath hydrogen study is that it is so sensitive that it may identify carbohydrate malabsorption that is not clinically significant. For the specific use of this test to detect small bowel bacterial overgrowth, see Chap. 20.

D-Xylose Test

D-Xylose is a pentose minimally metabolized in humans and totally and readily absorbed by the upper small bowel. D-Xylose absorption test is thus an unspecific test useful to assess the absorptive integrity of the small intestinal mucosa. After 6 h of fasting, administer a standard dose of 5 g, or alternatively 14.5 g/m^2 (maximum 25 g) of D-xylose orally as a 10% solution in water. In children less than 30 kg of weight, failure of serum level to exceed 25 mg/dL 1 h after the ingestion suggests malabsorption due to proximal small bowel mucosal lesion. In children heavier than 30 kg, 5 h

urinary excretion of <15% has the same meaning. It should be noticed that the test suffers from both false positives (reduced absorption due, for instance, to delayed gastric emptying) and, less frequently, false negatives.

FOOD ALLERGY

See Chap. 14. for a detailed analysis of available tests and their rational use.

GASTROESOPHAGEAL REFLUX DISEASE (GERD)

Gastroesophageal reflux (GER) is a common disorder in infants and older children due to inappropriate transient relaxation of lower esophageal sphincter (LES). Most babies with frequent spit ups who are otherwise healthy do not require any investigation and only reassurance for parents. However, when GER becomes pathogenic (GERD), it may lead to complications and should be approached accordingly. Tests are not always necessary, but they may be useful in certain situations (see Chap. 13 for a recommended approach to the patient suspected of having GERD and a rational use of diagnostic tests, here described.)

The following recommendations are based on the North American Society for Pediatric Gastroenterology, Hepatology, and Nutrition (NASPGHAN) guidelines for GERD.

Barium Contrast Radiography

The upper gastrointestinal series is useful to detect anatomic abnormalities, such as pyloric stenosis, malrotation, hiatal hernia, and esophageal stricture. When compared to esophageal pH monitoring, the upper GI series is neither sensitive nor specific for the diagnosis of GERD. The brief duration of the upper GI series results in false negative results, while the frequent occurrence of nonpathologic reflux (particularly seen in the postprandial period, such as after a barium swallow) results in false positive results. Thus, the upper GI series *is not a* useful test to determine the presence or absence of GER; however, it is useful when anatomic abnormalities are suspected.

Esophageal pH Monitoring

Esophageal pH monitoring measures the frequency and duration of episodes of acid reflux. The test is performed by the transnasal placement of a microelectrode into the lower esophagus, which measures and records intraesophageal pH. Abbreviated studies of fewer than 12 h are less reproducible than longer studies.

The percentage of the total time that the esophageal pH is <4, also called the reflux index, is considered the most valid measure of reflux because it reflects the cumulative exposure of the esophagus to acid. The mean upper limit of normal of the reflux index is 11.7% in infants 0–11 months, 5.4% in children 0–9 years old, and approximately 6% in normal adults. NASPGHAN recommended that the upper limit of normal of the reflux index be defined as up to 12% in the first year of life and up to 6% thereafter.

Esophageal pH monitoring can determine if a patient's symptom is temporally associated with acid reflux by calculating the symptom index. The symptom index is the ratio of the number of episodes of a symptom (e.g., heartburn or apnea) that occur concurrent with acid reflux divided by the total number of episodes of that symptom. Symptom index scores ≥0.5 suggest a relationship between symptom and gastroesophageal reflux.

Esophageal pH monitoring is also useful to assess the adequacy of the dosage of acid suppression therapy in children being treated with a proton-pump inhibitor.

It is also useful to determine if a patient's unexplained pulmonary symptoms (like nocturnal cough, asthma, and recurrent pneumonia) are due to GERD. For example, approximately 60% of children with asthma, poorly responsive to conventional treatment, have abnormal esophageal pH monitoring studies. In adults with chronic hoarseness there is a high incidence of abnormal GERD. The pH probe is often used for evaluation of infantile apnea although its use for establishing GERD

as a cause of apnea remains controversial. It should be reserved for cases where GERD is suspected but not clinically apparent as a cause of obstructive apnea.

Esophageal pH monitoring does not detect nonacidic reflux episodes such as occur postprandially in infants. In some patients, esophageal pH monitoring may be within the range of normal but brief episodes of GERD may cause complications such as apparent life-threatening event (ALTE), cough, or aspiration pneumonia.

Endoscopy and Biopsy

Endoscopy enables both visualization and biopsy of the esophageal epithelium. Endoscopy and biopsy can determine the presence and severity of esophagitis, strictures, and Barrett's esophagus, as well as exclude other disorders, such as Crohn's disease, webs, and eosinophilic or infectious esophagitis. A normal appearance of the esophagus during endoscopy does not exclude histopathologic esophagitis. The subtle mucosal changes of erythema and pallor may be observed in the absence of esophagitis.

Because there is a poor correlation between endoscopic appearance and histopathology, esophageal biopsy is recommended when diagnostic endoscopy is performed. Basal zone hyperplasia (>20–25% of total epithelial thickness) and increased papillary length (>50–75% of epithelial thickness) have been found to correlate with increased acid exposure. It has been proposed that a high number of eosinophils in the esophageal epithelium (>7–24 per high power field) suggest the diagnosis of eosinophilic esophagitis (see Chap. 16).

Helicobacter pylori Gastritis

Serologic Testing to Detect H. Pylori Antibodies

Enzyme-linked immunosorbent assays to detect *H. pylori* antibodies are relatively inexpensive and easy to use. However, when compared with histology the sensitivity and specificity of serologic assays are poor in both adults and children. In general, the accuracy of serum-based immunoassays in children in developed countries is poor, with a range of sensitivity of only 60–70%. Accordingly, treatment regimens based on the results of these tests cannot be recommended. Serologic tests may not be used reliably to verify eradication of *H. pylori*, because antibody titers can remain positive for many months, despite resolution of infection.

Endoscopy

The definitive diagnosis of *H. pylori* and the assessment of extent of gastritis can be made reliably only by endoscopy with multiple biopsy specimens obtained in one or more regions of the stomach including antrum, body, and transition zones (i.e., cardia and incisura). *H. pylori* gastritis in children is associated in approximately 50% of cases with nodularity of antral mucosa, endoscopically evident. Biopsies are absolutely necessary therefore to confirm the disgnosis, as histology is the golden standard for diagnosis, and in addition provides information on the severity and topographic distribution of gastritis.

Rapid Urease Testing of Biopsy Tissues

Urease testing (CLO, TriMed, Kansas City, MO) provides indirect identification of *H. pylori* infection within a few hours of endoscopy. *H. pylori* produces urease that hydrolyzes urea to ammonia (a base) detected by change in color of a pH sensitive dye. The color change may occur as soon as 30 min after inoculation, however, if bacterial load in the specimen is small, the reaction may take up to 24 h to develop. The accuracy of the test is dependent on the number of tissue specimens tested, the location of biopsy sites, bacterial load, and previous usage of antibiotics and proton-pump inhibitors.

Urea Breath Testing (UBT)

Urea breath tests are noninvasive and have high sensitivity and specificity (>95%) both in adults and children. The test requires the ingestion of either radiolabeled ^{14}C-urea or urea tagged with the stable isotope ^{13}C. Breakdown of urea by *H. pylori* urease causes production of labeled CO_2 which is measured in the expired air. Test results may be influenced by concurrent use of antibiotics and acid-suppressing medications and by the presence of other urease-producing organisms present in the oral cavity. Following treatment, the UBT is 100% sensitive and specific in assessing *H. pylori* status and has replaced endoscopy as investigation of choice for assessing treatment success in children. Breath test should not be carried out for at least 1 month after the completion of treatment.

Saliva and Urine Tests for H. pylori Antibodies

Similar to serologic tests, saliva-based tests also detect the presence of *H. pylori*-specific IgG antibodies. The tests are easy to perform, painless, and inexpensive; however, these tests are less sensitive than assays of serum or whole blood.

Stool Test for H. pylori Antigens

Testing of *H. pylori* antigens in stools has shown promising results for the noninvasive diagnosis of gastric infection and monitoring the success of eradication therapy. In adults test is 94% sensitive and 92% specific for the diagnosis of infection; however, patients may be reluctant to collect stool specimens. In addition, refrigerated stools are more difficult to test.

Gastrointestinal Manometry

Anorectal Manometry

Anorectal manometry is used for evaluation of children with defecation abnormalities, in particular those suspected with Hirschsprung's disease and fecal incontinence. It evaluates the response of the internal anal sphincter to inflation of a balloon in the rectum. When the rectal balloon is inflated, there is normally a reflex relaxation of the internal anal sphincter. In Hirschsprung's disease this rectoanal inhibitory reflex (RAIR) is absent; there is no relaxation, or there may even be paradoxical contraction, of the internal anal sphincter. In a cooperative child, anorectal manometry represents a sensitive and specific diagnostic test for Hirschsprung's disease. It is particularly useful when the aganglionic segment is short and results of radiologic or pathologic studies are equivocal. If sphincter relaxation is normal, Hirschsprung's disease can be reliably excluded. In the presence of a dilated rectum, it is necessary to inflate the balloon with large volumes to elicit normal sphincter relaxation. In the child with retentive behavior, there may be artifacts caused by voluntary contraction of the external anal sphincter and the gluteal muscles. Sedation, which does not interfere with the rectoanal inhibitory reflex, may be used in newborns and uncooperative children. If manometry results are abnormal, diagnosis should be confirmed with a biopsy.

Antroduodenal Manometry

During fasting, the stomach and small bowel show a cyclic pattern known as the migrating motor complex (MMC). Phase III of MMC consists of rhythmic regular contractions at three times per minute in antrum and 11–12 times per minute in small bowel. Absence of phase III activity, abnormal propagation of MMC, sustained uncoordinated pressure activity, and lack of fed response correlate well with neuropathic disorders of intestinal motility. Myopathic disorders are associated with low amplitude contractions. Antral hypomotility correlates with delayed gastric emptying.

Esophageal Manometry

NASPGHAN recommends esophageal manometry in the following situations:

- To evaluate symptoms or signs of esophageal dysfunction, such as dysphagia, odynophagia, chest pain, aspiration, and recurrent food impaction.
- To diagnose motility disorders of the esophagus such as achalasia as well as to detect esophageal manifestations of disorders

of connective tissue (such as scleroderma) and chronic intestinal pseudoobstruction.
- Esophageal manometry is generally not useful in the diagnosis or medical management of gastroesophageal reflux disease or structural lesions of the esophagus.

In achalasia, there is increased LES pressure, absence of esophageal peristalsis, and abnormal LES relaxation.

PEDIATRIC GASTROINTESTINAL ENDOSCOPY

Endoscopy in children was first reported in late 1960s using fiberoptic bronchoscopes and grew rapidly during the next two decades. The production and widespread distribution of small-diameter endoscopes and accessories contributed to this expansion. Flexible endoscopy allows direct inspection and selective nonsurgical tissue sampling of the alimentary tract. As a result, diagnoses can be established earlier and with greater accuracy. Treatments previously restricted to open surgical intervention are now performed via endoscopy with considerable efficacy and safety.

Esophago-Gastro-Duodenoscopy

Examination of the upper gastrointestinal tract by esophago-gastro-duodenoscopy (EGD) is the most frequently performed endoscopic procedure in children. EGD can be safely performed in nearly all children including very small infants (1.5–2 kg).

Diagnostic EGD—Indications

Dysphagia or Odynophagia

Dysphagia, odynophagia, and aversive feeding behavior may be due to esophagitis (acid reflux or allergic), stricture, dysmotility, or an impacted foreign body. Each of these problems requires endoscopic evaluation to confirm or treat the disorder. Some causes of esophagitis are associated with specific endoscopic findings like cheesy white exudates in *Candida* esophagitis, volcano ulcers with herpes esophagitis, and aphthous ulcers with Crohn's disease; however, in many cases biopsy with histology is required for definitive diagnosis. Esophagitis due to GER and eosinophilic esophagitis can have similar endoscopic appearance including vertical lines and circular rings.

Unexplained Vomiting

Unexplained vomiting warrants endoscopic evaluation to exclude inflammatory disease such as allergic or eosinophilic gastroenteritis, *H. pylori*-associated gastritis or ulcer disease, and Crohn's disease.

Unexplained Abdominal or Chest Pain

Substernal pain may be due to esophagitis, while unexplained abdominal pain may be due to *H. pylori* gastritis, ulcer, eosinophilic gastroenteritis, or Crohn's disease.

Malabsorption Syndromes

Small bowel biopsy identifies enteropathies (i.e., diseases of the small intestine) involving the mucosa of the proximal small intestine. As such, it is invaluable in diagnosing disparate conditions such as celiac disease, abetalipoproteinemia, lymphangiectasia, congenital microvillus inclusion disease, eosinophilic gastroenteritis, infectious disorders, and Whipple's disease (rare in children). At the time of biopsy, in addition to mucosa, it is possible to collect aspirates for examination for *Giardia* or bacterial culture. Mucosal samples can be frozen to assay for disaccharidase activities later. Depression of activities of all enzymes tested suggests a secondary deficiency associated with mucosal damage. Reduction of a specific enzyme or group of enzymes is consistent with a specific deficiency (lactase or sucrase-isomaltase deficiency).

Caustic Ingestion

Endoscopy performed within 24–48 h of caustic ingestion can help assess the damage and plan treatment.

Removal of Foreign Bodies

Coins are the most common foreign body ingested by young children. Of the foreign bodies that come to medical attention, 80–90% pass through the gastrointestinal tract without difficulty. Ten to 20% require endoscopic removal, whereas 1% or less requires surgical intervention. Once in the stomach, 95% of all ingested objects pass without difficulty through the remainder of the GI tract. Perforation after foreign body ingestion is estimated to be less than 1% of all objects ingested. Perforation tends to occur in areas of physiologic sphincters (pylorus and ileocecal valve), acute angulation (such as the duodenal sweep), congenital gut malformations (webs, diaphragms, or diverticula), or areas of previous bowel surgery. In older children and adults, oval objects greater than 5 cm in diameter or 2 cm in thickness tend to lodge in the stomach and should be endoscopically retrieved. Thin objects greater than 10 cm in length fail to negotiate the duodenal sweep and should also be removed. In infants and toddlers, objects longer than 3 cm or larger than 20 mm in diameter usually do not pass through the pylorus and should be removed. Open safety pins should also be endoscopically retrieved, but other small sharp objects can be managed conservatively.

Therapeutic EGD—Indications

Dilatation (Strictures/Achalasia)

Peptic strictures generally form in mid or distal esophagus, while strictures secondary to esophageal atresia occur at the anastomotic site.

Tools available to dilate strictures include rubber bougies (Maloney), wire-guided PVC bougies (Savary), and balloon dilators. No more than three dilators of increasing size (total 3 mm) should be passed in a single session. Pneumatic dilatation is useful in treatment of achalasia.

Upper Gastrointestinal Hemorrhage

Endoscopy is useful in finding the cause of bleeding like gastritis, erosions, ulcers, Mallory-Weiss tears, or varices. Endoscopic techniques such as electrocoagulation, injection of sclerosants, and band ligation are used to control the bleeding.

Placement of Enteral Feeding Tubes

Percutaneous gastrostomy (PEG) tubes can be placed endoscopically in children requiring prolonged nasogastric (NG) feeding eliminating the need to perform surgical gastrostomy. Endoscopy can also be used to place jejunostomy and cecostomy tubes.

Colonoscopy

Flexible colonoscopy allows direct inspection and histologic confirmation of mucosal abnormalities as well as therapeutic options like polypectomy or hemostasis.

Indications

Lower GI bleeding. Colonoscopy is essential for diagnosing persistent or recurrent lower GI bleeding for which no obvious cause like anal fissure or infectious colitis is found. Colonoscopy is invaluable in diagnosing causes of rectal bleeding like colitis, polyps, AV malformation, foreign body, and anastomotic ulcer. In case of colitis, histologic examination of biopsy samples will help in identifying the cause of colitis whether due to inflammatory bowel disorder or infectious or allergic in nature.

Chronic diarrhea. Colonoscopy is sometimes useful in finding the cause of chronic diarrhea due to microscopic colitis, Crohn's disease, or ulcerative colitis. However, when diarrhea is clearly of the secretory type and no evidence of colonic inflammation (e.g., blood and mucus in the stool, presence of excessive leucocytes) is obtained, its diagnostic yield is minimal.

Cancer surveillance. Colonoscopy is used for surveillance for polyps and possible malignancy in familial adenomatous polyposis and ulcerative colitis.

Therapeutic Colonoscopy—Indications

Various therapeutic procedures including polypectomy, balloon dilation of strictures, and hemostasis can be performed during colonoscopy.

Endoscopic Retrograde Cholangiopancreatography

Indications

Biliary. Endoscopic retrograde cholangiopancreatography (ERCP) may be needed for diagnosis of choledocholithiasis, choledochal cyst, biliary stricture, and sclerosing cholangitis.

Pancreatic. ERCP is indicated in suspected gallstone pancreatitis, recurrent or chronic pancreatitis, pancreatic trauma, and pancreas divisum.

Therapeutic. ERCP is used for sphincterotomy, stone extraction, stent placement, and dilation of strictures.

Major complication of ERCP is pancreatitis reported in 3–8%.

Bibliography

Rudolph CD, et al. Guidelines for evaluation and treatment of gastroesophageal reflux in infants and children: recommendations of the North American Society for Pediatric Gastroenterology and Nutrition. *J Pediatr Gastroenterol Nutr* 32(Suppl 2):S1–S31, 2001.

Walker WA, Durie PR, Hamilton JR, Walker-Smith JA, Watkins JB (eds.), *Pediatric Gastrointestinal Disease*, 3rd ed., 2000.

Walker WA, Goalet O, Kleinman J, Sherman P, Shneider B, Sanderson J (eds.), *Pediatric Gastrointestinal Disease*, 4th ed., 2004.

GASTROINTESTINAL DISORDERS

CHAPTER

11

ACHALASIA

Annamaria Staiano, Erasmo Miele, and Ray E. Clouse

INTRODUCTION

Achalasia is the most recognized motor disorder of the esophagus and is the hallmark example of hypermotility, i.e., motor dysfunction produced by a reduction in inhibitory neural influence or an imbalance between contraction and inhibition of contraction. The term achalasia means "failure to relax." The disorder is characterized by (1) partial or incomplete lower esophageal sphincter (LES) relaxation and (2) loss of esophageal peristalsis. An increase in LES resting pressure may also be present. A variety of diseases can produce the clinical, radiographic, and manometric features that characterize achalasia; however, it is generally accepted that use of the unqualified term be restricted to the idiopathic form of the disease.

Numerous theories exist regarding pathogenesis, but a degenerative lesion involving inhibitory neurons appears to be central to the disease. This neural degeneration cannot be corrected, and treatment is directed at palliation of symptoms and prevention of complications. Three palliative treatments are available: pharmacotherapy including botulinum toxin injection, dilatation, and myotomy. The complications of achalasia are related to retention and stasis in the esophagus and include esophagitis, aspiration of esophageal contents, and increased risk for the development of squamous carcinoma.

EPIDEMIOLOGY

Achalasia remains an uncommon but worldwide disorder. The incidence of the disease is about 1/200,000 per year with a prevalence of about 8/100,000 population. A striking variability in international prevalence has been reported, as have significant differences across regions within countries. The disease occurs with equal frequency in men and women and is seen in all age groups; however, fewer than 5% of all patients with achalasia manifest symptoms before the age of 15 years.

ETIOLOGY AND PATHOPHYSIOLOGY

Achalasia results from a loss of intramural nitric oxide-containing inhibitory nerves in the distal esophagus and LES. Lack of inhibitory influence prevents the normal sequencing of distal contractions (resulting in aperistalsis) and normal relaxation of the LES with swallowing. The etiology remains unknown, but both genetic and immunologic factors presumably are relevant.

Genetic predisposition has been suggested in that HLA-DQ alleles DQA1*0103 and DQB1*0603 are detected more frequently in achalasics than in normal controls. These HLA-DQ alleles also are associated with higher likelihood of autoantibodies against the myenteric plexus. An achalasia-like picture also accompanies a variety of genetically based syndromes, wherein the pathophysiologic mechanisms responsible for the esophageal manifestations may vary but reveal a genetic basis. For example, achalasia is associated with adrenal insufficiency and alacrima in an autosomal recessive disorder called the "triple A syndrome" (for "achalasia, alacrima, and adrenal insufficiency"). Sjogren's syndrome with xerostomia has now been described as one of the variant components of this disorder. Mutations of a novel gene in chromosome 12q13, termed AAAS, encoding a 546 amino acid polypeptide have been identified as being potentially responsible for the triple A syndrome. Achalasia also occurs in conjunction with Down's syndrome, a recent small study suggesting a prevalence of approximately 1 in 30 afflicted subjects. Despite the possibility revealed by these syndromes that genetic factors are relevant in the expression of achalasia, familial clustering in typical idiopathic achalasia is very uncommon.

Other data support an immunogenic basis for achalasia. Myenteric inflammation resulting from an immunologic process may be the major cause of myenteric neuronal degeneration in this disorder. The inflammatory infiltrate has been characterized immunohistochemically as a predominance of both CD3 and CD8-positive T cells expressing TIA-1 and granzyme B, two markers for the activation of T-cell subpopulations. Additionally, the process is focused on intramural inhibitory neurons. The stimulus for this inflammatory reaction is not completely understood but may be driven by autoimmune factors. Presumably participating in the process, autoantibodies against M2 muscarinic acetylcholine receptors have been found in patients with either achalasia from Chagas' disease or idiopathic achalasia. These antibodies increase the contractile activity of the LES through specific activation of the receptors.

The features of achalasia can also be produced by malignancy, a condition termed *malignant secondary achalasia* or *pseudoachalasia*. Malignant secondary achalasia enters into the differential diagnosis in adults and occasionally in children when the symptoms are of short duration and weight loss is greater than expected from the degree

TABLE 11-1

CLASSIFICATION OF ACHALASIA FOLLOWING ANTIREFLUX SURGERY

Type 1	Primary achalasia is misdiagnosed as reflux disease and inappropriate antireflux surgery is performed
Type 2	Secondary iatrogenic achalasia results from stenosis and scar formation at the site of the wrap
Type 3	Primary idiopathic achalasia follows antireflux surgery after a symptom-free period

of dysphagia and regurgitation. Secondary achalasia can also result from benign causes. The most common form encountered today follows antireflux surgery. The problem is sufficiently prevalent and a classification has been suggested (Table 11-1).

CLINICAL SIGNS/SYMPTOMS

Idiopathic achalasia presents at all ages and has been diagnosed even within the first 6 months of life. The pediatric presentation includes weight loss, recurrent pneumonia, and "vomiting" as dominant features, especially in younger children (Table 11-2). The mean age at the time of diagnosis

TABLE 11-2

CLINICAL SYMPTOMS AND SIGNS IN CHILDREN WITH ACHALASIA

Age	
"Younger" children	Weight loss
	Refusal to eat
	Symptoms resembling gastroesophageal reflux
	Recurrent pneumonias
	Nocturnal cough
"Older" children	Dysphagia
	Regurgitation
	Retrosternal pain

in the pediatric patients is 8.8 years with a mean duration of symptoms prior to diagnosis of 23 months. Younger children tend to have food avoidance or refusal to eat, while some may present as if they have gastroesophageal reflux. Respiratory symptoms can dominate the presentation and include choking, recurrent pneumonias, and nocturnal cough. Older children have symptoms that are similar to those in adults with dysphagia, regurgitation, and retrosternal pain being the most prominent. When present, retrosternal pain can be aggravated by food ingestion or occur in between meals.

The adult presentation can vary markedly across patients with dramatic variation in symptom type and severity. Although dysphagia is reported by only about 40% of patients at symptom onset, it is present in nearly all patients at the time of diagnosis. Dysphagia initially may occur with solid foods but typically is reported for both solid foods and liquids as the disease progresses. Stereotyped movements to assist swallowing, including arching of the neck and shoulders, standing, sitting straight, and walking, have been reported by 60% of subjects. Slow, deliberate swallowing during a meal also may enhance emptying by taking advantage of the 10–20 mmHg increment in intraesophageal pressure that occurs with swallowing from the poorly compliant esophagus. These often-subtle symptoms are important in that they may suggest the diagnosis when classical symptoms are less evident. Although the mean number of achalasia-related symptoms increased from <2 at onset to >5 at diagnosis, the severity or number of symptoms did not correlate with the severity of radiographic findings in one investigation.

COMPLICATIONS

Complications of achalasia primarily are related to retention and stasis in the esophagus and are more likely in patients with markedly dilated esophagi. Bacterial growth from stasis is thought to contribute to pulmonary infections, infectious complications following invasive endoscopic procedures, and even neoplastic changes in the esophagus. Irritation of the mucosal lining results in an endoscopically evident esophagitis. A more serious complication is the aspiration of esophageal contents. It is also accepted that achalasia is a risk factor for the development of squamous carcinoma, the complication possibly being more likely in patients who have had unsatisfactory or no treatment, dilated esophagi, and long-standing retention of esophageal contents. These latter observations suggest that stasis and mucosal irritation may be precipitating factors for this complication.

DIAGNOSIS

The diagnosis can be suspected from a compatible clinical history, findings at endoscopy, and the appearance and behavior of the esophagus during barium x-ray imaging. The diagnosis is established with manometry (Table 11-3).

Endoscopy

Endoscopy is a crucial diagnostic tool in the patient with symptoms of achalasia and should be performed even if radiographic evaluation findings are typical. The primary use of endoscopy is to exclude a malignancy or another cause of secondary achalasia. Suspicious endoscopic findings include retained esophageal contents, a dilated esophageal body, and a closed LES region through which the endoscope passes with gentle pressure. Endoscopy also provides information about the esophageal mucosa before treatment is undertaken, particularly to assess the presence of inflammation or infection.

Radiography

Although insensitive to less significant motor disorders, the barium swallow with videofluoroscopy can accurately detect achalasia in >90% of cases when typical features are systematically assessed. Unfortunately, the accuracy is much lower in prospective clinical use. Typical radiographic findings include absence of meaningful peristalsis in the smooth-muscle portion of the esophagus, a dilated esophageal body, and poor opening of the LES with swallowing. The LES does open periodically, but,

TABLE 11-3

DIAGNOSTIC TECHNIQUES IN ACHALASIA

Diagnostic Technique	Findings
Endoscopy	Retained esophageal contents
	Dilated esophageal body
	Closed LES region
Barium radiography	Absence of meaningful peristalsis
	Dilated esophageal body
	Poor opening of the LES with retention of a barium column on standing
	"Bird's-beak" appearance
Manometry (the diagnostic standard)	Aperistalsis[a]
	Inadequate relaxation of the LES[a]
	Elevation of intraesophageal pressure with respect to intragastric pressure
	Isobaric pressure phenomena in the esophageal body
	Increased LES basal pressure

[a]Essential criteria for manometric diagnosis. LES = lower esophageal sphincter.

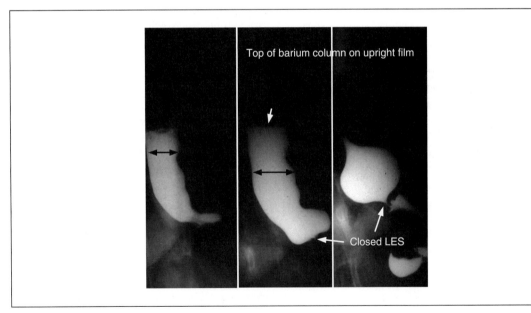

FIGURE 11-1

THREE IMAGES FROM BARIUM ESOPHAGOGRAMS IN PATIENTS WITH ACHALASIA
The esophageal body is dilated (black arrows), and the barium ends in a beak-like configuration at the closed lower esophageal sphincter (LES; seen in the second and third panels). Retention of the barium is demonstrated as an air-fluid level at the top of the barium column in an upright film (second panel).

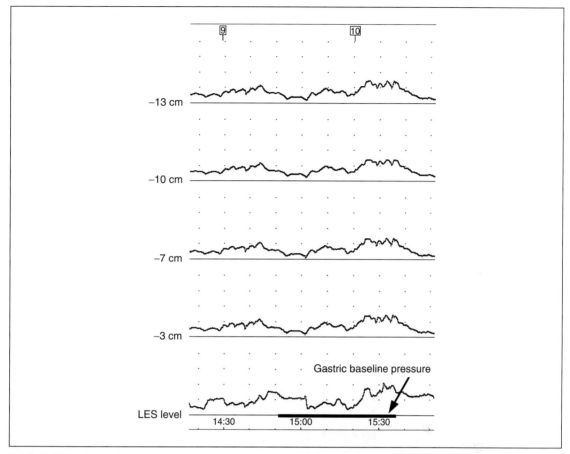

FIGURE 11-2

TWO SWALLOWS AS RECORDED MANOMETRICALLY IN A PATIENT WITH ACHALASIA

The sensors are spaced at 3 cm intervals, and the most distal sensor is in the lower esophageal sphincter (LES). Although some LES movement is seen with swallowing, relaxation to intragastric pressure does not occur. Identical wave forms are noted in the esophageal body tracings reflecting the isobaric pressure changes within the organ.

when closed, the barium column terminates in a smooth "bird's-beak" appearance (Fig. 11-1). Loss of peristalsis and some indication of LES dysfunction are required for establishing the diagnosis. A plain chest radiograph may show a widened mediastinum and an air-fluid level—providing a clue to the diagnosis.

Manometry

Esophageal manometry remains the gold standard for the diagnosis of primary achalasia. Two features

are characteristic and should be present before the diagnosis is offered with any certainty: aperistalsis in the esophageal body and inadequate relaxation of the LES (Fig. 11-2). Exceptions are encountered rarely. Sporadic segmental peristaltic activity is occasionally observed, especially after treatment with pneumatic dilatation or surgery, and brief complete relaxation of the LES can be seen in 20–30% of patients. Much of the latter is an artifact related to cephalad movement of the closed LES off the sensor, thereby mimicking relaxation. Other common manometric findings in achalasia include elevation of intraesophageal pressure over intragastric pressure (a reverse of normal) and increased resting LES pressure (seen in more than 50% of untreated patients).

High-resolution manometry using closely spaced sensors over a distance that spans the majority of the esophageal body and LES continues to show promise as a superior diagnostic method. This approach, along with three-dimensional topographic plotting of the pressure data, has proved highly accurate in detecting incomplete LES relaxation associated with achalasia by avoiding the pitfalls related to axial sphincter movement. An abnormal transsphincteric pressure gradient during the swallow (>5 mmHg) determined with these methods and reflecting incomplete LES relaxation has demonstrated high sensitivity and specificity (each >0.95) and appears superior to conventional analysis methods using point-pressure sensors. Although initially described only in adult

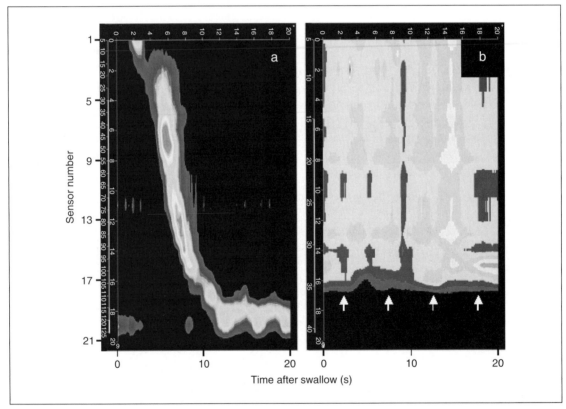

FIGURE 11-3

CONTOUR MAPS FROM SINGLE SWALLOWS GENERATED FROM HIGH-RESOLUTION MANOMETRY AND TOPOGRAPHIC PLOTTING METHODS IN A NORMAL SUBJECT (PANEL a) AND A PATIENT WITH ACHALASIA (PANEL b)

The 21 pressure recording sensors are spaced at 1 cm intervals, and the catheter has been positioned in the distal esophagus, across the lower sphincter, and into the proximal stomach in each case. Note the normal segmental architecture of progressive peristalsis in the normal subject. The proximal striated-muscle region is just visible at the top of the map and the two smooth-muscle segments end in lower sphincter contraction following swallow-induced relaxation. The differences in achalasia are readily apparent: normal peristaltic architecture is absent, intraesophageal pressure is elevated (brighter contour regions) compared with intragastric pressure (black), and intraesophageal pressure ends abruptly at a dam effect at the level of the nonrelaxing lower sphincter (arrows).

subjects, high-resolution manometry and topographic plotting is beginning to be used in pediatric subjects and likely will be a superior manometric method for achalasia diagnosis in this population (Fig. 11-3).

DIFFERENTIAL DIAGNOSIS

Idiopathic achalasia must be differentiated from other organic causes of esophageal obstruction, particularly benign or malignant neoplasms and benign structures. In some children suspected of having achalasia, leiomyomas of the distal esophagus have been found. Usually, endoscopy with biopsy is able to exclude such conditions. In adults, adenocarcinoma of the stomach is the most common tumor presenting as achalasia, although a variety of extraintestinal tumors have been reported. Most neoplasms produce the achalasia picture from direct invasion or compression of the gastroesophageal junction. Esophageal dysmotility resembling achalasia also can accompany malignancies that are remote from the esophagus through an immunologic reaction to the tumor. Diagnosis of such paraneoplastic syndromes requires a high index of suspicion.

Chagas' disease belongs to the differential diagnosis in areas where this disorder is endemic, particularly South America. Chagas' disease results from neuronal damage by the parasite *Trypanosoma cruzi*. Usually, damage to esophageal intramural nerve plexus occurs late in the disease, and a correlation between severity of the ganglion cell destruction and symptoms has been noted.

TREATMENT

Treatments for achalasia do not reverse inhibitory nerve damage, must be considered palliative, and can be classified as pharmacologic and nonpharmacologic (Table 11-4).

Pharmacologic Treatment

Pharmacologic treatments, including botulinum toxin injection, produce short-term benefits that

TABLE 11-4

TREATMENTS FOR ACHALASIA

Pharmacologic Treatments	
Per oral smooth-muscle relaxants	Nifedipine
Botulinum toxin injection	Isosorbide dinitrite
Nonpharmacologic Treatments	
Pneumatic dilatation	Open technique
Surgical myotomy	Minimally invasive technique (usually via laparoscopy)

may be helpful in the management of achalasia. Nifedipine (in standard, not extended- or slow-release preparations) and short-acting nitrates are the most studied oral pharmacologic agents. Nifedipine has a better side-effect profile, whereas nitrates may be more effective. In one study, 70% of patients with achalasia and minimal esophageal dilatation (<5 cm) treated with sublingual nifedipine before meals demonstrated a good to excellent initial clinical response without severe side effects. Oral pharmacologic agents are considered best used in those with early disease not accompanied by esophageal dilatation or when there are contraindications to pneumatic dilatation or surgery. Acute dosing with nifedipine (10–20 mg) can significantly decrease LES pressure and improve esophageal emptying, but a satisfactory long-term effect on emptying, prevention of eventual esophageal luminal dilatation, and avoidance of a more definitive treatment with pneumatic dilatation or myotomy are not expected outcomes from oral nonpharmacologic therapy.

Intrasphincteric botulinum toxin injection is a popular form of therapy with adult patients who have achalasia because of its simplicity and low risk, and this approach is efficacious in the majority for short-term symptom management. However, similar to oral pharmacologic treatment, botulinum toxin has a greater effect on symptoms than on LES pressure esophageal emptying. Consequently, it is not considered a suitable alternative to pneumatic dilatation or myotomy in the average patient with this disease. Duration of treatment response typically is brief. The duration of symptom relief appears to lengthen with subsequent injections, and treating patients on an as-needed basis may be the most acceptable management plan for patients who cannot tolerate pneumatic dilatation or surgery. The approach is not cost-effective and may actually interfere with the success of subsequent myotomy, if needed. Information on botulinum toxin injection in children is restricted to case reports.

Nonpharmacologic Treatment

Pneumatic Dilatation

Pneumatic dilatation remains an important management option for achalasia. The trend is to begin with smaller balloons and shorter inflation times; the response can be as good as with more aggressive approaches and complication rates are reduced. Most balloons used today have a predetermined size and are made of a modified polyethylene polymer mounted on a flexible polyethylene catheter. In children, the most common balloons are ≤30 mm in diameter when inflated. If necessary for older children, 35 and 40 mm diameter balloons are available. A reduction in LES resting pressure by more than 40% typically identifies the symptomatic responder to pneumatic dilatation. Likewise, and in contrast to observations with oral pharmacologic therapy or botulinum toxin injection, reduction in symptoms after treatment is associated with improvement in esophageal emptying. In fact, the combination of improved symptoms and improved emptying is an excellent predictor of a durable treatment response. In clinical practice, emptying can be assessed in a standardized way by measuring the height of the barium column 1 and 5 min after the patient ingests the barium in the upright position.

Like adults, many children require more than one pneumatic dilatation to attain or maintain response. Results in children have been variable and are difficult to compare across studies because of differences in technique used. For example, reported response rates have ranged from as low as 35% to as high as 100%. Esophageal perforation following pneumatic dilatation occurs in 1–12% of pediatric cases. In adults, the risk approaches 3% and at an older age, presence of a hiatus hernia or epiphrenic diverticulum, esophagitis, malnutrition, high amplitude esophageal contractions, and one or more previous dilatations may increase this number.

Surgical Therapy

The efficacy of surgical myotomy for achalasia is well established, whether the procedure is performed through an open or a minimally invasive approach—most information being derived from cohorts of surgically-treated adults. In one recent report, open myotomy and partial fundoplication via left thoracotomy (Belsey Mark IV repair) resulted in durable resolution of obstructive symptoms with improved esophageal emptying and reduced LES pressure over an average observation period of 7.2 years. However, it is the laparoscopic Heller myotomy that has gained wide acceptance as the primary surgical treatment of choice in achalasia, with outcomes equivalent to that from open operation. Partial fundoplication using the floppy-Toupet or floppy-Dor technique complements the procedure by providing an effective barrier against reflux; some investigators report low postoperative esophageal acid exposure even without an antireflux procedure. Laparoscopic myotomy can be performed safely in children, providing minimally invasive but definitive surgical options in the pediatric age group. Because the overall results after myotomy in children have been quite good, some authors have recently suggested that the primary treatment for children with achalasia should be surgical.

Intraoperative endoscopy during laparoscopic myotomy may be advantageous in guiding extent and verifying completion of the myotomy, possibly allowing preservation of natural antireflux mechanisms by directing precise dissection. However, data available to date on the specific use of intraoperative endoscopy are limited and uncontrolled, and more studies are required before the approach can be endorsed as routine.

The most common causes for surgical failure are incomplete myotomy and sclerosis of the myotomy site. Durable treatment options after surgical failure include pneumatic dilatation and repeat myotomy; the latter can be accomplished laparoscopically with good results in most instances.

PROGNOSIS

Complications from untreated achalasia include weight loss, malnutrition, and pulmonary disorders. Treatments that produce satisfactory esophageal emptying should prevent these complications. However, some disease progression can occur and result in further esophageal dilatation, anatomic changes around the LES region, and poorer esophageal emptying. The reason for this progression is not fully understood but may result from gradual advancement of the degenerative myenteric plexus process.

Squamous cell carcinoma can occur in patients with long-standing achalasia, a recent report suggesting an incidence of 1 cancer per approximately 175 patient-years of follow-up, equating to a cancer risk 140 times that of the general population. Barrett's metaplasia also has been reported in patients with long-standing achalasia, typically in association with gastroesophageal reflux after definitive therapy but also in untreated patients. Despite the amount of information establishing achalasia as a risk for subsequent esophageal carcinoma, the role of surveillance endoscopy remains debated. Some are recommending annual endoscopy for patients with achalasia of more than 15–20 years duration, regardless of symptoms.

Bibliography

Azizkhan RG, Tapper D, Eraklis A. Achalasia in childhood: a 20 year experience, *J Pediatr Surg* 15:452–456, 1980.

Clouse RE, Staiano A, Alrakawi A, Haroian L. Application of topographical methods to clinical esophageal manometry. *Am J Gastroenterol* 95(10):2720–2730, 2000.

Dunaway PM, Wong RK. Risk and surveillance intervals for squamous cell carcinoma in achalasia. *Gastrointest Endosc Clin North Am* 11(2):425–434, 2001.

Houlden H, Smith S, De Carvalho M, et al. Clinical and genetic characterization of families with triple A (Allgrove) syndrome. *Brain* 125(Pt 12):2681–2690, 2002.

Hussain SZ, Thomas R, Tolia V. A review of achalasia in 33 children. *Dig Dis Sci* 47(11):2538–2543, 2002.

Khoshoo V, LaGarde DC, Udall JN. Intrasphicteric injection of botulinum toxin for treating achalasia in children. *J Pediatr Gastroenterol Nutr* 24:439–441, 1997.

Mayberry JF. Epidemiology and demographics of achalasia. *Gastrointest Endosc Clin North Am* 11(2): 235–248, 2001.

McCord GS, Staiano A, Clouse RE. Achalasia, diffuse spasm and non-specific motor disorders. *Ballieres Clin Gastroenterol* 5:307, 1991.

Ruiz-de-Leon A, Mendoza J, Sevilla-Mantilla C, et al. Myenteric antiplexus antibodies and class II HLA in achalasia. *Dig Dis Sci* 47(1):15–19, 2002.

Staiano A, Clouse RE. Detection of incomplete lower esophageal sphincter relaxation with conventional point-pressure sensors. *Am J Gastroenterol* 96(12): 3258–3267, 2001.

Zaninotto G, Costantini M, Portale G, et al. Etiology, diagnosis, and treatment of failures after laparoscopic Heller myotomy for achalasia. *Ann Surg* 235(2): 186–192, 2002.

12

INFANTILE HYPERTROPHIC PYLORIC STENOSIS

Donald Liu and Stuart Zwang

INTRODUCTION

Infantile hypertrophic pyloric stenosis (IHPS) is a condition resulting from hypertrophy of the pylorus muscle. The lumen becomes obstructed by mucosa, resulting in a blockage of the lumen that extends from the stomach to the duodenum. The pyloric ring is no longer identifiable as a clearly definable separation between the normally distensible pyloric antrum and the duodenal cap. Instead, a channel of variable length (1.5–2.0 cm) corresponding to the pyloric canal separates the normally distensible portion of the antrum from the duodenal bulb. When viewed endoscopically, the mucosa protrudes as a nipple-like projection, likened to a cauliflower.

Although the cause of IHPS is still unknown, it is clearly associated with a failure of nitric oxide synthetase, resulting in a deficiency of nitric oxide and an inability of the smooth muscle of the pylorus to relax. Research has also indicated that when compared with control specimens, the muscular layer is deficient in the quantity of nerve terminals, markers for nerve-supporting cells, and peptide containing nerve fibers.

IHPS leads to several metabolic abnormalities, including metabolic alkalosis, hypochloremia, and hypokalemia. Frequent projectile vomiting in the infant leads to loss of stomach hydrochloric acid. The loss of hydrogen ions by vomiting causes cells to excrete potassium ions in an attempt to preserve electrolyte equilibrium; this condition can lead to hypokalemia. The loss of chloride ions may also lead to hypochloremia. Metabolic alkalosis results from a loss of acidic protons and an increased concentration of bicarbonate ion in response to a loss of chloride ions.

EPIDEMIOLOGY

IHPS is a common cause of gastric outlet obstruction in infants. It occurs in between 1.5 and 4.0 per 1000 live births (see Schwartz, 1998). The typical case is a first-born male infant presenting recurrent vomiting between 3 and 5 weeks of age; IHPS is more common in males than in females, for unclear reasons. Some evidence indicates a genetic predisposition to IHPS. Although there are reports suggesting that IHPS may be genetically inherited, it is most likely a multifactorial disease, not resulting from any congenital defect.

DIAGNOSIS

Clinical Symptoms

IHPS generally occurs in infants between 2 and 8 weeks of age. The main symptom is nonbilious projectile vomiting. Pyloric obstruction prevents the contents of the stomach from entering the small intestine; the contents of the stomach are ejected after several feedings. Due to gastric outlet obstruction, the presence of bile in the emesis is unlikely. The emesis may also have a coffee-ground appearance as a result of gastritis or esophagitis. Although affected infants remain hungry after vomiting, they generally are not febrile or ill appearing. The onset of dehydration, however, can produce lethargy. Diarrhea and jaundice are relatively uncommon symptoms. Vomiting often leads to hypokalemic alkalosis.

Physical examination reveals peristaltic waves in the upper right quadrant of the abdomen. The pylorus is palpable as a small, hard mass, or olive. The examiner should be able to roll the hypertrophied pylorus under the fingertips. Physical examination can be time-consuming and requires a cooperative infant. It has been less used and hence less successful in the past quarter-century as physicians have increasingly relied more heavily on ultrasonography.

Metabolic signs include hypochloremia and hypokalemic metabolic alkalosis (see Introduction). Weight loss and dehydration coupled with an insatiable appetite lead to a characteristic facies, with a furrowed brow, wrinkled appearance, and prominent sucking pattern. In emaciated infants, the distended stomach may be identifiable in hypochondrium, with active peristaltic activity visible through the thin abdominal wall.

Ultrasonography and Barium Upper Gastrointestinal (UGI) Examination

Ultrasonography has become the gold standard for diagnosis of IHPS. While standards for ultrasound interpretation vary slightly, the most commonly used criteria for positive identification are a pyloric muscle thickness of 4 mm or more, a pyloric channel length of 16 mm or more, and a pyloric diameter greater than 14 mm. Recent evidence suggests that the pyloric muscle appears thicker than normal in a state of water deprivation; these findings suggest that ultrasound examination should be performed when the infant is hydrated.

Barium upper gastrointestinal examination is also a useful diagnostic tool. A positive diagnosis requires that barium leave the stomach and form a "string sign" through the pylorus. This is required to differentiate IHPS from pylorospasm. If UGI is performed, residual barium should be aspirated from the stomach prior to surgery. There are several concerns with UGI, however. First, the barium meal may aspirate into the patient's lung. Secondly, it involves radiation exposure. Thirdly, it provides only indirect evidence of IHPS, while ultrasonography provides direct evidence. Fourthly, it requires time for the barium meal to reveal a string sign. For these reasons ultrasonography is preferable to UGI.

TREATMENT

Preoperative Treatment

Metabolic alkalosis in the infant can lead to hypoventilation and respiratory arrest after recovery from anesthesia. Thus, it is crucial that the infant's condition be stabilized prior to surgery. The infant should be rehydrated and normal electrolyte levels should be restored.

Operative Treatment

Prior to anesthesia, the infant's stomach must be aspirated. The standard operative procedure is the Ramstedt pyloromyotomy. This involves an incision of the serosa on the anterior wall of the hypertrophied pylorus just proximal of the pyloric vein to the antrum just proximal to the area of the hypertrophied muscle. The serosa is then spread by using a spreading clamp (see Figs. 12-1 and 12-2). It is important to avoid both an incomplete myotomy and a perforation of the mucosa.

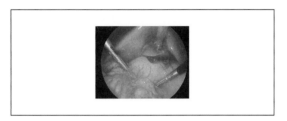

HYERTROPHIED PYLORUS PREPYLOROMYOTOMY

Laparoscopic pylorotomy has gained increasing acceptance in recent years. Studies suggest that laparoscopy produces a better cosmetic result, seems to produce less postoperative discomfort, and results in the absence of conversion in a shorter hospital stay. It is likely that average procedure lengths will decrease as laparoscopy is used more frequently.

Postoperative Treatment

Most infants can begin feedings about 6 h after surgery. Infants who present with hematemesis from gastritis may benefit from delaying feedings for an additional 6–12 h. Although more aggressive feeding schedules allow for earlier discharge, they increase the incidence of vomiting. Table 12-1 represents a general postoperative feeding schedule.

OUTCOME

Mortality rates are low. They most commonly result from perforation or infection. Furthermore,

TABLE 12-1

POSTPYLOROMYOTOMY FEEDING SCHEDULE

Pedialyte, 30 mL orally every 3 h × 2
Half-strength formula, 30 mL orally every 3 h × 1
Full-strength formula, 30 mL orally every 3 h × 1
Full-strength formula, 45 mL orally every 3 h × 2
Full-strength formula, 60 mL orally every 3 h × 2
Full-strength formula, 90 mL orally every 3 h × 2
Full-strength formula as desired

the long-term sequelae from pyloromyotomy are minimal.

Bibliography

Kobayashi H, Puri P. Selective reduction in intramuscular nerve supporting cells in infantile hypertrophic pyloric stenosis. *J Pediatr Surg* 29:651–654, 1994.

Malmfors G, Sundler F. Peptidergic innervation in infantile hypertrophic pyloric stenosis. *J Pediatr Surg* 21:303–306, 1986.

Okazaki T, Atsuyuki Y, Fijiwara T, et al. Abnormal distribution of nerve terminals in infantile hypertrophic pyloric stenosis. *J Pediatr Surg* 29:655–658, 1994.

Schwartz MZ. Hypertrophic pyloric stenosis. In: O'Neill, James A Jr, Rowe MI, Grosfeld JL, et al. (eds.), *Pediatric Surgery*, 5th ed. Mos by-Year Book Inc. St. Louis, MO, 1998, p. 112.

Sitsen E, Bax NMA, van der Zee DC. Is laparoscopic pyloromyotomy superior to open surgery? *Surg Endosc* 12:813–815, 1998.

Starinsky R, Klin B, Siman-Tov Y, et al. Does dehydration affect thickness of the pyloric muscle? An experimental study. *Ultrasound Med Biol* 28:421–423, 2002.

Wattchow D, Cass D, Furness J, et al. Abnormalities of peptide-containing nerve fibers in infantile hypertrophic pyloric stenosis. *Gastroenterology* 92:443–448, 1987.

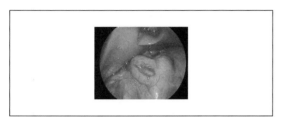

FIGURE 12-2

HYERTROPHIED PYLORUS POSTPYLOROMYOTOMY

13

GASTROESOPHAGEAL REFLUX

Francesca Cavataio and Stefano Guandalini

INTRODUCTION

For many years, the esophagus has been considered as an inactive tube suitable only for the passage of food and beverages from the mouth to the stomach. Only recently it has been demonstrated that transportation is only one of the several functions that characterized esophageal physiology. A great number of anatomic structures maintain the integrity of this organ and several mechanisms, some of which are still not well defined, are involved in its well functioning.

Gastroesophageal reflux (GER) can be considered the most common esophageal disorder both in children and in adults and typical symptoms of reflux are by far the most frequent complaints leading infants to the pediatric gastroenterologist's observation.

Though incidence, clinical presentation, and natural history of GER have been well characterized in recent years, no evidence-based guidelines for the diagnosis and treatment of the disease in the pediatric age exist in the literature; however, clinical practice guidelines with definitions for the categories of evidence have been published in 2001 by the GER Guideline Committee of the North American Society for Pediatric Gastroenterology, Hepatology, and Nutrition (NASPGHAN).[1]

By definition, GER is the retrograde passage of gastric contents into the esophagus and is quite a physiologic event; GER episodes occur several times a day in infants, children, and adults.

GER can be symptomatic or asymptomatic; symptomatic reflux presents with a great variety of symptoms (but regurgitation, vomiting, or respiratory symptoms generally prevail in the pediatric age); when reflux does not extend above the distal esophagus or when it does not affect the integrity of esophageal mucosa, it can occur in absence of symptoms. This latter condition has received recently great attention because it seems to expose patient to the risk of GER complications and to severe adult's disease.

Reflux becomes pathogenic when it occurs too frequently and when those defensive mechanisms that prevent esophageal mucosa to be damaged by noxious refluxate are defective. Under these circumstances, it results in gastroesophageal reflux disease (GERD), also named pathogenic GER.

Consequently, GERD cannot be considered an "all or none" phenomenon; it can be defined as symptomatic GER with associated complications. The most important complications of GER are esophagitis, malnutrition, and severe respiratory disease.

GERD differs from symptomatic GER in epidemiology, diagnostic approach, and natural history.

GER prevails in the first years of life and, at that age, is common and self-limited. It is also simply indicated as "spitting up" (babies who present this are referred to as "happy spitters") and resolves as lower esophageal sphincter (LES) and esophageal functions mature and the child passes from liquid to solid foods and from supine to upright posture. It does not need any diagnostic procedure; conservative measures and parental reassurance are usually all that is required while waiting for the condition to resolve.

GERD on the other hand may present at any age, sometimes following more severe forms of symptomatic GER that do not tend to recover after anti-GER therapy. GERD has often to be investigated by the means of one or more of several diagnostic procedures that are available; it has to be vigorously treated with pharmacologic therapy or, in refractory cases and in particular situations, with surgical intervention.

EPIDEMIOLOGY

The prevalence of GER depends on patients' age. In infants, epidemiologic data concerning GER are affected by the favorable outcome of the condition. Since reflux may be asymptomatic by definition, not all the babies with GER come to the attention of the pediatrician—only one-third of symptomatic infants receive medical attention. Excessive maternal anxiety is the first cause of over-estimation of the problem. Prevalence rates are variable in different population studies but it is clear that GER is a very common event in the first year of life. About 50% of 2-month-old infants regurgitate twice a day or more; the highest prevalence (67%) is reached around the fourth month and then the prevalence drops to 1% at 1 year; the sharpest drop is around 6 months and is probably related to the development of both improved neuromuscular control and infant's sitting up. The condition resolves in nearly all the patients within the first 12 months with no diagnostic evaluation and minimal intervention.[2]

There are no certain data on gender predilection or on peak age of onset beyond infancy.

Only a small percentage of infants will develop GERD; prevalence data are almost unknown, especially after the first year of life. GERD, as it happens for GER, is more frequent in infants than in children; it seems to affect 1:300 infants in the first year but, after this period, very little is known about its prevalence and natural history. Little is known about the prevalence of GERD in children or adolescents.

Interestingly, GER clusters in families, suggesting that a genetic component may be involved; some studies shared that maternal history of GER is significantly related both to infant spitting and to GER at 9 years, others described a higher frequency of GER in siblings; others showed a genetic component.

The possible existence of a gene for severe pediatric GERD mapping to chromosome 13q14 has also been reported (12, 13). This genetic locus has not been confirmed in another study and this seems to suggest genetic heterogeneity in familial pediatric gastroesophageal reflux disease.

PATHOGENESIS OF GER

GER pathogenesis is multifactorial, but the main mechanism is represented by inappropriate transient relaxations of the lower esophageal sphincter (TLESRs).[3]

TLESR is described as a reduction of LES tone to the level of gastric pressure lasting 5–35 s not associated with swallowing or with peristalsis; during this fraction of time the anatomic structures of the "antireflux barrier" remove their contribution to gastroesophageal competence so that gastric material, eventually contained in the stomach, may pass in the distal esophagus. These relaxations are mediated by a vagal reflex pathway. TLESRs can be physiologic. In fact, they occur with a frequency of five times in the first postprandial hour, causing brief episodes of reflux.

Physiologic reflux episodes are brief because esophageal clearing rapidly removes the refluxate

TABLE 13-1

THE THREE PHYSIOLOGIC LINES OF DEFENSE
OPERATING IN PREVENTING GERD

1. Antireflux barrier
   LES → limits the frequency and volume of
   refluxed gastric contents
2. Esophageal clearing
   Esophageal peristalsis, gravity and secretions →
   limit the duration of contact between luminal
   contents and esophageal epithelium
3. Tissue or esophageal mucosal resistance
   Quality of refluxate, mucosal intrinsic factors →
   limit the damage of gastric contents on
   esophageal mucosa

TABLE 13-2

MECHANISMS INVOLVED IN THE PATHOGENESIS
OF GER

Increased Frequency of Reflux Episodes
Abnormalities of antireflux barrier
TLESR
Reduced basal LES tone
Perisphincteric factors (hiatal hernia)
Increased gastric volume
Large/liquid meals
Delayed gastric emptying
Increased intraabdominal pressure
Contracture of the abdominal wall
   Cough, crying
    Externally applied abdominal pressure
    Obesity
Environmental factors
Drugs
Diet

Decreased Esophageal Clearing
Disorders of peristalsis (primary and secondary)
Gravity effects
Saliva

Reduced Mucosal Resistance to Refluxate
Increased noxiousness of refluxate
Mucosal intrinsic factors

from the mucosa, preventing tissue to be damaged by gastric material; even in those cases when the refluxate cannot be removed rapidly, other protective mechanisms (described in Table 13-1) help preventing esophageal damage.

In pathologic conditions, these defensive lines break down; several mechanisms (Table 13-2) may be responsible for increased frequency of reflux episodes, decreased esophageal clearing, and reduced mucosal resistance to refluxate.

Increased Frequency of Reflux Episodes

Children with GERD show increased frequency and/or duration of reflux episodes especially during fasting periods and during sleep. This phenomenon may result from

1. *Alteration of the antireflux barrier*—Hypotonic LES leads to inappropriate TLESRs that account for more than 90% of reflux episodes in children and adults.
2. *Increased gastric volume*—Gastric volume is determined by the ingested meal, gastric secretions, and gastric emptying. An association exists between GERD and delayed gastric emptying, as 50% of infants affected with GERD have delayed gastric emptying.

3. *Increased intraabdominal pressure*—In pediatric age increases in intraabdominal pressure are common and may be detected in more than 50% of reflux episodes.
4. *Environmental factors*—They include medications (i.e., diazepam, theophylline), dietary habits (i.e., overeating, eating late at night, assuming a supine position shortly after eating), type of foods (i.e., chocolate, peppermint, fatty or highly acidic foods, caffeine), food allergies, smoking, alcohol, and so on.

Decreased Esophageal Clearing

In GERD, reflux episodes are also increased in duration. This probably indicates a dysfunction of esophageal clearance due to

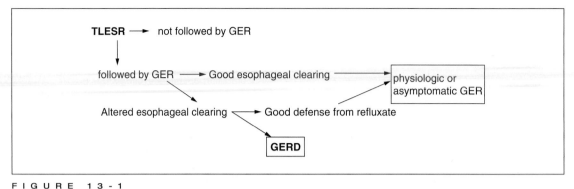

FIGURE 13-1

SEQUENCE OF EVENTS LEADING TO GER/GERD

1. *Abnormalities in peristalsis*—Nonspecific esophageal motility disorders may result in simultaneous and repetitive contractions that may decrease esophageal clearing.
2. *Gravity*—In the upright position gravity plays a key role by preceding the peristaltic waves in carrying the bolus down by the esophagus.
3. *Saliva*—Saliva helps the esophageal transport. A reduced production may be responsible for decreased buffering of acidic material present in the esophagus.

Reduced Mucosal Resistance to Refluxate

It is due to the increased noxiousness of refluxate and to the reduced activity of mucosal intrinsic factors such as mucosal barrier to ions' passage, mucosal blood flow, mucus, prostaglandins, and epithelial growth factors.

The factors described earlier are some of those involved in the pathogenesis of GERD and they operate in a complex and sequential net of events that is simplified in Fig. 13-1.

CLINICAL PRESENTATION

GER may present with a wide variety of symptoms, regurgitation and vomiting being the most frequent in the pediatric age. In recent years, several new clinical pictures have been described and thus symptoms of presentation may to date be divided into esophageal (usual) and extraesophageal (unusual).

GERD is characterized by complications of GER (especially esophagitis, malnutrition, or respiratory disease) and hence, in the pediatric age, it presents with substernal pain or heartburn, anemia, severe respiratory symptoms, or failure to thrive. Esophagitis may develop even in absence of symptoms. The most important symptoms of presentation of GERD are listed in Table 13-3.

In general, regurgitation/vomiting, airway obstruction, and feeding difficulties are more common in infants, whereas adult-like symptoms and airway irritation are more frequent in children older than 2 years.

In a clinical setting it is useful to divide patients in two subsets according to age: infants and children older than 2 years.

GER/GERD in Infants

Regurgitation and Vomiting

These are considered the main presenting symptoms of GER in infancy. Regurgitation can be defined as the effortless passage of refluxed gastric contents into the oral pharynx; vomiting is a forced expulsion of the refluxed gastric contents from the mouth with the participation of gastric muscles.

A high percentage of infants suffering from GER present as "happy spitters"—they regurgitate

TABLE 13-3

SIGNS AND SYMPTOMS OF GERD

Esophageal (usual symptoms)	Regurgitation/vomiting with
	Poor weight gain
	Anemia
	Dysphagia
	Heartburn/chest pain
	Hematemesis
Extraesophageal (unusual symptoms)	Pulmonary
	Chronic cough
	Asthma
	Wheezing
	Recurrent pneumonia
	Airway obstruction
	Aspiration
	Otolaryngologic problems
	Otitis media, "glue ear"
	Chronic sinusitis
	Laryngospasm/recurrent croup
	Laryngitis
	Laryngomalacia
	Stridor (chronic or recurrent)
	Hoarseness and voice disorders
	Subglottic stenosis
	Subglottic edema
	Others
	Distressed behavior
	Feeding problems
	Apnea (obstructive or reflex)
	ALTE
	Sandifer's syndrome
	Dental erosion

small amounts of food in absence of other symptoms and look otherwise healthy, happy, and well-thriving. Vomiting episodes may be present at medical history. This physiologic condition, though harmless and spontaneously resolving as the baby grows older, is responsible for parental anxiety especially when regurgitation is frequent, when large amounts of food are vomited or when the infants cry frequently.

Physiologic GER is characterized by postprandial regurgitation; on the contrary, it is advisable to consider suspected for GERD: episodes of regurgitation immediately before a new feeding, evidence of regurgitated material on the pillow after sleep, and episodes of crying that interrupt feeding or sleep (equivalent of heartburn in adults).

The quantification of the number of episodes of regurgitation or vomiting as long as the calculation of the amount of food regurgitated gives poor evidence of the severity of the disease. In fact, not all the reflux episodes are followed by regurgitation: some AA have demonstrated that fewer than 10%

of scintigraphically detected episodes of reflux to the upper esophagus were regurgitated from the mouth; nonetheless, there is evidence that even "silent refluxers" may show a certain degree of esophagitis at endoscopic examination.

Esophagitis

Esophagitis is the most important complication of GERD; in infancy, apart from hematemesis or anemia, it is responsible for food refusal and consequent poor weight gain and for distressed behavior. Anemia may be caused by continuous small losses of blood (that can be detected as occult blood in the stools). Food refusal is the result of a strong aversion to food caused by acute pain arising after the passage of ingested materials through an inflamed structure; feeding progressively transforms in a "negative experience" that, if not treated, may lead to total refusal. Poor weight gain is not always due to esophagitis; if large amounts of food are vomited, adequate daily caloric intake may not be maintained and failure to thrive may ensue. Respiratory problems are due to airway responsiveness to refluxate and are not necessarily associated with esophagitis.

Distressed Behavior

The infant with distressed behavior (caused by the discomfort due to acidic reflux episodes) looks like associating feeding with a disturbing situation: he/she becomes irritable, cries while arching the back, and refuses to feed. In addition, he/she may suffer from evening colic and/or alterations in sleeping pattern. In recent years, infantile colic has been used as a quantifiable measure of irritability: normal infants were considered those who fussed or cried intermittently for an average of 2 h per day. Actually, wide individual variations occur. Variable also is parental perception of the event. Similarly, the sleeping patterns of infants show such a great individual variation in maturation that it is still not possible to establish what is normal. Evidence concerning the relationship between reflux and irritability in infancy is still controversial and a certain overlap with cow's milk-allergic infants can be supposed.

In a recent study some peculiar behaviors, described as "discomfort" (crying or frowning), "emission" (of liquid or gas, i.e., regurgitation, drooling, or burping), yawning, stridor, stretching, mouthing, hiccupping, sneezing, thumb-sucking, coughing, or gagging, have been associated temporally with the onset of reflux events. The cause-effect relationship is however unclear, as some of these behavioral changes appeared to be the cause rather than the consequence of reflux.

Apneic Spells

Apneic spell is defined as the cessation of breathing for a period sufficient (at least 20 s) to produce bradycardia and cyanosis; usually the infant stops breathing, is flushed, presents staring eyes, and becomes progressively more hypertonic and cyanotic. As the apneic spell ends, the infant looks extremely pale and hypotonic.

The relationship between apnea and GERD is controversial; while there are reports of simultaneous recordings of esophageal pH, heart rate, chest wall movement, and nasal airflow demonstrating that reflux could precede apnea, in other studies this temporal relationship is not convincing suggesting a primary impairment in the regulation of respiration. Some AA reported that the majority of prolonged apnea episodes are not associated with regurgitation, but gross emesis or oral regurgitation can be correlated with either prolonged apnea (>20 s) or with shorter apnea and bradycardia. Other studies reported an occasional correlation of GER with short mixed apneas (5–15 s).

Apnea may be central or obstructive in pathogenesis; in GER-induced apnea both mechanisms may be involved: airway obstruction by refluxates and laryngospasm mediated by the stimulation of laryngeal receptors.

Apparent Life-Threatening Event

An apparent life-threatening event (ALTE) is defined as an episode of prolonged infant apnea, associated with change in skin and lips color (first redness, then cyanosis or even pallor), change in muscle tone (muscle weakness and limpness), choking, and gagging in an attack frightening to the caregiver.

ALTE was once defined "near miss syndrome," but the relationship with sudden infant death syndrome (SIDS) is still not definite. ALTE is observed in approximately 2–3% of the general pediatric population, the first event usually occurring between 1 and 2 months, rarely after 8 months of age. ALTEs can recur. One suggested mechanism by which GERD may trigger an ALTE is acid stimulation of laryngeal, pharyngeal, or esophageal chemoreceptors with resultant laryngospasm and prolonged apnea. Other causes of ALTE may be central apnea, obstructive apnea, cardiac arrhythmia, and seizure disorders. Children who experienced ALTEs are known to have vagal hyperactivity.

Respiratory Symptoms

The most frequent respiratory complaint due to GERD in infancy is recurrent wheezing; wheezing generally occurs in an infant whose airways are predisposed to hyperrespond to common inflammatory stimuli such as viral infections; recurrent wheezing is common in infancy and is particularly difficult to manage because of parental anxiety and lack of response to conventional therapy; in around two-thirds of infants affected by recurrent wheezing the disturbance is transient, while in one-third asthma will develop after months or years. The term "happy wheezier" applies to an infant with persistent or intermittent wheezing who shows chronic recurrences of the symptom for weeks and months especially when teething and at night, but who is active, happy and smiling, and not at all distressed. GERD is sometimes involved in infant wheezing but cow's milk allergy is more often associated.

GER/GERD in Children Older than 2 Years

Adult-like Symptoms

In this category dysphagia, odynophagia, heartburn, and substernal pain are included; also abdominal pain (especially epigastric), regurgitation or reswallowing and vomiting, anorexia, and other dyspeptic symptoms. Dyspepsia is a term used in adults but it actually encompasses age-dependent symptoms such as feeding-associated irritability in the infant, periumbilical pain in the younger child, and heartburn, nausea, and digestive discomfort in older child and in adults.

Heartburn (or substernal pain) is typical of older children and adults while in younger children the localization may be referred more as epigastric pain; these symptoms are caused by GERD irrespectively from presence or absence of endoscopic esophagitis.

Rumination, another symptom of presentation of GER, is the return of sour fluids into the mouth with reswallowing of the material; the child/teenager affected presents with repeated mastication movements. Rumination is more frequent in neurologically impaired subjects.

Esophagitis may be also responsible for problems with deglutition: discomfort or pain (odynophagia) or difficulty (dysphagia); it is also the cause of chronic blood loss (with consequent anemia), hematemesis, melena, or hypoproteinemia.

Respiratory Disturbances

Wheezing and airway obstruction are typical manifestation of GER in infancy, whereas asthma and recurrent pneumonia are the most frequent manifestations of GER in children and adolescents.

The true incidence of GER in children with asthma is not known and the relationship between gastroesophageal reflux and asthma is complex. It is not clear if GER is a concomitant finding in asthma, if it induces or exacerbates asthma.

There are three mechanisms proposed to explain how GER may cause asthma:

1. Macroaspiration of gastric contents into the lungs resulting in irritational bronchospasm
2. Microaspiration of gastric contents into the upper airway leading to stimulation of upper airway receptors and bronchospasm
3. Stimulation of esophageal chemoreceptors resulting in vagally mediated bronchoconstriction

Symptoms of GER may be present in children with asthma while in high percentage of children with persistent asthma gastroesophageal reflux may be detectable only by abnormal esophageal pH monitoring, the reported prevalence of pH monitoring abnormalities ranging from 25 to 75% at any age.

GER may be responsible for recurrent pneumonia following aspiration; recurrent pneumonia may arise in the absence of esophagitis. The incidence of GER and recurrent pneumonia in otherwise normal infants and children is difficult to establish since reported studies have included among patients a large number of children with neurologic disabilities and anatomic disorders of the upper intestinal tract. Several reports show that pediatric patients with recurrent pneumonia and GER improve after receiving medical or surgical GER therapy. Repeated small episodes of aspiration of gastric contents can eventually cause chronic pulmonary fibrosis.

Otolaryngologic Problems

Gastroesophageal reflux is an important factor in otolaryngologic problems. Symptoms of GER localized in the head and neck are not as obviously linked to reflux as in the case of the typical epigastric and substernal complaints.

Even though the symptoms are very noticeable (Table 13-4) physical findings can be subtle or absent; the diagnosis is clear even without special diagnostic measures when the regurgitation of

TABLE 13-4

OTOLARINGOLOGIC SYMPTOMS

Chronic sinusitis
Chronic cough
Reflux laryngitis, hoarseness, and throat clearing
Globus pharyngeus
Oropharyngeal dysphagia
Chronic sore throat
Otalgia/otitis media
Vocal cord granulomas and ulcers
Recurrent croup/spasmodic croup
Laryngomalacia
Pseudolaryngomalacia (GER-induced stridor)
Subglottic stenosis

gastric juice causes choking, burning, and laryngospasm. Gastronasal reflux and laryngotracheal reflux are probably the mechanisms by which GER is implicated in the pathogenesis of otolaryngologic symptoms. There is a mix between microaspiration, which may represent inadequate airway protection mechanisms and reflexive responses to esophageal refluxate, which may represent over-effective airway protection mechanisms.

GER plays a causative role in subglottic stenosis, recurrent croup, apnea, and chronic cough. It is an important inflammatory cofactor in laryngomalacia and possibly in true vocal cord granulomas and ulcers. GER is also thought to be an important inflammatory cofactor in chronic sinusitis and otitis (but its relationship with chronic otitis is still not defined) but in the older patients there are problems of differential diagnosis with chronic illness. Oropharyngeal dysphagia (i.e., impaired passage of food from the mouth to the upper esophagus) is sometimes described as GER-related; though evidence exists that vagal-mediated reflexes, triggered by the stimulation of esophageal chemoreceptors with consequent esophageal dysmotility, may be responsible for oropharyngeal dysphagia, a primitive or secondary swallowing dysfunction may also be at the basis of the disturbance.

In the case of complaints such as hoarseness, chronic laryngitis, globus sensation, and chronic sore throat, when other inflammatory causes have been excluded, diagnostic measures to rule out GER are recommended.

Sandifer's Syndrome

Sandifer's syndrome is characterized by stereotypical, repetitive stretching, and arching movements of the head and neck that are mistaken for atypical seizures or dystonia; the child's head tends to bend on the shoulder probably to avoid noxious refluxate to reach the upper portion of the esophagus.

Dental Erosions

Evidence suggesting GER-related dental erosions in the pediatric age is controversial; one study suggested that adolescents with GER had an increased incidence of erosion of enamel on the lingual surfaces of their teeth but another study showed no increased incidence of dental erosions in adolescents with abnormal esophageal pH monitoring.

Neurologically Impaired Children

Almost all neurologically impaired children (NIC) suffer from GERD and GER-related symptoms. The pathophysiology of reflux in these subjects is particularly complicated and multifactorial: (1) the neurologic disease itself may be responsible for delayed esophageal clearance and delayed gastric emptying and also for swallowing disorders; (2) the almost always recumbent position is a factor that prevent gravity to exert its beneficial function on the esophageal clearance thus exposing esophageal mucosa to higher degree of acidic contact; (3) constipation contributes to increase abdominal pressure. NIC are known to have high incidence of recurrent respiratory infections and malnutrition; GER in these patients may be responsible for both aspiration (that may aggravate respiratory symptoms) and regurgitation (that may decrease caloric intake with consequent worsening of malnutrition). It has to be emphasized that GER may not always be present in NIC (as it has been demonstrated by the persistence of symptoms after surgical treatment); sometimes isolated swallowing dysfunctions without GER are the prevalent cause of aspiration. In these cases, nasogastric tube feeding is necessary to restore acceptable clinical conditions. When GER is poorly recognized on the basis of clinical symptoms, NIC are exposed to the development of severe complications such as esophageal strictures or Barrett's esophagus.

Children with "Silent GERD"

Apart from infants, who may present with esophagitis even if asymptomatic or in the absence of severe degree of pHmetric reflux but who resolve spontaneously their disease, the term "silent GERD" applies to children who undergo instrumental examinations (pH monitoring and endoscopy) for reasons other than the detection of GER (i.e., the diagnosis

of celiac disease) and who are discovered affected by severe esophageal lesions.

The intensive use of pediatric endoscopy, especially after the recent reports of high proportion of organic abnormalities found in recurrent abdominal pain and after the increasing number of diagnosis of *Helicobacter pylori* infection, has led to the discovery of GERD in larger series of subjects.

Diagnosis

Assessing the infant or young child with symptoms or signs suspicious for GERD is largely guided by history and physical examination. In fact, in most infants with recurrent regurgitations and occasional vomiting, history and physical examination are often sufficient to reliably diagnose GERD, recognize complications, and initiate management.

A vast array of diagnostic tests and procedures are available to diagnose GERD and to assess the patient for its complications, but only a few need to be considered.

Upper GI X-Ray Series

This test is neither sensitive nor specific enough to diagnose GERD. In fact, sensitivity, specificity, and positive predictive value of the upper GI series range from 31 to 86%, 21 to 83%, and 80 to 82%, respectively when compared to esophageal pH monitoring.

However, it should be used whenever the infant or child being evaluated is suspected—in addition of GERD—of other possible disorders such as pyloric stenosis, malrotation, annular pancreas or, in the older child, hiatal hernia or advanced complications of GERD such as esophageal strictures. If the indication is only to rule out GERD, then the test should *not* be obtained.

Esophageal pH Monitoring

This remains the best and most direct way to assess the presence of GERD. The pH monitoring must be conducted for 24 h, obviously in the absence of any antacid treatment since at least 72 h, and will provide a valid, reliable, and reproducible measure of acid reflux. The test is performed by placing calibrated microelectrodes in the distal esophagus to detect intraluminal pH changes below 4.0; the pH probe is connected to a small device about the size of a portable recorder; the probe is inserted through the nose and the tip is located at 87% of the distance between the nares and the LES, calculated manometrically or using the Strobel formula:

Esophageal length

$$= 6.7 + [0.226 \ \text{height (cm)}] \quad \text{(oral)}$$

or

Esophageal length

$$= 5 + [0.252 \ \text{height (cm)}] \quad \text{(nasal)}$$

Intraluminal pH values are determined every 4–8 s and recorded during day and night with patients fully carrying out their physiologic activities; a reflux episode is defined as esophageal pH <4 for at least 15 s; computerized analysis calculate some parameters. This test is now indicated as the "silver," rather than the golden standard, as it may miss the rare instances of GERD where the refluxate is not acidic. Age-appropriate standards are available from reference populations, usually infants and children with other GI complaints, so that the pH probe can yield results regarding the frequency of GER episodes, the duration of episodes (related to clearance from the esophagus), and the relationship of episodes of GER to other symptoms (e.g., pain, posturing, coughing, hiccups, and wheezing). Table 13-5 reports the limits

of normal, on which the interpretation of the 24-h pH monitoring is based. Of the three indexes indicated in the table, the single one most used to conclude on the presence of GER and on its severity is the "reflux index," i.e., the percentage time that the probe read a pH below 4.0.

The usefulness of esophageal pH monitoring in infants with apnea or ALTEs has not been demonstrated. Heart rate, chest wall movement, nasal airflow, and oxygen saturation must be recorded simultaneously to esophageal pH monitoring to provide meaningful information on patients with ALTEs.

It should be finally stressed that the technique has some limits: it has a poor interobservers reproducibility, it does not detect nonacidic reflux (e.g., postprandial reflux in infants), it does not measure the volume of refluxed fluid in the esophagus and the distance covered by this fluid, and it cannot detect GERD complications (i.e., esophagitis) that may develop despite normal acid reflux. Furthermore, esophageal pH monitoring may be normal in some patients with GERD, particularly those with respiratory complications.

Upper GI Endoscopy with Biopsy

This procedure can assess the presence and severity of esophagitis (thus indirectly establishing the diagnosis of GERD), strictures, and Barrett's esophagus. It must be stressed however that normal endoscopic and histologic findings *do* not rule out GERD, as esophagitis is only a complication of this condition, and as such by definition is not present in all cases. Endoscopy may be very useful in patients with GERD resistant to common treatment practices (see below), as it may disclose the presence of an otherwise hidden eosinophilic esophagitis or of other diagnoses (e.g., gastritis and peptic ulcer).

Endoscopic esophageal damage is graded using different classifications: Savary-Miller grading of esophagitis use a scale of 1–4 with increasing severity of damage (Table 13-6).

In every endoscopy, even when the visual appearance of the esophageal mucosa is normal, mucosal biopsies should be obtained, as it is known

T A B L E   1 3 - 5

24-HR PH-PROBE MONITORING: MAIN UPPER LIMITS OF NORMAL VALUES

	Infants	Children	Adults
No. of daily episodes of reflux	73	25	45
No. of episodes of reflux ≥5 min	9.7	6.8	3.2
Reflux index (% of time pH < 4)	11.7%	5.4%	6%

TABLE 13-6

SAVARY-MILLER GRADING OF ESOPHAGITIS

Grade 0	Normal esophagus with no macroscopic damage
Grade 1—Erythema	Few areas of erythema, mucosal friability, and contact bleeding; linear, nonconfluent erosions
Grade 2—Linear erosions	Small superficial linear erosions, confluent and noncircumferential, associated with exudative lesions
Grade 3—Circumferential erosions	Erosions extending to the whole circumference of the esophagus; cobblestone appearance created by islands of edematous tissue between the erosions
Grade 4—Stricture	Extensive mucosal damage with deep ulcers. Strictures and possible metaplasia (Barrett's esophagus)

that a normal appearance at endoscopy is often seen in cases where a well-documented microscopic esophagitis exists. In addition, histologic findings are extremely important in determining the nature of esophagitis (peptic, allergic, eosinophilic, or infectious). Histologic classification of esophagitis may vary from center to center, an example being shown in Table 13-7.

Two categories of histologic changes are suggestive of esophagitis: reactive epithelial changes (including basal hyperplasia and papillary elongation) and inflammatory changes (infiltration by neutrophils, lymphocytes, and eosinophils). The exact role of eosinophils in reflux esophagitis is debated; it was once believed that eosinophils were the hallmark of peptic esophagitis; today, however, a high number of eosinophils seem to suggest allergic rather than peptic etiology especially when they are found in the proximal or middle esophagus. Moreover, the higher the number of eosinophils (>10 per high power field), the higher the possibility of eosinophilic esophagits (see Chap. 16).

Ultrasonography

Its use in the diagnosis of GER is controversial. Though not sensitive or specific in detecting pathologic reflux, it has been demonstrated to be particularly useful in evaluating gastric emptying in infants less than 6 months.

TABLE 13-7

HISTOLOGIC CLASSIFICATION OF ESOPHAGITIS

Grade	Histologic Criteria	Clinical Diagnosis
0	Normal	Normal
1	Basal zone hyperplasia Elongated stromal papillae Vascular ingrowth	Reflux
2	Polymorphonuclear (PMN) cells in the epithelium, the lamina propria or both	Esophagitis
3	PMN cells with epithelial ulcerations	Esophagitis
4	Aberrant columnar epithelium	Esophagitis + Barrett's esophagus

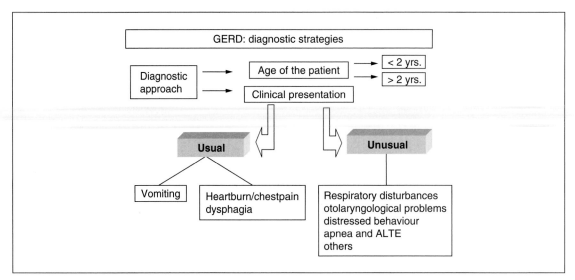

FIGURE 13-2

DIAGNOSTIC STRATEGIES IN APPROACHING GER

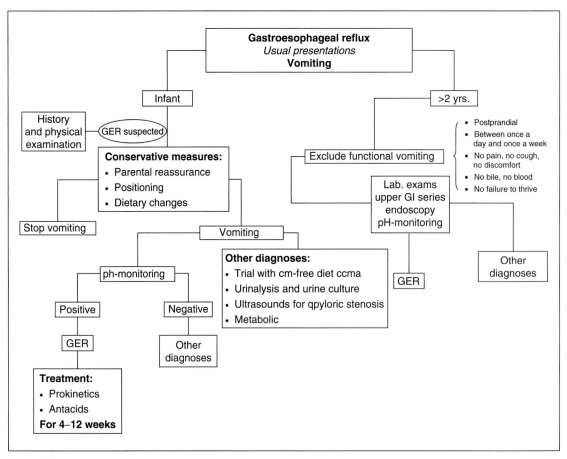

FIGURE 13-3

ALGORITHM I

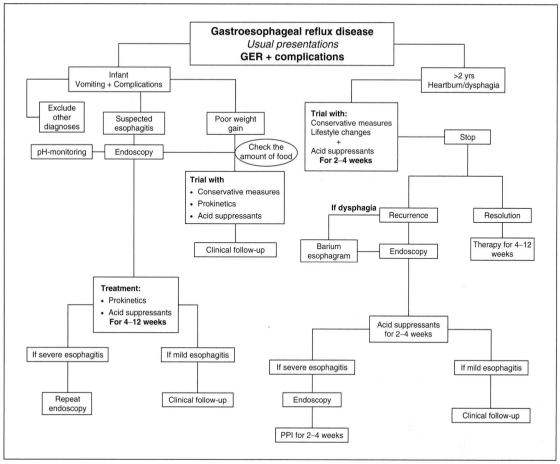

FIGURE 13-4

ALGORITHM II

Intraluminal Esophageal Impedance Technique

pH-independent intraluminal esophageal impedance technique has recently been used to measure fluid movements rather than luminal pH changes: it relies on the higher conductivity of a liquid bolus compared with esophageal muscular wall or air; so far, the technique has been validated in adults.

The technique has strong limitation because recording is limited to short periods during which the children are not in physiologic conditions (supine and motionless). It is likely that in the next few years a combination of pH monitoring and impedance data will provide the best accuracy in the diagnosis of GER.

Recommended Diagnostic Approaches

Figure 13-2 illustrates the diagnostic strategies to be implemented when approaching a patient with GER. The algorithms I–III reported in Figs. 13-3–13-5 present in a schematic way the suggested diagnostic and therapeutic steps to be undertaken when approaching patients presenting, respectively, these clinical situations

- Recurrent vomiting in either an infant or a child older than 2 years, uncomplicated (algorithm 1)
- Recurrent vomiting in either an infant or a child older than 2 years, with signs or symptoms of complicated reflux (algorithm 2)

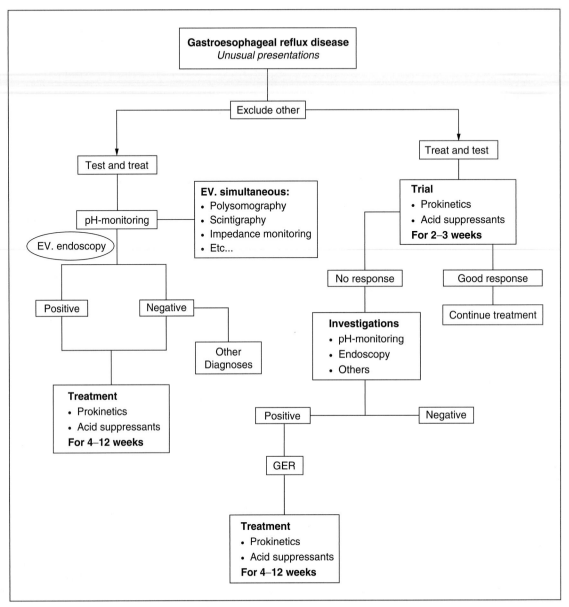

FIGURE 13-5

ALGORITHM III

- Unusual presentations (i.e., distressed behavior and unexplained feeding problems; apnea and ALTE; asthma; recurrent pneumonia; an otolaryngologic problems (algorithm 3)

The algorithms are self-explanatory.

Treatment

Removing the cause of the disease, the ideal of all pediatric intervention, is clearly rarely possible in GERD, as this condition has a multifactorial pathogenesis. For this reason, a correct therapeutic approach is the one that aims at improving the quality of life of young patients while preventing the occurrence of major complications.

An initial trial of medical therapy, for a well-defined time, is indicated in the majority of infants with GERD, also in order to determine if GERD is indeed the cause of the specific symptom(s). Initial therapy of infants with GER should be aimed at proper positioning of the baby and feeding techniques. Although esophageal pH studies have demonstrated that infants in the prone position have less GER, since it has been found that such position is associated with an increased risk of SIDS, prone positioning during sleep is only considered in the occasional case where the risk of death from GERD complications outweighs the risk of SIDS. Positioning of toddlers and children has not been adequately studied, though elevation of the head of the bed is likely to be beneficial.

Other recommendations for infants include frequent burping, and smaller and more frequent feedings. Thickened formula feeding (adding a tablespoon of rice cereal to 2 oz of formula) does not improve reflux index score, but does decrease the number of vomiting episodes. In the older child, avoiding caffeine, chocolate, spicy foods, and reducing the intake of foods that by prolonging gastric emptying contribute to GER (fried, fatty foods) is recommended.

Pharmacologic management is best initiated with antisecretory therapy based on H2 receptor antagonists. Use of over-the-counter antacids is not recommended, as they may mask and delay the diagnosis and also are ineffective in healing esophagitis, if present. Prokinetic agents such as cisapride have been shown to be effective,[4] but are no longer available. Among them, metoclopramide (Reglan) is widely used, but convincing proofs of its efficacy for GERD treatment are indeed lacking. In addition, it has significant adverse effects in about a third of the patients, that in rare cases even include dystonic movements and other extrapyramidal reactions, and so it is not recommended.[1] Thus in essence, we currently have no prokinetic available for GERD.

Proton pump inhibitors (PPIs) are the most effective acid suppressants, and they are superior to H2 antagonists in healing esophagitis. Their use is indicated in the presence of documented esophagitis,

TABLE 13-8

PHARMACOLOGIC AGENTS USED FOR GERD

H2 Antagonists	
Cimetidine	40 mg/kg per day divided tid or qid
Ranitidine	5–10 mg/kg per day divided tid or bid
Famotidine	1 mg/kg per day divided bid
Nizatidine	10 mg/kg per day divided bid
Proton-Pump Inhibitors	
Omeprazole	1–3.3 mg/kg per day
Lansoprazole	1.4 mg/kg per day

or in patients shown to have GERD who fail to respond to H2 antagonists. Although their use in pediatrics is relatively recent, data on safety of prolonged use of PPI in children are now available.[5] It should be noted, however, that omeprazole and lansoprazole[6] are the only PPIs approved by Food and Drug Administration (FDA) for use in pediatric patients.

Table 13-8 reports dosage for gastric antisecretory agents used in children.

Surgical Therapy

Surgical treatment of GERD has been available for children for several decades now. Its advantages, however, have to be weighed against risks of complications such as dumping syndrome, intractable gagging, and retching. Different types of operations may be performed for antireflux surgical treatment: Boix-Ochoa, Nissen, Thal-Ashcraft, Toupet, Rossetti, and Lortat-Jacob, but two procedures are most commonly performed: the Nissen fundoplication (2/3) and the Thal-Ashcraft procedure (1/3). Nissen fundoplication[7] is the most popular; laparoscopic procedures have also become popular in recent years—the results and complication rates are similar to those of the open procedure, but hospitalization is shortened.

Ninety percent of patients remain free from significant reflux symptoms after laparoscopic Nissen fundoplication, although side effects occur in up to 22%. Failure rates of 5–20% have been found after objective postoperative follow-up. In addition, as the children grow, many fundoplications "unwrap." If symptoms recur, the procedure has to be redone. Thus, surgery is now essentially used for infants and children with severe complications that do not resolve with medical management. Children with underlying neurologic disorders are particularly prone to GER and sequelae. If these children require surgery, a two-stage procedure is employed because the complication rate in these patients approaches 50%. The first step is to place percutaneoulsy a gastrostomy (PEG) and then assess whether the GERD and its complications improve with better nutrition support. Many of these children can thus avoid a fundoplication and its consequent problems. If GERD remains active, the surgeon can subsequently perform a fundoplication. More recently, a new procedure using a radiofrequency treatment for gastroesophageal reflux disease (the Stretta procedure) has been introduced and is rapidly gaining popularity in the adult population. To date, however, there are no published studies in pediatrics.

COMPLICATIONS OF GERD

Barrett's Esophagus

Metaplasia is the squamous epithelium of the esophagus that transforms in specialized columnar epithelium. Predisposing factors are: gender (males more commonly affected), severe gastroesophageal reflux, severe central nervous system damage, chronic pulmonary disease, esophageal atresia, and chemotherapy. The extent of intestinal metaplasia correlates strongly with the degree of esophageal acid exposure and inversely with the lower esophageal sphincter pressure and length. It is a premalignant condition that exposes to the risk of dysplastic degeneration and adenocarcinoma.

The percentage of Barrett's esophagus in children is not well known. It is asymptomatic and is diagnosed by endoscopy, unusually red color in areas of the lower esophageal mucosa. Radiography is inadequate but deep esophageal ulcers and midesophageal strictures are signs that are often associated.

Response of Barrett to antireflux therapy (including fundoplication) is controversial. Regression is possible. Yearly endoscopic surveillance to try and detect metaplasia before it becomes adenocarcinoma is recommended in adults but data in the pediatric age are still limited.

Peptic Strictures

They are usually found in cases of severe but asymptomatic esophagitis; strictures present as dysphagia and, when severe, with regurgitation of undigested liquids and drooling of saliva. Diagnosis is obtained radiologically—narrowing of the esophageal lumen usually about one-third of the esophageal length above the diaphragm. Endoscopy is necessary to diagnose the type of stenosis, to evaluate for Barrett's epithelium, and to treat by balloon dilation. Fundoplication is sometimes advisable to arrest reflux.

References

1   Rudolph CD, et al. Guidelines for evaluation and treatment of gastroesophageal reflux in infants and children: recommendations of the North American Society for Pediatric Gastroenterology and Nutrition. *J Pediatr Gastroenterol Nutr* 32(Suppl 2):S1–S31, 2001.

2   Nelson SP, Chen EH, Syniar GM, Christoffel KK. One-year followup of symptoms of gastroesophageal reflux during infancy. *Pediatrics* 102:E67, 1998.

3   Kawahara H, Dent J, Davidson G. Mechanisms responsible for gastroesophageal reflux. *Gastroenterology* 113:399–408, 1997.

4   Vandenplas Y, et al. The role of cisapride in the treatment of pediatric gastroesophageal reflux. The European Society of Pediatric Gastroenterology,

Hepatology and Nutrition. *J Pediatr Gastroenterol Nutr* 28:518–528, 1999.

5   Hassall E, et al. Omeprazole for treatment of chronic erosive esophagitis in children: a multicenter study of efficacy, safety, tolerability and dose requirements. International Pediatric Omeprazole Study Group. *J Pediatr* 137:800–807, 2000.

6   Tolia V, et al. Safety of lansoprazole in the treatment of gastroesophageal reflux disease in children. *J Pediatr Gastroenterol Nutr* 35:S300–S307, 2002.

7   Bergmeijer J, Harbers J, Molenaar J. Function of pediatric Nissen-Rosetti fundoplication followed up into adolescence and adulthood. *J Am Coll Surg* 184: 259–261, 1997.

14

COW'S MILK ALLERGY

Francesca Cavataio and Stefano Guandalini

INTRODUCTION

Hippocrates, the "Father of Medicine," first recorded adverse reactions to cow's milk (CM) in the fifth century BC when he described gastric upset and urticaria following the ingestion of cow's milk.

Nevertheless, only in recent years has cow's milk allergy been studied in depth. New concepts about the disease have been described by leading experts and researchers to define cow's milk protein allergy (CMPA)—a "dynamic" condition always evolving in its multiple aspects.

A new profile of CMPA has evolved from new acquisitions in these areas:

- *Epidemiology:* CMPA, once occasionally reported, is at present the leading cause of food allergy in the first 2 years of age; its prevalence has been increasing in the last decade but is now becoming stable.
- *Pathogenesis:* For years allergy has been considered synonymous with reaginic reaction; it is now clear that other immune mechanisms, apart from those IgE mediated, are involved in the pathogenesis. For this reason some cases, once believed to be "intolerance," are now included in CMPA.
- *Clinical presentation:* It ranges from classical enteropathy presenting as chronic diarrhea, vomiting, and failure to thrive to atypical symptoms such as constipation. It varies from

mild skin eczema, to infant wheezing, and up to severe anaphylaxis; every organ or system may apparently become the target of cow's milk-allergic reaction.
- *Treatment:* The "ideal" substitute for CM has to be nutritionally balanced and absolutely anallergic; though many good products are actually available, none has both these characteristics and the search on the best replacement diet is ongoing.
- *Natural history:* Not all the CMPA-affected infants become tolerant within 2 years, as it was once believed. Different mechanisms operating in the pathogenesis determine different evolutions of the disease.

Some of the features listed above justify the "dynamism" of CMPA; they are also responsible for some lack of agreement in the classification of the disease.

For example, the terms CM-allergy and CM-intolerance (CMI) are sometimes used interchangeably and this may generate certain confusion both in clinical practice and in research reports. To complicate the matter further, it is common among lay people and occasionally even among health care providers to use the term "lactose intolerance" (that refers to the clinical consequences of the lack of adequate digestive activity toward lactose by the enzyme lactase) to actually indicate CMPA.

Indeed, CMPA is an adverse reaction to food—this generic term indicates any untoward clinical reaction that follows the ingestion of a certain food, independently from the pathogenic mechanism.

Food allergy is an adverse reaction to food caused by an immune mechanism, while food intolerance is an adverse reaction to food not mediated by an immune mechanism (or, preferably, an adverse reaction for which an immune mechanism cannot be demonstrated).

Consequently, CMPA can be defined as an adverse reaction resulting from the interaction between one or more of cow's milk proteins (typically either beta-lactoglobulin or casein) and one or more immune mechanisms. CM-intolerance, on the other hand, is another adverse reaction to cow's milk proteins for which an immunologic mechanism cannot be demonstrated.

The semantic issue is irrelevant in daily clinical practice: CMPA and CMI are among the leading causes of adverse reaction to food in infants, no differentiation between allergy and intolerance is possible on the basis of symptoms or of laboratory tests commonly available for the diagnosis and, above all, the therapeutic approach is the same.

Laboratory tests are not helpful in distinguishing between allergy and intolerance because only skin prick test (SPT) and radio allergo sorbent test (RAST) (indicative of IgE-mediated reactions) can be routinely performed, and allergy cannot be ruled out unless extensive diagnostic tests for type II-III-IV reactions have proved to be negative.

To avoid confusion and for practical reasons, in this chapter the term CMPA will be used from a clinical point of view and will include both immune-mediated reactions and reactions that are "likely" to be determined by the immune system.

Complaints about adverse reactions to cow's milk are very common in the first 12 months of life, since parents blame the formula (milk-derived) as a cause of symptoms in their infants; sometimes performing a confirmatory challenge test is the only way to avoid the risks of both inappropriate elimi-nation diets (with their potential nutritional and psychosocial consequences) and unrecognized dangerous allergic reactions.

Summary

- The terms CM-allergy and CM-intolerance may be used interchangeably since no differences between these two conditions exist in terms of clinical presentation, severity of symptoms, or treatment.
- A correct diagnosis is the best way to avoid unnecessarily restricted diets.

EPIDEMIOLOGY

The prevalence of food allergy has increased worldwide in the last century becoming a serious health problem in industrialized countries. Food allergy affects genetically predisposed subjects when they are exposed to certain foods under influencing factors. Alimentary habits, early exposure to offending foods, and reduced incidence of infectious diseases are probably the most important factors of this increasing trend.

CMPA represents the most common type of food allergy in infancy. Following the general trend described for food allergies the prevalence of CMPA has increased enormously in the second half of the last century. The reduced prevalence of breast-feeding and the improved socioeconomical conditions ("hygiene hypothesis") have greatly contributed to this phenomenon.

Prevalence of Breast-feeding

The prevalence of breast-feeding varies very much throughout the world: it is rather low in many industrialized countries and in urban areas of many developing countries and relatively high in rural areas. Bottle-fed babies are precociously exposed to cow's milk proteins and this may increase, in genetically susceptible subjects, the risk of sensitization.

Epidemiologic data confirm the protective role of breast-feeding—the frequency of CMPA in the last decades has been inversely proportional to the prevalence of breast-feeding.

Hygiene Hypothesis

The ameliorated socioeconomical conditions and the consequent minor degree of exposition of newborns to bacteria and infectious agents in general seem to lead their immune system to a derangement from the acquisition of natural oral tolerance (see section PATHOGENESIS). This is confirmed by epidemiologic evidence of higher prevalence of CMPA in industrialized rather than in developing countries.

What is the real prevalence of cow's milk allergy? During the last decades several studies have described varying rates of incidence. The percentage ranged from 1.8 to 7.5% and this broad gap is reflective of differences in diagnostic criteria and study design.

Moreover, it is often a familial disorder. A family history of atopy and/or food allergies is one of the most important risk factors for CMPA in infancy and might be an indicator for preventive measures. The use of strict diagnostic criteria will probably make these percentages more homogeneous. It is a fact well known that parents blame milk as a cause of symptoms in their children. Symptoms suggestive of CMPA are seen in 5–15% of infants, but reproducible clinical reactions to CM have been reported in a less minor percentage. Bock and coworkers, in a study conducted on 480 infants, described adverse reaction to milk in 83% of the cases as perceived by parents but only 8% were reproducible on a second exposure to milk.

Other factors influencing the prevalence rate are: different clinical presentations, different dietary habits, age of patients included in the study, inclusion or exclusion of cases of CM-intolerance, and differences related to geographic area.

Thus, 2–3% seems to be the most acceptable estimate of CMPA incidence in infants in developed countries (0.5% in breast-fed infants).

Very little is known about CMPA prevalence after the first 1–2 years of life. It is now evident that CMPA may persist in later childhood and indeed even well in adulthood. The frequency of sensitization to cow's milk in adults has recently been estimated by RAST to be 0.7–1.2% in Scandinavian countries.

Summary

- In the first 2 years of life CMPA prevalence is about 2–3%.
- Since milk allergy is often a familial disorder, its presence in a patient can assist the physician in possibly discovering it in other members of the family.
- The major risk factors for cow's milk allergy are positive family history of atopy and early exposure to cow's milk proteins.

PATHOGENESIS

Under specific circumstances, some of which are inherited, tolerance to milk protein breaks down and the allergic sensitization starts.

In this perspective, CMPA may be considered the consequence of an imbalance between systemic tolerance and intestinal mucosal immunity.

Mechanisms of Oral Tolerance

Oral tolerance can be defined as antigen-specific systemic unresponsiveness induced by food (ingested by mouth). Oral tolerance represents the normal immune response to dietary antigens and it is also responsible for the absence of immune response to common mucosal flora.

Soon after birth the neonate's intestine must achieve the capability

- To absorb ingested nutrients
- To *train* mucosal immunity in preventing infectious agents from penetrating through the intestinal wall
- To develop tolerance toward numerous antigens (particularly food antigens)

This third step is a very complex process based on active mucosal immunologic mechanisms that are still partially unknown. Food antigens represent non-self-antigens and as such they are potentially able to induce an immune reaction.

In the intestinal lumen, food proteins undergo a digestion process that reduces them to small peptides ready to be absorbed; the presence of undigested or partially digested proteins in the intestinal lumen is a common event but their penetration through the intestinal wall is largely prevented by an intestinal defensive barrier consisting of two branches: anatomo-physiologic and immunologic (Table 14-1).

Nevertheless, even in normal conditions a certain number of dietary antigens, escaped to secretory IgA, are able to cross the epithelial layer via three pathways.

1. *By endoexocytosis.* The enterocytes modify the antigenic characteristics of the ingested molecules lowering their immunogenic power.
2. *Through specialized cells.* M cells (special epithelial cells found on Peyer's patches) offer samples of the antigens present in the intestinal lumen to the lymphoid tissue.
3. *Through intercellular junctions.* In this case, the molecule passes through without modification, so its immunogenic power remains unchanged.

TABLE 14-1
INTESTINAL DEFENSIVE BARRIER

Anatomic and Functional
Factors preventing antigen penetration
Intestinal motility
Mucus layer
Epithelium (enterocyte membrane and tight
junctions)
Factors involved in degrading protein
Gastric acidity
Enzymes (duodenal, pancreatic)
Immunologic
Factors counteracting the entry of antigens
(immune exclusion)
Antigen-specific secretory IgA
Factors clearing antigens after their penetration
through the intestinal wall
Antigen-specific circulating IgA and IgG
Reticuloendothelial system

Food antigens then interact with gut associated lymphoid tissue (GALT)—the gastrointestinal (GI) immune system. GALT is a huge complex of lymphoid structures and consists of as many as 10^{12} lymphocytes and of more antibodies—secretory IgA—than any other lymphoid districts.

Food antigens brought into contact with lymphoid cells cause an intense immune response especially at submucosal level where the macromolecules that have passed through intestinal defense barrier may stimulate lamina propria T lymphocytes toward a specific immune unresponsiveness that forms the basis of oral tolerance.

Both the enterocytes and the lamina propria lymphocytes (Th and CD8+) are involved in these mechanisms that have as an end-point the organization of a Th1-oriented immune response.

The different Th cytokine profiles are as follows:

- Th1 (IL-2, IFN-γ, TNF-β, TNF-γ) → defense against infectious agents
- Th2 (IL-4, IL-5, IL-10, IL-13) → allergic reactions
- Th3 (TGF-β) → anti-inflammatory action

At birth, the neonate's immune system is characterized by prevalence of Th2-type lymphocytes (with an "atopic" cytokine profile). It seems that environmental factors such as the intestinal bacterial colonization and the antigenic load of breast milk are responsible for an immunodeviation process that causes a Th2 → Th1 shift with prevalence of a cytokine profile typical of tolerogenic responses.

Tolerance is an active process causing suppression of IgE- and cell-mediated response and enhancement of antibodies synthesis (IgG, IgA, and IgM).

The ingestion of a new food is always accompanied by the secretion of antibodies, even in absence of allergic reaction. The formation of specific IgG, IgA, and IgM antibodies against food proteins is a natural phenomenon that indicates exposure rather than sensitization, i.e., antibodies specific for cow's milk rise after introduction of this food and fall during infancy; they are responsible for immune memory and tolerance and are not responsible for inflammatory phenomena.

TABLE 14-2

RISK FACTORS FOR DEVELOPMENT OF CMPA

Genetic predisposition
Age
Intrauterine sensitization
Environmental factors (hygiene hypothesis)
IgA deficiency
Lack of breast-feeding
Type, dose, and frequency of exposition to the
  antigen load
Alteration of common mucosal flora
Occurrence of infections in the GI tract

The Allergic Reaction

Under certain conditions the intestinal barrier breaks down, oral tolerance is lost, and the allergic response starts. The development of allergic reaction is a consequence of disequilibrium between "risk factors" (Table 14-2) and "protective factors."

Genetic Predisposition

Genetic predisposition is the most important among the risk factors, although not yet characterized. At present, we have only epidemiologic evidence for a genetic component of atopy; babies of atopic parents develop atopic diseases more frequently and atopic manifestations seem to cluster in family members.

Age

The "gut closure" is incomplete in the first few months of life; macromolecules may more easily pass through the intestinal wall resulting in alteration of the Th1/Th2 balance.

Intrauterine Sensitization

The fetus is able to synthesize IgE by the 11th week of gestation; specific IgE for food allergen are detected in amniotic liquid and in cord-blood; elevated cord-blood IgE indicates the intrauterine sensitization.

Environmental Factors

Better socioeconomical conditions are responsible for the "hygiene hypothesis" and the shift toward a Th2 response due to minor exposure to infectious agents; the exposure to tobacco smoke and air pollution are able to condition the development of allergies.

IgA Deficiency

This condition that affects approximately 1:600 individuals may alter the achievement of oral tolerance, since IgA are mostly involved in counteracting the antigen passage through the intestinal wall.

Breast-feeding

It has a protective effect on respiratory allergy and asthma but it seems to become a risk factor in atopic mothers. Breast milk contains an elevated number of immune stimulating cytokines [interleukin (IL)-1 beta, IL-6, IL-8, IL-10, granulocyte colony stimulating factor, macrophage-colony stimulating factor (M-CSF), tumor necrosis factor-α (TNF-α), interferon-gamma (IFN-γ), epithelial growth factor (EGF), transforming growth factor-α (TGF-α), and TGF-$\beta2$], but mothers whose babies expressed early CMA have higher levels of IL-4 and IL-8 and lower levels of TNF-α and TGF-$\beta2$ in their milk thus showing how the cytokine pattern of breast milk could be responsible, in the predisposed subject, for the development of CM-allergy.

Type, Dose, and Frequency of Exposition to the Antigenic Load

Massive antigen load is responsible for the formation of circulating immunocomplexes (Ic) in excess (especially IgE and IgG).

Alteration of Common Mucosal Flora

Atopic subjects have a higher prevalence of *E .coli*-like bacteria if compared to nonallergic subjects in whom Lactobacilli and Bifidobacteria prevails. Occurrence of infections in the GI tract—the higher frequency of gastroenteritis in the first year of life—may be a cause of altered intestinal permeability with consequent passage of macromolecules.

Mechanisms of Hypersensitivity Reactions

In the pathogenesis of cow's milk allergy, abnormal immune-mediated reactions play a basic role. Abnormal immune responses to circulating non-self-antigens in hypersensitivity reactions to food are able to cause real dysfunction in different organs. Four mechanisms are known to operate in hypersensitivity reactions.

Type I (IgE-mediated, Reaginic, Immediate)

Allergen binding to IgE previously attached to mast cell or basophil surface cause liberation of chemokine and inflammatory mediators, such as histamine and granulocyte chemotactic factors. These immediate reactions arise no later than 2 h after the ingestion of the offending protein. Symptoms are related to the organ or system where the reactive mast cells are located: acute vomiting and/or diarrhea, rhinitis, wheezing, urticaria, and anaphylaxis.

Type II (Cytotoxic)

Circulating antibodies bind the allergens thus activating the complement cascade with consequent destruction of the cell to which the antigen is attached.

Type III (Ic-mediated)

Circulating immunocomplexes (Ic) are usually cleared by reticuloendothelial system. Higher concentrations of Ic (of IgG type) are responsible for their deposition in tissues and endothelia. The activation of vasoactive amines may generate severe histologic lesions. Type III reactions are usually delayed and symptoms present hours or days after the contact with the allergens.

Type IV (Cell-mediated)

Antibodies are not involved in this type of allergic reaction. Allergens contact T lymphocytes directly activating liberation of cytokines and starting of an allergic cascade. This is also a delayed reaction since the cascade starts within 36–72 h from the antigen exposure.

Most cases of CMPA are mediated by any one of these three mechanisms: type I, type III, and type IV. Whatever the mechanism involved, the final pathway is represented by an inflammatory amplification circuit that starts with the attraction of mast cells, eosinophils, and other cells and develops with the liberation of cytokines and chemokines and consequent damage of the intestinal mucosa. If the specific homing of lymphocyte involves other organs, symptoms different from the gastrointestinal ones may also arise.

There is evidence that in the first year of life the vast majority of cases are not IgE-mediated and the possibility exists that more than one mechanism may be active in the same subject.

Allergenic Fractions in Cow's Milk

Cow's milk contains more than 20 different proteins: 80% are caseins, 20% whey proteins (the most common of them being β-lactoglobulin, α-lactalbumin, and immunoglobulins). Although β-Lactoglobulin is the most common allergen, the allergic reaction may also involve more than one protein.

Summary

- CMPA is responsible for allergic reactions in genetically susceptible infants exposed to some risk factors.
- All four hypersensitivity mechanisms described by Gell and Coombs may be relevant in the determinism of CMPA.
- CMPA may activate one or more than one pathogenic mechanism in the same subject.
- With the exception of temporal correlation between exposure to antigen and onset of symptoms there is a poor correlation between

any one specific mechanism and clinical presentation.

CLINICAL PRESENTATION

Clinical presentation of CMPA largely varies in terms of onset, severity, and kind of symptoms.

In recent years, many new clinical presentations of CMPA have been described in the literature and this has led to the conviction that almost every organ can be affected by the allergic reaction.

The age at onset of the disease may range from few days to several months after the introduction of CM in the diet, somehow the onset can be even during breast-feeding. Though the majority of cases occur in the first year of life, CMPA may become symptomatic at every age from birth to adulthood.

Data from the literature reported the onset of the disease within 1 week in 41–70% of the cases and within the first month in 69–85%. Early onset cases support the concept of intrauterine sensitization.

Allergic reactions to CM proteins typically involve the gastrointestinal, cutaneous, and respiratory systems but generalized reactions such as anaphylaxis are also common (Table 14-3).

Each patient may show one or more symptoms from one or more organs or systems. Skin and gastrointestinal symptoms are described in approximately 50–60% of patients, while 20–30% shows respiratory symptoms.

In addition to these typical symptoms of CMPA, a number of "new" clinical pictures such as infantile colic, chronic constipation, apnea, and sleeping disorders have—both in the past and more recently—been attributed to or probably caused by CMPA (Table 14-4).

Gastrointestinal Symptoms

Milk-induced Gastroesophageal Reflux and Reflux Esophagitis

Recently, a form of gastroesophageal reflux (GER) associated or secondary to CMPA and clinically indistinguishable from primary GER has been described. Typical symptoms of presentation are recurrent vomiting, respiratory symptoms, such as wheezing or recurrent pneumonia, and when complications arise anemia and failure to thrive. The

TABLE 14-3

CLINICAL PRESENTATION OF CMPAN INFANTS

| **Gastrointestinal Symptoms** |
| Nausea/vomiting |
| Diarrhea |
| Abdominal pain |
| Feeding disorders |
| Oral pruritus |
| **Cutaneous Symptoms** |
| Erythematous rash |
| Urticaria/angioedema |
| Eczema |
| Atopic dermatitis |
| **Respiratory Symptoms** |
| Bronchitis/asthma |
| Wheezing |
| Rhinitis, conjunctivitis |
| Cough |
| Stridor |
| **Systemic Symptoms** |
| Failure to thrive |
| Iron-deficiency anemia |
| Anaphylactic shock |

TABLE 14-4

OTHER CLINICAL PRESENTATIONS OF CMPA IN INFANTS

Caused by CMPA	Possibly Caused by CMPA[a]
GERD	Recurrent otitis media
Eosinophilic	Migraine
gastroenteropathy	Arthritis
Colitis	Nephrotic
Pulmonary	syndrome
hemosiderosis	Autism
Constipation	Enuresis
Infant colic	Sleeping disorders
	Apnea, ALTE

[a]No strong evidence-based data exist on these associations.

frequency of association between GER and CMPA in the first year of life is around 30% and often the reflux is CMPA-dependent. CMPA-sensitive esophagitis is characterized by infiltrates of eosinophils with focal T-lymphocyte activation and upregulation of basal and papillary epithelial expression of the chemokine eotaxin. Differential diagnosis can be obtained on the basis of pHmetry characteristics (phasic tracing in CMPA-induced reflux) or with intestinal permeability tests (IPT). In common clinical practice, however, this is rarely necessary. More commonly, when an infant fails to respond as expected to conventional antireflux therapy (see Chap. 13), a trial excluding CM antigens from the diet is recommended. In some cases where other signs of allergy exist (e.g., eczema and asthma) or family history is suggestive of food allergy, the dietetic trial may be the first line of treatment.

Eosinophilic Esophagitis

It is diagnosed frequently during infancy through adolescence and it is not necessarily associated with GER. Vomiting, dysphagia, anorexia, abdominal pain, and irritability are among its main presenting symptoms. It fails to respond to conventional antireflux therapy and is sometimes complicated by esophageal strictures. Total serum IgE are normal to slightly increased and peripheral eosinophilia is uncommon. The diagnosis is achieved by means of histologic examination that shows eosinophilic infiltration of mucosa and submucosa, not always associated with papillary elongation and basal zone hyperplasia. Characteristically, these changes are present not only in the distal esophagus as in GERD, but also in the middle and upper esophagus. Treatment is based on food elimination diets (young infants may respond to extensively hydrolyzed formula, but older patients require AA-based formulas) or on systemic steroids. Ingested fluticasone has also been shown to be efficacious (see Chap. 16).

Eosinophilic Gastroenteritis

It is characterized by the infiltration of eosinophils into the GI tract wall and may affect pediatric patients at all ages (see Chap. 16).

Cow's Milk-sensitive Enteropathy

The mucosa of the small intestine is the hotbed of the immunologic events that lead to CMPA. For this reason, in the gut of infants with cow's milk allergy, inflammation is probably always present irrespective of symptoms. CM-sensitive enteropathy is a typical malabsorption syndrome presenting with vomiting, chronic diarrhea, and failure to thrive; the patients look dystrophic and show abdominal distention. This syndrome usually affects infants older than 4 months and can be differentiated from celiac disease by the absence of antiendomysium or antitissue transglutaminase antibodies. The pathogenic mechanism involves a T-cell-mediated reaction. Malabsorption is due to the damage of the jejunal mucosa—varying villous atrophy and crypt hyperplasia associated with inflammation in surface epithelium and lamina propria. The density of eosinophils may be moderately increased.

Milk-induced Enterocolitis

It is an eosinophilic colitis that can affect neonates aging 1 week up to 3 months; the patients show diarrhea with mucus and blood in the stools; failure to thrive and malabsorption are not always present; skin prick tests are often negative but allergic colitis should always be considered in the differential diagnosis of every newborn with hematochezia after having excluded infectious and anatomic disorders.

Milk-induced Constipation

Recent reports underline the high prevalence of CM-induced constipation in infants and children who do not outgrow CMPA after the second year. CMPA should be considered as a cause of chronic refractory constipation in children especially when family history of atopy or personal history of concomitant allergic symptoms is evident. The pathogenic mechanisms seem to involve an alteration of mucus quality. As functional constipation (see Chap. 5) is an exceedingly common disorder, patients with possible CMPA as a cause should be selectively identified. It is therefore recommended to search for multiple markers such as anal fissures, perianal erythema, and edema, as well as for concomitant CMPA symptoms, positive RAST, histologic evidence of proctitis. Among typical histologic findings, we described infiltration of lymphocytes, lymphoid nodules, interstitial edema and, above all, eosinophilic infiltration of the lamina propria, sometimes associated with intraepithelial "eosinophilic abscesses." The diagnosis is confirmed by the resolution of constipation and the prompt healing of anal and perianal lesions in response to a CMP-free diet.

Eosinophilic proctitis

It occurs in the first few months of life in an otherwise healthy infant that presents blood-streaked, soft-to-loose stools; the majority are breast-fed infants. Blood loss may be responsible for anemia; the diagnosis is endoscopic and it is based on the demonstration of linear erosions, edema of the mucosa of distal large bowel, and on histologic findings of eosinophilic infiltration. Appropriate dietetic measures have to be taken since a certain percentage of infants also react to the extensively hydrolyzed formula.

Other Symptoms

Atopic Dermatitis

It should be regarded as a manifestation of food allergy; it is a particular kind of chronic eczema that shows a typical progression of skin lesions (erythema → itchiness → papules → infection → lichenification) and a typical distribution of such lesions on the body surface (face, extensor surfaces of arms and legs in infancy, flexor surfaces of arms and legs during childhood, hands, feet, and flexor surfaces in adolescence and adulthood). The role of CMPA in the pathogenesis of the disease is still debated but CMP exclusion from the diet is somehow advisable.

Respiratory Symptoms

We consider infants' wheezing and asthma among the most important symptoms of CMPA. Other symptoms are rhinitis, chronic cough, and stridor. Asthma often occurs in children that do not outgrow CM-allergy, as a manifestation of "pathomorphism" (see section NATURAL HISTORY).

Infantile Colic

Sudden, inconsolable fits of crying associated with fussiness and irritability (distressed behavior): the infant is hyperactive and vigorously bends his legs onto the abdomen. Severe colic is seen when an infant cries more than 3 h a day for more than 3 days in a week. In these cases, underlying CMPA must be ruled out, as it may be responsible for severe colic in 10–15% of cases.

Urticaria and Angioedema

Erythematous wheals cover the body surface and they are sometimes associated with angioedema of face, hands, and external genitals.

Anaphylactic Shock

Shock is not always IgE-mediated; it is caused by rapid and massive liberation of inflammatory mediators such as histamine, prostaglandins, and leukotrienes from tissue mast cells and circulating basophils. As a consequence, the cardiovascular system undergoes a severe vasodilatation associated with a drop in blood pressure and followed by shock.

Some other symptoms have occasionally been reported in association with CMPA: recurrent otitis media, pulmonary hemosiderosis, iron-deficiency anemia, headache, sleep disturbances, hyperactivity, nephrotic syndrome, even autism. For none of these disorders has the association proved to be one of cause/effect.

This clinical heterogeneity seems to reflect the different mechanisms involved in the pathogenesis of the disease; indeed it is conceivable that diverse mechanisms elicit different clinical manifestations in CMPA.

An attempt at classifying gastrointestinal manifestations of food allergy according to pathogenic mechanisms has been done during a workshop held

TABLE 14-5

CLASSIFICATION OF GASTROINTESTINAL REACTIONS TO FOOD ACCORDING TO PATHOGENIC MECHANISMS

IgE	Non-IgE
Immediate gastrointestinal hypersensitivity	Dietary protein enterocolitis
Oral allergy syndrome	Dietary protein proctitis
Allergic eosinophilic esophagitis	Dietary protein enteropathy
Allergic eosinophilic gastritis	
Allergic eosinophilic gastroenterocolitis	

in Washington, DC in 1998. The results are shown in Table 14-5.

A more useful differentiation that can be made concerns the relationship between pathogenic mechanism and clinical presentation. Hill and coworkers[1] have recently divided CMPA-affected infants in three groups:

- *Immediate reactors*. Patients who show allergy few minutes (<45 min) after the ingestion of even small quantities of CM, mainly as cutaneous eruptions (urticaria and angioedema) or anaphylactic shock; in this group an IgE-mediated mechanism is demonstrable.
- *Intermediate reactors*. Patients who react to CM within hours (1–20 h after challenge) of ingestion of moderate quantities of CM; in these cases the symptoms are mainly gastrointestinal (i.e., vomiting, regurgitation, and diarrhea) and IgE are uncommonly involved in the pathogenesis. Antibody-dependent cell-mediated cytotoxicity to β-lactoglobulin has been demonstrated in some of these cases.
- *Late reactors*. Patients who show gastrointestinal, respiratory, or cutaneous symptoms several hours or days after the ingestion of CM—in these patients an IgE-mediated mechanism is seldom

demonstrated, while an elevated T-cell reactivity *in vitro* can be revealed; diagnostic tools for these reactions are still under development (i.e., lymphocyte stimulation and cytokine generation on incubation of lymphocytes with cow milk proteins).

Summary

- Always consider the possibility of CMPA when facing an infant with whatever symptom emerging soon after the ingestion of CM.
- Pay attention to unusual clinical presentation especially if symptoms are late onset-type.
- Remember that different mechanisms may form the basis of the same clinical presentation.

DIAGNOSIS

Laboratory investigations are of limited value in the diagnosis—when positive, they are not enough to confirm diagnosis, while when negative, CMPA may still be present[2] Thus, when CMPA is suspected, the patient must undergo a period of CM-free diet. A definitive diagnosis will be done once the patient responds to the elimination diet and a subsequent challenge with milk is followed by a clinical relapse.

The "golden standard" for the diagnosis remains the double-blind, placebo-controlled food challenge that must be performed in a hospital setting. In practice, the challenge is almost never done in a blind fashion, and since it is typically postponed after the age of about 1 year,[3] this results in many "apparently nonconfirmed diagnoses."

The diagnostic work-up consists of several steps, outlined in Fig. 14-1.

Case History and Physical Examination

A thorough history taking is the first and most important step of the diagnostic process and provides very valuable data. Great attention has to be paid in the evaluation of all the risk factors involved in the pathogenesis of the disease (see section

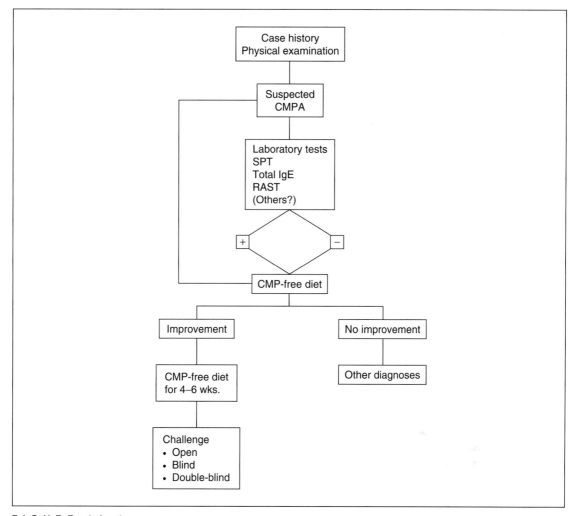

FIGURE 14-1

DIAGNOSTIC ALGORITHM

PATHOGENESIS). All the information listed in Table 14-6 should be collected.

Physical examination must include measurement of height and weight (to look for possible growth deficiency) and all signs associated with the various clinical manifestations of CMPA, such as pallor, skin lesions, wheezing, and perianal lesions.

Laboratory Tests

Laboratory tests may be helpful in the diagnosis of CMPA, all have a low predictive positive value; they cannot substitute for clinical evaluation. No single laboratory test is diagnostic of CMPA. Due to the multiple mechanisms involved, one would have to explore all the four mechanisms of hypersensitivity but, unfortunately, at present most available tests only explore the IgE-mediated type. It is obviously possible to assess circulating antibodies other than IgE directed against cow's milk protein, but their presence (up to certain levels) is quite physiologic and does not indicate sensitization to CM. The most common laboratory tests for the diagnosis of CMPA are as follows.

TABLE 14-6

INFORMATION USEFUL IN SUSPECTING CMPA

History of atopy and allergic diseases (personal and familiar)

Socioeconomic conditions

Type of feeding and alimentary habits (possible breast-feeding)

Age at introduction of CM in the diet and age at weaning

Age at onset of symptoms

Time elapsed between CM ingestion and the beginning of symptoms

Concomitant infectious diseases or history of recurrent infections (particularly infections of the GI tract)

History of previous symptoms consistent with the diagnosis of CMPA

Skin Prick Test

This test is simple, not invasive, and inexpensive. SPT detects skin IgE directed against food allergens. The results of SPT may be helpful in selecting patients to treat with an elimination diet but their accuracy in diagnosing allergy is controversial. Once again, while they are of great value in patients with immediate reaction (IgE-mediated), delayed-type reactions are not detected. In addition, even positive tests do not always indicate symptomatic reactivity. As a consequence, it is unjustified to start a CMP-free diet in a patient only on the basis of a positive SPT. A negative SPT rules out only IgE-mediated mechanisms—making unlikely the appearance of immediate reactions after a CM challenge. SPT's accuracy does not vary with the age of the patients, while higher accuracy is recorded if they are carried out with fresh milk rather than with commercial allergen extracts.

SPT may be also performed with hydrolyzed formulas when selecting "hypoallergenic" formulas for CMPA management.

Radio Allergo Sorbent Test

This test evaluates serum levels of specific IgE. When CMPA is suspected, RAST for the three main protein fractions (β-lactoglobulin, casein, and α-lactalbumin) can be performed. The test has the same indications mentioned for SPT but it is more expensive. It is useful in screening patients with suspected IgE-mediated allergies but it is not 100% diagnostic; it has the same limitations as SPT (low sensitivity and high specificity; low positive predictive accuracy and high negative predictive accuracy for IgE-mediated reactions). Therefore, its results should be cautiously interpreted especially when symptoms are mild. RAST is selectively used in those subjects who suffer from harmful IgE-mediated reactions or when the subject is treated with antihistaminic drugs.

Patch Test

This test is generally used in contact dermatitis. It has recently been tested in the diagnostic work-up of pediatric patients with atopic dermatitis, and it has been shown that, when combined with SPT, patch test enhances the accuracy of the diagnosis of CMPA in atopic dermatitis.

Tests Exploring Hypersensitivity Mechanisms of Type II and III

These mechanisms are responsible for circulating antibodies different from IgE and so the laboratory tests must detect circulating levels of IgG, IgA, and Ic. As mentioned earlier high levels of antibodies against food allergens are not diagnostic of allergic reaction to food. In the same way the occurrence of IgG anti-β-lactoglobulin is a physiologic phenomenon without diagnostic significance. The shorter the breast-feeding period and the earlier the introduction of cow's milk formula, the higher the antibody levels. Recently, it has been shown that high titers of IgG anti-β-lactoglobulin in patients less than 1-year-old might be used to confirm CMPA. If confirmed by further evidence, this test would be of great use in diagnosing CMPA in the first year of life, when as indicated, the vast majority of CMPA patients is not SPT or RAST-positive.

Tests Exploring Hypersensitivity Mechanisms of Type IV

These mechanisms seem to be involved in cow's milk-sensitive enteropathy. The tests available (immune-cell proliferation test and leukocyte migration inhibition test) measure the late phase of the allergic reaction. They are, however, rarely used as routine tests because their sensitivity and specificity are low and clinical significance is still debated.

Tests Evaluating Mucosal Damage (rarely used)

Tests evaluating the small intestinal mucosa damage are useful whenever an enteropathy results from CMPA.

1. *Intestinal permeability tests (IPT).* They provide a noninvasive means for assessing intestinal mucosal integrity. Intestinal permeability is altered in CMPA as a result of the inflammatory process; this alteration is responsible for the increased mucosal passage of disaccharides, such as lactulose and cellobiose, while the damage to the absorptive surface causes the decreased absorption of monosaccharides, such as mannitol, rhamnose, and xylose. After a reasonable time (a few weeks) on a CMP-free diet, normal permeability is restored. IPT are not specific for CMPA but they might be used in the differential diagnosis (i.e., in an infant presenting vomiting, IPT may be used in differentiating CMPA from primary GER). IPT show the highest accuracy at ages 6–12 months and when CMPA presents with gastrointestinal symptoms.
2. *Fecal tests.* In patients with atopic dermatitis, challenge with cow's milk results in an increase in the fecal excretion of eosinophil cationic protein (ECP) and TNF-α, while in CMPA patients with digestive symptoms, only fecal TNF-α (but not ECP) is increased. Individual serial follow-up of fecal IgA and ECP can be used to estimate the degree of inflammation in the gut and an appropriate time for a challenge test, but are not diagnostic for CMPA.
3. *Duodenal biopsy.* Since this is an invasive test, it should be limited to those severe conditions

in which a definitive diagnosis is necessary. Pathologic changes resemble those found in celiac disease (villus atrophy and crypt hyperplasia); infiltration of T lymphocytes and macrophages that secrete IFN-γ and other cytokines is responsible for mucosal damage and consequent malabsorption.

Cow's Milk Protein (CMP) free Diet

Once CMPA is suspected independently from the results of the laboratory tests, the patient must undergo a period of strict and well-defined diet devoid of cow's milk proteins. This is achieved by replacing the infant formula and, in addition, avoiding any CMP-containing foods (see Chap. 31 for details on the diet).

If the diagnosis of CMPA is correct, within about 2–3 weeks, depending on the severity of symptoms, a clear clinical response is usually seen. If the symptoms persist despite the CMP-free diet, the diagnosis of CMPA is excluded.

Cow's Milk Challenge Test

When symptoms regress the diagnosis of CMPA is likely, but not conclusively proven, as the improvement might have been coincidental. Thus, from an academic point of view, the diagnosis remains to be established by a milk challenge procedure ("diagnostic challenge").

A challenge followed by the reappearance of symptoms is considered diagnostic. Although a "double-blind, placebo-controlled" challenge is regarded, in adult medicine, as the "golden standard"; in pediatric clinical practice this procedure is too cumbersome and rarely followed outside of research purposes. Open, controlled challenges in infants are typically done under professional observation in a hospital setting, and they have been shown to be reliable.

It should be stressed that challenges are unsafe because they expose the patients to the risk of harmful reaction such as anaphylaxis, especially when SPT or RAST are positive (IgE-mediated reactions!). Thus, in patients with history of previous anaphylaxis, the challenge is best avoided.

PROFILE OF THE PATIENT SELECTED FOR HOME CHALLENGE

Age: at least 18 months
Non-IgE-mediated reactions (negative SPT)
Negative history of anaphylaxis
Negative history of family atopy
Mostly digestive symptoms

How long after beginning the CMP-free diet should the challenge be performed? There are two options:

1. Challenge may be performed to confirm the diagnosis of CMPA (diagnostic challenge) 4–6 weeks after the CMP-free diet and in a hospital setting. A milk-based infant formula is administered at increasing doses or as a single dose. Clinical reaction is the only valuable parameter in considering the challenge positive, but changes in blood leukocyte distribution at 6 or 12 h after challenge may be taken as supportive evidence.

2. Challenge may be postponed until sometime after the first birthday. In this scenario, which in clinical practice is by far the most common, the procedure should actually be seen not so much as a diagnostic test, but rather as a way of assessing the acquisition of tolerance to CM ("recovery challenge," see Table 14-7). This late challenge may be done in medically supervised settings and with the same modalities of the former. Whenever there is no reason to expect an immediate-type reaction this may also be conducted at home. In this case, a progressive introduction of foods containing modified CMP (such as aged cheese or yogurt) is recommended, followed by the administration of CM. If no adverse clinical reactions are seen after a total of 3–4 weeks on this regimen, the challenge may be taken to indicate that the child has acquired tolerance.

Summary

1. In the first year of life:
   - Non-IgE-mediated forms prevail by far → SPT and RAST generally not useful

   - Each individual patient must be assessed for the need of performing challenge:
     a. Severe and immediate symptoms associated with positive SPT and/or RAST → no challenge
     b. Delayed reaction and SPT and/or RAST negativity → good response to CM-free diet → no challenge
     c. Delayed reaction and SPT and/or RAST negativity → doubtful response to CM-free diet → open controlled challenge (even "blind," if necessary)
2. After the first year:
   - IgE-mediated reactions become more common
   - Laboratory tests are more useful and can also be used as a prognostic guide for adverse reaction on challenge
   - Pediatric gastroenterologists should create their own personal standard of laboratory tests

TREATMENT

Obviously, the treatment of CMPA is a complete avoidance of cow's milk proteins. This means the complete elimination of cow's milk from the diet of the affected child or maternal elimination diets in breast-fed infants.

If the breast-fed infant shows severe symptoms, the nursing mother has to exclude from her diet not only CM and dairy products but also other foods such as egg, gluten, and fish.

Apart from resolving symptoms, antigen elimination preserves the barrier function of the intestine and reverses some disturbances of the humoral and cell-mediated immune responses to CM, preventing aberrant antigen absorption.

However, as milk is an important source of nutrients in childhood, a milk-free diet may not adequately meet the child's nutritional needs especially in the first few months of life, when milk is the only constituent of the diet.

When infants grow older, the exclusion of dairy products and other food that may represent hidden sources of CM is necessary. In fact, the inadvertent ingestion of even small amounts of cow's milk allergens hidden in foods may result in severe clinical reactions.

What is the best replacement for milk-based formulas? During the past century, a wide range of protein sources have been used to replace cow's milk, the better known being soy (and, particularly in Europe, soy hydrolyzed formulas), extensively casein and whey hydrolyzed formulas, and amino acid formulas (only the latter true "elemental" diets) (see Chap. 31 for a detailed analysis of the composition of formulas available in the United States).

Cow's milk ideal substitute should be

- Balanced in composition (to meet the child's nutritional needs)
- Good in taste (to ensure baby's compliance)
- Anallergic (to avoid allergic reactions)

In clinical practice, probably the most commonly used substitutes are soy milk and CMP hydrolysates. For both of these formulas, their ability to result in normal somatic development of children is well described. As for soy-based formulas, their palatability, widespread commercial availability, and low cost have made them one of the most popular CM substitutes. However, the well-known and repeatedly demonstrated possibility that a large percentage of infants sensitized to CMP will develop a secondary allergy to soy proteins (that are just as allergenic as CMP) makes the use of soy-based formulas not justified for infants with suspected or proven CMPA.

Formulas Based on Protein Hydrolysates

Their protein components (casein or whey proteins) have undergone a more or less extensive hydrolysis. Hydrolysates have been developed for the purpose of reducing the allergenicity of cow's milk proteins. They can be divided in extensively hydrolyzed formulas (E-HF) and partially hydrolyzed formulas (P-HF).

E-HF (as defined by the European Society of Paediatric Allergy and Clinical Immunology) are based on hydrolyzed proteins with fragments small enough to fulfill the criteria of 90% clinical tolerance in infants with proven IgE-mediated CMPA (95% confidence interval) as specified by the American Academy of Pediatrics Nutritional Committee.

P-HF contain peptides large enough to cause allergic reactions to CM protein and are not recommended for the treatment of CMPA (their use in prevention is still debated).

Residual allergenicity of E-HF has been demonstrated and it is clinically relevant since 5–10% of the children who are allergic to cow's milk proteins do not tolerate E-HF. These infants will tolerate elemental diets.

Natural Milks

The term "natural milks" is applied to milks that are derived from mammals other than cow (e.g., goat, sheep, and donkey)—all such milks have been used in CMPA elimination diet.

One of their limitations is their unbalanced composition: for example, goat milk is responsible for folate-deficiency anemia and donkey milk has a low fat content.

Another weak point is the immunologic cross-reactivity between protein from cow, sheep, and goat; these proteins are in fact highly homologous and thus cross-react in approximately 80% of subjects with CMPA.

Elemental Diets

Synthetic amino acid-based formulas have been used for a subgroup of patients who do not tolerate casein or whey E-HF. These patients often demonstrate severe allergic symptoms (severe atopic eczema or delayed type of gastrointestinal reactions) and multiple food allergies (MFA). As a consequence, they require highly restricted dietary regimens. In these formulas no protein fraction is detectable since they only contain a mixture of individual free amino acids.

These formulas are therefore the only ones really anallergic. Their limitations are the high cost and typical bad palatability, although recently their taste has been definitely improved.

PREVENTION

At present, preventive strategies have the aim to avoid the occurrence of CMPA risk factors in genetically predisposed subjects. In other words, prevention is based on (1) identifying the population at risk of food allergy and (2) reducing the food allergenic exposure of such atopy-prone infants and children.

Family history of atopic conditions and elevated cord-blood IgE are the best predictive elements for development of allergic disease available at birth.

Once the population at risk has been selected, the prevention is feasible by means of the following dietary interventions.

Breast-feeding

Breast-feeding is a time-honored practice, recommended for infants at high risk of allergy in order to prevent altogether or at least delay the development of food allergies and atopic eczema. The fact that even breast-fed infants may develop CMPA has led to the speculation that the composition of breast milk in some mothers is abnormal and may increase the risk for the baby to develop CMPA. In fact, milk from mothers whose babies were affected by CMPA compared to that from mothers with infants without CMPA (1) has significantly less macrophages; (2) has a higher proportions of neutrophils (>20%); and (3) contains eosinophils in percentages higher than 1% of total cells. Moreover, inadequate quantities of maternal IgA antibodies to food allergens may have a permissive role and seem to be more closely associated with symptoms than parental atopic history.

Hydrolyzed Formulas

Both E-HF and P-HF have been used in the prevention of CMPA; however, it is now very clear that only extensively hydrolyzed formulas have a role in CMPA prevention.

Delayed Introduction of Solid Foods

Sensitization is related to the level of allergen exposure during early life; delayed introduction of solid foods aims at allowing immature immune system to mature.

In conclusion, breast-milk should remain the feed of choice for all babies. In infants with at least one first degree relative with atopy, extensively hydrolyzed formula for a minimum of 4 months combined with dietary restrictions and environmental measures may reduce the risk of developing asthma or wheeze in the first year of life.

Summary

A guide to the choice of the alternative milk:

- Exclusive breast-fed infants → exclusion diet to nursing mother
- In the first 3 months E-HF have to be preferred; if severe forms → amino acid-based formulas
- After the third month and after weaning, soy milk has to be preferred
- If the infant refuses to assume the substitutive food (and he is older than 6 months) → natural milk or homemade preparations
- In MFA
  a. Severe forms → amino acid-based formulas and or oligoelemental diet
  b. Mild forms → ass milk
- If the infant shows enteropathy and consequent malabsorption → E-HF with low lactose and high MCT content

NATURAL HISTORY

In the past two decades, it was general opinion that every infant affected with CMPA was able to outgrow it by the age of 2 years. In 1990, a seminal paper by Bishop et al.[4] showed that allergy is outgrown by the age of 2 only in 28% of CMPA patients, 56% become tolerant at 4 years, and 78% at 6 years. Moreover, the higher incidence of persistent CMPA was typical of both, patients with multiple food allergies and immediate reactors who show anaphylaxis or urticaria within 45 min from the ingestion of CM. After this report, these observations were basically confirmed, with widely different percentages of remission. Host et al.[5] showed percentages of recovery of 56% at 1 year, 77% at 2 years, and 87% at 3 years.

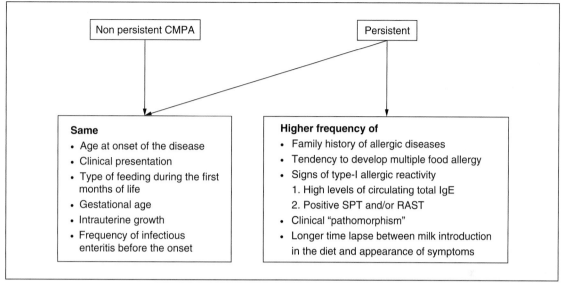

FIGURE 14-2

COMPARISON BETWEEN PATIENTS AFFECTED WITH EITHER "PERSISTENT" OR "NONPERSISTENT" CMPA

Some useful hints come from the study of Iacono et al.[6] These authors demonstrated that patients who do not overgrow CMPA by 4 years showed some peculiar characteristics (Fig. 14-2). In fact, their clinical manifestations may change over months ("pathomorphism") and symptoms after repeated challenges are different from those at presentation. Typical gastrointestinal manifestations were the most frequent at the onset, whereas at the last—still positive—challenge there was a prevalence of wheezing and constipation. In addition, the delay between CM ingestion and clinical reaction was prolonged, with symptoms becoming evident 3 or 4 weeks later, even in those patients who at onset had immediate-type reactions.

Further information is necessary to fully understand what causes the observed differences in the natural history of CMPA.

MULTIPLE FOOD ALLERGIES

Multiple food allergies can be defined as allergy to more than one basic food. As mentioned earlier, there are some infants affected with CMPA that develop allergy to other foods, especially those used as substitute of CM. Cow's milk, egg, peanut, and soybean are the foods most commonly responsible for allergic reactions in children.

MFA is a potentially harmful condition—when an infant becomes progressively intolerant to the most common foods like milk, wheat, and egg, in the absence of adequate dietary advice, the infant may experience inadequate nutrition and failure to thrive.

The risk factors for MFA are somehow similar to those described for CMPA—early sensitization with consequent early onset of symptoms (MFA occurs in up to 40% of infants with early onset CMPA), early weaning in genetically predisposed infants, IgE-mediated mechanism, history of pathomorphism, and persistent CMPA.

The treatment of MFA is challenging especially in the earlier months because patients are typically malnourished and often have a severe malabsorption syndrome. Synthetic amino acid-based formulas have been shown to be the best dietetic/nutritional resource for children with MFA.

If the patients are older and MFA develops after weaning, it is necessary to eliminate all the offending foods from the diet and test the achieved tolerance for each single food 6–12 months after the elimination.

In severe MFA, oligoantigenic diets are used but they cannot be prolonged for more than 4 weeks. The reintroduction of different foods in the diet has to be performed one by one every 7 days.

Regarding the prognosis of MFA, it has to be noticed that allergies to cow's milk, egg, and soy frequently remit whereas allergies to peanut, nuts, and fish typically persist in adulthood.

Summary

- Oral tolerance is frequently acquired in about 50–90% of children with CMPA within the first 6 years of life.
- Severe CMPA may persist in adulthood.
- CMPA presenting in infancy tends to run a prolonged course when the following hallmarks are present:
  a. Family history of allergic diseases
  b. Early onset disease
  c. IgE-mediated reactions
  d. Tendency to develop multiple food allergy
  e. Clinical "pathomorphism" (change in CMPA manifestations over time)
  f. Prolonged delay between CM intake and manifestation of symptoms
- In the follow-up of a CMPA patient after a period of CM-free diet of about 1 year (6 months if the patient is older than 8 months at onset), the acquisition of tolerance has to be checked by a recovery challenge.

- When SPT for cow's milk is positive, postponement of reevaluation is indicated.
- Children with persistent CMPA frequently develop asthma, dermatitis, and constipation. They should repeat challenge yearly and need to be followed by a medical staff familiar with the management of these problems.
- During the recovery challenge, patients should undergo an accurate follow-up and frequent outpatient observation, particularly if they are older than 2 years; every unusual manifestation has to be regarded as a relapse and tested with a period of CM-free diet.

References

1   Hill DJ, Hosking CS, Heine RG. Clinical spectrum of food allergy in children in Australia and South-East Asia: identification and targets for treatment. *Ann Med* 31(4):272–281, 1999.
2   Sampson HA. Improving in-vitro tests for the diagnosis of food hypersensitivity. *Curr Opin Allergy Clin Immunol* 2(3):257–261, 2002.
3   Stern M. Allergic enteropathy/food allergy. In: Walker W, et al. (eds.), *Pediatric Gatsrointestinal Disease.* Hamilton, ON: BC Decker, pp. 746–761.
4   Bishop JM, Hill DJ, Hosking CS. Natural history of cow milk allergy: clinical outcome [see comments]. *J Pediatr* 116(6):862–867, 1990.
5   Host A, et al. The natural history of cow's milk protein allergy/intolerance. *Eur J Clin Nutr* 49(Suppl 1):S13–S18, 1995.
6   Iacono G, et al. Persistent cow's milk protein intolerance in infants: the changing faces of the same disease. *Clin Exp Allergy* 28(7):817–823, 1998.

15

GASTROINTESTINAL AND FEEDING PROBLEMS OF THE NEUROLOGICALLY HANDICAPPED CHILD

Antonino Tedeschi

INTRODUCTION

Disabled children can face problems in any step of successful feeding. Some handicapped children have little appetite, do not perceive hunger, or are unable to communicate that they are hungry. They may lack motor abilities for appropriate feeding. Severe hypotonicity is an interfering factor that makes the neurologically impaired child unable to support head, shoulder girdle, and trunk and actively move arm and hand for self-feeding. Normal tone in the tongue, cheeks, and lips allows food to be kept in the mouth while eating and allows bolus organization and movement. This tone may be lacking in disabled children. The tongue, lips, and jaw move with rhythm and coordination in taking food into the mouth in preparation for swallowing. The neurologically handicapped child is unable to sustain a sucking rhythm and has difficulties in moving the food from the front to the back of the mouth. Moreover, this child may lack the coordination between sucking, swallowing, and breathing that is

required for feeding without choking and aspirating. *Gastroesophageal reflux* (GER) can occur in up to 75% of children with cerebral palsy.[1] It contributes significantly to dysphagia and can be another cause of recurrent aspiration pneumonia. Abnormality of sensitivity and motor tone of disabled children make mealtimes stressful and frustrating. Children with cerebral palsy may be unable to maintain a normal nutritional status; they may even take up to 15 times longer than normal children to eat a mouthful of food, but the actual quantity may not be sufficient.[2]

EPIDEMIOLOGY

Cerebral palsy occurs in 2–4 births per 1000 live births.[3] Feeding disorders have been reported in up to 90% of children with cerebral palsy.[4] Children affected by cerebral palsy constituted 49% of neurodevelopmentally disabled children referred for treatment for feeding disorders[5] and 45% of children with severe mental retardation who underwent a fundoplication for severe gastroesophageal reflux.[6] The other etiologies of cerebral dysfunction are made up of highly heterogeneous, mainly genetic, rare diseases, such as genetic syndromes and inborn error of metabolism which, because of their global incidence, represent both an important cause of morbidity and mortality in childhood and a growing challenge for the health care system due to increased life expectancy.[7] Therefore, it is likely that the prevalence of feeding problems in neurodevelopmentally disabled children is about 1/200–250 live births. Feeding is the most time-consuming of basic care for individuals with spastic tetraplegia.[8] After reduced mobility, poor feeding ability is the best single predictor of early death in profoundly neurologically handicapped individuals.[9] Pneumonia is the leading cause of death in profoundly retarded individuals.[10] This observation is not surprising considering that oral-motor dysfunction clearly predisposes to aspiration.

ETIOLOGY AND PATHOPHYSIOLOGY

Swallowing is a complex sequence of contraction-relaxation of 22 muscle groups, regulated at cortical, medullary, and peripheral levels[11] in order to carry food from the mouth to the stomach and protect the airways from aspiration.

Functional Anatomy

Anatomically, the pharynx is made up of three parts: the nasopharynx, the oropharynx, and the hypopharynx. The nasopharynx and hypopharynx are part of both the alimentary and respiratory tracts. The nasopharynx is the section of the pharynx between the nasal chonae and the roof of the soft palate. The oropharynx extends from the palate above to the base of the tongue below and includes the vallecules, which are bilateral "pockets" formed by the base of the tongue and the epiglottis. The mouth is in continuity with the oropharynx. The hypopharynx or laryngeal pharynx extends from the valleculae to the cricopharyngeal sphincter. The anterior wall of the hypopharynx includes the laryngeal inlet and the cricoid cartilage. The piriform sinuses are bilateral "pockets" located laterally

below the inlet of the larynx. When a swallow is triggered, the cricopharyngeal sphincter (upper esophageal sphincter) relaxes and allows passage of the bolus into the esophagus. Structural anomalies of the oropharynx, isolated or as part of a complex syndrome, can hinder the various phases in swallowing with the risk of aspiration and insufficient assumption of nutrients. Both the anatomy and physiology of swallowing evolve with a child's growth, adjusting the structures and functions to the type of food.

Newborns and Infants

At birth the mouth is filled by the tongue. The lateral walls of the oral cavity are stabilized by fat pads. The larynx is elevated so that the epiglottis almost touches the soft palate. This position of the epiglottis helps protect against aspiration. As the head and neck grow, the oral cavity enlarges, the tongue descends and moves back into the mouth, the neck elongates and the larynx descends to its adult position. The anatomic relationships of the infant mouth and pharynx are ideal for feeding from a breast or a bottle. The early *suckle* pattern is characterized by a rhythmic in-out movement of the tongue and up-down movement of the jaw. The regular rhythm is approximately one up-down cycle per second.[12] The tongue forms a median groove to direct liquid to the back of the oral cavity and provides a peristaltic action which compresses the nipple. Lips form an anterior seal around the nipple. Cheeks provide stability and lateral boundaries for the food. A negative pressure is created in the oral cavity to extract fluid. The jaw provides a stable base and assists in enlarging the oral cavity by moving downward. As the infant matures and the oral cavity increases in size, usually by 6 months of age, sucking becomes prominent. During the "suck" the tongue moves up and down in conjunction with the mandible. In conjunction with this, a tighter lip seal leads to a more negative pressure in the oral cavity. Acquiring this tongue movement is necessary not only for swallowing, but also for the articulation of sounds. Therefore, the impaired development of the normal oral phase of swallowing is associated with irregularities in the articulation of sounds.[12] Sucking rate, size, and speed of bolus affect frequency and timing of swallowing.[13] Nutritive and nonnutritive sucking occured. There is a 1:1 ratio for nutritive sucking and swallowing and this ratio becomes higher at the end of a feed. A stable pattern of rhythmic sucking and swallowing is present by 34–36 weeks gestation.[14] As a protective mechanism, respiration is suppressed during swallowing. During infant feeding the suck, swallow, and breath are in a 1:1:1 relation. Given their small oropharynx and the presence of a nipple the infants are necessarily nose breathers during feeding. Reflexes which make certain oral movements automatic are present in the newborn infant. The rooting reflex, used to locate food, disappears at 3–4 months, later if the infant is breast-fed. The suck-swallow reflex is elicited by stroking the anterior third of the tongue or the center of the lips, and disappears at 4 months. Feeding development results in the disappearance of rooting and other primitive reflexes (e.g., Moro, asymmetric tonic neck reflex, and positive support reflex) and maturation of more volitional components of the process.

Steps of Feeding Development

- Between 6 and 8 months of age, tongue mobility increases and the capacity to push food to one side or the other, which is necessary for chewing, is acquired.
- The capacity to bite relatively soft foods or crackers comes at about 1 year. This ability requires sufficient jaw stability and incisors.
- The ability to bite food with consistency (e.g., an apple) is usually developed by 18 months.
- Chewing development is fully complete at 24 months with enough strength in the child's jaws to chew food, perform rotatory movements of the jaw, and control the opening and bite-strength appropriately for different food bolus sizes and consistency.[15]

Mealtime requires a set of motor abilities that develop parallel to swallowing development, such as the ability to support the head, to hold a sitting position with a straight trunk, to hold objects and bring them to the mouth, and to hold a teaspoon and glass correctly. In addition, there is a sensorial component which, in a disabled child, can be very important. A child can develop a marked dislike for a particular taste or food, if associated, even temporarily, with a painful or unpleasant sensation. If a child has a choking or aspiration crisis during mealtimes, or feels pain due to a problem with motility or an infection of the mouth or esophagus, the child may develop a dislike for food. Infants who have been intubated and tube-fed for a long period, experience a series of unpleasant sensations connected to the face and mouth and show resistance to all movements which concern these parts of the body. The concept of "critical sensitive period" for acquisition of new skills[16] is a possible explanation for some feeding problems. Premature infants, and those with central nervous system dysfunction, may require prolonged enteral or parenteral feeding and thus do not experience feeding during a particular portion of the developmental sequence. These children, deprived of oral stimulation for a prolonged period of time, have great difficulty learning to eat.

Mature Swallowing

This takes place in two voluntary phases, preparatory and oral, followed by two reflex phases, pharyngeal and esophageal (Fig. 15-1). Each phase depends on the earlier one.

- A bolus is formed in the *preparatory phase*. During preparation the lips are kept closed and the food is held along a longitudinal groove of the tongue, while the close contact between the tongue and soft palate forms a closure and hinders progression before the bolus is ready for the next phase.
- In the *oral phase* the bolus is pushed toward the retropharynx by a coordinated, sequential contact of the tongue against the palate which moves backward like a wave. When the bolus passes to the pharynx a swallowing reflex is activated and from this moment the process becomes involuntary.

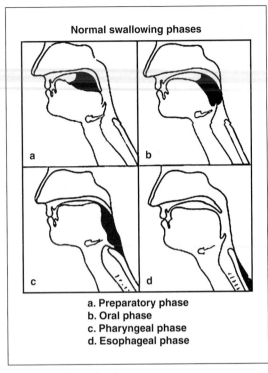

Normal swallowing phases

a. Preparatory phase
b. Oral phase
c. Pharyngeal phase
d. Esophageal phase

F I G U R E   1 5 - 1

SCHEME OF NORMAL SWALLOWING PHASES

- In the *pharyngeal phase* the soft palate rises and adheres to a muscular protrusion of the posterior nasopharynx wall, thus preventing nasal reflux. The bolus is pushed by the peristaltic contractions of the constrictor muscles of the pharynx toward the cricopharyngeal sphincter. At the same time, the larynx is lifted and pushed forward to the base of the tongue; the epiglottis and the vocal chords close, protecting the airway from penetration by food or liquid. This movement increases the pharyngeal lumen and opens the esophagus releasing the cricopharyngeal sphincter. Respiration stops briefly to allow the bolus to move to the upper esophageal sphincter.
- Thus, the *esophageal phase* starts. The bolus is pushed down by the peristalsis until, with the release of the inferior esophagus sphincter, it passes into the stomach. The patency of the airway can be affected by the degree of neck

flexion or extension—with increasing neck flexion the airway is more prone to collapse; when the neck is extended, there may be a mechanical advantage in keeping the airway open. Therefore, craniocervical posture and pharyngeal airway stability are interconnected.

Neural Control

The swallow motor pattern is generated by the medullary swallowing center and is completed in just over 1 s. The center is more a functional system than an anatomicus locus; it integrates and processes input signals from oropharyngeal sensory fibers and higher cortical and subcortical centers and generates the swallowing process via efferent motor fibers in the cranial nerves. Afferent sensory fibers are contained in four cranial nerves (V$_3$, VI, VII, X); efferent motor fibers are contained in five cranial nerves (V$_3$, VII, IX, X, XII) and two cervical peripheral nerves (C$_1$, C$_2$). Sensory feedback from the mouth and intact muscular strength and coordination are required for an effective oral phase of swallowing and progression of feed. Progressing from reflex-effected suckling to independent eating ability, at about 24–30 months, does not happen in children with cerebral palsy or other neurologic disorders. The normal process may be disrupted by various anatomic, neurologic, physiologic, and social factors. Failure of normal development progression of feeding ability may lead to inadequate intake of calories and malnutrition. Moreover, disordered feeding and swallowing patterns predispose children with neurologic damage to the development of recurrent respiratory disease.

CLINICAL SIGNS/SYMPTOMS

Children with neurologic handicaps and severe feeding problems have some common characteristics. Two or more of the following physical and sensory behaviors are usually observed: hyperextension, disorganized sucking patterns, swallowing disorders, respiratory difficulties, abnormal or aversive responses to oral stimulation, gastroesophageal reflux, and constipation.[12]

Physical Examination

A physical examination usually reveals hyperextension of the neck, accompanied by scapular adduction and shoulder girdle elevation. A probable reason for this pattern is that the child compensates for the lack of head and trunk stability in a sitting position by bringing the scapulae together in adduction, elevating the shoulder girdle, and resting the head back to this stable support. Moreover, neck hyperextension may be used to increase the diameter of the pharyngeal airway to compensate for respiratory difficulties; however, this compensatory position constitutes a major risk of aspiration.

Tongue

High muscle tone tends to accompany bunched, retracted, or humped tongue. The *lower tone* tongue is protruded, flat, and wide. It is very common to observe a neurologically handicapped child attempting to compensate retraction of the tongue by fixing it against the midportion of the hard palate. A strong protrusive movement may be used to counteract tongue retraction. This protrusion is called *tongue thrust* and is generally associated with increased tone. It is very difficult to maintain the fixed tongue position or its protrusive movement and eat successfully at the same time—the ability of the tongue to form an adequate central groove, to form and hold the bolus in the posterior portion of the mouth, may be lacking. Food, particularly liquid, may spill prematurely into the vallecular or piriform sinuses, when the larynx is not closed, and aspiration may occur. Moreover, a strongly elevated tongue can block adequate spoon or nipple placement and can be a cause of feeding difficulties.

Jaw, Cheeks, Lips, and Palate

Neurologically disabled children usually lack normal jaw movement which should be smooth, in small excursion, and rhythmic. Their mouth and jaws are often open, and there is a large excursion of the jaw, indicating a poorly graded movement that may interfere with lip seal, resulting in fluid loss and difficulty

in closing the mouth for chewing. The overall increased extensor tone is often associated with *jaw thrust*, a forceful opening of the jaw to the maximal extent during eating, drinking, attempts to speak, or general excitement. Jaw thrusting is often accompanied by tongue thrusting. Oral stimulation may elicit the *tonic bite reflex*, a strong jaw closure when teeth and gums are stimulated. Such patterns interfere with all aspects of feeding. Too high or too low tone of cheeks can compromise suction and decrease feeding efficiency. With generalized hypotonia, lips are loose, floppy, and do not seal well, so liquid can leak from the mouth. Lip retraction may occur at the approach of the spoon or cup toward the face when the underlying tone is increased. An abnormally shaped hard palate is often observed. It may be narrow, grooved, high-arched with clefts, and interfere with an efficient feeding process. Food routinely escaping through the nose during feeding or emesis may indicate abnormal soft palate movement.

Oral-motor Problems

Sucking, swallowing, and breathing coordination. The well-coordinated, nonnutritive sucking rhythm is approximately two sucks per second with bursts of 6–10 sucks. The rate of nutritive suck is one suck per second. The major clinical indications of swallowing dysfunction are respiratory symptoms.

- Coughing and choking during swallowing are a sign of aspiration.
- Excessive pooling of secretion is generally the result of poor swallowing. It may lead to aspiration. Normally, oral feeding is not safe for a child who is unable to handle secretions.
- Noisy breathing suggests swallowing dysfunction. If the noise arises during feeding, insufficient velar elevation should be considered. Residual food in the pharynx following feeding produces wet-sounding breathing. Aspiration can occur if the food falls into the open airway.
- Frequent unexplained respiratory infection, including pneumonia, suggests the presence of aspiration, even if oral feeding and sucking pattern are normal. *Videofluoroscopic*

swallowing study (VFSS) can confirm a silent aspiration.
- Multiple swallows suggest difficulties in organizing bolus and faulty pharyngeal peristalsis.

A prolonged sucking pattern (of at least 5–20 sucks) without breaths, in a full-term infant, can be a hallmark of a coordination problem between swallowing and breathing and could be the first sign of future neurologic problems. The long burst of sucking often ceases only when the baby coughs or becomes cyanotic and bradycardic with apnea.

Gastrointestinal Dysfunction

Gastroesophageal reflux. GER is very common in neurologically handicapped children (Table 15-1). The following four causes may be found in the same child, in addition to the direct effect of central nervous system dysfunction on the *lower esophageal sphincter* (LES):

- Dysmotility of the esophagus
- Lowered esophageal sphincter pressure
- Gastric emptying abnormalities

- Increased abdominal pressure because of spasticity, seizures, scoliosis, constipation, and abnormal posturing[17]

Reflux esophagitis, recurrent vomiting, recurrent aspiration pneumonia, and malnutrition are more commonly associated conditions. GER may not be associated with vomiting. Recurrent laryngospam, broncospasm, irritability, and anemia may be the only symptoms. Sandifer's syndrome, the association of unusual posturing with extension of the neck and rotation of the head, during or immediately after meals, and iron deficiency anemia and esophagitis, is a manifestation of GER. In disabled children the syndrome may not be recognized and may instead be diagnosed as a movement disorder.

Constipation. Constipation and fecal impaction are frequent and distressing complaints in neurologically impaired children (Table 15-1). Several mechanisms may be involved in the pathogenesis of chronic constipation:[18]

- Inadequate food and liquid intake
- Inadequate dietary fiber intake
- Lack of conscious urge to defecate
- Immobilization

TABLE 15-1

SYMPTOMATOLOGY OF CHILDREN WITH DEVELOPMENTAL DISABILITIES (ALL CHILDREN (A), CHILDREN WITH SEVERE HANDICAP (B))[a]

	Patient A		Patient B	
	No. 22	%	No. 13	%
Vomiting	12	54	9	75
Hematemesis	8	36	8	62
Feeding problems[b]	16	72	13	100
Recurrent respiratory infection	9	41	9	69
Malnutrition[c]	15	68	8	61
Anemia	4	19	4	31
Pain/irritability	9	43	7	54
Constipation	15	68	13	100

[a]Profound mental retardation, severe motor and speech language handicap.
[b]Tongue thrust, coughing or choking, fluid or food loss during eating, excessive time required for meals, difficulties in consuming textured foods.
[c]Weight for height

- Motor paralysis of the abdominal and perineal muscles
- Disruption of the neural modulation of colonic motility

Constipation is associated with early satiety and is an additional reason for poor feeding in neurologically handicapped children.

COMPLICATIONS

Nutritional Problems

Neurologically handicapped children have a high level of risk for malnutrition. Oral-motor dysfunction, GER, and aversive feeding behavior all affect food intake and nutrient requirements. Most of these children remain undernourished despite the efforts of their caregivers. There is evidence that nutritional factors have a role in growth failure and mortality in children with cerebral palsy. Anthropometric indicators of undernutrition were found in 43% of children with cerebral palsy, and of overnutrition in 9%, in a study by Thommessen.[19] A higher prevalence of malnutrition was found in the population of children with neurodevelopmental disorders reported in Table 15-1. On the other hand, an improvement in nutritional status may determine a reduction in the number of GER episodes,[20] an improvement in mood,[2] and even a reduction in spastic contractions.[21] Early nutritional management of children with severe cerebral palsy is effective in reverse nutritional deficit both in length and in weight.[22] A nutritional intervention 8 years or more after the central nervous insult improved weight but not length. As a result of physical deformity and growth abnormality, reduced weight for height cannot be relied on in the usual way as an indicator of wasting. Even weight measurement may be difficult. Measurements of the mid-arm muscle circumference are usually lower because of muscle atrophy, but may be relatively higher in spastic children as an effect of constant contraction (like athletic training). On the other hand, skin-fold thickness, which measures adipose tissue, is not affected by the neurodevelopmental handicap *per se* and should be normal unless undernutrition has occurred.[23] Thus, most research considers skin-fold measurement the most useful method of assessing nutritional status.[24] For clinical purposes measurement of triceps skinfold is considered as a useful method to assess the child's adipose store and his nutritional status. Total daily energy needs are affected by activity levels. Thus, the energy needs of children with neurologic disease who, with rare exception, have limited activity, are lower than the recommended nutrition intakes. The only useful biochemical data in assessment of nutritional status in these children are iron and hemoglobin values. However, children receiving long-term anticonvulsivant therapy with phenytoin or phenobarbital are at risk for vitamin D and folate deficiency. The vitamin D requirement in nonambulatory handicapped patients with seizure is probably 1200 IU per day; also chronic treatment for constipation with mineral oil may induce fat-soluble vitamin deficiency.

Respiratory Complications

Aspiration pneumonia is the most common cause of death in patients with dysphagia due to neurologic disorders.[25] Children with impaired swallowing are at high risk of aspiration.

- Aspiration *before* swallowing may be due to poor tongue control or delay in or absence of the triggering of the swallow reflex. If the bolus rolls back from the mouth to the pharynx when the airway is still open, it may produce aspiration. We can imagine that a liquid bolus brings more risk of aspiration than a mush one.
- Aspiration *during* swallowing is considered a result of reduced laryngeal closure, often as a result of vocal cord paralysis.
- Aspiration *after* swallowing may be due to the food that remains in the valleculae or in the piriform sinuses as a result of inefficient swallowing and enters the airway when the larynx reopens after swallowing. Moreover, gastroesophageal reflux may result in aspiration after swallowing.

In a disabled child aspiration is possible without coughing if there is impaired cough reflex. Silent aspiration, without cough, occurred in 71% of children with ataxia-teleangiectasia.[26] Aspiration can result in chronic lung disease and *Pseudomonas aeruginosa* infection in patients with frequent hospitalizations.

DIFFERENTIAL DIAGNOSIS

A diagnostic work-up includes history, physical examination, and direct observation of feeding. Instrumental assessments can be useful in selected patients.

History

The first step of the evaluation process should be to interview the parents or caregiver to determine specific concerns regarding feeding and current feeding methods.

The following questions should help to clarify the problems and to formulate treatment strategies.

- *Do the feeding problems vary with food texture?* Children with lack of coordination in oral and pharyngeal functions are at greater risk of aspiration with liquids than with thicker textures.
- *What is the child's position during mealtime?* The risk of aspiration may be increased either with extensor arching of the trunk or with a "floppy" neck and excessive flexion of the oropharynx.
- *Does the child have emesis? Is he/she irritable?* GER is a common problem; also consider GER if the child is often agitated, cries a lot, draws knees to chest with crying, and sleeps poorly.
- *Does the child refuse food?* It could be a way of communicating problems with oral-motor function, pain in the gastrointestinal tract, and/or parent-child interaction abnormalities. Reported lethargy during meals may result from excessive fatigue or sedating medication.
- *Does the child have cough, choking, apnea, noisy breathing, with feeding? Does he/she have excessive drooling, history of respiratory illness (pneumonia, asthma)?* All these signs could be caused by problems with coordination of sucking, swallowing, and breathing.

- *How long is the meal?* In general, mealtimes should take no more than 30 min. Longer mealtime could indicate difficulties in consuming the required calories.
- *What is the weekly defecation frequency?* A good result, which does not require treatment, for the disabled child is a pain-free, spontaneous defecation, with minimum effort, every 2–3 days.[27]

It is useful to ask about the use of drugs—benzodiazepames induce reduced pharyngeal constrictor function, lack of cricopharyngeal coordination, and drooling;[28] phenytoin and barbiturates may precipitate deficiency in serum folate and vitamin D. The use of mineral oil for the treatment of chronic constipation could induce fat-soluble vitamin deficiency.

Physical Examination

A physical examination could help identify signs of a genetic syndrome. Actually, dysphagia is very common in a number of genetic syndromes (Table 15-2). An assessment of muscle tone, primitive reflex activity, and habitual postural control should be carried out before a feeding evaluation. Particular attention should be paid to the child's posture and to the support that is provided to the child for efficient feeding. The child should be observed for at least 15–20 min to evaluate signs of fatigue as feeding progresses. Difficulties in oral-motor capacity are indicated by the presence of the following signs:

- Tongue thrust
- Fluid or food loss during eating
- Cough, choking during eating
- Marked prolongation of mealtimes
- Difficulty in consuming textured food

A more impaired function is indicated by association of these signs.[29]

Instrumental Assessment

Cardiorespiratory Monitor

This monitor gives information about the child's heart rate status. If there is a dramatic increase in

TABLE 15-2

MISCELLANEOUS DISORDERS ASSOCIATED WITH FEEDING AND SWALLOWING DIFFICULTIES AND NEURO-MOTOR HANDICAP

Prader-Willi syndrome	Beckwith-Wiedermann
Coffin siris	Trisomy 18
Smith-Lemli-Opitz-syndrome	Trisomy 21
De Lange syndrome	Arnold-Chiari malformation
Dubowitz	Degenerative diseases of white and gray matter
Rubenstein-Taybi	Multiple sclerosis
Spinocerebellar disorders	Amyotrophic lateral sclerosis
Dystonia musculorum deformans	Metabolic encephalopathies
Syringobulbia	Traumatic encephalopathies
Infantile spinal muscular atrophy	Infections of central nervous system
Miastenia gravis	Hypossic-ischemic encephalopathy
Metabolic myopathies	Cerebral palsy
Congenital myopathies	
Duchenne's muscular dystrophy	

heart rate with feeding, the work of feeding may be excessive for the child. A bradycardia with feeding could be a sign of a possible life-threatening event.

Oximetry

Normal oxygen saturation values are above 95%. Low saturation values during feeding could be a sign of lack of coordination between swallowing and breathing.

Radiologic Procedures

Technetium scan. Images made over a 1-h period after feeding provide information regarding the number of reflux episodes and the height of reflux. It measures both acid and alkaline reflux. Gastric emptying may be assessed. Delayed images can be used to detect pulmonary aspiration of the technetium.

Barium swallow. This identifies structural abnormalities such as esophageal strictures, duodenal obstruction, and malrotation syndrome. It can detect the presence or absence of GER; however, the predictive value of a positive result is very low and it gives a limited evaluation of swallowing.

Videofluoroscopic swallowing study. This is designed to evaluate the pharyngeal swallow. Liquid barium is mixed with milk or pureed food. Supplementary information may be gained by giving barium paste or crackers coated with barium. In the lateral projection it is possible to evaluate the tongue shape, position and movements, nasal escape, and laryngeal penetration by contrast medium. It is also possible to evaluate the response to treatment technique. Typical problems that indicate the need for a VFSS include coughing or choking between or during meals, profuse drooling, recurrent pulmonary infection (to exclude possible silent aspiration), and history of nasopharyngeal reflux.

Ultrasound

This is a technique that does not involve ionizing radiation, so it could be particularly useful in pediatric age. Observation over several swallows allows detection of abnormal movements of the tongue, hyoid bone, and coordination of the phases of swallowing. However, the procedure does not permit vision of the last movement and the detection of nasal escape. Moreover, larynx aspiration during swallowing is not well assessed by this technique.

Esophageal pH Monitoring

This is considered the gold standard for diagnosis of GER (see Chap. 13); however, it can be unreliable in disabled children with scoliosis where accurate positioning of the probe is more difficult. Nevertheless, a number of reports testify to the value of esophageal pH monitoring in cases where an antireflux procedure is required.

Esophagoscopy—Esophageal Manometry

Esophagoscopy helps determine the need for antireflux procedures in the event that GER does occur and symptoms are not controlled by drug treatment. Esophageal manometry is used to measure the pressure in the upper and lower esophageal sphincter to assess their competence.

GUIDELINES TO TREATMENT AND FOLLOW-UP

The complexity of the processes of feeding should involve many different professionals: speech and language therapist, occupational therapist, physiotherapist, dietitian, dentist, pediatrician, respiratory specialist, radiologist, gastroenterologist, and surgeon. However, some items of treatment are so obviously effective and are so simple to apply that an informed physician, without the support of a team of specialists, can give a great deal of help to these children.

Compensatory Strategies

They involve controlling[30]

- The position of the patient's head and body
- The food texture
- The volume of food
- The rate at which food is given

There is no ideal position useful for all children with motor disorders. Nevertheless, the position of the head and neck in eating and drinking is critical. Tilting the child's head forward narrows the airway;

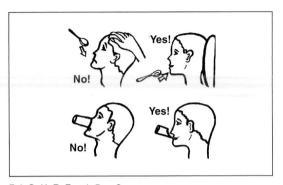

FIGURE 15-2

METHODS TO PREVENT FOOD ASPIRATION

tilting the head backward can promote the passage to the pharynx prior to triggering the swallow reflex and increase the risk of aspiration. The neck should be aligned in a neutral position. Liquids move rapidly by gravity and have a high risk of splashing into the airway if there is a delay in triggering the pharyngeal swallow. It has been shown that some patients are able to manage bolus volume of a certain size, but have problems with larger volumes. Aspiration can result if food is presented faster than the child can clear it from the pharynx. Figures 15-2 and 15-3 show some practical suggestions regarding the best positions for preventing aspiration of food. Having an aspirator at home is advisable, to be used in case of abundant secretions in the mouth which are not

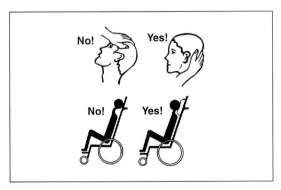

FIGURE 15-3

PRACTICAL SUGGESTIONS TO PREVENT ASPIRATION OF FOOD

removed by coughing. Indirect therapy strategies are suggested in which the child manipulates something in the mouth without actually swallowing it. Such therapy could improve oral-motor and laryngeal control. Maintaining sensorial stimulation of the lips, tongue, and cheeks during enteral or parenteral nutrition could help prevent future aversive response to sensory oral stimulation.

Gastrostomy Feeding

The *American Academy for Cerebral Palsy and Developmental Medicine* (AACPDM) considers gastrostomy as an alternative to exclusive oral feeding of disabled children in the following situations:[31]

- Nasogastric feeding beyond the short-term, acute care period
- A long time to feed
- Inadequate weight gain
- Unsafe swallowing (i.e., significant risk of aspiration of food)

The overall rates of major complications were reported to be from 17 to 39.3%. These included bowel obstructions, gastrointestinal bleeds, ulceration, and peritonitis. High rates of minor complications were also reported, such as leakage around the tube, dislodgment, disconnection or blockage, site irritation, infection, and granulation tissue. Although tube feeding has been associated with an approximately doubled mortality rate among children with less severe disabilities in a retrospective analysis of a large population of children with disabilities and mental retardation,[32] the report of AACPDM underlines the consistency of results in favor of gastrostomy. On the other hand, it should be considered that some parents take several hours each day to feed their disabled child by mouth. A study has shown that initiation of tube feeding improved the quality of life for both the child and family in 90% of cases, despite frequent minor complications.[33]

Energy Requirements

Once patients entirely fed by gastrostomy have reached an adequate nutritional status, as judged by fat-fold thickness, they require only 700–1100 kcal/die.[34] This makes providing their other nutrient needs a problem. For this reason the use of pediatric or even infant formulas has been recommended, since they have a higher nutrient to energy ratio. On the other hand, extraordinarily high energy requirements have been observed in children with athetosis. Adjusting energy intake for triceps skinfolds represents a valid method of determining energy requirements. The nutritional intervention should result in restoration of the child's adipose store (usually the 25th centile for age of triceps skinfold). The weight to use as a basis for the child's subsequent growth is obtained when skin-fold measurement is normal. The difficulty is in choosing a starting point from which to determine caloric intake. The *resting metabolic rate* (RMR) of patients with severe impairment of the central nervous system is overestimated by the World Health Organization equation used to calculate RMR.[35–37] Nevertheless, the use of such formulas to calculate energy requirement, adjusted by an activity factor of 1.3 for well-nourished spastic children and 1.5 for malnourished children, is recommended.[10] As a starting point of daily energy requirements the author uses the WHO equation adapted by Prof. Paul Pencharz, kindly given for use, adjusted by an activity factor of 1.2–1.5 for children with spastic quadriplegia and 1.7–2.0 for children with athetosis (Table 15-3).

Formulas

The formulas available for gastrostomy feeding fit into four categories: home-liquidized, polymeric, elemental, and modular.

- *Home-liquidized formulas* cost less than other formula foods and offer a psychologic benefit. Nevertheless, there is a greater potential for bacterial contamination, it is difficult to calculate the actual given nutrients, and food preparation is time-consuming. The disadvantages, especially that of contamination, outweigh the advantages.[37]
- *Polymeric formulas* may be useful. Many formulas contain fiber that is of benefit in

TABLE 15-3

BASAL METABOLIC RATE[a]

Age (years)	Females (kcal/kg per day)	Males (kcal/kg per day)
1	56.4	57
2	54.3	53.65
3	53.0	53.60
4	51.0	50.80
5	50.9	48.43
6	47.4	46.72
7	44.7	44.80
8	42.0	41.5
9	39.1	40.30
10	37.1	38.3
11	35.2	36.6
12	32.0	35.1
13	30.0	33.4
14	27.0	30.9
15	26.0	29.5
16	25.5	28.4
17	24.8	27.6
18	24.5	27
19	24.3	26.5
20	24.2	26.4

[a]Determination of total daily energy requirements: MB × 1.2—patient confined to bed; MB × 1.5—patient sedentary; MB × 1.7—normal activity; MB × 2.0—athlete.

constipation, which is so common in these patients; however, the high density of the formulas may also result in slower emptying. Such an effect would be dangerous in patients at risk of reflux.

- *Elemental formulas* might be more useful. A decrease in gastric emptying time and a lower incidence of GER has been seen in children with severe neurologic impairment fed a whey-based formula.[38,39] Therefore, the use of such a formula has been recommended in children with severe neurologic impairment.
- *Modules.* Usually, modules, adjusted to individual patient's needs of protein, fat, and carbohydrates, are not used.

Formula Delivery

- Bolus feeds via syringe over a few minutes carry the risk of causing bloating, cramping, nausea, diarrhea, and aspiration.
- Intermittent feeds are given by gravity drip or pump. The rate can be adjusted to the patient's tolerance. This method of food delivery is considered more physiologic and is recommended.[40]
- Continuous feed may be the only way to feed patients with delayed gastric and/or abnormalities of intestinal transit which in some patients may be so severe as to determine intestinal pseudoobstruction.

Decrease Reflux

The presence of GER before PEG, and its possible aggravation after PEG, led some surgeons to always perform antireflux surgery at the time of gastrostomy. Nevertheless, evidence has been gathered about the efficacy, safety, and tolerability of *proton-pump inhibitors* (PPIs) in children, including children in whom antireflux surgery or other medical therapy has failed.[41,42] Doses of omeprazole required for healing chronic erosive esophagitis in a population of 57 children, including patients with neurologic impairment, were 0.7–3.5 mg/kg per day (maximum 80 mg per day).[43] Long-term use for up to 7 years has been associated with a reduction in antireflux surgery from 50 per year to fewer than 5 per year.[41] Considering the complications of antireflux surgery in disabled children the following statements have been proposed:[44]

- Systematic prophylactic fundoplication associated with PEG placement should be ruled out. Obviously, a detailed evaluation of the importance of GER disease (GERD) should be done beforehand.
- If GERD occurs or worsens after PEG, PPIs treatment should be adapted/adopted first and bolus feeding should be replaced by continuous enteral nutrition. A whey-based formula might be useful.

- If severe GERD is not controlled by medical treatment and is associated with impaired pulmonary function, before PEG is decided, fundoplication or esophagogastric dissociation[45] should be considered.

Efficiency and tolerance of percutaneous gastrojejunostomy, a possible alternative to surgery, need to be confirmed.[44] H2 antagonists are less effective than PPIs in the treatment of GERD.[46] Randomized studies of the effect of sodium alginate have given contrasting results on symptoms and on pH metric values.[46] There are insufficient data on the efficacy and security on the use of sucralfate in children.[46] Baclofen, a structural analog of the inhibitory neurotransmitter GABA, is used for the therapy of spasticity of cerebral origin when given for 1 month to GER disease patients, 10 mg four times daily for 4 weeks Baclofen reduced esophageal acid reflux and the percentage of time with esophageal pH <4, and significantly reduced symptoms.[47]

How many neurologically handicapped children need surgery (PEG, fundoplication, or Bianchi procedure) for the treatment of feeding problems? How many are cured by the compensatory strategies and PPI? An answer comes from the following data of the study by Schwarz.[5] Fifty-one out of 79 (65%) disabled children, with moderate-to-severe motor or cognitive dysfunction, responded to medical treatment of GER with ranitidine showing improved nutrition and decreased morbidity, thus avoiding surgical intervention for gastrostomy tube placement or fundoplication.[5] Perhaps a greater proportion of children could be treated without surgery using PPIs instead of ranitidine.

Treatment of Constipation

The basic principles for the treatment of constipation are the same for children with neurologic disabilities as for normal children.

Goal

A good result of treatment is to produce an easy pain-free defecation, at least every 3 days.

Prevention

- Provide a diet with adequate fluids and fiber
- Early recognition of anal discomfort given by fissure and/or perianal skin infection with group A *Streptococcus*

Softening

Sometimes to reach the liquid requirement the addition of extra fruit juice may be sufficient. For people who are tube-fed it may be useful to give a formula with fiber to reach the recommended intake for age. Various laxatives and stool softeners can be used. Recent reports[48,49] have demonstrated that polyethylene glycol is an effective, safe, and palatable treatment for constipation. The effective dose for chronic treatment was 0.75–1 g/kg per day given in two divided doses of the solution obtained with 17 g in 240 mL of water, juice, or other clear liquid.[48] A dose up to 1.5 g/kg per day of a solution obtained with 0.15 g/mL was used for three consecutive days for the treatment of fecal impaction.[50]

Treatment of Chronic Respiratory Infections

Many neurologically handicapped children develop chronic lung infection. In most cases, bypassing the pharynx by tube feeding and preventing aspiration by reflux with an operation, even the most impaired lungs improve. Nevertheless, in some cases, structural damage of lung parenchyma and/or aspiration of mucus and secretion maintain chronic pulmonary infection. *P. aeruginosa* is the predominating organism isolated from the sputum of hospitalized patients.[25] The treatment strategies in such cases are very similar to those adopted in cystic fibrosis. Physiotherapy may be useful. Antibiotic therapy according to the results of sputum culture is useful for infection control. Continuous low dose of active antibiotics[10] or cyclic use of anti-*Pseudomonas* therapy may be useful even if it has not been demonstrated by controlled studies. Broncho-dilators and oral steroid may suppress wheeze symptoms.

CASE STUDY 15-1

Exemplary

C.G. was a 19-year-old boy at the first nutritional evaluation, affected by spastic quadriplegia.

He was hospitalized for pneumonia and respiratory failure. His weight was 18 kg and height was not measured because of scoliosis and leg deformity. He had been fed only milk for a long time because he was unable to eat any solid food. He had been hospitalized many times for the same reason, i.e., aspiration pneumonia. In addition, he had a long history of vomiting, often with blood, coughing, and choking with feeding. He suffered from severe constipation and epilepsy treated with phenobarbital. *P. aeruginosa* was found in the culture of the sputum.

Treatment

- Ceftazidime and tobramicyn
- Omeprazole
- Nasogastric tube feeding (with a polyurethane tube) with a polymeric formula with fiber

The caloric supply was initially 2100 kcal per day which was about 70% of recomended dietary allowance (RDA) for age.

Follow-up

- After 2 months his weight was 34 kg (>16 kg)
- After 5 months his weight was 60 kg (10–25th centile), triceps skinfold was >90th centile, and mid-arm muscle circumference was <5th centile.
- With a caloric supply of 1500 kcal per day, his weight was down to 42 kg <5th centile, but triceps skinfold was at 25–50th centile and mid-arm muscle circumference at <5th centile.
- C.G. has not had an operation for reflux, has not been hospitalized for respiratory problems in 8 years of follow-up, but has received several cycles of anti-*Pseudomonas* IV and tobramicyn aerosol treatment at home. Parents refused PEG.

Comment

The quality of life for this boy changed after recognizing his feeding problems and the relationship with respiratory problems. His caloric needs are much lower than expected requirements for age. Omeprazole was sufficient to control GERD without surgery for reflux. Enteral nutrition by nasogastric tube may be sufficient for treatment, but frequent tube dislodgment has been a considerable problem. The treatment of chronic lung infection using protocols very similar to those used for other chronic lung diseases such as cystic fibrosis has been effective.

References

1   Couriel JM, Bisset R, Miller R, et al. Assessment of feeding problems in neurodevelopmental handicap: a team approach. *Arch Dis Child* 69:609, 1993.

2   Gisel EG, Patrick J. Identification of children with cerebral palsy unable to maintain a normal nutritional state. *Lancet* 1:283, 1988.

3   Behrman RE, Kliegman RM. *Nelson Textbook of Pediatrics*. Philadelphia, PA: WB Saunders, 2000.

4   Reilly S, Skuse D, Poblete X.: Prevalence of feeding problems and oral motor dysfunction in children with cerebral palsy: a community survey. *J Pediatr* 6:877, 1996.

5   Schwarz SM, Corredor J, Fisher-Medina J, Cohen J, et al. *Pediatrics* 108:671, 2001.

6   Spitz I, Roth K, Kiely EM, et al. Operation for gastro-oesophageal reflux associated with severe mental retardation. *Arch Dis Child* 68:47, 1993.

7   Dionisi-Vici C, Rizzo C, Burlina AB, et al. Inborn error of metabolism in the Italian pediatric population:

a national retrospective survey. *J Pediatr* 140:321, 2002.

8   Edebol-Tysk K. Evaluation of care-load for individuals with spastic tetraplegia. *Dev Med Child Neurol* 31:737, 1989.

9   Eyman RK, Grossman HJ, Chaneey RH, et al. The life expectancy of profoundly handicapped people with mental retardation. *N Engl J Med* 323:584, 1990.

10 Sullivan PB, Rosenbloom L. *Feeding the Disabled Child.* London: Mac Keith Press, 1996.

11 Cook IJS. Normal and disordered swallowing: new insights. *Baillieres Clin Gastroenterol* 5:245, 1991.

12 Morris SE. Development of oral-motor skills in the neurologically impaired child receiving non oral feeding. *Dysphagia* 3:135, 1989.

13 Wolf LS, Glass RP. *Feeding and Swallowing Disorders in Infancy Assessment and Management.* San Antonio, TX: Therapy Skill Builders, 1992.

14 Rudolph CD. Feeding disorders in infants and children. *J Pediatr* 125:S116, 1994.

15 Cloud H. Feeding problems of the child with special health care needs. In: Ekvall SW (ed.), *Pediatric Nutrition in Chronic Diseases and Developmental Disorders, Prevention, Assessment and Treatment.* New York, NY: Oxford University Press, 1993, p. 203.

16 Illingworth RS, Lister J. The critical or sensitive period, with special reference to certain feeding problems in infants and children. *J Pediatr* 65:839, 1964.

17 Sullivan PB. Gastrostomy feeding in the disabled child: when is an antireflux procedure required? *Arch Dis Child* 81:63, 1999.

18 Staiano A, Simeone D, Del Giudice E, et al. Effect of the dietary fiber glucomannan on chronic constipation in neurologically impaired children. *J Pediatr* 136:41, 2000.

19 Thommessen DM, Rasmussen M, Selberg T: Feeding and nutritional characteristics in children with moderate or severe cerebral palsy. *Acta Paediatr* 86:336, 1997.

20 Lewis D, Khoshoo V, Pencharz PB, et al. Impact of nutritional rehabilitation on gastroesophageal reflux in neurologically impaired children. *J Pediatr Surg* 29:167, 1994.

21 Patrick J, Boland M, Stoski D, et al. Rapid correction of wasting in children with cerebral palsy. *Dev Med Child Neurol* 28:724, 1986.

22 Sanders KD, Cox K, Cannon R, et al. Growth response to enteral feeding by children with cerebral palsy. *J Parenter Enteral Nutr* 14:23, 1990.

23 Dietz WH, Bandini L. Nutritional assessment of the handicapped child. *Pediatr Rev* 11:109, 1989.

24 Patrick J, Pencharz PB. Undernutrition in neurodevelopmental disability. A statement of the Nutrition Committee of the Canadian Paediatric Society. *Can Med Assoc J* 151:753, 1994.

25 Marik PE. Aspiration pneumonitis and aspiration pneumonia. *N Engl J Med* 344:665, 2001.

26 Lefton-Greif M, Crawford TO, Winkelstein JA, et al. Oropharyngeal dysphagia and aspiration in patients with ataxia-telangectasia. *J Pediatr* 136: 225, 2000.

27 Eicher PM. Feeding the child with disabilities. In: Batshaw ML, Perret YM (eds), *Children with Disabilities*, 3rd ed. Baltimore, MD: Paul H. Publishing, 1992, p. 197.

28 Arvedson JC, Rogers BT. Swallowing and feeding in the pediatric patient. In: Perlman AL, Schulze-Derieu KS (eds), *Deglutition and its Disorders, Anatomy, Physiology, Clinical Diagnosis, and Management.* San Diego, CA: Singular Publishing Group, 1997, p. 419.

29 Stallings VA, Cronk CE, Zemel BS, et al. Body composition in children with spastic quadriplegic cerebral palsy. *J Pediatr* 126:833, 1995.

30 Logeman JA. Approaches to management of disordered swallowing. *Baillieres Clin Gastroenterol* 5:269, 1991.

31 Fang LS, O'Donnel M. Effects of gastostomy feeding in children with cerebral palsy: an AACPDM evidence report. *Dev Med Child Neurol* 45:415, 2003.

32 Strauss D, Kastner T, Ashwal S, et al. Tube-feeding and mortality in children with severe disabilities and mental retardation. *Pediatrics* 99:358, 1997.

33 Smith SW, Camfield C, Camfield P. Living with cerebral palsy and tube feeding: a population-based follow-up study. *J Pediatr* 135:307, 1999.

34 Fried MD, Pencharz PB. Energy and nutrient intakes of children with spastic quadriplegia. *J Pediatr* 119:947, 1991.

35 Bandini LG, Puelzi-Quinn H, Morelli JA, et al. Estimation of energy requirements in persons with severe central nervous system impairment. *J Pediatr* 126:828, 1995.

36 World Health Organization. *Energy and Protein Requirements: Report of a Joint FAO/WHO/UNU Meeting.* Geneva: World Health Organization, 1985.

37 Grunow JE, Chait P, Savoie S, et al. Gastrostomy feeding. *Recent Adv Paediatr* 12:23, 1993.

38 Fried MD, Khoshoo V, Secker DJ, et al. Decrease of gastric emptying time and episodes of regurgitation in children with spastic quadriplegia fed a whey-based formula. *J Pediatr* 120:569, 1992.

39 Khoshoo V, Zembo M, King A, et al. Incidence of gastroesophageal reflux with whey and casein based formulas in infants and in children with severe neurological impairment. *J Pediatr Gastroenterol Nutr* 22:48, 1996.

40 American Gastroenterological Association Patient Care Committee. American Gastroenterological Association Medical Position Statement: Guidelines for the use of enteral nutrition. *Gatroenterology* 108:1280, 1995.

41 Hassal E. Antireflux surgery in children: time for a harder look. *Pediatrics* 101:467, 1998.

42 Pashankar D, Blair GK, Israel DM. Omeprazole maintenance therapy for gastroesophageal reflux disease after failure of fundoplication. *J Pediatr Gastroenterol Nutr* 32:15, 2001.

43 Hassal E, Israel D, Shepherd R, et al. Omeprazole for treatment of chronic erosive esophagitis in children: a multicenter study of efficacy, safety, tolerability and dose requirements. *J Pediatr* 137:800, 2000.

44 Gottrand F, Michaud L. Percutaneous endoscopic gastrostomy and gastro-esophageal reflux: Are we correctly addressing the question? *J Pediatr Gastroenterol Nutr* 35:27, 2002.

45 Bianchi A. Total esophagogastric dissociation: an alternative approach. *J Pediatr Surg* 32:1291, 1997.

46 Rudolph CD, Mazur LJ, Liptak GS, et al. Guidelines for evaluation and treatment of gastroesophageal reflux in infants and children: recommendations of the North American Society for Pediatric Gastroenterology and Nutrition. *J Pediatr Gastroenterol Nutr* 32(S2):1, 2001.

47 Ciccaglione AF, Marzio L. Effect of acute and chronic administration of the GABA B agonist baclofen on 24 hour pH metric symptoms in control subjects and in patients with gastro-oesophageal reflux disease. *Gut* 52:46, 2003.

48 Pashankar DS, Bishop WP: Efficacy and optimal dose of daily polyethylene glycol 3350 for treatment of constipation and encopresis in children. *J Pediatr* 139:428, 2001.

49 Pashankar DS, Loening-Baucke V, Bishop WP. Safety of polyethylene glycol 3350 for the treatment of chronic constipation in children. *Arch Pediatr Adolesc Med* 157:661, 2003.

50 Youssef NN, Peters JM, Henderson W, et al. Dose response of PEG 3350 for treatment of childhood fecal impaction. *J Pediatr* 141:410, 2002.

16

EOSINOPHILIC GASTROENTEROPATHY

John M. Russo

INTRODUCTION

Eosinophilic gastroenteropathy is an idiopathic, chronic, and relapsing disease characterized by an eosinophilic inflammatory infiltration of the tissues of the *gastrointestinal* (GI) tract. Kaijser was the first to describe this disease in 1937.[1] There is a broad spectrum of disease with various manifestations based on the region of the gastrointestinal tract involved. Due to its variable presentation, eosinophilic gastroenteropathy may go undiagnosed or misdiagnosed for extensive periods prior to making the correct diagnosis.

EPIDEMIOLOGY

Eosinophilic gastroenteropathy is a rare disorder that may occur at any age, from infancy through adulthood. It may be underdiagnosed secondary to clinicians being unfamiliar with its varied presentations. It affects all races and has a slightly higher incidence in males. A personal or family history of allergy or atopy is present in many cases.

ETIOLOGY AND PATHOPHYSIOLOGY

The cause of eosinophilic gastroenteropathy remains uncertain. Food sensitivity may play a role in some patients, but the cause is often undetermined. Total IgE may be elevated in some patients, while it is normal in others. In addition, variable IgE responses to food challenges are observed. This implies that both IgE- and non-IgE-dependent factors are involved in the disease process.

Eosinophils normally exist in the gastrointestinal tissue where they are involved in proper host defense. They are present in excess in eosinophilic gastroenteropathy, in which their infiltration and degranulation lead to tissue damage. The cytokines IL-3, IL-5, and *granulocyte-macrophage colony stimulating factor* (GM-CSF) are involved in eosinophil recruitment and activation. Desreumaux et al. compared duodenal and colonic biopsies from 10 patients with eosinophilic gastroenteropathy to sex and age-matched controls and found IL-3, IL-5, and GM-CSF in 9 out of 10 patients with eosinophilic gastroenteropathy and in none of the 10 controls. This provides support that these cytokines may be behind the recruitment of eosinophils to the gastrointestinal tract.[2] Eotaxin, an eosinophil chemoattractant, has also been implicated in the recruitment of eosinophils.[3]

CLINICAL SIGNS AND SYMPTOMS

The clinical signs and symptoms are related to the location within the gastrointestinal tract and the depth of the eosinophilic infiltration. Eosinophilic gastroenteropathy is commonly divided into *mucosal*, *muscular*, and *serosal* subtypes, but there may be considerable overlap between subtypes. In addition, the disease can present with periodic flares that can further confuse the clinical picture.

Mucosal eosinophilic gastroenteritis commonly presents with abdominal pain, nausea, vomiting, and diarrhea. Symptoms depend on the site of the GI tract involved—dysphagia and heartburn are more common with eosinophilic esophagitis; emesis and abdominal pain prevail with eosinophilic gastropathy; diarrhea and even a frank malabsorption syndrome with small intestinal eosinophilic inflammation; and a dysenteric picture with mucus and streaks of blood in eosinophilic colitis[4] (see Chap. 14). The ingestion of specific food antigens may, whenever the syndrome is triggered by food allergy, worsen the symptoms. In addition, when an enteropathy is present, tissue damage can result in enteric protein loss with hypoalbuminemia leading to peripheral edema.

Eosinophilic esophagitis deserves a special mention, as it has emerged in recent years as a separate entity. It presents with symptoms similar to gastroesophageal reflux, such as dysphagia, chest pain, irritability, vomiting, and poor weight gain. Patients are often referred because of failure to respond to reflux therapy. This entity is characterized by a dense eosinophilic infiltrate of the esophagus in the absence of gastroesophageal reflux disease. Typically, peripheral eosinophils are not increased and skin tests are negative.

Muscular eosinophilic gastroenteritis may be localized or diffuse. The inflammation can be prominent, especially in the antral region of the stomach, causing obstructive symptoms. In infants, this may be mistaken for hypertrophic pyloric stenosis. Diffuse inflammation resulting in extensive thickening of

the stomach and small intestine may mimic Crohn's disease. If the eosinophilic infiltration occurs in the appendix, it may be mistaken for appendicitis.

Serosal eosinophilic gastroenteritis is the least common form. Eosinophilic ascites is present and the patient could have symptoms of peritonitis or abdominal distention.

DIAGNOSIS

The diagnosis of eosinophilic gastroenteritis requires

1. Gastrointestinal symptoms as described earlier
2. Eosinophilic infiltration of the gastrointestinal tissue as demonstrated on biopsy (usually >20–25 per high power field)
3. Absence of eosinophilic involvement of multiple organs outside the gastrointestinal tract
4. Absence of parasitic infection

There is no consensus on the number of eosinophils per high power field to be considered diagnostic, the threshold ranging between 10 and 30 cells. The inflammatory cell infiltrate should in any case be mainly eosinophilic and may be described as sheets of eosinophils.

Peripheral blood eosinophilia is seen in approximately 70–80% of patients, but these counts may vary over time. Patients with serosal disease tend to have even higher levels of eosinophilia.[5] Elevated total and food-specific IgE levels by *radioallergosorbent test* (RAST) or skin testing may be present. Protein-losing enteropathy with resulting hypoalbuminemia is recognized through increased fecal α-1 antitrypsin levels. Low immunoglobulin levels can also be a result of the protein-losing enteropathy. Iron deficiency anemia results from chronic blood loss. Finally, ascitic fluid containing high numbers of eosinophils supports the diagnosis of serosal eosinophilic gastroenteropathy.

Radiologic evaluation may reveal enlarged gastric folds and, with muscular involvement of the antrum and pylorus, an obstructive picture may result. Thickened mucosal folds and nodularity of the small bowel may also be present and in severe cases result in obstruction. Upper GI studies may reveal esophageal strictures and stenosis in the case of eosinophilic esophagitis.

Endoscopic examination may be normal or it may show erythema, edema, nodularity, ulcerations, or erosions.

In the case of eosinophilic esophagitis, the mucosa may appear furrowed or ringed with linear exudates. Because of the patchy distribution of the disease, multiple biopsies from multiple sites, especially the stomach and small bowel, should be obtained.

DIFFERENTIAL DIAGNOSIS

The differential diagnosis of eosinophilic gastroenteritis (see Table 16-1) includes other diseases that may produce eosinophilia. Parasites and drug reactions can present with peripheral eosinophilia. With thickened bowel and tissue eosinophilia, inflammatory bowel disease, especially Crohn's disease, must be considered. Histologic features, such as crypt architectural changes, help guide in the diagnosis of Crohn's disease. Collagen vascular diseases, such as polyarteritis nodosa and Churg-Strauss syndrome,

TABLE 16-1

DIFFERENTIAL DIAGNOSIS

Allergies—milk protein
Connective tissue disease—dermatomyositis, scleroderma
Parasites—*Ascaris, Strongyloides, Toxocara canis, Schistosoma, Anisakis*
Inflammatory bowel disease—Crohn's disease, ulcerative colitis
Celiac disease
Medications—gold, azathioprine
Vasculitis—Polyarteritis nodosa, Churg-Strauss syndrome
Malignancy—lymphoma, gastric adenocarcinoma, hypereosinophilic syndrome, irritable bowel syndrome, hypertrophic pyloric stenosis, appendicitis

may have tissue eosinophilia, but commonly also have extraintestinal symptoms. Malignancies, such as lymphoma or gastric cancer, may also produce eosinophilia. The hypereosinophilic syndrome typically involves multiple organs outside of the gastrointestinal tract.

Cow's milk and soy protein intolerance must be considered in infants and children and should respond to removal of the inciting antigens. While, as repeatedly stated, a food-allergic condition may underlie eosinophilic gastroenteropathy, it should also be clearly stated that food allergies can exist without any eosinophilic infiltrate at all.

MANAGEMENT

Given the complexity of this syndrome and its variable manifestations, as well as the fluctuating course of the disease, the management of eosinophilic gastroenteritis is based on a patient's individual presentation and symptomatology.

Dietary manipulation can be very effective therapy, especially in the presence of specific food allergies. Elimination of specific foods identified by allergy testing or the simple removal of those foods that provoke the typical symptoms can lead to significant improvement. If a patient does not respond to an elimination diet and/or if specific offending foods cannot be identified, an elemental diet may be more effective. Elemental diets consist of amino acid-based formulas, thus eliminating by definition any possibility of triggering or perpetuating an immune response. They, however, are often not well tolerated in children beyond infancy, secondary to their unpleasant taste and smell. Nutrition may need to be given via *nasogastric* (NG) or *gastric* (G) tube if this diet is to be maintained.

If symptoms persist despite dietetic treatment, the use of corticosteroids at 1–2 mg/kg per day for a short course has been effective in most children. Unfortunately, some children have a relapse of symptoms as doses are tapered or discontinued, and the dosage may need to be modified or the medication restarted. In addition, steroids have well-known long-term side effects and so the use of topical steroids, as well as other steroid-limiting or steroid-sparing agents, are desirable alternatives.

For those patients with eosinophilic esophagitis, the topical steroid fluticasone propionate has been used with success. It is administered via a metered dose inhaler without the use of a spacer and it is swallowed. Teitelbaum et al.[6] showed that fluticasone propionate relieved patients' symptoms and reduced mucosal inflammation. Doses were based on age and given as two puffs twice daily.

The use of oral cromolyn sodium, a mast cell stabilizer, alone and in combination with steroids, has also been proposed for resistant cases. It may be more effective in those patients with elevated IgE levels.[4]

Leukotrienes are inflammatory mediators released from mast cells and eosinophils. Montelukast is a leukotriene receptor antagonist that has primarily been used in the treatment of asthma. In 1999, there was a report of improvement in a single teenage patient with the use of montelukast.[7] More recently, Vanderhoof described eight children with eosinophilic gastroenteropathy who did not respond well to other therapies and showed improvement with montelukast.[8]

Ketotifen, an H1 antihistamine that acts as a mast cell stabilizer, has been shown to improve symptoms and eosinophilia,[9] but is currently not available in the United States.

Surgical intervention is rarely required, but may be necessary in a patient with obstructive symptoms.

References

1   Kaijser R. Allergic disease of the gut from the point of view of the surgeon. *Arch Klin Chir* 188:36–64, 1937.

2   Desreumaux P, Bloget F, Seguy D, Capron M, Cortot A, Colombel JF, Janin A. IL-3, GM-CSF and IL-5 in eosinophilic gastroenteritis. *Gastroenterology* 110:768–774, 1996.

3   Bischoff SC. Mucosal allergy: role of mast cells and eosinophil granulocytes in the gut. *Baillieres Clin Gastroenterol* 10(3):443–459, 1996.

4   Whitington PF, Whitington GL. Eosinophilic gastroenteropathy in childhood. *J Pediatr Gastroenterol Nutr.* 7(3): 379–385, 1988.

5   Talley HJ, Shorter RG, Phillips SF, Zinsmeister AR. Eosinophilic gastroenteritis: a clinicopathological study of patients with disease of the mucosa, muscle layer, and subserosal tissues. *Gut* 31(1):54–58, 1990.

6   Teitelbaum JE, Fox VL, Twarog FJ, Nurko S, Antonioli D, Gleich G, Badizadegan K, Furuta GT. Eosinophilic esophagitis in children: immunopathological analysis and response to fluticasone propionate. *Gastroenterology* 122:1216–1225, 2002.

7   Neustrom MR, Friesen C. Treatment of eosinophilic gastroenteritis with montelukast. *J Allergy Clin Immunol* 104(2 Pt 1):506, 1999.

8   Vanderhoof JA, Young RJ, Hanner TL, Kettlehut B. Montelukast: use in pediatric patients with eosinophilic gastrointestinal disease. *J Pediatr Gastroenterol Nutr* 36(2):293–294, 2003.

9   Melamed I, Feanny SJ, Sherman PM, Roifman CM. Benefit of ketotifen in patients with eosinophilic gastroenteritis. *Am J Med* 90(3):310–314, 1991.

17

HELICOBACTER PYLORI GASTRITIS AND GASTRODUODENAL ULCERS

Giuseppina Oderda

INTRODUCTION

Helicobacter pylori (*H. pylori*) is a gram-negative spiral bacterium residing in the human stomach where it is the major cause of gastritis. No natural reservoir of the infection is known but the human stomach, and transmission is mainly from person-to-person by close contact or by sharing non-well-sterilized nasogastric tubes, endoscopes, or pH- monitoring probes.

Gastritis (i.e., mononuclear inflammatory infiltration with or without polymorphs of the gastric mucosa) may be more or less severe, usually becomes chronic unless treated, and may evolve in gastric or duodenal ulcer or, later in life, in gastric carcinoma in a small minority of subjects. The World Health Organization has classified *H. pylori* as a group 1 carcinogen. Determinants of evolution are both host-dependent and bacterium-dependent, but dietary factors may play an important role. There is no evidence demonstrating a link between *H. pylori*-associated gastritis and *any* clinical picture;

indeed, in the majority of children the infection can occur without any symptoms or signs, except in cases where gastric or duodenal ulcer disease is present. Prevalence of peptic ulcer in *H. pylori*-infected children is variable in different populations. Screening with noninvasive test for *H. pylori* infection should not be performed routinely in children with upper gastrointestinal (GI) symptoms including abdominal pain. In population with a high prevalence of infection, such screening will lead to treatment of unacceptably too many children.

EPIDEMIOLOGY AND TRANSMISSION

Prevalence

It is one of the commonest bacterial infections worldwide. How and when the infection is acquired remains largely unknown. There are great differences in the prevalence of infection in different populations and in ethnic groups originating from high-prevalence regions; high prevalence is related to lower level of hygienic conditions and sanitation. In developing countries, infection occurs at a much earlier age, usually in the first 2 years of age, where about 40% of children are already infected and up to 90% are infected in adulthood. In developed countries, prevalence of infection in school children varies from 6 to 20% and is related to poor socioeconomic conditions, where high density of living and bed-sharing are risk factors for acquiring the infection. Clustering of infection in families confirms that close contacts with infected parents or older siblings favors person-to-person spread. Prevalence of infection increases with age and reaches about 50% of the population around the fifth decade of life.

Acquisition

Humans seem to be the only reservoir of *H. pylori* which spreads by oral-oral, fecal-oral, or gastro-oral routes. Most infections are acquired in childhood possibly from parents or other children living as close contacts (siblings, school mates). Infection from the environment or from animals cannot be entirely excluded. Iatrogenic transmission through sharing of nasogastric tubes, pH electrodes, and endoscopes or biopsy forceps is well documented. Breast-feeding from infected mothers with high-specific IgA titers in their milk may protect from or at least delay infection. Poor nutritional status, particularly low serum protein or vitamin C levels, could have a facilitating role in spreading the infection. Volunteers infected by oral ingestion develop acute transient dyspeptic symptoms for a few days but in the majority of subjects symptoms at acquisition may be absent, and the symptoms at acquisition are not known. This accounts for the difficulty of studying the naturally occurring mode of transmission.

Transmission

The pathway followed for person-to-person transmission is still an unsolved problem.

The oral-oral route is suggested by some observations: (1) higher prevalence of *H. pylori* is found in Chinese-Australian using chopsticks used also to share food; (2) *H. pylori* DNA encoding 16S rRNA is found by *polymerase chain reaction* (PCR) in dental plaque and saliva of infected patients; (3) viable

H. pylori was cultured from dental plaque; and (4) about half of infected spouses harbor the same ribopattern of their partner. Other studies do not confirm these findings.

The other possible pathway is the fecal-oral route. Infections transmitted by fecal-oral route spread more readily among young children, the age group of subjects where *H. pylori* is most commonly acquired. Some findings favor this route of transmission: (1) *H. pylori* was cultured from human feces, (2) the *ureA* and *cagA* gene can be detected in the feces of infected patients, and (3) there is a positive association with hepatitis A virus infection known to be spread by the fecal-oral route.

An intriguing hypothesis is that the infection could be transmitted through a gastro-oral route via refluxed gastric content or vomitus. Indeed, attempts to culture *H. pylori* from feces or saliva have met with difficulties, the infection is easily transmitted by gastric intubation, and acute infection is characterized by achlorhydric vomiting. Mucus may serve as vehicle for transmission in refluxate or vomitus. A high prevalence of infection with the same strain has been found in mentally retarded cohabiting children with frequent gastroesophageal reflux.

Waterborne transmission could occur, since coccoid forms of the microorganisms have been found to survive for up to 1 year in river water and spiral forms for up to 10 days in cold river water. In Peruvian children drinking water from cisterns the prevalence of infection is much higher than in children drinking tap water. In Chile an increased prevalence of infection is associated with the consumption of uncooked vegetables. The possibility of zoonotic transmission is suggested by the increased prevalence of infection in abattoir workers and veterinarians and by the detection of *H. pylori* in domestic cats. Houseflies could be a vector for transmitting the infection from individual to individual.

In conclusion, how transmission of *H. pylori* occurs is still largely unknown. Infection is acquired at a young age. The infection is transmitted by different pathways: person-to-person transmission potentially occurs by the fecal-oral and/or gastro-oral routes in children, and by oral-oral route in adults. In developing countries it could be a waterborne infection. Cultural practices and environmental factors may well influence the mode of transmission in different human populations.[1]

PATHOPHYSIOLOGY

Gastric Inflammation

H. pylori infection causes chronic inflammatory infiltration in the gastric mucosa and can be associated with gastric and duodenal ulcer disease in a minority of children. Eradication of *H. pylori* leads to healing of chronic gastritis and to long-term healing of ulcer disease.

The bacterium has four to six polar flagella that help it penetrate the gastric mucus barrier and adhere to gastric epithelial cells though it never penetrates the epithelium. Production of toxins and bacterial enzymes contributes to epithelial damage; recruitment and activation of immune cells in the gastric mucosa involves *H. pylori* chemotaxins, epithelial-derived chemokines (IL-8), and proinflammatory cytokines (TNF-α, IL-1, IL-6). Antigen-specific cellular immunity results in predominant Th1 lymphocyte response with increased interferon-gamma (IFN-γ) secreting T-helper cells; humoral responses lead to production of anti-*H. pylori* antibodies and complement activation. T regulatory lymphocytes may be activated with production of IL-10 to downregulate the inflammation that becomes chronic and decrease in antitumoral immunity predisposing to gastric cancer.[2] The bacterium colonizes exclusively the gastric epithelium of the stomach or areas of gastric metaplasia in the duodenum, the esophagus, or in Meckel's diverticula.

Histologic Changes

According to the updated Sydney classification[3] gastritis can be

- Active (with polymorph infiltration, either neutrophils or eosinophils) or nonactive (with plasma cells and lymphocytic infiltration without polymorphs)
- Superficial (with intact glandular epithelium)
- Atrophic (with decrease or loss of glandular epithelium)

- Follicular (with lymphoid follicles)
- With intestinal metaplasia

Infiltration and epithelial damage can be mild, moderate, or severe, without any relationship with symptom severity. In children, gastritis is usually superficial or follicular and active. Atrophy and intestinal metaplasia are rare. The mucosal changes may be mild and only an experienced pathologist may recognize it, but the *H. pylori*-colonized gastric mucosa is almost never normal.

Endoscopic Changes

The endoscopic picture may be macroscopically completely normal or show a mild hyperemia, edema or friability, and erosions or ulcers. In about half of infected children a characteristic nodularity of the gastric mucosa is present, usually at the antrum, but it can extend to the fundus. This is a very specific endoscopic picture; up to 95% of nodular gastric mucosa are colonized by *H. pylori*. However, up to half of the children may have a normal appearing gastric and duodenal mucosa; therefore antral biopsies are always necessary to search for the infection.

Gastric Acid Secretion

Gastric acid secretion influences density of *H. pylori* colonization, its distribution within the stomach, and severity of mucosal inflammation. In addition, *H. pylori* gastritis alters gastric acid secretion. In subjects with predominant *antral* gastritis, increased gastrin secretion stimulates gastric hyperacidity predisposing to duodenal ulcer; whereas in subjects with predominant *body* gastritis, acid secretion is impaired with an increased risk of gastric cancer. Age of acquisition of infection may influence distribution of gastritis.[4]

CLINICAL SIGNS AND SYMPTOMS

Both the *North American Society of Pediatric Gastroenterology, Hepatology, and Nutrition* (NASPGHAN) and the *European Society of Paediatric Gastroenterology, Hepatology, and Nutrition* (ESPGHAN) Consensus Conferences on *H. pylori* in children issued a statement saying that in the pediatric age group there is no specific clinical picture of this infection, indicating a need to screen children with dyspeptic symptoms for *H. pylori* with noninvasive tests. There is no evidence demonstrating a link between *H. pylori*-associated gastritis and abdominal pain except in the rare cases where gastric or duodenal ulcer disease is present and no data demonstrate that *H. pylori* eradication in infected children without ulcer disease is superior to placebo or nontreatment for symptom relief.

Dyspepsia

Dyspeptic symptoms frequently reported in *H. pylori*-infected children are as follows:

- Ulcer-like dyspepsia, with epigastric pain, often relieved by food ingestion
- Reflux-like dyspepsia, with heartburn and acid regurgitation
- Dysmotility-like dyspepsia, with nausea, bloating, and recurrent vomiting

However, a cause and effect relationship, as previously stated, is still controversial. Up to now the only way to ascertain whether dyspeptic symptoms are due to *H. pylori* is to eradicate the infection and follow the child: about one-third of children will improve, some will not, and in some patients the symptoms will become worse, particularly when gastritis is associated with esophagitis. On the other hand, *recurrent abdominal pain* (RAP) is not usually associated with *H. pylori* infection[5] because RAP is usually due to irritable bowel syndrome[6] where gastritis does not seem to play a role.

Extraintestinal Manifestations

Helicobacter pylori has been reported in association with iron-deficient refractory anemia, chronic urticaria, and more recently with thrombocytopenic purpura.[7] In these three instances data are convincing because a higher prevalence of infection is present in cases than in controls, and signs and symptoms disappear with eradication of the infection. A causal relationship of other signs and symptoms reported as associated with the infection like short stature, acute diarrhea, chronic diarrhea and malnutrition, protein-losing enteropathy, and failure to thrive, is less convincing and still to be demonstrated by interventional studies.

Gastric and Duodenal Ulcer

In a register established on the ESPGHAN web site in 2000–2002 prevalence of ulcer in infected children undergoing upper GI endoscopy for dyspeptic symptoms was found to be 12%. Signs and symptoms in children with ulcer do not usually differ from dyspepsia. However, pain may be more severe, nocturnal, and awaking the child; occult bleeding with progressive, occasionally severe, anemia may occur; gross hemorrhage with hematemesis and melena is rare. In children with gastric or duodenal ulcer associated with *H. pylori*, symptoms greatly improve or disappear with eradication of the infection.

COMPLICATIONS

The most severe complication of *H. pylori* gastritis is gastric carcinoma. Such complication, however, usually occurs in the fourth to fifth decade of life, and in a small minority of infected subjects. Best estimate of long-term risk for noncardia gastric cancer in *H. pylori*-infected subjects is 5.9 as compared to noninfected subjects.[8] The link between *H. pylori* infection and gastric cancer can be summarized as follows: *H. pylori* infection acquired at a very early age (probably before the age of 2 years), associated with genetic predisposition (IL-1β polymorphism) and to a diet poor in antioxidant vitamins and rich in salts and reactive nitrogen, can cause, over the long run, DNA damage, increased cell proliferation, increased apoptosis, and mutations. These changes can lead to glandular atrophy, metaplasia, dysplasia, and eventually cancer. Whether eradication of the infection can stop this slow process and at what stage it may be still effective is not known.

DIAGNOSIS WITH DIFFERENTIAL

A "test and treat policy" with the use of a noninvasive test has been recommended for young adults with dyspepsia without alarming symptoms (i.e., malabsorption and/or bleeding) but the relation of benefits to risks and costs of such a policy differ between adults and children, since *H. pylori*-related ulcer disease occurs with a much lower frequency in children. However, assessment of *H. pylori* status could be performed as part of the evaluation when symptoms are suggestive of organic disease such as peptic ulcer or esophagitis and the child therefore requires an upper gastrointestinal endoscopy with antral biopsy.

Importance of Performing Endoscopy

Children should only be investigated for *H. pylori* when their symptoms are severe enough to justify the risks of therapy. Endoscopy is the preferred method of investigation in children with upper digestive symptoms suggestive of structural dis-

ease after exclusion of other causes with noninvasive methods (i.e., lactose maloligestion celiac disease; constipation; pancreas, liver, and biliary system disease).[9]

Endoscopy provides complete information on the disease process. It allows the identification of other causes of pain such as esophagitis and peptic ulceration. It is the only method by which biopsies can be obtained in order to diagnose gastritis, eosinophilic gastroduodenitis, or esophagitis (Fig. 17-1). It also allows obtaining small intestinal biopsies to look for celiac disease.

A gastric biopsy can be cultured to grow *H. pylori* and subsequently to test for resistance to antibiotics. In fact, antibiotic susceptibility is a growing problem—in Europe more than 20% of strains are resistant to clarithromycin or metronidazole. The necessity to carry out an endoscopy, which has to be justified by symptoms indicating organic disease,

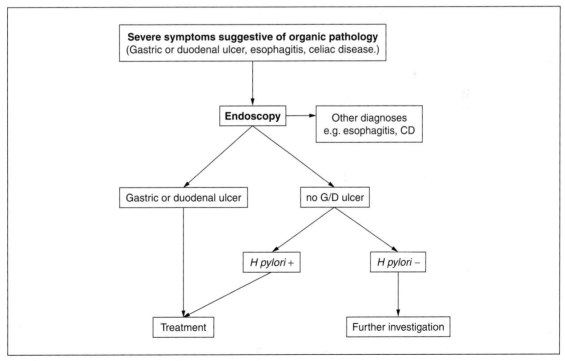

F I G U R E   1 7 - 1

FLOW CHART SUGGESTED BY THE ESPGHAN GUIDELINES TO DIAGNOSE AND TREAT *H. PYLORI*-INFECTED CHILDREN

would attenuate the misuse of noninvasive tests and the prescribing of anti-*H. pylori* therapy in children with nonspecific symptoms. Compliance with *H. pylori* eradication therapy may be better after endoscopy compared to diagnosis of the infection by noninvasive testing. Better compliance results in a lower rate of treatment failures and, therefore, a reduced risk of therapy-induced antibiotic resistance.

Endoscopy must always be completed with gastric biopsies in the antral area and at the fundus. Biopsy specimens can be used for rapid urease test ("CLO" test) to demonstrate the infection in the endoscopy room. If the CLO test is positive in the first hour (with the yellow urea medium, liquid or solid, turning violet) the diagnosis is almost 100% sure and treatment can be started. If CLO test is positive only after a few hours or the day after,

treatment should be postponed until the results of histology are known, for the possibility of slow urease-producing bacteria giving a false-positive result.

Other biopsy specimens are to be processed for histology, with *Giemsa* staining for the microscopic demonstration of the bacterium, and hematoxylin and eosin staining for the diagnosis and the characterization of gastric mucosa damage. If available in the laboratory, another biopsy should be cultured in a highly selective and blood-enriched medium in a microaerophylic atmosphere to test for antibiotic sensitivity to clarithromycin and metronidazole. Culture is only suggested at first diagnosis, but becomes mandatory when a first treatment fails, particularly in children with a previous peptic ulcer (Fig. 17-2).

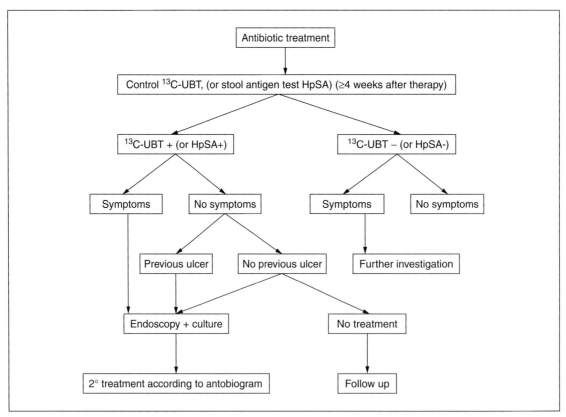

FLOW CHART SUGGESTED BY THE ESPGHAN TO FOLLOW THE CHILDREN AFTER TREATMENT

Use of Noninvasive Tests

Serologic tests (ELISA, Immunoblot), especially quick tests, are not as reliable in children as in adults. In young children or when acquisition is very recent, the serologic response may be weak or still absent. Most commercial kits have not been validated in children. The cut off point validated in adults may be too high for children resulting in a low sensitivity of the test. Furthermore, serology does not distinguish between actual and previous infection since the antibody titer decreases very slowly after cure, therefore it is not appropriate for monitoring the response to treatment. False-positive results can occur after spontaneous eradication that can occur in very young children.

The ^{13}C urea breath test and measurement of the stool antigen test (HpSA) are reliable diagnostic tests; however, they should not be used to screen children before endoscopy. Their use is recommended only for epidemiologic studies or to test children after therapy. Indeed, in children treated for *H. pylori* infection the response to treatment should be monitored with a reliable noninvasive test. Their accuracy is better if the test is performed at least 4–6 weeks after the end of treatment (Fig. 17-2).

GUIDELINE TO TREATMENT AND FOLLOW-UP

Evidence-based data to construe suggestions on treatment schedules in children are scanty. Good placebo-controlled randomized trials are completely lacking. NASPGHAN has suggested treating children with a *proton-pump inhibitor* (PPI, such as omeprazole, lansoprazole, pantoprazole, or exomeprazole) plus two antibiotics (triple therapy) for 2 weeks. Antibiotics most commonly used are: amoxicillin, metronidazole, clarithromycin, and bismuth salts. However, a recent systematic review on all available data in children[10] showed that dual therapies with bismuth plus one antibiotic (either amoxicillin or nitroimidazole) or 2 antibiotics when administered for two or more weeks are as effective as triple therapies either bismuth-based or PPI-based. Triple therapies are less effective in children than in adults; bismuth-based triple therapies

are more effective when given for 2 weeks than for 1 week and PPI-based triple therapies have a similar efficacy irrespective of the duration. So in children, dual therapies are as effective as triple therapies and longer courses of PPI-based triple therapies are not better than shorter ones. The overall eradication rate to be expected after therapy is around 60–70% (Fig. 17-3).

Dosage of omeprazole should be 1 mg/kg (1.5 mg/kg for lansoprazole) in one dose early morning before breakfast, whereas antibiotics should be given at meals (breakfast and dinner) at 12 h intervals: 50 mg/kg per day for amoxicillin, 20 mg/kg per day for metronidazole or tinidazole, 15 mg/kg per day for clarithromycin, and 1 mg/kg per day for bismuth salts that seem to be more effective when administered in 3 or 4 doses a day. Antibiotics and PPI or bismuth can be given in various combinations for 1 or 2 weeks (Fig. 17-2). Treatment can be continued for 1–2 weeks and 4–6 weeks later eradication has to be tested with a noninvasive test (either ^{13}C urea breath test or stool antigen test).

Long-term remission of duodenal ulcer can be achieved with antimicrobial regimens that eradicate the infection, but in children with ulcer a second endoscopy has to be performed 4–6 weeks after the end of therapy to monitor ulcer healing.

Response to treatment cannot be evaluated by symptoms response. In a great proportion of children symptoms continue despite eradication due to the persistence of gastric mucosa inflammation that takes several months to heal. In the meantime antacids given on demand or antisecretory drugs (either PPI or H2 blockers like ranitidine or famotidine) may help. Quite often symptoms disappear irrespective of persistent infection.

SHORT- AND LONG-TERM PROGNOSIS

If treatment has been effective in eradicating the infection, gastritis and/or duodenal ulcer will heal in time, and symptoms due to the infection will disappear after a few months. One possible problem arising after eradication is the worsening of symptoms due to peptic esophagitis. *H. pylori* urease generate ammonia in the stomach with an

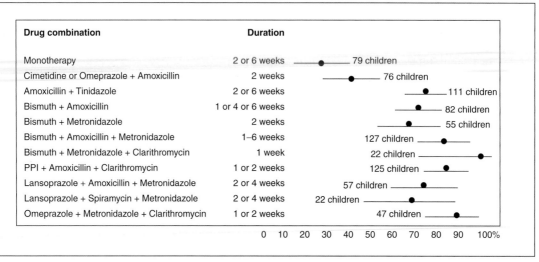

FIGURE 17-3

OVERALL ERADICATION RATES (95% CI) OF THE MOST COMMONLY USED TREATMENT
Source: Schedules extracted from 30 full articles published from 1987 to October 1999; total reported children are 870.

antacid effect. After eradication, gastric acid hyper-acidity can occur, and peptic esophagitis, already present but more or less silent, can worsen. A course of PPI or H2 blockers has to be considered.

If treatment has not been effective in eradicating the infection, the child can still have symptoms, and a second endoscopy should be considered to test for antibiotic sensitivity. Alternatively, the child can be symptomless, and a long-term follow-up can be considered. *H. pylori*-infected individuals have a lifetime risk of 10–15% to develop *H. pylori*-associated serious organic diseases, like peptic ulcer or gastric carcinoma. Since in a given patient the individual risk for complications cannot be estimated, a proven infection should not be left untreated.

References

1   Oderda G. Transmission of *Helicobacter pylori* infection. *Can J Gastroenterol* 13:595–597, 1999.
2   Bodger K, Crabtree JE. *Helicobacter pylori* and gastric inflammation. *Br Med Bull* 54:139–150, 1998.
3   Dixon MF, Genta RM, Yardley JH, et al. Classification and grading of gastritis—the updated Sydney system. *Am J Surg Pathol* 20:1161–1181, 1996.
4   McColl KEL, ElOmar E, Gillen D. Interactions between *H. pylori* infection, gastric acid secretion and anti-secretory therapy. *Br Med Bull* 54:121–138, 1998.
5   Macarthur C, Saunders N, Feldman W. *Helicobacter pylori*, gastroduodenal disease, and recurrent abdominal pain in children. *JAMA* 273:729–734, 1995.
6   Hyams JS, Treem WR, Justinich CJ, et al. Characterization of symptoms in children with recurrent abdominal pain: resemblance to irritable bowel syndrome. *J Pediatr Gastroenterol Nutr* 20:209–214, 1995.
7   Hashino S, Mori A, Suzuki S, et al. Platelet recovery in patients with idiopathic thrombocytopenic purpura after eradication of *Helicobacter pylori*. *Int J Hematol* 77:188–191, 2003.
8   Webb PM, Law M, Varghese C, et al. Gastric cancer and *Helicobacter pylori*: a combined analysis of 12 case control studies nested within prospective cohorts. *Gut* 49:347–353, 2001.
9   Drumm B, Koletzko S, Oderda G, European Paediatric Task Force on *Helicobacter pylori*. *Helicobacter pylori* infection in children. Report of a Consensus Conference held in Budapest, September 1998. *J Paediatr Gastroenterol Nutr* 30:207–213, 2000.
10 Oderda G, Rapa A, Bona G. A systematic review of *Helicobacter pylori* eradication treatment schedules in children. *Aliment Pharmacol Ther* 14(Suppl 3):56–60, 2000.

CHAPTER

18

CELIAC DISEASE

Stefano Guandalini

INTRODUCTION

Celiac disease (CD) is an enteropathy that occurs in genetically susceptible individuals triggered by the ingestion of gluten. Three cereals are toxic for celiac patients: wheat, rye, and barley. Gluten causes intestinal damage in individuals whose antigen-presenting cells express either the heterodimer DQ2, produced by individuals who are HLA DR3 (or DR5/DR7) or the heterodimer DQ8, produced by those who are HLA DR4.

EPIDEMIOLOGY

When the prevalence of celiac disease is estimated based on the florid cases presenting with overt *gastrointestinal* (GI) manifestations, a low prevalence (around 1:1000) is reported in most studies. However, it is now well known that CD is a protean disorder that can present in many different ways (see clinical preparation) and at times can even be totally asymptomatic. The availability of tests for malabsorption, but most importantly the recent availability of sensitive and specific serologic tests, has made it possible to assess a truer prevalence of CD by detecting minimally symptomatic or even asymptomatic cases with typical mucosal changes. With this type of tool, screening

studies have shown a very high prevalence of CD, occurring in about 1 in 150 of the European general population.

Until recently CD was generally believed to be a rare disorder in the United States, and prevalences lower than 1:10,000 were often quoted. However, a recent vast screening—a multicenter study throughout the United States that screened more than 13,000 healthy individuals with *antiendomysium antibody* (EMA)—found a prevalence of 1:133,[1] that is, identical to that found in Europe. In spite of similar rates of prevalence, it is clear that the current rates of diagnosis of CD in the United States are much below those in Europe, possibly due to the fact that CD in North America presents less frequently than in Europe as a GI disorder.

PATHOPHYSIOLOGY

CD is an autoimmune disorder. The initial event in the pathogenesis of the celiac lesion is thought to be an abnormal permeability allowing the entry of gliadin peptides not entirely degraded by the intraluminal and brush-border bound peptidases. Indeed, the most toxic amongst the many fractions of gliadin that have been shown to be harmful to celiac mucosa are incredibly resistant to digestion by gastric, pancreatic, and mucosa-associated enzymes.

Under normal circumstances, the intestinal epithelium acts as a barrier to the passage of such macromolecules; but in CD, a well-documented loosening of the intestinal tight junctions, possibly even triggered by gliadin itself, leads to an increased permeability to macromolecules.

There are then two pathways involved in the pathogenesis of CD: an early one, involving mainly the innate immune system, and a subsequent one, involving the T cells. Soon after reaching the serosal side of the intestinal epithelium, some of the toxic—but not immunodominant—gliadin peptides elicit an early response by the innate immune system that causes crucial modifications of the mucosal microenvironment that precede and actually "set the stage" for the subsequent involvement of the pathogenic T cells.[2] During the first phase, there is a marked increase of HLA-DR expression on both the epithelium and the adjacent lamina propria macrophages; this is followed by overexpression of the intercellular adhesion molecule 1 (ICAM-1). Finally, CD8+ T cells invade epithelial cells (intraepithelial lymphocytes).

About 95% of all celiac patients belong to the DR3 (or DR5/DR7 heterozygous) genotype and express the DQ2 α,β-heterodimer, encoded by DQA1*0501/DQB1*0201, while the remaining 5% are DR4 and show the DQ8 α,β-heterodimer, encoded by DQA1*0301/DQB1*0302. This strong association implies that the adaptive branch of the immune system, and in particular CD4+ T lymphocytes, must play a crucial role in the pathogenesis. In fact, DQ2 and DQ8 molecules are located on the surface of antigen-presenting cells and bind peptides to be presented to CD4+ T lymphocytes. The autoantigen in CD, major target of all autoantibodies, has been found to be the ubiquitarious enzyme tissue transglutaminase (tTG). This enzyme, among other functions, selectively converts glutamine residues within gluten peptides to glutamic acid. Such deamination increases the negative charges on the gliadin peptides with consequent strong enhancement of DQ binding and T cell recognition.

From a morphologic point of view, small bowel mucosal damage occurs as a result of gradual change from normal mucosa to overt mucosal atrophy with crypt hyperplasia. At least three distinctive patterns of mucosal changes can be recognized:

- The infiltrative (type 1) lesion, seen in the latent phase is characterized by morphologically normal mucosa and is not usually associated with gastrointestinal symptoms. It is characterized by an increase in the number of *intraepithelial lymphocytes* (IEL), followed by infiltration of the lamina propria with plasma cells and lymphocytes.
- The hyperplastic (type 2) lesion is similar to type 1, but with elongation of crypts due to a marked increase in undifferentiated crypt cells.
- The destructive (type 3) lesion is the most advanced pathologic change, synonymous with total or subtotal villous atrophy, i.e., the classical lesion originally considered the landmark of CD.

CLINICAL PRESENTATION: CELIAC DISEASE CAN TAKE MANY FORMS

Gastrointestinal Manifestations

The classic form of CD presents with gastrointestinal symptoms between 6 and 24 months of age. Symptoms begin at various times after the introduction of weaning foods containing gluten. Infants and young children typically present with chronic diarrhea, anorexia, abdominal distention, abdominal pain, poor weight gain or weight loss, and vomiting. Severe malnutrition can occur if the diagnosis is delayed. Behavioral changes are common and include irritability and a sad and introverted attitude. Rarely, severely affected infants present with a "celiac crisis" characterized by explosive watery diarrhea, marked abdominal distention, dehydration, hypotension, and lethargy, often with profound electrolyte abnormalities including severe hypokalemia. Older children with CD presenting with gastrointestinal manifestations may have onset of symptoms at any age. The variability in the age of onset of symptoms is possibly dependent on the amount of gluten in the diet and other environmental factors such as duration of breast-feeding. Gastrointestinal symptoms in older children include diarrhea, nausea and vomiting, abdominal pain, bloating, weight loss, and constipation.

Extraintestinal Manifestations

In recent years, however, an increasing number of patients are being diagnosed without typical gastrointestinal manifestations at an older age,[3] and it is currently believed that almost 50% of patients with newly diagnosed CD do not present with gastrointestinal symptoms. There is also a relationship between age of onset and type of presentation: in infants and toddlers, gastrointestinal symptoms and failure to thrive clearly predominate, while during childhood minor GI symptoms, inadequate rate of weight and height gain, and delayed puberty tend to be more common. In teenagers and young adults anemia is the most common form of presentation. In adults and in the elderly, again GI symptoms, though often minor, are more prevalent. Table 18-1 reports the main extraintestinal manifestations of celiac disease.

Dermatitis Herpetiformis

This variant of CD presents with blistering skin rash involving elbows, knees, and buttocks associated with dermal granular immunoglobulin (Ig) A

TABLE 18-1

MAIN EXTRAINTESTINAL MANIFESTATIONS OF CELIAC DISEASE

- Dermatitis herpetiformis
- Permanent dental enamel hypoplasia
- Iron-deficient anemia resistant to PO Fe
- Short stature
- Delayed puberty
- Chronic hepatitis with hypertransaminasemia
- Arthritis
- Osteopenia/osteporosis
- Epilepsy with occipital calcifications
- Primary ataxia
- Psychiatric disorders
- Women infertility

deposits. Rash as well as mucosal morphology improve on a *gluten-free diet* (GFD). It should be stressed that dermatitis herpetiformis is an exceedingly rare occurrence in childhood, being described almost exclusively in adults.

Dental Enamel Hypoplasia

Dental enamel defects may be the only presenting manifestation of celiac disease. These patients may have no or minimal gastrointestinal symptoms.

Iron-deficiency Anemia

Iron-deficiency anemia, resistant to oral iron supplementation, has been found to be the most common extraintestinal manifestation of celiac disease in adults in some studies. In one study, 5% of all patients with anemia had celiac disease and prevalence rose to 8.5% when only patients with microcytic anemia resistant to iron therapy were considered.[4]

Short Stature and Delayed Puberty

Short stature may be the only manifestation of celiac disease. As many as 8–10% of children with "idiopathic" short stature may have CD that can be detected on serologic testing. Some cases of CD with short stature have also impaired growth hormone production following provocative stimulation testing which return to normal on a gluten-free diet. Adolescents with untreated celiac disease may have delayed onset of menarche.

Chronic Hepatitis and Hypertransaminasemia

Elevated transaminase levels are a frequent finding in untreated patients with celiac disease. In the majority of cases liver enzymes normalize on a gluten-free diet. As many as 9% of patients with elevated transaminase levels of unclear etiology may have silent celiac disease. Liver biopsies in these patients show nonspecific reactive hepatitis. Recently, celiac disease has been described as causing, in adult patients, severe liver disease, indeed hepatic failure, that was further shown to regress with a gluten-free diet.[5]

Arthritis and Arthralgia

Arthritis can be a common extraintestinal manifestation in adults with celiac disease including those on a gluten-free diet. Two to three percent of children with juvenile chronic arthritis may have celiac disease.[6]

Osteopenia/Osteoporosis

Patients with CD are at high risk for developing low bone mineral density and osteoporosis. Bone mineral density improves in a majority of patients on gluten-free diets, and is back to normal as soon as 1 year after starting the diet.

Neurologic Problems

A number of neurologic conditions have been attributed to CD in adults and, to a lesser extent, in children. Celiac disease may cause occipital calcifications and intractable epilepsy; these patients can be resistant to antiseizure medicines but can benefit from a gluten-free diet if started soon after onset of seizures.[7] The association with cerebellar ataxia is well described in adults, where the term "gluten-induced ataxia" has been proposed.

Psychiatric Disorders

Although in recent years a large number of behavioral problems and disorders, such as autism and attention deficit-hyperactivity disorder, have been thought to be caused by CD, there is no evidence so far that this is the case. CD nevertheless can present with some psychiatric disorders, such as depression and anxiety. These conditions can be severe and usually will respond to the GFD.

Infertility

Celiac disease may be responsible for unexplained infertility in women. Ciacci et al.[8] reported that the relative risk of miscarriage in women affected by CD is nine times higher than in healthy subjects,

and that a GFD substantially reduced its relative risk.

Associated Diseases

In addition to causing the extraintestinal signs and symptoms described previously, CD is also known to be strongly associated with a number of other disorders (see Table 18-2). It is evident that many of these disorders are also of the autoimmune type. The association of CD with autoimmune conditions is in fact well established. A strong positive correlation is known to exist between the age at diagnosis of CD and the prevalence of autoimmune disorders, such as type 1 diabetes, thyroiditis, and alopecia, thus suggesting that it is indeed the presence of CD that acts as a trigger to the development of other autoimmune conditions.[9]

Type 1 (Insulin-dependent) Diabetes

Approximately 10% of patients with type 1 or insulin-dependent diabetes mellitus have been

TABLE 18-2

CONDITIONS ASSOCIATED WITH AN INCREASED PREVALENCE OF CELIAC DISEASE

Condition	Approximate Prevalence of Celiac Disease (%)
Insulin-dependent (type 1) diabetes mellitus	10
First degree relatives of patients with type 1 diabetes	2
Thyroiditis	3
Sjögren's syndrome and other connective tissue diseases	5
Down's syndrome	12
Turner's syndrome	
Williams syndrome	
Selective IgA deficiency	3
First degree relatives of celiac patients	5–10

found to have typical features of CD on duodenal biopsy. The real percentage is even higher. Studies of such patients in serial screening over a period of years have documented that many individuals who initially had negative serologic tests eventually developed positive tests and characteristic intestinal changes. Typically, diagnosis of diabetes precedes by years that of celiac disease, which most commonly presents with none to only mild gastrointestinal symptoms.[10] As some of these symptoms are also seen in patients with diabetes (e.g., bloating or diarrhea), diagnosis of CD may be missed, unless a screening is performed. Laboratory abnormalities such as anemia (iron and folate deficiency) are also common.

Although there is no convincing evidence that the GFD has any obvious effect on diabetes, it is thought that these patients will have to follow the diet, in order to prevent all long-term complications of CD. Thus, the case for screening type 1 diabetics for CD seems well founded.

Down's Syndrome

The best documented and widely reported association of CD with a nonautoimmune disorder is that with Down's syndrome. The prevalence of Down's syndrome in CD, as assessed by screening methods, has been found to be between 5 and 12%. Unlike type 1 diabetes patients, the majority of Down's patients with CD have some gastrointestinal symptoms, such as abdominal bloating, intermittent diarrhea, anorexia, and failure to thrive. However, it is also known that about one-third of all Down's patients with CD had no gastrointestinal symptoms. Therefore, it seems highly desirable that Down's patients get screened for CD and whenever found positive start the diet.

As CD may start at any age, Down's patients testing negative at the serologic markers (see celiac serology) would have to be retested again and again. To avoid this, since CD only occurs in specific HLA haplotypes (see Epidemiology), an algorithm based on determining first the HLA haplotypes (thus leaving out of the rescreening process all those whose HLA haplotypes are inconsistent with CD) has been proposed. An analogous strategy should be applied to screen for CD in patients with the rarer Turner's and Williams syndromes, where also an increased incidence of CD has also been reported (see under *celiac genes* for a complete list of conditions to be first screened for the HLA haplotypes).

DIAGNOSIS

Diagnosis of celiac disease is based on a biopsy of the mucosa of proximal small bowel. Histology characteristically shows a dramatic flattening or blunting of villi, crypt hyperplasia, and increased number of lymphocytes in lamina propria and within the epithelium. Marsh classified the histologic changes of CD in more detail as

- Type 0 or preinfiltrative stage (normal)
- Type 1 or infiltrative lesion (increased intraepithelial lymphocytes)
- Type 2 or hyperplastic lesion (type 1 + hyperplastic crypts)
- Type 3 or destructive lesion (type 2 + villous atrophy of various degree)

Biopsies are obtained now almost universally by endoscopy. It is recommended that multiple biopsies are obtained[3,4] as it is known that CD may be patchy and areas of villous atrophy may be adjacent to normal areas. It is also recommended that the biopsy site be as distal as possible (third portion of the duodenum), as the presence of Brunner's glands in the bulb and second portion may render interpretation more difficult. Although endoscopically visible changes have been described (e.g., scalloping of the mucosa and sparse duodenal folds), such changes are neither constant nor specific and diagnosis of CD should never be based on their presence or absence. Although the features most characteristic of CD are those of class 3, the presence of a positive serology and consistent clinical findings in lesions of stage 2, and even 1, is suggestive of CD. It should be noted that none of these changes are, however, specific for CD, seen also in other enteropathies, such as cow's milk protein allergic enteropathy (see Chap. 14), advanced malnutrition, *Giardia* infections, and autoimmune enteropathy. For this reason, it was considered initially necessary to document the gluten-dependency of such changes. Thus, a cumbersome diagnostic itinerary involving three biopsies was followed: one at the florid stage, the second after 1 year of gluten-free diet to document the normalization of the mucosa, and the third and last one after reintroducing gluten to observe the recurrence of the changes.

With the increasing availability of serologic tests for diagnosis, new diagnostic, simplified criteria were introduced and widely followed.[11] According to them, the diagnosis of celiac disease can be established on a definitive basis when the characteristic changes of the duodenal mucosa are found in a child with signs and/or symptoms consistent with CD, provided that a full and unequivocal clinical remission after withdrawal of gluten is seen, associated with the disappearance of circulating antibodies. These criteria are currently universally used, and it can be seen that, although the emerging role of serology testing was recognized and taken into crucial consideration, diagnosis still clearly relies on the intestinal biopsy findings.

Given the fact that serology is now widely used to screen for celiac disease, and also to monitor dietetic compliance, the following sections will describe how to correctly request and interpret celiac serology.

Celiac Serology

Antigliadin Antibodies (AGA)

These are food protein-directed antibodies. Interlaboratory variations for AGA have been wide, as pointed out by more than one well-conducted multicenter study. Antigliadin antibodies have been widely used since the early 80s, being widely available and inexpensive. Two classes are typically measured: IgG and IgA. AGA-IgG, even though considered of good sensitivity (85–98% in most large series), has been repeatedly shown to be extremely unspecific. Indeed, AGA-IgG can be found in a stunning 30% of control populations, and thus their positive predictive value is of no use. AGA-IgA, on the other hand, are known to be

generally more specific (90–95%), but are unfortunately also less sensitive (sensitivities reported range between 70 and 90%). Although in clinical practice AGA are often measured in conjunction with either antiendomysium or antitissue transglutaminase antibody (in the so-called "celiac panel"), their added value is doubtful. Indeed, the only reason why presently one should continue to test for AGA is to monitor the compliance to the gluten-free diet in an already-established celiac patient, as it is known that AGA antibodies are more prompt to reappear in the presence of even minimal dietary transgressions. Thus, currently it is not recommended to test children suspected to have CD with AGA.

Antiendomysium Antibodies

The antiendomysium antibodies are detected by assessing immunofluorescence of sections of monkey esophageal or human umbilical cord smooth muscle exposed to sera from patients being tested. Although the test relies on subjective operator assessment of fluorescence, its sensitivity and (even more) specificity in detecting untreated celiac disease are quite good. A recent study conducted with strict criteria by the European working group on Serologic Screening for Celiac Disease showed that EMA had, among seven laboratories, a remarkable mean specificity of 99% (93.9–99.9%), while the mean sensitivity proved to be 90% (82.7–92.5%)[12]; also the interlaboratory reliability proved to be quite good for this test, unlike the poor reproducibility of AGA. This assay is however relatively costly and its use of monkey esophagus further limits its use for the screening of large populations. In essence, EMA should be regarded as the most specific test currently available for celiac disease.

Tissue Transglutaminase Antibodies

In 1997, tissue transglutaminase was identified as the autoantigen of celiac disease. Soon, an *enzyme linked immunosorbent assay* (ELISA) for guinea pig immunoglobulin A (IgA) tTG antibodies was developed and found to be highly sensitive and specific. Numerous studies have since confirmed the high sensitivity and specificity of tTG antibodies in the diagnosis of celiac disease. Sensitivity and specificity were further improved by using human antigen instead of guinea pig antigen. Currently, most laboratories are using only the human tTG antibody assay. Although tTG sensitivity is reportedly very high, in the range of 99–100%, they are occasionally positive in individuals who are not celiacs. Indeed, they are known to be falsely positive especially in patients who have other autoimmune conditions, like type 1 diabetes.

Celiac Disease Serology: Conclusions

In summary:

1. AGA should never be employed to screen for celiac disease, given their poor specificity.
2. EMA remain the most specific serologic test, but its sensitivity is not 100% (otherwise one would not need the biopsy).
3. tTG have become the gold standard for screening celiac disease. Their sensitivity is very close to 100%, but their specificity of about 98% makes them still unable to replace the biopsy.

As both EMA and tTG are measured as IgA antibodies, false-negative tests can occur in the occasional IgA-deficient celiac. In practice, to avoid this possibility, when screening a patient for CD, one should also always obtain total IgA, along with EMA or tTG. If total IgA are below 5 mg/dL, then EMA-IgG or tTG-IgG should be sought.

Figure 18-1 suggests a diagnostic algorithm to be followed for patients presenting with GI symptoms consistent with CD.

The "Celiac Genes": HLA DQ2 and DQ8

As stated earlier, susceptibility to celiac disease is restricted to individuals possessing the major histocompatibility complex class II genes HLA-DQA1*0501-DQB1*02 (expressing the molecule DQ2) and HLA-DQA1*0301-DQB1*0302 (expressing the molecule DQ8). These antigens can be easily detected with polymerase chain reaction

(PCR) techniques on a blood test. However, they are of very limited diagnostic use, because the same haplotypes are found in about 35% of Whites. Thus, the presence of these antigens has a very weak positive predictive value, but their absence on the other hand carries a 100% negative predictive value. In clinical practice, it is recommendable to obtain these determinations only in the following circumstances:

- When assessing a patient who has not had a formal diagnosis of CD (i.e., no biopsy) but is already on a GFD longer than 3 months, mostly—again—to rule out CD. If positive, no diagnosis can obviously be made without further work-up.
- When screening asymptomatic first-degree relatives of known celiac patients. In fact, a negative test will allow ruling out CD in that individual not simply at that point in time, but rather for life, thus making repeat testing for antibodies unnecessary.
- When screening asymptomatic patients who belong to groups known to be at-risk for CD. Again, a negative test allows ruling out CD for life, avoiding further testing for this condition. The groups are the following:
  a. Type 1 diabetics
  b. Down's syndrome patients
  c. Turner's syndrome patients
  d. Williams syndrome patients

TREATMENT

Total lifelong avoidance of gluten ingestion is the cornerstone treatment for celiac disease. Wheat, rye, and barley are the grains containing toxic peptides. When children with symptomatic CD adhere to a gluten-free diet, they can be expected to resolve their gastrointestinal symptoms typically within a few weeks, showing additionally normalization of nutritional measures, improved growth in height and weight (with resultant normal stature), and normalization of hematologic and biochemical parameters. Furthermore, treatment with a GFD reverses the decrease in bone mineralization and

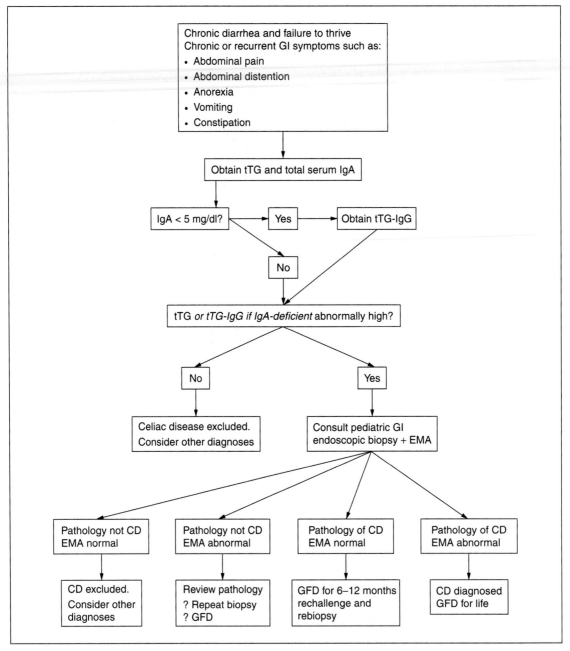

FIGURE 18-1

DIAGNOSTIC APPROACH TO CHILDREN PRESENTING WITH GASTROINTESTINAL SYMPTOMS CONSISTENT WITH CELIAC DISEASE

the risk for fractures. Symptomatic children treated with a GFD also improve in their sense of physical and psychologic well-being.

For a long time, oats were considered toxic too and their elimination from the diet had been recommended. However, during the past decade or so, a growing body of scientific evidence obtained from *in vitro* studies as well as from clinical investigations particularly in adults but also, more recently, in children, allows us to conclude that oats are indeed totally safe. This also makes sense based on the genetics of the grains, as oats are genetically entirely unrelated to the group of wheat, rye, and barley. However, because of uncontrolled harvesting and milling procedures, as well as the possibility that manufacturing lines used for wheat-based flours are also used in the preparation of oats-based foods, cross-contamination of oats with gluten is still a concern.

Often in the initial phases of dietary treatment, lactose is eliminated too. This has its basis in the lactase deficiency that is thought to accompany the flat mucosa. However, it should be pointed out that, as we have seen, today most new celiacs are diagnosed in the absence of overt malabsorptive symptoms, and in these circumstances clinically significant lactose malabsorption or intolerance is rarely seen. Furthermore, even in cases with obvious malabsorption, the recovery of lactase activity is typically fast, so that the use of a lactose-free diet even in these cases must be on a short-term basis only.

The possibility of an association between celiac disease and milk protein allergy has been repeatedly raised in the past, but is now very clear that the two conditions may simply coexist as a result of a statistical association, so that again there is no need to recommend avoidance of "dairy products."

A commonly asked question is "how strict must the diet be?" This implies that there could be a threshold, below which "some gluten" might be tolerated. In reality, there is no scientific answer. It is well known that tolerance is highly variable between celiac individuals, making predictions in single cases impossible. Furthermore, no data are available to suggest what might be the lowest amount of gluten that all celiacs would not show

any reaction to. That's why "zero tolerance" is recommended. The National Food Authority has recently redefined their term for "gluten-free." Previously, <0.02% gluten was accepted as being gluten-free, but now "gluten-free" means no gluten and <0.02% is regarded as "low gluten." The *American Dietetic Association* (ADA) publishes guidelines for the dietary treatment of CD. They are a reliable source of information for a GFD. However, given the dynamics of this field, the diet requires ongoing collaboration between patients, health care providers, and dietitians.

References

1 Fasano A, Berti I, Gerarduzzi T, et al. Prevalence of celiac disease in at-risk and not at-risk groups in the United States. *Arch Intern Med* 163:286–292, 2003.

2 Maiuri L, Ciacci C, Ricciardelli I, et al. Association between innate response to gliadin and activation of pathogenic T cells in coeliac disease. *Lancet* 362:30–37, 2003.

3 Bottaro G, Cataldo F, Rotolo N, Spina M, Corazza GR. The clinical pattern of subclinical/silent celiac disease: an analysis on 1026 consecutive cases. *Am J Gastroenterol* 94:691–696, 1999.

4 Corazza GR, Valentini RA, Andreani ML, et al. Subclinical coeliac disease is a frequent cause of iron-deficiency anaemia. *Scand J Gastroenterol* 30:153–156, 1995.

5 Kaukinen K, Halme L, Collin P, et al. Celiac disease in patients with severe liver disease: gluten-free diet may reverse hepatic failure. *Gastroenterology* 122:881–888, 2002.

6 Lepore L, Martelossi S, Pennesi M, et al. Prevalence of celiac disease in patients with juvenile chronic arthritis. *J Pediatr* 129:311–313, 1996.

7 Gobbi G, Bouquet F, Greco L, et al. Coeliac disease, epilepsy, and cerebral calcifications. The Italian Working Group on Coeliac Disease and Epilepsy [see comments]. *Lancet* 340:439–443, 1992.

8 Ciacci C, Cirillo M, Auriemma G, Di Dato G, Sabbatini F, Mazzacca G. Celiac disease and pregnancy outcome. *Am J Gastroenterol* 91:718–722, 1996.

9 James M, Scott B. Coeliac disease: the cause of the various associated disorders? *Eur J Gastroenterol Hepatol* 13:1119–1121, 2001.

10 Holmes G. Coeliac disease and type 1 diabetes melli-
    tus: the case for screening. *Diabet Med* 18:169–177,
    2001.
11 Walker-Smith J, Guandalini S, Schmitz J,
    Shmerling D, Visakorpi J. Revised criteria for
    diagnosis of coeliac disease. Report of Working
    Group of European Society of Paediatric
    Gastroenterology and Nutrition. *Arch Dis Child*
    65:909–911, 1990.
12 Stern M. Comparative evaluation of serologic tests
    for celiac disease: a European initiative toward stan-
    dardization. Working Group on Serologic Screening
    for Celiac Disease. *J Pediatr Gastroenterol Nutr*
    31:513–519, 2000.

19

SHORT GUT SYNDROME

Fernando Navarro

INTRODUCTION

A normal absorption of nutrients is essential throughout life, and becomes critical especially during infancy and childhood, periods in which proper nutrition is required for normal growth and development. *Short gut syndrome* (SGS) is a functional term, defining a condition in which the normal absorptive capacity of the small intestine is compromised as a result of surgical resection of a significant portion of the small intestine.[1]

The prognosis of patients after an extensive bowel resection, especially newborns, was poor in the past. However, the advent of *parenteral nutrition* has changed the outcome in the last two decades, by allowing infants and children with SGS to grow normally during the period required for intestinal adapaption.

The impact of SGS on the normal absorption of nutrients is determined not only by the extension of small bowel resected, but also by the intestinal adaptation of the remaining normal intestine. The minimum remaining intestinal length necessary for complete bowel adaptation is shorter for children than adults, suggesting better bowel adaptation in the younger population.[2]

Basic information that will help the resident-in-training to have a better understanding of SGS will be provided in the following sections.

EPIDEMIOLOGY

The exact prevalence and incidence of SGS is unknown in adults and children Epidemiologic estimates based on the use of parenteral nutrition (PN) have been reported. However, given that not all patients on PN have SGS and not all of them permanently require it, the prevalence and incidence of these two are not identical.

The dynamic nature of SGS makes epidemiologic calculations difficult. For instance, experience in *necrotizing enterocolitis* (NEC) has shown that close to 20% of neonates with NEC develop SGS after surgery; however, this percentage decreases significantly at mid- and long-term follow-up, as a consequence of the complete functional gut adaptation that many patients achieve.

ETIOLOGY AND PATHOPHYSIOLOGY

The etiology of short bowel syndrome in children differs from that in adults. In adults short bowel is more commonly secondary to mesenteric infarction, inflammatory bowel disease, and radiation. Other causes include major abdominal trauma, resection of tumors, and complications of abdominal surgery.

In children, the most common causes of SGS are necrotizing enterocolitis, abdominal wall defects, jejunal ileal atresia, and mid-gut volvulus.

These patients develop short bowel as complication of extensive intestinal resections. Enterocolitis is an important cause of short bowel especially in preterm neonates.[3]

In children the length of the intestine varies with age.[4] Pediatric SGS can be classified based on the remaining intestinal length. Standardized normal intestinal lengths for neonates and infants until 1 year of age are available. In the remaining age groups, the intestinal length can be estimated by extrapolation of these normalized values.

The length of the small intestine in a full-term newborn is between 200 and 300 cm and increases up to 700 cm in adults. The normal mean small intestine length in adults is 550 cm, ranging from 350 to 700 cm. The length of the intestine also depends on the race, body weight, and size of the patient.

During gestation, the intestine experiences a rapid elongation that starts during the last trimester of pregnancy and lasts until the crown-heel length of 60 cm is reached. After this point, the rate of intestinal growth decreases until reaching the adult length, which occurs approximately when the individual's height is between 100 and 140 cm.

Short bowel syndrome is a malabsorptive state acquired after an intestinal resection, which decreases the normal intestinal absorptive area. The degree of malabsorption depends on several factors such as the location and extent of resection, and the preservation of the *ileocecal valve* (ICV).

Pathophysiologically, resection of different sections of the small intestine causes loss of site-specific transport systems. These affect nutrient absorption, as well as water and electrolyte balance in the intestine.

Jejunal Resection

More than 90% of the digestion and absorption of nutrients is completed within the first 100 cm of jejunum. Therefore, patients who have at least 100 cm of remaining jejunum can maintain proper nutrition on oral feedings.[5]

The malabsorption resulting from extensive jejunal resection involves all nutrients as well as minerals, electrolytes, trace elements, and most of the vitamins. Severe diarrhea following extensive jejunal resection is associated with steatorrhea. The degree of malabsorption is proportional to the length of jejunum resected and will be compensated, to some extent, by the ileum and/or by the process of adaptation in response to loss of intestinal surface. Loss of part of jejunum will compromise nutrient absorption more than loss of an ileal segment of similar length, not only because of the taller villi and deeper crypts in the jejunum, but also because this part of the intestine has more active microvillus enzymes and higher nutrient absorptive capacity per unit length of intestine than the ileum.[6]

Ileal Resection

Even if most nutrients are absorbed in the proximal jejunum, as we have just seen, the residual ileum is able to adapt and to increase substantially its role of macronutrient absorption. However, the specialized cells of the terminal ileum, where vitamin B_{12}/intrinsic factor receptors are located and where bile salts are reabsorbed, cannot be replaced by jejunal hypertrophy. Thus, the ileum has specific functions which the jejunum cannot substitute. In addition, resection of the distal ileum usually includes the ICV. Finally, malabsorption of bile salts is responsible for specific complications:

- Watery diarrhea may be severe and is related to the excess of bile salts within the colon. The consequences are proportional to the concentration and dehydroxylation of bile salts into the lumen.
- Circulating pool of bile acids is reduced as a consequence of their malabsorption. This causes lipid malabsorption and steatorrhea.
- Fat-soluble vitamins (A, D, E, and K) are prone to be malabsorbed, as bile salts concentration in the lumen is not enough to create micelles.
- Bile lithogenicity is increased, as bile acids concentration in the bile is reduced.

An extensive loss of the ileum also reduces transit time as the so-called "ileal brake" is lost.

Has the Ileocecal Valve Been Removed?

Notice should always be taken, when caring for patients with SGS, about the preservation of the ileocecal valve or its removal at resection. In fact, the ICV regulates the flow of fluid and nutrients from the ileum into the colon and prevents bacteria from entering the small bowel. The resection of the ICV thus accelerates transit time (no more ileocecal brake) and allows colonic bacteria to enter and colonize the small intestine. Bacterial overgrowth (see Chap. 20) negatively impacts digestion and nutrient absorption. Thus, ICV resection constitutes an additional major cause of malabsorption of nutrients, water, and electrolytes; deconjugation of bile salts; mucosal injury; and motility disorders. Furthermore, the lack of the ICV influences markedly the period required to achieve intestinal autonomy following efficient small bowel adaptation. Finally, ICV resection increases the risk of sepsis of intestinal origin that is known to occur much more frequently in infants without the ICV than in those with an intact cecum.

Is the Colon in Place?

The colon has the capacity to absorb water and electrolytes, not nutrients. However, in patients with SGS, the preservation of partial or full colonic function at surgery is highly beneficial for nutrient absorption, because the colon may salvage nutrients by absorbing *short chain fatty acids* (SCFA). These SCFA that come from degradation, by bacterial enzymes, of malabsorbed carbohydrates and proteins, are absorbed by the colonic epithelium. It has been estimated that this process can generate up to 1000 kcal per day in energy supply.

Effects on Motility

Gastrointestinal motility may also be affected in patients with SGS due to abnormal levels of enteric hormones. For instance, faster gastric emptying and rapid small bowel transit are found in patients with jejunostomy. Lower peptide YY levels may explain these changes. This peptide as well as other hormones such as *glucagon-like peptide 1 and 2* (GLP1 and GLP2) and neurotensin are produced in the terminal ileum and colon and are released in the presence of luminal nutrients such as fats and carbohydrates. These hormones slow gastric emptying and gastrointestinal transit. In addition, GLP1 and GLP2 are increased in patients with intestinal resection in which the colon has been preserved; in these patients the gastric emptying is normal.[7,8]

The Process of Intestinal Adaptation

The initial postoperative malabsorption improves due to adaptive changes in the remaining intestinal mucosa occurring as early as 48 h. Intestinal adaptation after massive small bowel resection is a slow process accompanied by a gradual increase in absorption capacity of nutrients, electrolytes, and minerals. The process involves muscular hypertrophy (increased bowel diameter and wall thickness) and hyperplasia of the intestinal mucosa. Microscopically, there is crypt and villous hyperplasia. Macroscopically, there is dilatation, lengthening, and thickening of the bowel. The intestinal hyperplasia is thought to be the result of increased crypt cell production mediated by several growth factors. They include hormonal mediators such as enteroglucagon, glucagon-like peptides neurotensine, peptide YY, growth hormone, and insulin-like growth factor. Additionally, oral or enteral feeding stimulates the release of enterotrophic hormones such as gastrin, cholecystokinin, and neurotensine, which may further improve the process of gut adaptation. The process leads to an increased number of enterocytes per unit of intestinal length, an increased rate of enterocyte proliferation, and an increased villous height and crypt depth.

Intraluminal substrates and nutrients, provided by oral or enteral feeding, are essential for achieving intestinal adaptation after extensive resection.

The process of intestinal adaptation may require as long as 2 years to complete.[9] For instance, after jejunal resection there is a gradual improvement in absorption as the ileum undergoes adaptation with significant growth in length, diameter, and function of villi.

From a clinical standpoint, intestinal adaptation is aimed at allowing the gradual transition from *total parenteral nutrition* (TPN) to enteral feeding and eventually to the resumption of full oral feeding. It should be stressed however that not all children with SGS do reach this outcome, as it depends on several factors; in particular the extent of the resection, the age at resection, and the part of the small gut that was resected.

CLINICAL SIGNS AND SYMPTOMS

The diagnosis of short bowel syndrome is suspected after the patient has undergone resection of a "significant" length of intestine. However, the exact remaining bowel length at which the clinical manifestations of SGS appear has not been determined.[10]

During a laparotomy for intestinal resection, the surgeon clearly attempts to preserve as much viable intestine as possible. During surgery the amount of intestine resected and the length of the remaining small and large intestine are measured. Radiographic estimation of the length of short bowel correlates well with the measured length at surgery, and can therefore be used whenever information on surgery is scanty.

In adults, less than 200 cm of remaining jejunoileal length is considered the length at which clinical manifestations of SGS may develop. Diarrhea and short-term malabsorption may occur when 30–50% of jejunoileal length is resected. However, the loss of more than 70% of jejunoileal length causes long-term malabsorption and a significant impact in nutrition.[11]

The clinical manifestations of short bowel syndrome are primarily determined by the extent of the intestinal resection. Diarrhea and steatorrhea are the predominant clinical symptoms. Patients may also develop hypovolemia, hyponatremia, and hypokalemia due to the increased stool losses. Malabsorption of nutrients, vitamins, and trace elements can lead to weight loss and nutrient deficiencies.[12]

COMPLICATIONS

In patients with SGS, the loss of absorptive surface can result in carbohydrate malabsorption and protein loss. Depending on the type of intestinal resection, they may also have bacterial deconjugation of bile acids which interferes with absorption of monoglycerides and fatty acids.

Carbohydrate malabsorption can be estimated directly by testing the stool or ostomy fluid for reducing substances (e.g., with a Clinitest tablet) and indirectly by calculating stool pH. A pH below 5.5 is considered indirect evidence of carbohydrate malabsorption. The use of breath tests to diagnose malabsorption is less informative in patients with SGS because of their more rapid intestinal transit.

Malabsorption of nutrients can lead to nutrient deficiencies especially after patients have been weaned off parenteral nutrition. In patients with SGS, especially those with extensive intestinal resections in which the intestinal adaptation process is difficult to predict, serum levels of vitamins and minerals need to be frequently monitored.

The combination of SGS and long-term PN exposes patients to these main complications:

- Catheter-related sepsis and thrombosis
- Bone disease
- Peptic acid disease
- Liver damage
- Urolithiasis
- D-Lactic acidosis

Daily catheter care and prevention of septic complications are essential (see Chap. 31).

Phosphorus and calcium status should be assessed and, if necessary, supplies should be given to prevent PN-related bone disease.

Patients with SGS may develop hypergastrinemia due to the loss of negative feedback mechanism for inhibiting gastrin secretion. Secondary acid hypersecretion predisposes these patients to peptic ulcer disease and esophagitis.[12,13] In addition, pancreatic enzymes are inactivated in the presence of a low pH. This state of gastric hypersecretion usually resolves within the first few months after resection.

Liver function tests should be performed on a regular basis because of the risk of cholestasis and liver injury. If initial surgery did not include a gallbladder resection, an ultrasonography aiming to look for sludge or cholelithiasis should be repeated every 3 months. Gallstones are formed because of alteration in the bile content and flow. The lack of enterohepatic circulation alters the cholesterol content in bile and the absence of enteral stimulation of intestinal hormones decreases the bile flow.[14] Liver disease is certainly the most frequent and the most severe complication in short bowel patients. Premature babies and/or small for gestational age babies with severe necrotizing enterocolitis are especially at high risk to develop liver disease and rapid end-stage liver failure, because of the combination of prematurity, subocclusion, gram-negative sepsis, and repeated catheter-related sepsis. In general, liver disease is mostly related to the impaired small intestine and is further aggravated by inadequate PN.

Patients with SGS, especially those who have fat malabsorption, are at risk of oxalate urine stones. Nonabsorbed bile salts induce an increased colonic permeability to small molecules such as oxalate. This complication only occurs in those patients in which, after the resection, the colon and the small intestine have been already anastomosed. The risk of urolithiasis is increased when patients have a high stool output and metabolic acidosis. A decreased urine output, acidic urine pH, and decreased citrate secretion all promote the formation of calcium oxalate and uric acid stones.

Hyperoxaluria is treated with a low oxalate diet, a high fluid intake, and correction of the metabolic acidosis if present. Cholestyramine, which binds bile acids and oxalate, can also be used if tolerated. A low-fat diet, in addition, may be helpful by reducing the quantity of fatty acids and free oxalate in the colon; however, a low-fat diet may be inadequate to fulfill the caloric requirements of patients with SGS.[15]

D-Lactic acidosis is another metabolic complication of short bowel syndrome most commonly seen in patients with preserved colon. Gram-positive anaerobes or lactobacilli produce D-lactate when nonabsorbed carbohydrates reach the colon and produce organic acids whose reabsorption leads to a metabolic acidosis that could be severe. Patients may develop slurred speech, confusion, and cerebellar ataxia.[16]

D-Lactic acidosis is treated by correction of the metabolic acidosis and the administration of oral antibiotics (e.g., vancomycin, gentamicin, and metronidazole) to decrease the concentration of D-lactate-producing organisms. Because carbohydrates, particularly simple sugars, are the substrate for the production of D-lactate, a low carbohydrate diet may be beneficial, especially if starch polymers are used.

MANAGEMENT

The medical management of SGS is typically exemplified by three consecutive phases.

- The first phase follows small bowel resection and is associated with massive losses of water and electrolytes, with a severe diarrhea worsened by gastric hypersecretion. During this period, total PN is required, but small amounts of organic substrates must be provided by the enteral route, per os or by continuous gastric infusion as soon as intestinal transit has recovered.

- In the second phase intestinal transit is reestablished, and intestinal function improves as a result of progressive adaptation of the remaining small bowel. PN is continued to allow the short gut to develop and to become functional. During this time, which can be several months or years before obtaining maximal adaptation, nutrients by the enteral route are cautiously and progressively increased and PN progressively reduced.

- The third phase starts when intestinal function is sufficiently resumed and allows absorbtion of nutrients, thus enabling PN to be ultimately completely withdrawn. All calories are eventually provided by the oral route, and oral intake can then be further liberalized according to the tolerance of the patient.

This long period requires special management and follow-up.

First Phase

After an intestinal resection, the predominant goals are the administration of parenteral nutrition and prevention of fluid and electrolyte abnormalities. During the immediate postoperative period, patients should remain nothing by mouth (NPO), to address the postsurgical ileus and to allow healing.

Medical therapy is aimed at compensating for the intestinal losses while attempting to reduce them and to achieve nutritional repletion. Stool output (stomal and fecal) must be measured to establish the baseline water and electrolytes losses. Depending on the type of surgery, the quality and amount of fluid loss differs. For instance, patients with jejunostomy may have significant sodium losses (up to 80–100 meq/L). Thus, replacement solutions not uncommonly require a very high sodium concentration in order to maintain fluid and electrolyte homeostasis. The requirements of massive intravenous fluids and the necessity to avoid multiple peripheral perfusions necessitate the early placement of a central venous catheter. Such vascular access allows the safe replacement of volumes of fluid according to the evaluation of intestinal losses. When losses stabilize, fluid and electrolyte losses can be added to the PN solution and administered through a single infusion device. Patients with proximal enterostomy require special trace elements supplementation. PN must provide adequate nutritional supply to the child allowing optimal growth: such nutritional support includes the use of 1.5–2.5 g/kg per day amino acids, a caloric intake consisting of 70–80% of non-protein-energy substrates such as dextrose, and 20–30% energy provided by a 20% intravenous fat emulsion. Maintenance amounts of vitamins and trace elements are added to the PN solution by using commercially available preparations. Calcium, phosphate, and magnesium are also added to the solution according to the patients' need and the stability of the solution (see Chap. 31).

During the early phases of therapy, serum electrolytes, glucose, urea, and calcium should be measured daily. When the patient's condition and the intestinal losses become stable, blood monitoring can be less frequent. During the first stage after resection, H2 blockers should be given intravenously in high doses to inhibit gastric hypersecretion: ranitidine, 10–15 mg/kg per day, can be added to, PN solution, the drug being delivered as a continuous infusion.

The first phase of management ends when the patient has recovered from the surgical procedure, is stable on PN, and has controlled intestinal losses.

Second Phase

The duration of this second stage (PN + oral or enteral feedings) depends on several factors including the length of the remaining total intestine, the conservation of the ICV, and the functional capacity of the remaining small intestine. The slow transition from TPN to full oral feeding requires time during which the nutritional status has to be maintained at the optimal level. In this regard, home PN is the best tool to maintain both nutritional status and to achieve bowel adaptation. Most patients who have been weaned from PN maintain some degree of malabsorption that is compensated for by a relative hyperphagia. Conversely, trying to wean an infant with neonatal short bowel syndrome (SBS) from parental antrition (PN) too rapidly increases the occurrence of metabolic complications.

During the initiation of enteral feedings, H2 blockers or proton-pump inhibitors still need to be administered, as the suppression of gastric hypersecretion, by alkalinizing the intestinal contents, may improve nutrient absorption and reduce fluid losses.

Supplementation of fat-soluble vitamins (A, D, E, and K) is required in patients with steatorrhea. In addition, vitamin B_{12} supplementation is required in those patients who have had a significant resection of the terminal ileum.[17] Water-soluble vitamin deficiency is not frequent in SGS, because they are absorbed in the upper parts of the small bowel (duodenum and upper jejunum) that are usually preserved.

The mode of administration of feedings (oral vs. enteral) varies in different centers. Oral feeding seems to be preferable in neonates because they are more physiologic, stimulate the motility of the gallbladder, and have been found to reduce PN-related liver disease. If breast milk is available, its use has the advantage of containing additional non-nutritive factors and it seems a logical choice, even if it contains lactose. Elemental or semielemental diets can be used, but if given orally they still increase stool volume and frequency. Oral feedings should be started at 50–80 mL per day, divided into six to eight meals. Thereafter, the amounts are progressively increased over several days or weeks. Diarrhea will develop when the amount of diet exceeds the digestive and absorptive capacities of the remaining small intestine.

Continuous enteral feeding (CEF) can be achieved using either a *nasogastric* (NG) tube or a *feeding gastrostomy* (G-tube). Whatever the gastric access, CEF allows gradual infusion of an appropriate liquid diet chosen depending on the estimated capacity or digestion and absorption of the remaining small bowel. Enteral nutrition is usually started slowly. The solution should contain no fiber, have an osmolality below 310 mOsm/kg, and contain substrates which are rapidly absorbed without leaving intraluminal residues. The caloric concentration is gradually increased from 0.6 to 1 kcal/mL according to digestive tolerance. It is also important to avoid excessive fluid administration which may result in patient fluid overload. Continuous enteral infusion enhances absorption by fully saturating the various gut transporters around the clock. If the child is managed by using CEF, oral feedings should be maintained. In particular, solid feedings should be introduced by 6 months of age to promote proper learning of chewing and swallowing habits at an appropriate age.

Protein hydrolysate and elemental formulas, because of their higher percentage of fat and hypoallergenicity, are widely employed. Their prolonged use is also often required in those patients with documented cow's milk protein allergy or lactose intolerance. In the majority of patients, however, long-term use of protein hydrolysate and elemental formulas is not recommended due to their high cost and poor palatability.

The addition of fiber to the diet should begin only after achieving some degree of intestinal adaptation. In addition to providing additional calories, especially in those patients with sufficient remaining colon, fiber may enhance the production of short chain fatty acids. The use of fiber can also help indirectly by reducing the amount of stools and secondarily preventing perianal skin deterioration.

In some cases, malabsorption makes the amount of calories taken enterally insufficient. For this reason, patients unable to maintain adequate caloric intake such as those who have inadequate weight gain or weight loss, or those who have stool losses in which enteral replacement is not possible may need a combination of cycled home parenteral nutrition and enteral feedings.

Third Phase

When the transition between total PN and full enteral/oral feeding is achieved, phase 3 begins with the discontinuation of artificial nutrition. Discontinuation of PN is attempted after the patient receives no more than 2 or 3 perfusions per week. If both protein-energy intake and intestinal function are adequate, normal weight gain and growth velocity must be achieved. After documenting that an adequate weight gain is shown for at least 3 months without PN, the central venous catheter can be removed. When all the necessary calories are provided by oral feeding, oral intake can be further liberalized both in volume and variety.

Surgical Management

Short gut syndrome may require surgical management. Different techniques of surgical bowel lengthening or bowel tapering are available that can sometimes enhance intestinal function among patients with short bowel syndrome. Intestinal tapering and lengthening have been performed especially in selected patients with dilated bowel segments. In fact, marked dilatation of the proximal intestine may occur secondary to chronic obstruction or adaptation. The ensuing stasis leads to bacterial overgrowth which further aggravates malabsorption.

SGS is considered the most common cause of intestinal failure leading to *small bowel transplantation* (SBTx). This "last resource" procedure is indicated in patients with severe forms of SGS who are thought to never be able to achieve adaptation (residual intestinal length <20 cm) and for those patients in which medical or surgical management of intestinal failure is unsuccessful. It should not be forgotten that SBTx may lead to complications such as sepsis, cytomegalovirus infection, lympho-proliferative disease, and rejection after transplantation. Currently, the long-term mortality of SBTx remains unfortunately very high, around 50% at 5 years posttransplant.

PROGNOSIS

The ultimate goal in the management of SGS is the achievement of intestinal autonomy and total independence from PN; however, this goal is not always achieved. In patients with SGS, the length of the remaining small bowel, site of resection and the presence or absence of colon in infants, the birth weight, and the gestational age are considered important determinants for establishing and maintaining intestinal autonomy.[18] However, the residual intestinal length is the main determining factor of the duration of PN.

The presence of the ileocecal valve, cholestatic jaundice, bacterial overgrowth, and the inability to institute early enteral feeding are other factors that also have been related to a prolonged PN duration. In addition, in infants, the duration of parenteral nutrition also depends on the gestational age and the birth weight. Therefore, in order to decrease the time of PN and subsequently diminish the incidence of its complications, early enteral nutrition and the prompt closure of diverting ostomies need to be important considerations.

In addition to the PN-related complications, there is a 10–15% reported incidence of neurologic and developmental complications in SGS.[19]

Finally, the reported overall mortality of SGS ranges from 15 to 20%. Clearly, however, advances in surgical techniques, postoperative care, and parenteral nutrition have positively impacted the survival of these patients and can be expected to provide further improvement in the outcome of SGS patients.[20,21]

References

1   Vanderhoof JA, Langnas AN. Short-bowel syndrome in children and adults. *Gastroenterology* 113:1767–1778, 1997.

2   Wasa M, Takagi Y, Sando K, Harada T, Okada A. Long-term outcome of short bowel syndrome in adult and pediatric patients. *JPEN J Parenter Enteral Nutr* 23:S110–S112, 1999.

3   Ford EG, Senac MO Jr, Srikanth MS, Weitzman JJ. Malrotation of the intestine in children. *Ann Surg* 215:172–178, 1992.

4   Weaver LT, Austin S, Cole TJ. Small intestinal length: a factor essential for gut adaptation. *Gut* 32:1321–1323, 1991.

5   Johansson C. Studies of gastrointestinal interactions. VII. Characteristics of the absorption pattern of sugar, fat and protein from composite meals in man. A quantitative study. *Scand J Gastroenterol* 10: 33–42, 1975.

6   Lennard-Jones JE. Review article: practical management of the short bowel. *Aliment Pharmacol Ther* 8:563–577, 1994.

7   Savage AP, Adrian TE, Carolan G, Chatterjee VK, Bloom SR. Effects of peptide YY (PYY) on mouth to caecum intestinal transit time and on the rate of gastric emptying in healthy volunteers. *Gut* 28:166–170, 1987.

8   Vanderhoof JA, Park JH, Herrington MK, Adrian TE. Effects of dietary menhaden oil on mucosal adaptation after small bowel resection in rats. *Gastroenterology* 106:94–99, 1994.

9   Kurkchubasche AG, Rowe MI, Smith SD. Adaptation in short-bowel syndrome: reassessing old limits. *J Pediatr Surg* 28:1069–1071, 1993.

10 Dudrick SJ, Latifi R, Fosnocht DE. Management of the short-bowel syndrome. *Surg Clin North Am* 71:625–643, 1991.

11 Tilson MD. Pathophysiology and treatment of short bowel syndrome. *Surg Clin North Am* 60:1273–1284, 1980.

12 Nordgaard I, Hansen BS, Mortensen PB. Colon as a digestive organ in patients with short bowel. *Lancet* 343:373–376, 1994.

13 Williams NS, Evans P, King RF. Gastric acid secretion and gastrin production in the short bowel syndrome. *Gut* 26:914–919, 1985.

14 Quigley EM, Marsh MN, Shaffer JL, Markin RS. Hepatobiliary complications of total parenteral nutrition. *Gastroenterology* 104:286–301, 1993.

15 Obialo CI, Clayman RV, Matts JP, et al. Pathogenesis of nephrolithiasis post-partial ileal bypass surgery:

case-control study. The POSCH Group. *Kidney Int* 39:1249–1254, 1991.

16 Bongaerts G, Tolboom J, Naber T, Bakkeren J, Severijnen R, Willems H. D-lactic acidemia and aciduria in pediatric and adult patients with short bowel syndrome. *Clin Chem* 41:107–110, 1995.

17 Thompson WG, Wrathell E. The relation between ileal resection and vitamin B12 absorption. *Can J Surg* 20:461–464, 1977.

18 Wilmore DW. Factors correlating with a successful outcome following extensive intestinal resection in newborn infants. *J Pediatr* 80:88–95, 1972.

19 Sigalet DL. Short bowel syndrome in infants and children: an overview. *Semin Pediatr Surg* 10:49–55, 2001.

20 Anagnostopoulos D, Valioulis J, Sfougaris D, Maliaropoulos N, Spyridakis J. Morbidity and mortality of short bowel syndrome in infancy and childhood. *Eur J Pediatr Surg* 1:273–276, 1991.

21 Cooper A, Floyd TF, Ross AJ 3rd, Bishop HC, Templeton JM Jr, Ziegler MM. Morbidity and mortality of short-bowel syndrome acquired in infancy: an update. *J Pediatr Surg* 19:711–718, 1984.

20

SMALL BOWEL BACTERIAL OVERGROWTH

Roberto Berni Canani, Pia Cirillo, and Maria Teresa Romano

INTRODUCTION

Small bowel bacteria overgrowth (SBBO) is defined as a proliferation in the upper gastrointestinal tract (stomach, duodenum, and jejunum) of bacteria, often changing from predominantly oropharyngeal to colorectal species. In a healthy child, bacteria do not inhabit the upper small intestine and stomach in significant numbers. The relative sterility of the upper small intestine depends on a number of nonimmunologic and immunologic factors that act to reduce bacterial load and prevent colonization. Epidemiology of SBBO in the pediatric population is scarce; however, it may still reflect predisposition. A recent retrospective study including 100 adult patients affected by SBBO suggests that the most common coexisting conditions include gastroparesis (37%), chronic pancreatitis (28%), Crohn's disease (6%), and ulcerative colitis (4%).

PATHOPHYSIOLOGY

At birth, the gastrointestinal tract is sterile. It is then colonized by bacteria coming from maternal intestinal microflora or from contact with surroundings. In this period there is a prevalence of facultative anaerobes, such as enterobacteria, coliforms, and lactobacilli, thereafter the composition of diet may condition microorganism species. In fact, in breast-fed infants bifidobacteria is the dominating strain, while in formula-fed infants there is a complex microflora composed of bifidobacteria, enterobacteria, lactobacilli, bacteroides, clostridia, and streptococci. After weaning, microflora composition becomes similar to that of adults and remains relatively stable throughout life. In the human intestine there are at least 500 different bacterial species even if 10–20 genera are predominant: *Bacteroides, Clostridium, Fusobacterium, Lactobacillus, Bifidobacterium, Escherichia coli*, and *Peptococcus*. The composition of intestinal microflora along the entire gastrointestinal tract is represented in Fig. 20-1. The total number of bacteria that can be cultured is in the order of 10–20%, while the remaining 80–90% are defined as "unculturable." The qualitative and quantitative microflora composition depends on the specific segments of the gastrointestinal tract which creates a complex and varied environment for microorganisms (Fig. 20-2). The esophagus

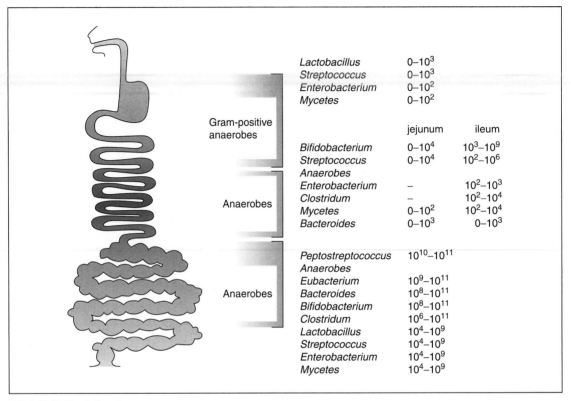

FIGURE 20-1

PREDOMINANT BACTERIAL SPECIES ALONG THE GASTROINTESTINAL TRACT

does not have a colonizing commensal flora, but it may have transient microorganisms coming from the oral cavity and from dietary sources. The stomach content presents very low levels of bacteria, in particular acid-resistant lactobacilli; also in the upper small intestine there is a low bacterial load because bile salts and pancreatic secretion destroy many orally acquired microorganisms, and peristalsis prevents adhesion and colonization. However, in this part of the gastrointestinal tract, aerobic bacteria typical of the oral cavity predominate and are present in number of 10^5 organisms/mL. On traversing the terminal ileum and into the cecum the microbial flora increases in number and diversity. Ultimately, in the large intestine, strict and facultative anaerobes, adapted to grow within the fecal mass where bacterial metabolism quickly deprives the environment of

oxygen, are most common and their total number reaches 10^{12} bacteria/g of luminal contents. It is estimated that bacteria constitute one-third of the dry weight of feces. The average person excretes between 10^{11} and 10^{14} bacteria in their feces everyday.

Intestinal microflora exerts several beneficial effects on human health such as inhibition of pathogenic microorganism colonization in the intestine and stimulation of the local and systemic immune response. Its importance is well shown by the germ-free animal model showing several intestinal abnormalities reported in Table 20-1.

Multiple mechanisms are involved in the control of gut microecology and in preventing excessive proliferation of intestinal bacteria. These defense mechanisms (summarized in Table 20-2) include both nonimmune and immune factors.

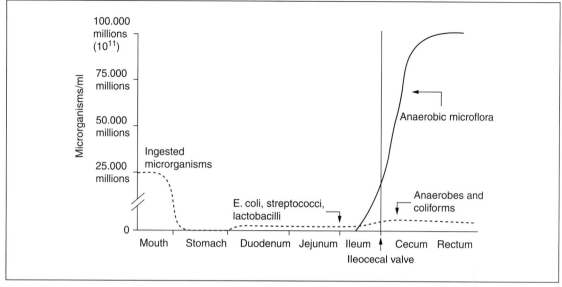

FIGURE 20-2

DIFFERENT MICROORGANISM CONCENTRATIONS ALONG THE ENTIRE GASTROINTESTINAL TRACT IN THE NORMAL CHILD

Nonimmune Factors

- *Mucosal surface.* It provides a protective interface between the internal environment and the constant challenge of food antigens and microorganisms. It produces important substances such as defensines and mucus. The latter is composed of glycoprotein and salts

and it is able to bind bacteria and to limit their access to the intestinal mucosa.
- *Gastric acidity.* A pH less than 4.0 has a bactericidal effect on most species of microorganisms. This is proved by the effects

TABLE 20-1

MAIN INTESTINAL ABNORMALITIES IN
GERM-FREE ANIMAL MODEL

Mucosal atrophy
Enzymatic brush-border activity deficiencies
Reduced mucosal blood flow
Impaired intestinal motility
Immunodeficiency
• Reduced cytokines production
• Reduced cellular immunity
• Reduced development of gut associated lymphoid tissue (GALT) and MVWSA associated lymphoid tissue (MALT)
High risk of infection

TABLE 20-2

MAIN IMMUNE AND NONIMMUNE ANTIBACTERIAL
DEFENSIVE FACTORS IN UPPER INTESTINE

Nonimmune
Substances produced by enterocytes (e.g., defensines, lactoferrin)
Mucus
Gastric acidity
Peristalsis
Pancreatic enzymes and bile salts
Ileocecal valve
Immune
sIgA
IgG
Activated B and T lymphocytes
Macrophages

of chronic inhibition of gastric acidity induced by antiacids drugs (ranitidine and/or omeprazole) that is able to increase the bacterial count in stomach and duodenum.

- *Peristalsis.* It prevents adhesion and colonization of ingested microorganisms, as suggested by a rise in bacterial count induced by pharmacologic inhibitors of migratory motor complexes.
- *Enzymatic digestion.* The antibacterial effect of pancreatic juice is based on its proteolytic and lypolitic enzymes, while bile and digestive secretions act by diluting bacteria and inhibiting the formation of stagnant niches.
- *Ileocecal valve.* It inhibits retrograde colonization of bacteria from distal to proximal bowel.

Immune Factors

The immune system (including sIgA, cytokines, and leucocytes) plays an important role in controlling gastrointestinal proliferation of bacteria as demonstrated by bacterial overgrowth in immunodeficiencies.

Small bowel bacteria overgrowth occurs when these normal defense factors against bacterial proliferation are reduced. In particular, etiologic factors in the development of SBBO include anatomic abnormalities, alterations of intestinal peristalsis, abnormalities of intestinal immune and nonimmune defence mechanisms (see Table 20-3).

CLINICAL MANIFESTATIONS

Excessive bacterial colonization may lead to a variety of defects that results in nutrient malabsorption and other clinical features (see Table 20-4).

In particular, bacterial overgrowth determines malabsorption of the following:

- *Fats.* Bacterial deconjugation and dehydroxylation of bile acids leads to their

TABLE 20-3

MAIN PREDISPOSING FACTORS FOR SBBO

Anatomic Abnormalities
Diverticulosis
Duplication
Blind loop
Stenosis and strictures (Crohn's disease, radiation, surgery)
Motility Disorders
Idiopathic intestinal pseudoobstruction
Absence of the migratory motor complexes
Autonomic neuropathy
Radiation enteritis
Crohn's disease
Excessive Bacterial Load
Hypoachloridria
Gastrocolic or jejunocolic fistula
Lack of the ileocecal valve
Abnormal Host Defense
Immunodeficiency
Hypoachloridria (atrophic gastritis medications)
Prematurity

TABLE 20-4

CLINICAL SYMPTOMS OF SBBO

Local
Chronic diarrhea
Steatorrhea
Anemia
Systemic
Nephritis
Hepatitis
Erythema nodosum
Papular rash
Raynaud's phenomenon
Arthritis
Tenosynovitis
Associated Symptoms
Weight loss
Short stature
Abdominal pain
Protein-losing enteropathy
Hypoalbuminemia
Osteoporosis
Night blindness
Ataxia

premature absorption in the jejunum and thus to their unavailability to perform micellar solubilization of fats. In addition, bacterial deconjugation determines the production of the lithocolic acid which may damage intestinal mucosa contributing to malabsorption of fat and other nutrients.

- *Carbohydrates.* Intraluminal bacterial consumption leads to reduction of their absorption, while free bile acids cause monosaccharide malabsorption via mucosal damage.
- *Proteins.* Bacteria degrade intraluminal protein, and free bile acids inhibit amino acids and dipeptide absorption and also lead to protein-losing enteropathy.
- *Vitamins.* Vitamin B_{12} is not only produced but also used by intestinal anaerobe bacteria, so the deficiency of this vitamin is frequently associated with SBBO.

Thus, bacterial overgrowth-related nutrient malabsorption is an important player in the pathogenesis of the following typical clinical picture:

- Abdominal distention and flatulence due to the gas produced by carbohydrate degradation (CO_2, methane, H_2)
- Steatorrhea and fat-soluble vitamin deficiency derived from fat malabsorption
- Watery diarrhea determined by numerous factors, including hydroxylated fatty acids, motility disorders, bacterial toxins, and inflammatory mediators
- Anemia and neurologic symptoms related to vitamin B_{12} deficiency
- Other symptoms including dyspepsia, abdominal pain, weight loss, intestinal dismotility, and less frequently ataxia and delirium due to absorption of neurotoxic fermentation-derived products, such as D-lactate

Finally, SBBO can cause cholestatic liver damage in a small percentage of patients (less than 10%). Obligate anaerobes such as *Bacteroides* spp. are considered to play an important role in the pathogenesis of these abnormalities, possibly by promoting increased small intestinal permeability to proinflammatory bacterial polymers.

In some children, symptoms of the primary disease predominate, and evidence of bacterial overgrowth may be found only on investigation. In others, the primary condition is symptomless, and the patient shows a typical malabsorption syndrome due to SBBO.

DIAGNOSIS

Small bowel bacterial overgrowth should be included in the differential diagnosis of any child presenting chronic diarrhea, steatorrhea, weight loss, macrocytic anemia, or other signs of intestinal malabsorption; however, establishing the diagnosis of SBBO is frequently problematic. An accurate medical history often provides crucial clues suggesting that more investigations, related to the possibility of underlying small intestinal bacterial contamination, are warranted. First of all, a history of previous intestinal surgery should always be sought. This is important because SBBO, due to either alterations of intestinal motility or the creation of anatomic regions of intestinal stasis or modification of the anatomic barrier for viable organisms that enter the proximal small intestine (i.e., lack of the ileocecal valve), can occur as a longterm adverse complication of gut surgery. Similarly, signs and symptoms suggestive of systemic disease (i.e., collagen vascular disease or longstanding diabetes mellitus-related autonomic neuropathy) should be explored in a detailed history. For these reasons, SBBO should be suspected if a barium meal with follow-through (as a part of routine evaluation of a child with malabsorption) shows hypomotility, partial obstruction, dilatation, diverticula, or other mechanical factors associated with delayed gastrointestinal motility. The Schilling test is also abnormal, because in patients with SBBO the bacteria combine with, or destroy, intrinsic factor and/or the vitamin B_{12} causing its malabsorption; however, after an antibiotic treatment the vitamin B_{12} absorption returns to normal. There are

TABLE 20-5

TESTS USEFUL IN THE DIAGNOSTIC APPROACH TO THE PATIENT WITH SUSPECT SBBO

Screening
Steatorrhea
Schilling's test with intrinsic factor
Folic acid dosage
Barium meal with follow-through

Diagnostic
Jejunal aspirate
  Culture
  Deconjugated bile salts dosage
  Short chain fatty acids dosage
Indicanuria
Serum bile acids
Breath tests
  Radioisotopes
    ^{14}C-D-xylose
    ^{13}C-D-xylose
  Breath hydrogen
    Fasting
    Lactulose
    Glucose

many laboratory or instrumental tests that can be used for the diagnosis of SBBO (see Table 20-5). Although the demonstration of a high bacterial concentration (>10^5 organisms/mL) in small intestinal secretion, obtained by esofagastroduodenoscopy or by per-oral jejunal intubation, is considered the gold standard for the diagnosis of SBBO, this approach is invasive and culture of aspirate is both time-consuming and dependent on sophisticated anaerobic techniques. In addition, contamination from oropharyngeal flora may occur during specimen collection, and bacterial overgrowth may be patchy and missed by a single culture, or located in relatively inaccessible sites. Multiple organisms are typically present in varying numbers. Common species include *Streptococci, Bacteroides, E. coli,* and *Lactobacillus.* Culture of unwashed mucosal biopsies facilitates the detection of subjects with SBBO when luminal secretions are scarce, but remains an invasive means of establishing this

diagnosis. Therefore, indirect measures of the bacteria presence within the intestinal lumen are frequently employed. Many of these measures, including serum folate and D-lactate or urinary indican levels, have inadequate diagnostic accuracy. Other methods, including measurement of unconjugated bile acids and short chain fatty acids (i.e., acetic, propionic, butirric, isobutirric, valeric, and isovaleric acids) in duodenal fluid or serum, require invasive techniques to obtain samples or sophisticated laboratory procedures for analysis, limiting their clinical utility. Various less invasive alternatives have been proposed, including measurement of luminal bacterial metabolism products in the breath in fasting state or following a fermentable substrate administration (the breath test). The principle of breath hydrogen testing is the administration of a test dose of carbohydrate (usually glucose), which in children with SBBO is associated with a rise in breath hydrogen levels. In humans, only bacteria (specifically, colonic anaerobic bacteria) are capable of producing hydrogen. The bacteria produce hydrogen when they are exposed to unabsorbed food, particularly carbohydrates. Some of the hydrogen produced by the bacteria is absorbed into the blood flowing through the intestinal wall and reaches the lungs where it is released into the breath and thus can be measured. Figure 20-3 is a schematic representation of the breath test principles. Glucose-breath hydrogen testing is safe and easy to perform; however, the usefulness of the test is limited by a lower sensitivity and specificity compared to ^{14}C-xylose test. This is due to the following factors: approximately up to 20% of children with SBBO harbor bacteria that do not produce hydrogen; the hydrogen peak occurring from bacterial overgrowth in the distal small intestine may be difficult to discriminate from the normal peak seen when the test substrate reaches the colon; finally, rapid delivery of the test substrate to the colon in patients with short bowel syndrome may lead to false-positive results. Because the administration of ^{14}C is associated with negligible radiation exposure, it is not recommended for children. A breath test, in which xylose is labelled with ^{13}C (a safe, nonradioactive isotope), has recently been developed. A list

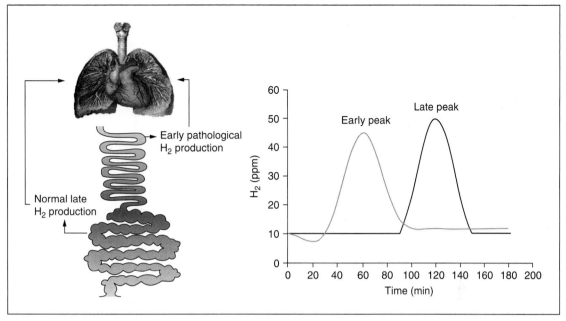

FIGURE 20-3

SCHEMATIC REPRESENTATION OF BREATH TESTING

In the healthy child a late-normal colonic peak is detected. On the contrary, an early peak and/or an elevated baseline hydrogen value are suggestive of small bowel bacterial overgrowth.

of factors useful to improve the diagnostic accuracy of the breath test is reported in Table 20-6.

TREATMENT

When suspicion for SBBO is high, some clinicians use empiric treatment as a diagnostic test. A major drawback to this approach is that treatment may require more than one antibiotic and sometimes cyclic treatment. Because many antibiotics may be associated with adverse effects, some of which may mimic symptoms of SBBO (such as diarrhea and abdominal pain), establishing a clear diagnosis is important. Another potential problem with empiric therapy is that symptoms of SBBO may mimic an exacerbation of an underlying disorder, such as an inflammatory bowel disease.

The optimal therapeutic approach to a patient with SBBO is reported in Table 20-7. The treatment

of SBBO involves removing the cause, when possible. The addition of broad-spectrum antibiotics may often induce a long-term remission. If the cause cannot be eliminated and symptoms recur, good

TABLE 20-6

RECOMMENDATIONS TO IMPROVE ACCURACY OF HYDROGEN BREATH TEST

During the 2 Days Before the Test

Avoid antibiotics, lactose, milk of magnesia, sorbitol or high-fiber foods, and supplements

Fast 12 h before the test

Wash mouth with an antiseptic

Two Hours Before and During the Test

The patient may not eat, drink, smoke, sleep, or do physical exercise

The patient with intestinal dismotility syndrome needs breath samples taken up to 3 h after the ingestion of substrate

THE FOUR PILLARS IN TREATMENT OF SBBO

1. Correction of underlying disease Surgery for diverticula and strictures Prokinetics for dismotility syndromes
2. Nutritional supplementation Enteral feeding Parenteral nutrition
3. Correction of micronutrient deficiencies Cyanocobalamin supplements Fat-soluble vitamins Iron
4. Antibiotic therapy

results can be achieved with intermittent use of antibiotics.

Correction of Underlying Disease

The underlying cause of SBBO is usually not easily treated and it may require surgery. In particular, surgical correction may resolve SBBO related to a large Meckel's diverticulum, bowel dilatation, gastrocolic or jejunocolic fistulae or intestinal strictures due to radiations, surgery, or Crohn's disease.

Pharmacologic agents such as cisapride or erythromycin may improve cases deriving from motility disorders (e.g., diabetes mellitus, scleroderma, and intestinal pseudoobstruction).

Nutritional Supplementation

Nutritional support is very important for patients affected by SBBO and in particular for those presenting a significant weight loss or evidence of micronutrient deficiency. When the caloric intake is limited by abdominal pain, malabsorption, or anorexia, nutritional supplements such as medium-chain triglycerides may be useful. Deficiencies of calcium, vitamins A, D, E, K, and B_{12} have been rarely reported and may be treated with the administration of fat-soluble vitamins and cyanocobalamin. In addition, dietary changes may improve some symptoms—lactose containing products

should be avoided since lactase deficiency may develop in many patients with SBBO and fats are better than carbohydrates in limiting bacterial fermentation which cause D-lactic acidosis, flatulence, and discomfort.

Antibiotics

They are used to modify intestinal microflora leading to an improvement of symptoms. Antibiotic selection must be based on the prevalent microorganisms, as bacterial culture and antibiotic sensitivity may not be helpful due to the presence of different bacterial species. Generally, antibiotic spectrum should cover aerobic and anaerobic bacteria such as *E. coli*, *Klebsiella*, and *Bacteroides*. No satisfactory controlled trial examining antimicrobial agent selection, length of therapy, or appropriate management of recurrence is available. The following antibiotics have been used with apparent success: tetracycline, amoxicilline-clavulanate, ciprofloxacin, combination of oral gentamicin and metronidazole, or combination of cephalosporin (cephalexin), trimethoprim-sulfamethoxazole, and metronidazole. In many cases a single course of therapy for 7–10 days is successful; but in some patients there is a need of a prolonged therapy (1–2 months). For the recurrence of the symptoms, cycles of therapy repeated each month on the first 5–10 days are requested. To prevent overgrowth-resistant organisms in these patients the broad-spectrum antibiotics should be rotated every 1–2 months (tetracycline or trimethoprim-sulfamethoxazole → ciprofloxacin → amoxiciline-clavulanate → metronidazole or ciprofloxacin → doxycicline → metronidazole).

Other Therapeutic Strategies

Patients presenting symptoms refractory to standard therapy could be treated with periodic gastrointestinal irrigations performed with polyethylene glycol solution, anti-inflammatory drugs, or probiotics. Intestinal irrigations reduce bacterial count by removing microorganisms embedded in mucus. Anti-inflammatory drugs, such as corticosteroid or mesalazine (5-ASA) preparations, may be used for patients presenting persistent unexplained intestinal or colonic inflammation.

Another potential adjunctive therapy for SBBO is probiotic administration. A recent formal definition of probiotic is 'living organisms, which, when ingested in certain numbers, exert health benefits beyond inherent basic nutrition.' In particular, lactobacilli such as *Lactobacillus casei* strain GG, *Lactobacillus plantarum*, and the yeast *Saccharomyces boulardii* have been shown to induce beneficial effects in SBBO. The main mechanisms of probiotic action are: inhibiting adhesion and growth of potentially pathogenic microorganisms; producing antimicrobial substances and nutrients, such as short chain fatty acids, with trophic and/or proabsorptive effects on water and ions intestinal transport; and removing potentially toxic agents from the intestine.

Bibliography

Borriello SP. The normal flora of the gastrointestinal tract. In: Hart AL, Stagg AJ, Graffner H, Glise H, Falk P, Kamm MA (eds.), *Gut Ecology*. London: Martin Dunitz, 2002, p. 3.

Bousvaros A. Intestinal flora. *Int Semin Paediatr Gastroenterol Nutr* 7:1, 1998.

De Boissieu D, Chaussain M, Badaul J, et al. Small-bowel bacterial overgrowth in children with chronic diarrhoea, abdominal pain, or both. *J Pediatr* 24:119, 1996.

Dellert SF, Nowicki MJ, Farrell MK, et al. The ^{13}C-xylose breath test for the diagnosis of small bowel bacterial overgrowth in children. *J Pediatr Gastroenterol Nutr* 25:153, 1997.

Vanderhoof JA, Young RJ, Murray N, et al. Treatment strategies for small bowel bacterial overgrowth in short bowel syndrome. *J Pediatr Gastroenterol Nutr* 27:155, 1998.

21

CROHN'S DISEASE AND INDETERMINATE COLITIS

Ranjana Gokhale

INTRODUCTION

Chronic *inflammatory bowel diseases* (IBD), which include *Crohn's disease* (CD), *ulcerative colitis* (UC), and *indeterminate colitis* (IC), are important causes of chronic *gastrointestinal* (GI) disease in children and adolescents. An increasing incidence of CD has been reported in recent years. The early age of disease onset in some children, variable clinical presentations, therapeutic challenges, as well as the emotional needs of children and their parents can pose a difficult challenge to the gastroenterologist.

The differentiation between CD and UC can be made in most patients based on clinical, endoscopic, radiologic, and pathologic criteria, but in approximately 10% of cases with colitis, the changes are not specific and are categorized as IC.

EPIDEMIOLOGY

Crohn's disease occurs worldwide, but is more prevalent in the Northern Hemisphere. Incidence rates vary from 1.6 to 5.4/100,000 person-years with prevalence rates of 27 to 48/100,000 person-years.[1] Few such epidemiologic studies are available from

the United States. A recent study from Olmsted County, Minnesota examining the years between 1940 and 1993 reported a dramatic increase in the incidence of CD during the 1960s and early 1970s with stabilization of the rate since.[2] The adjusted incidence rate was 5.8/100,000 person-years; however, the prevalence rate increased by 46% since 1980–133/100,000 person-years.

CD usually occurs with a peak incidence during the second decade of life. However, about 25–30% of all patients with IBD develop symptoms during childhood, before 20 years of age, with about 5% being diagnosed before 10 years of age.[3] Younger children often present with small bowel disease and are at increased risk for developing stricturing disease, increasing the risk for morbidity and surgical interventions needed.

ETIOLOGY

Although the exact etiology remains unknown, available evidence suggests that IBD results from immune-mediated bowel injury, triggered by environmental factors in a genetically predisposed individual. The inflammatory response is thought to be a result of an abnormal or a dysregulated mucosal response to normal luminal bacterial flora leading to persistent intestinal inflammation.

Genetic Factors

Genetic factors play a significant role in determining risk of developing CD, especially during childhood. Thirty percent of children diagnosed with IBD before the age of 20 years have a positive family history of IBD, as compared to about 13% in patients diagnosed after the age of 40 years.[4] The increased risk in early onset CD is thought to be from genetic anticipation. In families where multiple members are affected there is concordance seen in most members both for the disease type and for the location of involvement. Genetic influences are also apparent from high concordance rates for CD seen among monozygotic twins (42–58%) with no differences seen in dizygotic twins as compared to other siblings. The frequency of IBD in Ashkenazi Jews is two to four times higher as compared to the general population.

Genetic linkage studies using genome-wide scans have been used in multiplex-affected families for the purpose of identifying chromosomal regions shared in excess of statistical expectations. Studies in kindred from multiplex families with IBD have been successful in identifying an area of linkage on chromosome 16, in kindred with CD.[5] This locus, designated as IBD1, is linked only to CD and not seen in ulcerative colitis. The evidence for linkage at this region is largely accounted for by the association of three amino acid polymorphisms within the NOD2/CARD 15 (caspase activation and recruitment domain) gene. NOD2 is a cytoplasmic protein expressed in peripheral blood monocytes and mediates host resistance to bacterial lipopolysaccharides. Variants within NOD2 seen in CD result in reduced macrophage activation of nuclear factor κB in response to bacterial components.[6] The risk of developing CD in persons carrying one variant NOD2 allele is two- to fourfold, but increases dramatically to 20–40-fold in persons with two variant alleles. Carriage of NOD2 is also associated with earlier onset of disease, ileal location, and stricturing disease.[6] It is important to note that the overall population risk for CD due to NOD2 mutations is about 26%. Other loci have

also been described in smaller studies that contribute to susceptibility for CD. The IBD3 locus on chromosome 6p, which encompasses the major histocompatibility complex, has been associated in both CD and UC, with linkage especially in males.[7] IBD5 locus, described in Canadian families, on chromosome 5q31-q33 has been linked to early onset of CD.[7] This locus also contains genes for various cytokines, including interleukins 3, 4, 5, and 14; colony stimulating factor; and interferon regulatory factor, which may be important in the pathophysiology of CD.

Environmental Factors

No differences have been noted between children with IBD and normal children with regard to frequency of breast-feeding, formula intolerance, prior gastrointestinal illness, or emotional stressors. Smoking, especially in women with CD, is associated with a higher risk of developing severe disease. Increased intestinal permeability is seen not only in patients with CD but also in their asymptomatic first-degree relatives. Appendectomy may also increase risk for developing CD, with more aggressive disease seen in patients with a history of perforated appendix.[8] Mycobacterial infections and perinatal exposure to measles have been implicated, but not proven, in developing CD.

PATHOPHYSIOLOGY

Chronic, recurrent intestinal inflammation occurring in CD is thought to result from mucosal immune system stimulation from the products of commensal bacteria within the lumen. Any process which compromises the integrity of the mucosal barrier, including dietary antigens, environmental triggers, and increased permeability from genetic determinants, allows passage of bacterial antigens for interaction with the mucosal dendritic cells and lymphocytes. In patients with CD, the immune response is characterized by activation of CD4+ lymphocytes with a *type 1 helper T cell* (Th1) phenotype, which produce interferon-γ, interleukin-2, and cell-mediated immunity. Th1 cytokines in turn activate macrophages which secrete several proinflammatory cytokines, including *tumor necrosis factor* (TNF), interleukin-1, and interleukin-6, which trigger a wide nonspecific inflammatory response leading to a self perpetuating cycle of inflammation and tissue destruction.

Histologic findings can help establish the diagnosis of IBD, although the distinction between CD and UC can sometimes be difficult. The characteristic finding in CD, the epithelioid granuloma, can be identified in less than 50% of biopsy specimens and cannot always be relied on. The hallmark of CD is "skip lesions" with areas of normal mucosa seen adjacent to inflammatory areas in a single biopsy. Small superficial ulcerations over a Peyer's patch (aphthoid ulcer), along with inflammatory cells extending to the submucosa can be seen. Crypt architectural distortion may be present even with quiescent disease.

CLINICAL SIGNS AND SYMPTOMS

Intestinal Manifestations

Crohn's disease involves any part of the gastrointestinal tract from the oropharynx to the perianal area, and clinical presentation is dependent on the areas affected with CD. In children, the commonest location of disease is ileocolonic (42%), followed by diffuse small bowel (28%) and isolated colonic or anorectal disease (31%).[9] Younger children are more likely to present with diffuse small bowel disease as compared to colonic disease in older children.[4]

The presentation in CD can sometimes be vague or subtle, often leading to a delay in diagnosis. In patients with ileocolonic involvement, abdominal pain is usually postprandial and may be referred to the periumbilical area or the right lower quadrant. Diarrhea is frequently seen in these patients but may not always be bloody. Examination may localize tenderness to the right lower quadrant and an inflammatory mass, which represents thickening of the mesentery adjacent to the ileocecal region, may occasionally be felt. Gastroduodenal CD presents with early satiety, nausea, emesis, epigastric pain, or dysphagia. Delay in gastric emptying can occur

leading to discomfort following meals and children often limit their caloric intake to diminish their discomfort. Thus, patients with upper gastrointestinal CD may present with anorexia and weight loss rather than diarrhea, which frequently leads to delay in diagnosis. Extensive small bowel disease causes diffuse abdominal pain, anorexia, diarrhea, and weight loss. Lactose malabsorption may occur either secondary to extensive small bowel involvement or primarily due to disaccharidase deficiency. Physical examination reveals diffuse abdominal tenderness. Clubbing of the distal phalanges is rare, but seen most frequently in those children with extensive small bowel disease. Isolated colonic CD may mimic UC, presenting with diarrhea with blood and mucus, associated with crampy lower abdominal pain often relieved by defecation. Perianal disease is common and presents as anal skin tags, deep anal fissures, or fistulae.

Complications result from uncontrolled inflammation or due to the transmural nature of the disease. Extension of the inflammation to the sorosal surface may lead to perforations and intraabdominal abscess formation. Increasing abdominal pain, fevers, tenderness to palpation, or peritoneal signs should prompt urgent evaluation for this complication. Fistulae, either between intestinal loops or to adjacent organs, including urinary bladder, vagina, or skin, can occur especially in patients with ileocolonic disease. Abdominal distention, bilious emesis, and severe abdominal pain may indicate stricturing disease leading to obstruction which is usually managed surgically.

EXTRAINTESTINAL FEATURES

Extraintestinal manifestations (EM) are usually related to disease activity, may precede or develop concurrently with intestinal symptoms, and are common to both UC and CD. About 25–35% of all patients with CD will present with at least one EM.

Fever

Episodes of fever are seen in 40% of patients with CD at the time of presentation. Fevers are usually chronic, low grade, and occasionally associated with night sweats. They, however, may frequently go unrecognized.

Weight Loss/Delayed Growth and Sexual Maturation

Weight loss or a failure to maintain a normal growth velocity in children is the commonest systemic feature of IBD, and is observed more frequently with CD than with UC. It is important to plot serial weights and heights over time in order to appreciate deceleration of growth.

Weight loss occurs from suboptimal enteral intake due to anorexia and abdominal discomfort as well as from increased intestinal losses from diarrhea leading to a protein-losing enteropathy. Malabsorption of nutrients is rare and is seen only in patients with extensive intestinal resections leading to short gut syndrome. Other contributing factors include elevated levels of circulating cytokines, especially TNF-α, which cause anorexia and contribute to weight loss.

Growth failure and delayed sexual maturation may occasionally be the initial presentation of CD in children. Chronic undernutrition is considered the primary etiologic factor contributing to growth failure. There have been no abnormalities noted in growth hormone levels with CD. However, low circulating levels of *insulin-like growth factor* (IGF-1) or somatomedin C levels have been seen in CD, with return to normal levels following nutritional restitution. Patients also have concomitant delay in skeletal maturation, which is evaluated by obtaining a bone-age x-ray of the nondominant hand. Growth delay can also occur as a consequence of chronic *corticosteroid* (CS) use, which is shown to decrease type 1 collagen production that is important for linear growth. Female patients can experience secondary amenorrhea as a result of weight loss.

Arthralgia and Arthritis

Arthralgia and arthritis are the commonest EM seen with CD. They usually coincide with disease activity and improve with medical treatment of underlying intestinal inflammation. Two forms of involvement are seen—a peripheral form and an axial form, including ankylosing spondylitis or sacroileitis. The peripheral form is usually pauciarticular affecting large joints, such as knees, ankles, hips, wrists, and elbows in decreasing order of frequency. Joint deformity is rare, although a destructive granulomatous synovitis has been described in CD.

Less common presentations include *chronic recurrent multifocal osteomyelitis* (CRMO), which is characterized by aseptic inflammation of the long bones and clavicles. CRMO may precede IBD by up to 5 years and improvement is seen following immunosuppressive therapy used to control underlying bowel disease. Hypertrophic osteoarthropathy (digital clubbing, painful swelling of the limbs, arthralgia, and joint effusions) has been described in patients with proximal CD.

Mucocutaneous Lesions

Oral aphthoid ulcers occur commonly with CD (20%). Ulcers usually cause minimal discomfort although they may occasionally cause debilitating pain. They tend to parallel disease activity, and treatment is directed toward underlying disease. Granulomatous tonsillitis has also been described in a child with CD.

Erythema nodosum is characterized by the development of painful, indurated, purplish red, ovoid nodules 1–3 cm in diameter, most commonly seen over extensor surfaces. Erythema nodosum is more common in CD than in UC, but it is nonspecific, as it may also be seen in association with other chronic inflammatory disorders, such as tuberculosis. In CD, it usually occurs in association with active colonic disease; improvement coincides with treatment of the bowel disease. On histologic examination, a vasculitis or panniculitis is seen.

Metastatic cutaneous CD is a rare EM characterized by noncaseating granulomatous infiltration of the skin at anatomically distinct sites from gastrointestinal involvement. Lesions vary and may be in the form of ulcers, nodules, plaques, or papules. The lesions usually resolve with treatment of the underlying CD.

Ophthalmologic Complications

Ocular complications result from IBD itself or chronic CS therapy. Episcleritis is usually related to disease activity and presents with scleral and conjunctival erythema with a burning sensation and photophobia. Local CS drops are usually effective. Iritis and uveitis are associated with the presence of the human leukocyte antigen HLA-B27 and typically run a course independent of the bowel disease. They present with eye pain, headache, and blurred vision or may be asymptomatic. Asymptomatic uveitis has been described in patients with Crohn's colitis. The diagnosis is made by slit lamp examination, which shows cellular or proteinaceous exudates of inflammatory cells in the anterior chamber of the eye. Treatment consists of pupillary dilatation, covering the eye to decrease pain and photophobia, and local or systemic CS.

Corticosteroids (CS) increase the frequency of posterior subcapsular cataracts and increase intraocular pressure. Ophthalmologic evaluation should be performed at six monthly intervals in patients who are on long-term CS.

Hepatobiliary and Pancreatic Disease

Hepatobiliary diseases are more common in UC as compared to CD. *Autoimmune hepatitis* (AIH), *primary sclerosing cholangitis* (PSC), as well as granulomatous hepatitis have been described in CD. The differentiation between AIH and PSC can be made using a liver biopsy and an endoscopic retrograde cholangiopancreatography. Most patients with liver disease may be asymptomatic and liver function abnormalities may be found on routine liver function testing. Liver disease, especially PSC, follows a course independent of IBD.

Cholclithiasis is seen in patients with disease involving terminal ileum or following ileal disease. Increased fecal losses of bile salts causes depletion of the bile salt pool, leading to lithogenic bile with formation of cholesterol stones. Granulomatous cholecystitis and acalculous cholecystitis have also been described.

Pancreatitis occurs with duodenal CD (<1%), and may be from reflux of duodenal contents into the pancreatic duct or from stenosis of the ampulla from CD. Granulomatous inflammation of the pancreas leading to pancreatitis has also been described. Secondary pancreatitis may occur from immune suppressants or other drugs used to treat CD.

Renal Disease

Nephrolithiasis occurs as oxalate calculi in CD. Hypercalciuria from prolonged bed rest or CS therapy, ileostomy, or extensive ileal disease appear to be risk factors. Glomerulonephritis, from immune complex deposition, and primary chronic interstitial nephritis leading to renal failure have both been described with CD.

Obstructive complications may occur due to ureteral compression by inflammatory mass or enterovesicular fistula. Secondary amyloidosis is extremely rare, but has been reported in CD.

Bone

Osteopenia or reduced bone mass can occur both at onset of IBD and as a complication of prolonged CS use. Osteopenia is an important potential complication of pediatric IBD as more than 90% of peak bone mass is attained during childhood and adolescence. Failure to attain peak bone mass increases future fracture potential. Low *bone mineral density* (BMD) was seen in 33% of children with CD and about half of those patients had severely reduced BMD (*z* score >2 SD below mean).[10] Pubertal and postpubertal girls with CD were more likely to have low bone mass than pubertal children. CS use was a predictor of low BMD but other contributing factors remain to be determined.

Aseptic or avascular necrosis is rare, and although associated with CS use, the pathogenesis is unclear. Persistent joint pains, especially involving hip and knees, should prompt consideration of this complication.

DIAGNOSIS

CD is diagnosed based on clinical presentation, hematologic tests, and radiologic and endoscopic

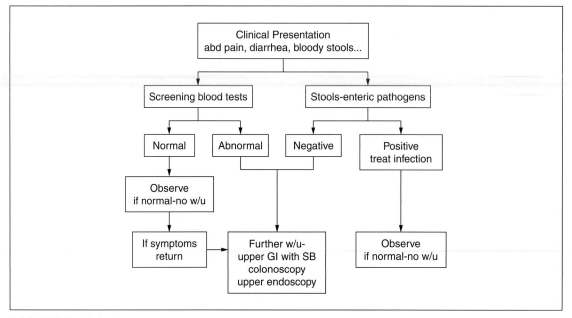

FIGURE 21-1

PARADIGM TO WORK-UP PATIENTS WITH SUSPECTED CROHN'S DISEASE

evaluation (Fig. 21-1). If the presenting symptom is diarrhea (bloody or nonbloody), prior to any further work-up, the presence of enteric infections must be excluded.

Unusual pathogens seen in association with IBD include *Salmonella, Shigella, Campylobacter, Aeromonas, Plesiomonas, Yersinia, Escherichia coli* O157:H7, *Clostridium difficile, Giardia lamblia, Histoplasma,* and *Entamoeba histolytica.* Patients with IBD may have concomitant infections at onset, but their symptoms fail to resolve with treatment of the infectious agent or recur within days to weeks.

Hematologic Tests

Screening tests for CD include a complete blood count, inflammatory markers, and a metabolic profile that includes liver enzymes. An elevated white blood count with increased band forms, microcytic anemia, and thrombocytosis is suggestive of CD (Table 21-1). Acute phase reactants like sedimentation rate and C-reactive protein may be elevated. Hypoalbuminemia and a low serum iron level may be seen. Elevated liver enzymes should prompt an evaluation for associated liver disease.

TABLE 21-1

TESTS TO DIAGNOSE CROHN'S DISEASE

Complete blood counts	Microcytic anemia
	Leucocytosis with band forms
	Thrombocytosis
Acute phase reactants	Elevated sedimentation rate
	C-reactive protein
Chemistries	Low serum iron level, hypoalbuminemia, elevated liver enzymes
Special serologic tests	ASCA titers, pANCA titers
Stool examinations	Occult blood, fecal leucocytes
Endoscopic evaluation	Esophagogastroduodenoscopy with biopsy
	Colonoscopy with biopsy
Radiologic evaluation	Upper GI with small bowel follow-through
	CT scan, MRI
	Barium enema, enteroclysis (rarely used)
	Scintiscan

Newer serologic tests include *anti-Saccharomyces cerevisiae antibodies* (ASCA) and *perinuclear antineutrophilic cytoplasmic antibody* (pANCA). These tests are not used to establish a diagnosis of CD, but may be useful as supportive criteria or in patients with IC to differentiate between UC and CD. ASCA is detected in 44–54% of children with CD, but when present is highly specific (89–97%). pANCA is detected in 14–19% of children with CD, especially in patients with predominantly colonic disease or "UC-like" presentation.[11]

Endoscopic Evaluation

Both upper endoscopy and colonoscopy are usually performed if CD is suspected. Microscopic involvement of the upper GI tract is found in about 20% of patients even in the absence of clear-cut symptoms. On colonoscopy, involvement is typically patchy with relative sparing of the rectum. Findings can vary from mild involvement, which consists of erythema, aphthous ulcerations, loss of vascular markings, increased friability to severe including deep linear or serpiginous ulcerations and cobblestoning. The ileocecal valve may be edematous or ulcerated and the terminal ileum may appear ulcerated and polypoid. Multiple biopsies are usually taken from inflamed and normal-appearing mucosa.

Radiologic Studies

An upper GI with small bowel follow-through is performed to assess involvement of small bowel loops and terminal ileum. Enteroclysis may provide better visualization of the small bowel mucosa but is seldom used in pediatrics due to pain and discomfort from passage of jejunal tube past the ligament of Treitz. Characteristic features of CD are rigid stenotic segments, skip areas, and sinus tracts or fistulae. Barium enemas are beneficial in CD only to delineate stenosis, fistulae, or sinus tracts.

Computerized axial tomography (CT scan) with oral and intravenous contrast is used for the diagnosis of extraintestinal manifestations of CD, including intraabdominal abscesses, fistulae, and

sinuses into surrounding soft tissues. *Magnetic resonance imaging* (MRI) is used mainly for assessment of fistulous perianal CD. Scintiscans, using technetium-HMPAO-labeled white blood cells, are used as adjunctive diagnostic tools in patients with active disease.

TREATMENT

The medical treatment for a child with CD should be individualized based on the degree and site of intestinal involvement, extraintestinal manifestations, and nutritional status (Table 21-2).

Corticosteroids

Corticosteroids are used for their anti-inflammatory effects and are effective in inducing remission

TABLE 21-2

MEDICATION DOSAGES IN PEDIATRIC CROHN'S DISEASE

Agent	Dosage
Corticosteroids	1.0–2.0 mg/kg per day prednisone equivalent IV or PO in divided doses (max 40–60 mg)
Budesonide	9 mg starting dose, 6 mg maintenance dose
Sulfasalazine	25–75 mg/kg per day (max 4 g)
Mesalamine	30–60 mg/kg per day (max 4.8 g per day)
Metronidazole	10–20 mg/kg per day
Azathioprine	1–2 mg/kg per day Adjust dose with 6-MP metabolite levels
6-Mercaptopurine	1–1.5 mg/kg per day Adjust dose with 6-MP metabolite levels
Methotrexate	15 mg/m^2 per week (max 25 mg)
Thalidomide	1–2 mg/kg per day single bedtime dose
Infliximab	5 mg/kg intravenous infusion

in about 80% of patients. CS can be used orally in children with mild-to-moderate disease activity but are used *intravenously* (IV) in children with severe disease who require hospitalization. Control of symptoms, fever, severe abdominal pain, and diarrhea, can be usually achieved within 7–10 days. Once clinical remission is achieved, CS can be used orally in the form of prednisone and the dose can be tapered to prevent long-term complications from CS use. Occasionally low dose CS ($\leq$5 mg per day) or alternate, days therapy may be effective in reducing disease activity and may not cause growth suppression, but CS should not be used for "maintenance therapy." Many patients may have a relapse of their symptoms when the dose is lowered below a threshold level and in these patients additional medications are usually used.

Budesonide, a CS with topical anti-inflammatory effects and low systemic side effects due to rapid first-pass metabolism in the liver, is now available for use in patients with ileocecal CD. However, in a recent pediatric study, although the response rate was 59% at 8 weeks, the remission rate at 8 weeks was about 30% with subnormal linear growth seen in patients who received the drug for 1 year.[12]

Sulfasalazine and Mesalamine

Sulfasalazine (SASP) is useful for colonic disease. SASP can be prepared as a liquid and is useful in children with colonic CD. The high incidence of side effects, especially to the sulfa component, limits the use of the drug. Some of the newer mesalamine preparations [active component *5-aminosalicylic acid* (5-ASA), Asacol and Pentasa, are formulated for release at a higher pH and may be useful for disease affecting the small bowel (jejunum, ileum)]. However, 5-ASA preparations are not commercially available as a liquid formulation and hence cannot be administered to a young child. Side effects are more common with SASP as compared to mesalamine and include headaches, nausea, abdominal pain, diarrhea, and hypersensitivity reactions (skin eruptions, hemolytic anemia). The long-term efficacy of SASP/mesalamine medications in maintaining remission of CD is unclear.

Antibiotics: Metronidazole and Ciprofloxacil

Metronidazole has been useful in the treatment of perianal disease, which may be seen in up to 40% of children. Long-term use may also be beneficial for closure of perineal fistulae. Side effects seen include nausea, metallic taste, furry tongue, and (rarely) sensory neuropathy, which resolves completely or improves after discontinuation of the drug. Ciprofloxacil has similar efficacy as metronidazole and can be used in patients who are intolerant of metronidazole.

Immunosuppressive Therapy

6-Mercaptopurine and Azathioprine

6-Mercaptopurine (6-MP) and *azathioprine* (AZT) are used in children with steroid-dependent or refractory CD, extensive small bowel disease or upper gastrointestinal CD, history of previous resections, and perianal and fistulous disease. 6-MP has also been used as initial therapy for moderate-to-severe CD.[13] In this study, use of 6-MP was found to lower the duration and cumulative dose of CS used, and remission was induced in 89% of children. Further relapse was seen in only 9% of patients on 6-MP as compared to 47% of controls. The long-term efficacy and safety of 6-MP/AZT use has been established in children on these drugs for up to 10 years with about 80% tolerating the drug with no side effects.[14] Patients need to be carefully monitored with routine blood monitoring for leucopenia and elevated transaminases, which are common and dose-dependent. 6-MP/AZT is discontinued in patients who develop hypersensitivity reactions (pancreatitis, high fever). Monitoring of 6-MP levels in blood may be useful to guide dosing and prevent toxicity.

Methotrexate

Methotrexate (MTX) is useful in maintaining long-term remission in both adults and children with CD. MTX is used in patients who are intolerant to 6-MP and in patients with significant joint disease. However, compliance limits its use as MTX has been found to be useful only if given subcutaneously, with poor efficacy if used orally. Patients on long-term MTX need careful monitoring of liver functions as hepatic fibrosis has been described with cumulative doses.

Cyclosporine and Tacrolimus

Cyclosporine (CSA) and tacrolimus are not found to be as useful in patients with CD, except in the management of fistulae. A recent study showed tacrolimus to be effective in improving fistulae in 43% patients, but only 10% achieved fistula remission.[15] Limited experience with tacrolimus is available in the treatment of CD in children.

Infliximab

Increased production of inflammatory cytokines, especially TNF-α, has been described both in histologically normal and in the inflamed mucosa in CD. Infliximab infusions have since been successfully used to maintain remission as well for the treatment of fistulas in patients with CD. Pediatric use of infliximab, initially strictly limited to severe disease, refractory to conventional therapies, and particularly to fistulizing forms, is now progressively being extended to other indications. Efficacy has been proven in short-term studies with clinical remission in 10 out of 15 patients at 10 weeks.[16] Complications are usually related to transfusion reactions on repeated administration of the drug, serum-sickness like delayed reaction, and infectious complications. Long-term safety data with regard to secondary lymphoma have not been described in children.

Thalidomide

Originally used for its sedative and antiemetic properties thalidomide has recently been shown to inhibit production of TNF-α, interleukin-12, and other proinflammatory cytokines. Thalidomide was shown to be efficacious in adults and in one pediatric study with chronically active, steroid-dependent CD and in patients with severe aphthous ulcerations from CD. Side effects were mild and dose-dependent,

with the most common being drowsiness, peripheral neuropathy, edema, and dermatitis.

NUTRITIONAL RESTITUTION

Nutritional deficiencies due to suboptimal caloric intakes, malabsorption, or increased losses are common in children and may cause devastating effects on growth and sexual maturation. Providing adequate calories is important to reverse growth failure but the child may not be able to take adequate calories orally due to his underlying disease. Semielemental or elemental formulae are used to optimize calories but compliance may be limited due to their unpleasant taste. *Nasogastric* (NG) infusions at night are useful but children are unable or unwilling to pass a NG tube daily. Polymeric formulae may be equally efficacious and better compliance is achieved, and are commonly used in our practice.

It should be mentioned here that the use of enteral nutrition, either with semielemental diets or with whole protein, has been found useful in children and teenagers with Crohn's disease localized in the small intestine, not only as a means of providing nutritional supplementation but also in reducing the activity of the disease. This form of treatment has indeed been found as effective as CS in inducing remission[17] and is widely used in Europe, but failed to find widespread support in the United States.

Mineral and iron deficiencies are also commonly seen in children with CD. All patients with IBD should be recommended a daily complete multivitamin with calcium supplementation, if their milk intake is suboptimal. Iron supplements are given if indicated. Restriction of dairy products, which provide an excellent source of protein, calcium, and calories, is not recommended unless the child is lactose intolerant.

SHORT- AND LONG-TERM PROGNOSIS

The course of CD can be variable, with disease activity remaining high in some patients, in spite of aggressive medical treatment. A long-term pediatric study in children with CD showed that about a third of children continue to have mild gastrointestinal symptoms while the remaining two-thirds will vary between severe exacerbations and remissions. About 17% patients have severe unremitting disease despite medical interventions.[18] Surgery is reserved for patients with medical intractability, suspected perforation or abscess, intestinal obstruction or hemorrhage, and growth failure, particularly if there is a localized area of resectable disease. However, there is a high incidence of recurrence after surgery with a 50–80% relapse within 3 years of surgery. Children with extensive CD, especially colitis, have an increased risk of colorectal cancer (relative risk 18-fold), if their CD was diagnosed before 25 years of age.[19]

References

1   Bernstein CN, Blanchard JF. Epidemiology of inflammatory bowel disease. In: Cohen RD (ed.), *Inflammatory Bowel Disease: Diagnosis and Therapeutics*. Totowa, NJ: Humana Press, 2003.

2   Loftus EV, Silverstein MD, Sandborn WJ, et al. Crohn's disease in Olmstead County, Minnesota, 1940-1993: incidence, prevalence, and survival. *Gastroenterology* 114:1161– 1168, 1998.

3   Baldassano RN, Piccoli DA. Inflammatory bowel disease in pediatric and adolescent patients. *Gastroenterol Clin North Am* 28:445–458, 1999.

4   Polito JM, Childs B, Mellits ED, et al. Crohn's disease: influence of age at diagnosis on site and clinical type of disease. *Gastroenterology* 111:580–586, 1996.

5   Hugot JP, Laurent-Puig P, Gower-Rousseau C, et al. Mapping of a susceptibility locus for Crohn's disease on chromosome 16. *Nature* 379:821–823, 1996.

6   Bonen DK, Cho JH. The genetics of inflammatory bowel disease. *Gastroenterology* 124:521–536, 2003.

7   Rioux JD, Silverberg MS, Daly MJ, et al. Genomewide search in Canadian families with inflammatory bowel disease reveals two novel susceptibility loci. *Am J Hum Genet* 66:1863–1870, 2000.

8   Andersson RE, Olaison G, Tysk C, et al. Appendectomy is followed by increased risk of Crohn's disease. *Gastroenterology* 124:40–46, 2003.

9   Farmer RG, Whelan G, Fazio VW. Long-term follow-up of patients with Crohn's disease. Relationship between the clinical pattern and prognosis. *Gastroenterology* 88:1818–1825, 1985.

10 Gokhale R, Favus MJ, Karrison T, et al. Bone mineral density assessment in children with inflammatory bowel disease. *Gastroenterology*. 114:902–911, 1998.

11 Ruemmele FM, Targan SR, Levy G, et al. Diagnostic accuracy of serological assays in pediatric inflammatory bowel disease. *Gastroenterology* 115:822–829, 1998.

12 Kundhal P, Zachos M, Holmes JL, et al. Controlled ileal release budesonide in pediatric Crohn disease: efficacy and effect on growth. *J Pediatr Gastroenterol Nutr* 33:75–80, 2003.

13 Markowitz J, Grancher K, Kohn N, et al. A multicenter trial of 6-mercaptopurine and prednisone in children with newly diagnosed Crohn's disease. *Gastroenterology* 119:895–902, 2000.

14 Kirschner BS. Safety of azathioprine and 6-mercaptopurine in pediatric patients with inflammatory bowel disease. *Gastroenterology* 115:813–821, 1998.

15 Sandborn WJ, Present DH, Isaacs KL, et al. Tacrolimus for the treatment of fistulas in patients with Crohn's disease: a randomized, placebo-controlled trial. *Gastroenterology* 125:380–388, 2003.

16 Hyams JS. Use of infliximab in the treatment of Crohn's disease in children and adolescents. *J Pediatr Gastroenterol Nutr* S33:36–39, 2001.

17 Zachos M, Tondeur M, Griffiths AM. Enteral nutritional therapy for the induction of remission in Crohn's disease. *Cochrane Database Syst Rev* (3): CD000542.

18 Griffiths AM, Nyugen P, Smith C, et al. Growth and clinical course in children with Crohn's disease. *Gut* 34:939–943, 1993.

19 Gillen CE, Walmsley RS, Prior P, et al. Ulcerative colitis and Crohn's disease: a comparison of the colorectal cancer risk in extensive colitis. *Gut* 35: 1590–1592, 1994.

CHAPTER

22

ULCERATIVE COLITIS

Ranjana Gokhale

INTRODUCTION

Ulcerative colitis (UC) is a chronic inflammatory disease involving the colon, and is an important cause of chronic gastrointestinal disease in children and adolescents. The disease can present at an early age with varying severity posing a therapeutic challenge to the gastroenterologist.

EPIDEMIOLOGY

Ulcerative colitis occurs throughout the world, but like *Crohn's disease* (CD) is commoner in the Western Hemisphere. Most of the available epidemiologic data comes from Northern Europe, where incidence rates vary between 6.3 and 15.1/100,000 person-years and prevalence rates vary between 58 and 157/100,000 person-years.[1] The trend is similar within the United States where UC is more prevalent in the northern as compared to the southern United States. In contrast to the increasing incidence of CD, the incidence of UC has remained stable throughout the 80s and 90s. Within the United States, in reports from Olmsted County, Minnesota, incidence rates of 15/100,000 person-years remained unchanged from 1960 to 1993, with prevalence rates of 225/100,000 person-years from 1960 to 1979 increasing slightly to 229/100,000 person-years from 1980 to 1993.[2]

UC is seen with a bimodal distribution, with peaks during the second through the third decade of life, and a second peak in the sixth through the seventh decade of life. The disease is also seen during childhood, about 25–30% of all presenting cases before age 20, with about 5% of cases occurring before age 10.[3] As in the adult population, the incidence of UC in children has remained stable through the last three decades, except for an annual 8% increase from 1993 through 1995 in Swedish children at age 15 years or less.[4]

ETIOLOGY

The etiology of UC is unknown, but is thought to result from immune-mediated bowel injury, which may be triggered by environmental factors in a genetically susceptible host, leading to chronic inflammation. In contrast to Crohn's disease, bacterial antigens are thought to play a limited role in the development of UC.

Genetic Factors

Although genetic factors play an important role, UC is thought to be "less genetic" than CD. First-degree relatives of a patient affected with *inflammatory bowel diseases* (IBD) have an increased risk of IBD that is 4–20 times higher than the background population.[5] The risk is higher with childhood IBD; 30% of children diagnosed with IBD before the age of 20 years have a positive family history of IBD, as compared to about 13% in patients diagnosed after the age of 40 years.[6] Concordance rates for UC among monozygotic twins are lower at 6–17% as compared to CD, with no differences seen in dizygotic twins as compared to other siblings. The frequency of IBD in Ashkenazi Jews is two to four times higher as compared to the general population.

Significant linkage has been shown between HLA class II and UC. A metaanalysis of 29 studies showed significant positive associations in UC to DR2, DR9, and DRB3*0301, with a negative association for DR4.[7] HLA class I and II genes have also been associated with disease location and *extraintestinal manifestations* (EM), such as the increased incidence of HLA-B27 with *ankylosing spondylitis* (AS). Patients with the variant HLA DR3*0301 are more likely to have extensive, severe colitis with increased risk of surgery. Smaller studies have shown greater linkage in UC as compared to CD, for the IBD2 locus on chromosome 12.[8] The IBD3 locus on chromosome 6p, which also encompasses the major histocompatibility complex, has been linked to both UC and CD especially in males.[9]

Environmental Factors

No differences have been noted between children with IBD and normal children with regard to frequency of breast-feeding, formula intolerance, prior gastrointestinal illness, or emotional stressors. Early appendectomy, prior to the age of 20 years, is associated with a decreased risk of UC.[10] Smoking decreases the risk of UC with disease flares seen in patients who discontinue smoking, the effect is due to the modulatory effect of nicotine on colonic mucous.

PATHOPHYSIOLOGY

As with CD, the chronic inflammation in UC is thought to result from an inappropriate immune response of the host to luminal bacterial antigens, with dietary and environmental factors serving as possible triggers. The mucosal response in UC is dominated by CD4+ lymphocytes with an atypical *type 2 helper T cell* (Th2) phenotype, which produces interleukin-4, IL-5, IL-6, IL-10, and transforming growth factor-β, and mediates humoral immunity. Elaboration of proinflammatory cytokines leads to activation of macrophages and recruitment of polymorphonuclear cells leading to an inflammatory response that causes tissue destruction.

Two autoantibodies appear to be more specific to UC and may play a role in the pathogenesis of the disease. *Perinuclear antineutrophilic cytoplasmic antibodies* (pANCA) are present in about 80% of patients with UC and are also seen in healthy relatives of patients with UC. Increased prevalence of pANCA has been associated with aggressive UC and pouchitis. Antibodies to tropomyosin, a cytoskeletal protein, have been isolated from colons of patients with UC; however, their relevance is still unclear.[11]

UC is a condition in which the inflammatory response and morphologic changes remain confined to the colon. The characteristic histologic findings are acute and chronic inflammation of the mucosa by polymorphonuclear leukocytes and mononuclear cells, crypt abscesses, distortion of the mucosal glands, and goblet-cell depletion. The degree of crypt architectural distortion and mucosal atrophy tends to be greater in UC as compared to CD.

CLINICAL SIGNS AND SYMPTOMS

Ulcerative colitis always affects the rectum and extends proximally in a symmetric fashion involving variable lengths of the colon. Involvement could be limited to the rectum (proctitis), extended to the distal colon (up to the splenic flexure or left-sided colitis), or to the entire colon (pancolitis). Children tend to have a higher likelihood of pancolitis at presentation and may also have proximal extension of disease over time.

Intestinal Manifestations

Ulcerative colitis is usually diagnosed earlier after the onset of symptoms than CD, as rectal involvement leads to the presence of gross blood in the stools alerting parents and physicians to a gastrointestinal problem. The most consistent feature of UC is the presence of blood and mucus mixed with stool, accompanied with lower abdominal cramping which is most intense during the passage of bowel movements. Patients may also experience tenesmus, which is a sensation of needing to evacuate stool. The location of abdominal pain depends on the extent of colonic involvement. Pain is in the left lower quadrant with distal disease and extends to the entire abdomen with pancolitis. Systemic symptoms including fever, anorexia leading to weight loss, and anemia which may occur with fulminant colitis.

The most feared intestinal complication of UC is *toxic megacolon*. This is heralded by increasing abdominal distention, guarding, and rebound tenderness to palpation with decrease in bowel sounds. Narcotics used for pain management and electrolyte imbalances, especially hypokalemia, increase risk of developing toxic megacolon. Management of this severe, acute complication is usually conservative, based on careful monitoring of the colon distention by x-ray films, repeated every 12 h, and supportive therapy with broad-spectrum antibiotics, steroids, IV fluids. Worsening of dilatation or of general status may require urgent surgical intervention.

Extraintestinal Manifestations

Extraintestinal manifestations are commonly seen with both UC and CD. They are usually related to disease activity and may precede or develop concurrently with intestinal symptoms.

Fever

Fevers are seen in 40% of patients with IBD at the time of presentation. Fevers are usually chronic, low grade, and hence may frequently be unrecognized.

Weight Loss/Delayed Growth and Sexual Maturation

Weight loss or a deceleration of growth velocity can be seen with UC although is much less common as compared to CD. It is important to obtain previous heights and weights for comparison to appreciate a fall from previous growth percentiles. Weight loss results from a suboptimal enteral intake due to anorexia, abdominal pain, and increased diarrheal losses.

Growth delay can occur from chronic undernutrition, but more often is a consequence of chronic *corticosteroid* (CS) use. No abnormalities have been demonstrated in growth hormone levels, but undernutrition can cause low circulating levels of *insulin-like growth factor* (IGF-1) or somatomedin C, which are important for linear growth. IGF-1 levels return to normal on nutritional restitution. Chronic CS therapy leads to slowing of linear growth due to decrease in type 1 collagen.

Delayed sexual maturation can occur in boys and girls and some girls may experience secondary amenorrhea from weight loss.

Arthralgia and Arthritis

Arthralgia and arthritis occur frequently and may occasionally precede intestinal manifestations of IBD. They usually parallel disease activity and improve with medical treatment of underlying intestinal inflammation. Arthralgia is usually pauciarticular affecting large joints, such as knees, ankles, hips, wrists, and elbows in decreasing order of frequency. Joint deformities are usually not seen.

Ankylosing spondylitis is more common with UC and is associated with HLA-B27 in 50–80% of cases. Progression is variable and does not appear to correlate with severity of bowel symptoms. Colectomy does not affect the course of AS. Sacroilitis is usually aymptomatic and may be detected on bone scans.

Chronic recurrent multifocal osteomyelitis (aseptic inflammation of the long bones and clavicles) and hypertrophic osteoarthropathy (digital clubbing, painful swelling of limbs, arthralgia, and joint effusions) are uncommon but have been described. Both these conditions are managed by treating the underlying colitis.

Mucocutaneous Lesions

Oral aphthoid ulcers occur less commonly with UC (5%). Ulcers usually cause minimal discomfort although they may occasionally cause debilitating pain. They tend to parallel disease activity, and treatment is directed toward underlying disease.

Pyostomatitis vegetans is rare and characterized by inflammatory vegetations on labial, buccal, and palatal mucosa.[11] Topical corticosteroids may be helpful in treating these lesions in addition to controlling colonic inflammation.

Pyoderma gangrenosum (PG) is a deep, severe ulceration of the skin, and is an unusual manifestation usually seen in association with UC (<1%). Lesions can be multiple in numbers and are typically located below the knee. Biopsy of the lesion shows neutrophilic infiltration with abscess surrounded by a lymphocytic vasculitis. PG usually parallels active colonic disease but on occasion may be refractory to treatment and may require intensive local therapy, corticosteroids, minocycline, dapsone, clofazimine, or tacrolimus (FK-506).

Erythema nodosum is characterized by the development of painful, indurated, purplish red, ovoid nodules 1–3 cm in diameter, most commonly seen over extensor surfaces. Erythema nodosum is less common in UC, improvement coincides with treatment of the bowel disease.

Ophthalmologic Complications

Iritis and uveitis are associated with the presence of the human leukocyte antigen HLA-B27 and typically run a course independent of the bowel disease. They present with eye pain, headache, and blurred vision or may be asymptomatic and detected by slit lamp examination. Treatment consists of pupillary dilatation, covering the eye to decrease pain and photophobia and local or systemic CS. Episcleritis usually is related to disease activity and presents with scleral and conjunctival erythema with a burning sensation and photophobia. Local CS drops are usually effective.

Chronic corticosteroid use is associated with increased frequency of posterior subcapsular cataracts and increased intraocular pressure, hence children on long-term steroids should undergo an ophthalmologic evaluation at six monthly intervals.

Hepatobiliary Disease

Primary sclerosing cholangitis (PSC) is usually seen in association with UC. PSC may be asymptomatic and is detected because of elevated alkaline phosphatase and γ-glutamyltransferase during routine blood screening. Patients may occasionally present with pruritis and PSC prior to the development of UC. The course of PSC appears to be unrelated to underlying bowel disease and may progress even after a colectomy. PSC is diagnosed either by liver biopsy or an *endoscopic retrograde cholangiopancreatogram* (ERCP) showing characteristic bile duct changes. Peripheral antineutrophilic cytoplasmic antibodies are positive in most patients with PSC and may be a marker for genetic susceptibility for this disease.

Autoimmune hepatitis (AIH) is also seen in association with UC. Diagnosis is made following a liver biopsy, which shows lobular inflammation with piecemeal necrosis. Treatment includes CS and immunosuppressive medications. As with PSC the course of AIH can be independent of UC.

Renal Disease

Nephrolithiasis occurs predominantly as uric acid calculi in UC, although the exact mechanism for development of calculi has not been elucidated. Hypercalciuria from prolonged bed rest or CS therapy appear to be risk factors. Immune complex glomerulonephritis has also been described in UC, can be progressive, and is unrelated to disease duration and severity.

Bone

Osteopenia is an important potential complication of pediatric IBD as more than 90% of peak bone mass is attained during childhood and adolescence. Failure to attain peak bone mass increases future fracture potential. Osteopenia is not as common in UC as CD but can be seen in up to 10% of patients, especially with disease in the prepubertal age group.[12] CS use is a predictor of low *bone mineral density* (BMD), but other contributing factors remain to be determined.

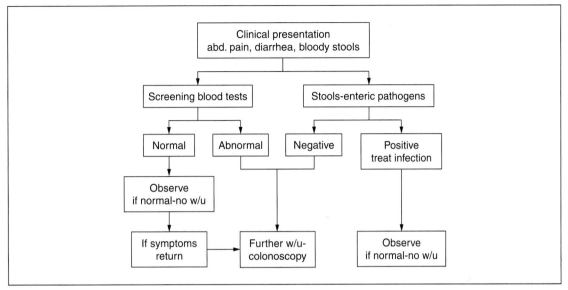

FIGURE 22-1

WORK-UP ALGORITHM FOR PATIENTS WITH SUSPECTED ULCERATIVE COLITIS

DIAGNOSIS

The diagnosis of UC is based on clinical presentation, hematologic screening tests, radiologic examination, endoscopic appearance, and histologic findings (Fig. 22-1).

The importance of excluding enteric pathogens before confirming the diagnosis of UC cannot be overemphasized. The presence of unusual infections like *Salmonella, Shigella, Campylobacter, Aeromonas, Plesiomonas, Yersinia, Eschericha coli O157:H7, Clostridium difficile, Giardia lamblia, Histoplasma,* and *Entamoeba histolytica* must raise the suspicion of an underlying colitis. Associated infections may be the presenting symptom of UC or may lead to flare of preexisting colitis.

Hematologic Tests

Screening tests for UC include a complete blood count, inflammatory markers, and a metabolic profile that includes liver enzymes (Table 22-1). An elevated white blood count with increased band forms, microcytic anemia, and thrombocytosis is

suggestive of UC. However, it must be remembered that the children with UC in contrast to CD are more likely to present with normal laboratory evaluations. Acute-phase reactants like sedimentation

TABLE 22-1

TESTS USED TO DIAGNOSE ULCERATIVE COLITIS

Complete blood counts	Microcytic anemia
	Leucocytosis with band forms
	Thrombocytosis
Acute phase reactants	Elevated sedimentation rate
	C-reactive protein
Chemistries	Low serum iron level, hypoalbuminemia, elevated liver enzymes (GGTP)
Special serologic tests	pANCA titers
Stool examinations	Occult blood, fecal leucocytes
Endoscopic evaluation	Colonoscopy with biopsy
Radiologic evaluation	Plain x-ray (suspected megacolon)

rate and C-reactive protein may be elevated. Hypoalbuminemia may result from a protein-losing enteropathy due to chronic diarrhea. Elevated liver enzymes, especially an increased GGTP should prompt an evaluation for associated liver disease.

The perinuclear antineutrophilic cytoplasmic antibody is detected in 66–83% of children with UC.[13] pANCA titers are also associated with chronic pouchitis.

Endoscopic Evaluation

Changes seen on colonoscopy are always more severe distally and extend in a continuous fashion proximally to varying levels. Changes may be mild, ranging from erythema, loss of vascular markings, and increased friability, to severe with ulcerations or inflammatory pseudopolyps.

Radiologic Studies

Barium enemas are not used anymore to diagnose UC, and in fact should not be used with moderate or severe colitis to avoid inducing toxic megacolon. Plain radiographs may be useful for suspected toxic megacolon or in excluding spontaneous perforations.

DIFFERENTIAL DIAGNOSIS

Exclusion of infectious etiologies as a reason for bloody diarrhea is of paramount importance. Acute infectious colitis is usually abrupt in presentation in a previously healthy child. Organisms that can mimic UC include *Salmonella*, *Shigella*, *E. coli* O157:H7, and *Campylobacter*. *E. histolytica* infections are acquired if there is a history of travel to endemic areas. Diagnosis is made by obtaining stool for cultures, ova, and parasites. *C. difficile* infections may occur following frequent antibiotic use or may be acquired nosocomially. Stools should be tested for toxin A and B, or pseudomembranes may be seen on sigmoidoscopy. Severe and usually painless bleeding can occur with a Meckel's diverticulum. Polyps, usually juvenile benign polyps,

present with rectal bleeding but diarrhea is not a feature of the latter two conditions.

Other unusual causes may be apparent based on the clinical setting, radiation enteritis, mucositis, or typhlitis following chemotherapy and radiation for childhood cancers, or rarely *graft versus host disease* (GVHD) may present with bloody diarrhea.

TREATMENT

Mild Disease

Oral sulfasalazine (SASP) alone or in combination with topical medications, is usually effective in the treatment of mild colitis (Table 22-2). SASP can be made into a solution and is especially useful to

TABLE 22-2

MEDICATION DOSAGES IN PEDIATRIC ULCERATIVE COLITIS

Agent	Dosage
Corticosteroids	1.0–2.0 mg/kg per day prednisone equivalent IV or PO in divided doses (max 40–60 mg)
Sulfasalazine	25–75 mg/kg per day (max 4 g)
Mesalamine	30–60 mg/kg per day (max 4.8 g per day)
Azathioprine	1–2 mg/kg per day Adjust dose based on 6-MP metabolite levels
6-Mercaptopurine	1–1.5 mg/kg per day Adjust dose based on 6-MP metabolite levels
Cyclosporine	4–8 mg/kg per day IV or PO Trough blood levels 200–250 µg/mL
Tacrolimus	0.15 mg/kg per day PO Trough blood levels 10–15 µg/mL
Infliximab	5 mg/kg intravenous infusion

treat younger children who are unable to swallow pills. Folic acid supplementation should be given to patients on SASP. SASP use is limited by side effects, mainly to the sulfa component, which include headaches, nausea, abdominal pain, diarrhea, and hypersensitivity reactions (skin eruptions, hemolytic anemia). Newer *5-aminosalicylic acid* (5-ASA) medicines: mesalamine, olsalazine, and balsalazide are useful in patients unable to tolerate SASP. Side effects seen with mesalamine are similar to SASP but are less common. Topical preparations are useful for patients with limited proctitis or left-sided colitis. Mesalamine enemas and suppositories, corticosteroid foam, and enemas are very useful, but compliance in the pediatric population is somewhat limited.

Moderate-to-Severe Disease

Children presenting with significant abdominal cramping, frequent bloody diarrhea, abdominal tenderness on palpation, anemia, and hypoalbuminemia need to be hospitalized for close clinical observation. *Intravenous* (IV) steroids are initiated, along with bowel rest, which consists of no oral intake or a clear liquid intake.

Hyperalimentation may be required if the child has had significant weight loss or has suboptimal intake due to colitis. Oral medications are held when oral intake is limited to avoid gastrointestinal distress. Most children respond by 7–10 days and can then be given prednisone at equivalent doses as outpatients. Response is judged by resolution of abdominal pain, and bloody diarrhea as well as improvement in acute inflammatory markers and stabilization of hemoglobin.

Once clinical improvement occurs, SASP/mesalamine can be introduced and attempts to wean the prednisone dose should be initiated to prevent long-term complications from chronic CS use.

Budesonide, a newer CS, undergoes rapid first-pass metabolism in liver and hence has limited systemic effects, has not yet been proven to be effective in the treatment of UC. Budesonide enemas have recently been used safely and effectively in patients with limited proctitis and distal UC.[14]

IMMUNOSUPPRESSIVE THERAPY

Azathioprine and 6-Mercaptopurine

Azathioprine (AZT) and *6-mercaptopurine* (6MP) are used increasingly at the onset of moderate-to-severe disease to prevent relapses as well as for their steroid-sparing effects. They are effective in suppressing disease activity in approximately 70% of steroid-dependent or refractory children. However, they require about 4–6 weeks for their beneficial effects and are thus not useful in acute episodes of severe colitis. Patients need careful monitoring for side effects, which include leucopenia and elevated transaminases, which are dose-dependent and resolve when the dose is lowered. Rarely, hypersensitivity reactions, pancreatitis, or skin rashes may occur which preclude further use of these agents.

Cyclosporine and Tacrolimus

Cyclosporine (CSA) is useful in children with acute steroid-refractory UC, when surgery seems inevitable. Clinical improvement occurs in 7–10 days in 60–70% of children who enter remission, but long-term remission (more than 6 months) is seen in less than half of those who respond, ultimately leading to colectomy. Concomitant administration of AZT or 6-MP, once the child is in remission, may facilitate weaning of CSA. Long-term use of CSA leads to undesirable cosmetic side effects, gingival hypertrophy and hypertrichosis, which limit use especially in female patients. Tacrolimus is as effective as CSA without the undesirable cosmetic side effects and may be preferred. Other side effects for both of these are similar and include increased risk of infections, hypertension, nephrotoxicity, seizures, insulin-dependent diabetes mellitus, and benign tumors. Long-term safety with regard to risk of *Epstein-Barr virus* (EBV)-induced lymphoproliferative disease remains to be seen.

Infliximab

Tumor necrosis factor-α is a potent proinflammatory cytokine found in serum and inflamed tissue in

IBD, and is involved in the pathogenesis of the disease. Infliximab, an antitumor necrosis-factor antibody, has been useful in the treatment of refractory CD. Its use in UC has been less well described. However, a recent pediatric study in nine patients showed decreased activity in seven of nine patients and CS could be discontinued in six of nine patients.[15] The long-term effects of infliximab on UC are not known.

SHORT- AND LONG-TERM PROGNOSIS

Among patients with severe UC, approximately 25–40% will eventually require colectomy. It is generally accepted that patients with extensive colitis require surveillance colonoscopy to detect dysplasia approximately 8 years after diagnosis. After initiating surveillance colonoscopy repeat examinations should follow every 1–2 years. The risk of developing colon cancer in Swedish patients diagnosed before 15 years of age was 1% after 15 years, 6.5% after 20 years, and 15% after 25 years.[16]

References

1 Bernstein CN, Blanchard JF. Epidemiology of inflammatory bowel disease. In: Cohen RD (ed.), *Inflammatory Bowel Disease: Diagnosis and Therapeutics*. Totowa, NJ: Humana Press, 2003.

2 Loftus EV, Silverstein MD, Sandborn WJ, Tremaine WJ, Harmsen WS, Zinsmeister AR. Ulcerative colitis in Olmsted County, Minnesota 1940-1993; incidence, prevalence and survival. *Gut* 46:336–343, 2000.

3 Baldassano RN, Piccoli DA. Inflammatory bowel disease in pediatric and adolescent patients. *Gastroenterol Clin North Am* 28:445–458, 1999.

4 Lindberg E, Lindquist B, Holmquist L, Hildebrand H. Inflammatory bowel disease in children and adolescents in Sweden, 1984-1995. *J Pediatr Gastroenterol Nutr* 30:259–264, 2000.

5 Orholm M, Munkholm P, Langholz E, Nielsen OH, Sorensen TIA, Binder V. Familial occurrence of inflammatory bowel disease. *N Engl J Med* 324: 84–88, 1991.

6 Baldassano RN, Piccoli DA. Inflammatory bowel disease in pediatric and adolescent patients. *Gastroenterol Clin North Am* 28:445–458, 1999.

7 Stokkers PC, Reitsma PH, Tytgat GN, van Deventer SJ. HLA-DR and DQ phenotypes in inflammatory bowel disease: a meta-analysis. *Gut* 5:395–401, 1999.

8 Satsangi J, Parkes M, Louis E, Hashimoto L, Kato N, Welsh K, Terwilliger JD, Lathrop Gm, Bell JI, Jewell DP. Two stage genome-wide search in inflammatory bowel disease provides susceptibility loci on chromosomes 3, 7, and 12. *Nat Genet* 14:199–202, 1996.

9 Rioux JD, Silverberg MS, Daly MJ, Steinhart AH, McLeod RS, Griffiths AM, Green T, Brettin TS, Stone V, Bull SB, Britton A, Williams CN, Greenberg GR, Cohen Z, Lander ES, Hudson TJ, Siminovitch KA. Genomewide search in Canadian families with inflammatory bowel disease reveals two novel susceptibility loci. *Am J Hum Genet* 66:1863–1870, 2000.

10 Das KM, Dasgupta A, Mandal A, Geng X. Autoimmunity to cytoskeletal protein tropomyosin. A clue to the pathogenetic mechanism for ulcerative colitis. *J Immunol* 150(6):2487–2493, 1993.

11 Chan SWY, Scully C, Prime SS, Eveson J. Pyostomatitis vegetans: oral manifestation of ulcerative colitis. *Oral Surg Oral Med Oral Pathol* 72:689–692, 1991.

12 Gokhale R, Favus MJ, Karrison T, Sutton MS, Rich B, Kirschner BS. Bone mineral density assessment in children with inflammatory bowel disease. *Gastroenterology* 114:902–911, 1998.

13 Ruemmele FM, Targan SR, Levy G, Dubinsky M, Braun J, Seidman EG. Diagnostic accuracy of serological assays in pediatric inflammatory bowel disease. *Gastroenterology* 115:822–829, 1998.

14 Hanauer SB, Robinson M, Pruitt R, Lazenby AJ, Persson T, Nilsson LG, Walton-Bowen K, Haskell LP, Levine JG. Budesonide enema for the treatment of active, distal ulcerative colitis and proctitis: a dose ranging study. *Gastroenterology* 115:525–532, 1998.

15 Mamula P, Markowitz JE, Brown KA, Hurd LB, Piccoli DA, Baldassano RN. Infliximab as a novel therapy for pediatric ulcerative colitis. *J Pediatr Gastroenterol Nutr* 34:307–311, 2002.

16 Ekbom A, Helmick GC, Zack M, Holmberg L, Adami HO. Survival and causes of death in patients with inflammatory bowel disease: a population based study. *Gastroenterology* 103:954–960, 1992.

23

CLINICAL MANAGEMENT OF GASTROINTESTINAL POLYPS IN CHILDREN

Jan Taminiau and Marc Benninga

INTRODUCTION

The presence of polyps in the gastrointestinal tract is these days easily detected by endoscopic investigation. Polyps have a stalk or have a broad basis. They might be single, but also occur multiply in the polyposis syndromes. Polyps are divided in two categories: hamartomas (juvenile polyps, Peutz-Jeghers' polyps, and hyperplastic polyps) and adenomas. Solitary polyps in children are most commonly hamartomas and predominantly of the juvenile type. Single Peutz-Jeghers' or hyperplastic polyps are extremely rare as are solitary adenomas in children. Multiple polyps are usually familial syndromes, such as *familial adenomatous polyposis* (FAP) and the much less common juvenile polyposis syndrome or Peutz-Jeghers' syndrome. Juvenile and hyperplastic single polyps do not proceed to malignancy, while rare solitary adenomas may lead to malignancy. The chance of malignancy is largely increased in polyposis syndromes.[1]

CLINICAL PRESENTATION

The most frequent symptom of a bowel polyp is painless rectal blood loss, usually separated from the stools, but might be mixed with stools. Differential diagnosis is with infectious colitis, allergic colitis (in very young children), Meckel's diverticulum, vascular anomalies, inflammatory bowel disease, and anal fissures. In about 4% of children referred for rectal blood loss, a colorectal polyp is detected, which in most cases is a juvenile polyp. If a gastrointestinal polyp causes abdominal pain, this nearly always is a sign of pending bowel obstruction. A large polyp causing intussusception might lead to ischemia of the bowel. In Peutz-Jeghers' syndrome polyps are large and truncated and prone to intussusception. Hyperplastic polyps in the duodenum in children might cause abdominal pain and obstruction. Spontaneous anal prolapse of a polyp is usually without symptoms. In polyposis syndromes (FAP and juvenile polyposis syndromes), mucus secretion with stools might precede rectal blood loss. Sometimes it is accompanied by diarrhea. In generalized juvenile polyposis of the newborn, the presenting symptoms are anemia, severe bleeding, severe diarrhea, and exudative enteropathy. Although it is commonly stated that juvenile polyps are located in the rectosigmoid tract, 25–60% of them are reported in the literature to be located proximal to the sigmoid colon. More than one polyp is noticed in between 40 and 50% of children with juvenile polyps. Therefore, only full colonoscopy and not limited flexible sigmoidoscopy are the investigations of choice in assessment of rectal bleeding in children. Visualizing techniques are unsuitable for children because histology is necessary to offer a proper treatment and follow-up guidance.[2]

HISTOLOGY OF POLYPS

Adenomas

Adenomas are by definition always dysplastic. In dysplasia three categories are distinguished: mild, moderate, and severe.

- In mild dysplasia, goblet cells and epithelial cells are distinguished but by lack of differentiation immature epithelial cells are increased with mucus-visible secretion. Nuclei are enlarged with numerous mitoses and dark-stained cytoplasm.
- In moderate dysplasia, nuclei are larger and more hyperchromatic, crypts are elongated with pseudostratification. Focal loss of polarity is seen.
- In severe dysplasia, nuclei are oval and prominent with a vesicular aspect. Crypts are branched and mucus production is absent stromal tissue is diminished.

Adenomas are distinguished histologically as tubular, tubulovillous, and villous adenomas. Cancer risk increases in this sequence. Villous adenomas usually have a broad base and are flat. When abnormalities reach the muscularis mucosa the carcinoma is called invasive.

Hamartomas

Juvenile polyps are nearly always stalked with a diameter of 1–3 cm with a smooth, red granular surface. Pathology shows dilated cysts with mucus, a prominent lamina propria with a clear inflammatory infiltrate. Polyps often have an ulcerated surface and abundant eosinophilia might be present. Dysplasia is rare, occurring in less than 5% of polyps. Peutz-Jeghers' polyps have a broad base but also might be stalked. Most of them are pedunculated with a lobulated surface and contain branched smooth muscle tissue in the lamina propria. They have less stroma and have less cystic changes than juvenile polyps. Dysplasia is noticed in less than 5% of cases.

Hyperplastic polyps have an increased crypt depth, enlarged vesicular nuclei with prominent nucleoli, increased migration of enterocytes from the crypts to the surface, and increased mitotic activity.

SINGLE POLYPS

Juvenile Polyps

Juvenile polyps represent 90% of single polyps in children. It is estimated that 1–2% of asymptomatic children have juvenile polyps. They are diagnosed in the first decade of life with a peak incidence between 2 and 5 years of age. Polyps in infants less than 12 months of age are exceedingly unusual but do occur. Polyps occur in all ethnic groups around the world, more frequently in boys than in girls. Probably a large deal of polyps is lost by autoamputation. In around 40% of children with juvenile polyps, more than one juvenile polyp is found on endoscopy and more than 60% of juvenile polyps occur in the proximal region to the rectosigmoid. The recurrence rate is between 5 and 7%. The risk of malignancy is essentially negligible. In the literature, only eight cases have been described in the age range of 1.5–67 years (mean age 24 years).

Each polyp should be removed by full colonoscopy and histologically investigated. Follow-up of these patients is not indicated but if the same symptomatology occurs, full colonoscopy should be performed again, because it is unclear which patient with a solitary juvenile polyp at diagnosis is actually having the first polyp which later develops into a juvenile polyposis syndrome.[3]

Hyperplastic Polyps

Single hyperplastic polyps account for 3% of the single polyps in children. They occur in the duodenum or antrum, and may cause abdominal pain due to intussusception.[4]

Adenomatous Single Polyps

Adenomas in children are extremely rare as a single polyp. They too may present with blood loss in stools. Adenocarcinoma of the colon is only seen in children who have predisposing diseases like ataxia-teleangiectasia, which is accompanied by lymphoproliferative malignancies. It is unknown if the premalignant adenoma phase is present in these children. Bowel cancer can occur in adults after FAP or hereditary non-polyposis colorectal cancer (HNPCC), but in childhood cancer development in these conditions is extremely rare.

JUVENILE POLYPOSIS SYNDROME

Juvenile polyposis is a collection of a heterogeneous group of rare autosomal-dominant inherited conditions characterized by multiple gastrointestinal hamartomatous polyps in the colon. This form of polyposis might be isolated without other clinical symptoms but could also be a part of a syndrome in combination with other symptoms. In general, juvenile polyposis is considered when three or more juvenile polyps are identified.[5] The common age of the initial symptoms is around 9 years and symptoms are rectal bleeding, anemia, or rectal prolapse due to the polyp.

A rare condition occurs in infancy characterized by anemia due to GI bleeding, severe watery diarrhea, and protein-losing enteropathy: this syndrome is called "infantile generalized juvenile polyposis." These infants have polyps throughout the whole gastrointestinal tract and are prone to multiple resections, end up with a short bowel, and die before the age of 2 years. Patients with juvenile polyposis syndrome gradually develop more polyps, slowly progressing to 50 or 100 polyps, mostly right-sided colonic polyps. Primarily they are found in the colon but later are also seen in the stomach and small intestine. Malignant degeneration has been estimated to be 15% at the age of 35 years, increasing to 68% at the age of 60 years.

Arbitrary cancer screening is indicated when three or more polyps are seen, which is based on a retrospective review in the juvenile polyposis syndrome. Colorectal neoplasia occurred when three or more polyps were present and was ex-tremely rare when there were only one or two polyps present.

A significant proportion of patients with juvenile polyposis syndrome also present associated morphological abnormalities. They include digital clubbing, microcephaly, alopecia, cleft lip or palate, congenital heart disease, genito-urinary abnormalities, and mental retardation. In addition, two other rare syndromes (see Fig. 23-1) are described in this group:

- Bannayan-Riley-Ruvalcabe syndrome: macrocephaly, pigmentation of the genitalia, and psychomotor delay in childhood
- Cowden's syndrome: multiple hamartomas of multiple organs, microcephaly, thyroid, and breast disease

Genetic Basis

Mutations in the SMAD4-gene and BNPR1A-gene have been found on chromosomes 18 and 10, respectively, in patients with juvenile polyposis syndrome. Some syndromes in this group have been associated with PTEN-gene abnormalities on chromosome 10q, but the frequency of these mutations is low in follow-up studies of these patients. Therefore, it is still unclear if isolated individuals with multiple polyps have the same risk for cancer as do patients presenting familiar forms.

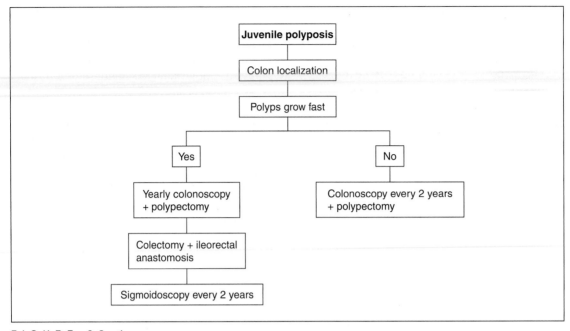

FIGURE 23-1

FOLLOW-UP OF PATIENTS WITH JUVENILE POLYPOSIS SYNDROME

Consequently, it is presently recommended to screen these patients every 2 years with colonoscopy and, if necessary, polypectomy at follow-up. If the occurrence of polyps is more rapid and symptomatology is increasing, colectomy with ileorectal anastomosis might be considered, followed every other year by a sigmoidoscopy and polypectomy. In first-degree relatives with juvenile polyposis syndrome, colonoscopic screening at the age of 12 and beyond is recommended at 3-year intervals.[6–10]

Peutz-Jeghers' syndrome is a rare autosomal-dominant disorder with an incidence of 1:120,000 births. It occurs in association with macular melanin pigmentation. This pigmentation is seen on the lips, buccal mucosa, and occasionally on hands, feet, and eyelids. Polyps arise in the small bowel and less frequently in stomach and colon. The main presenting symptom is small bowel obstruction by intussusception with complaints of vomiting and abdominal pain. Occasionally, intestinal bleeding leading to severe anemia might be the only presenting symptom. Peutz-Jeghers' syndrome

is associated with a significant increased risk for benign tumors and malignancies, located both in the intestine and in extraintestinal sites. Peutz-Jeghers' polyps may develop into carcinomatous lesions in stomach, small bowel, and colon. In 5–10% of girls with Peutz-Jeghers' syndrome, ovarian tumors leading to precocious puberty and irregular menstruations are seen. In prepubertal boys with Peutz-Jeghers' syndrome, Sertoli cell tumors might occur which lead to gynecomastia, accelerated growth, and advanced bone age. Malignancy in the gastrointestinal tract as well as gynecologic tumors, breast cancer, and other malignancies are usually not seen before the adult age. In two surveys, only five tumors occurred before the age of 18.[11]

Diagnosis and Screening

The diagnosis must be considered in family members of a known Peutz-Jeghers' case in whom typical oral pigmentation is noticed. When bowel obstruction with abdominal pain due to intussus-ception by a Peutz-Jeghers' polyp is the presenting symptom, the diagnosis will be made by histologic investigation; also, a follow-up after anal prolapse of a Peutz-Jeghers' polyp will give the diagnosis. Genetic investigation is possible; the mutated gene is a LBK1/STK11 (serine-threonine kinase) on chromosome 19p. This gene on occasion might be found in family screenings, even in patients with-out pigmentation. Screening for the benign tumors by ultrasound investigation in children with Peutz-Jeghers' syndrome is directed only at hormone-producing tumors until adulthood. During childhood no specific surveillance for gastrointestinal tumors in Peutz-Jeghers is indicated because of the rare occurrence of such malignancies in these children.

Treatment for bowel obstruction or pending obstruction with symptomatology indicating inter-mittent obstruction or obvious blood loss with anemia is an indication for laparotomy. This proce-dure will allow surgically guided pull-through endoscopic removal of all polyps larger than 3 cm from the anus to the esophagus. Only when the polyp has a broad base and perforation is a risk will a small resection be performed. Repeated laparo-tomies are only indicated for recurrent obstruction or severe blood loss and anemia. Following this plan ensures that patients do not end up with short bowels, as was often the case in the past when mul-tiple resections were performed. Clearly, however, this requires the availability of a well-suited service (see Fig. 23-2).

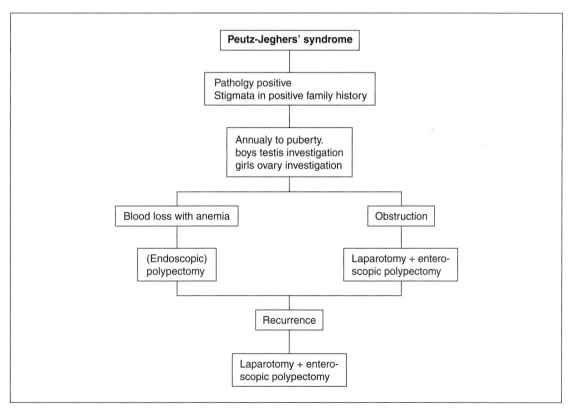

FIGURE 23-2

FOLLOW-UP OF PATIENTS WITH PEUTZ-JEGHERS' SYNDROME

Familial adenomatous polyposis is an autosomal-dominant syndrome occurring in 1:10,000 newborns. The defect is located in the APC-gene on chromosome 5q21. The condition is characterized by hundreds or thousands of adenomatous polyps in the colon. They first develop in childhood or in early adolescence and increase in number with time. Without treatment colon carcinoma occurs in all patients before the age of 50 years. In adulthood, malignancies also occur in the duodenum, thyroid, and pancreas. In children, only hepatoblastoma has been seen under the age of 5 years.

Genetic Basis

The *adenomatous polyposis coli* (APC) gene is localized on chromosome 5q21. It is a large gene with 50 exons coding for a protein of 2843 amino acids. At this point in time, 300 mutations have been discovered accounting for 80% of patients. In a large percentage of patients the mutation is *de novo*. A relation exists between the position of the mutation and the degree and severity of clinical symptoms; number of polyps, desmoid tumors, and congenital hypertrophy of the retinal pigment. These findings are of limited value for the individual patient. If the exact mutation in the family is established, other family members can be tested with 100% reliability. Usually, there are no symptoms when adenomas develop.[12,13]

Diagnostics and Screening

In young children in FAP-families, α-fetoprotein concentration and ultrasound of the liver might be performed to detect hepatoblastoma. Endoscopic surveillance should start at the age of 10–12 years or earlier when symptoms are present. This usually starts after genetic counseling in families. At the age of 11, a child is able to oversee the consequences of the positive result and understands endoscopic surveillance. The position and self-image of the child in relation to the family will change when the diagnosis is made and psychosocial care should be instituted in time before the investigations start. Polyps usually start in the rectosigmoid tract, so sigmoidoscopy every 2 years is sufficient for surveillance until the age of 18, when full colonoscopy has to start.[14,15]

Treatment

When polyps are detected, colectomy has to be performed and ileorectal anastomosis instituted. Patients have normal defecation frequency and normal sexual function. Only when the number of polyps in the remaining rectum is untreatable with laser coagulation, does not respond to *nonsteroidal anti-inflammatory drugs* (NSAIDs), and has a high degree of dysplasia, ileoanal anastomosis and institution of a pouch should be performed. Some FAP families have mutations associated with a severe phenotype, which leads to severe dysplasia and malignant degeneration in children even younger than 12 years. In these families the mutation might guide to early treatment. In other children it has to be discussed at what age they would like to have the colectomy and ileorectal anastomosis performed. Usually they prefer to have it done before the end of their adolescence, between 12 and 15 years. When the gene is not known only sigmoidoscopic follow-up can detect polyps—family members who do not have the unknown mutation have to undergo endoscopy frequently. After ileoanal anastomosis and pouches, surveillance should continue because a remnant carcinoma still occurs in up to 15% in these patients on long-term follow-up. Turcot syndrome is a combination of brain tumors and adenomatous polyposis. A PMS2 gene mutation is found linking it to HNPCC and also an autosomal recessive form of HNPCC. In patients with glioblastoma multiform and brainstem tumors with diarrhea, colonoscopic surveillance should be performed (see Fig. 23-3).[16–18]

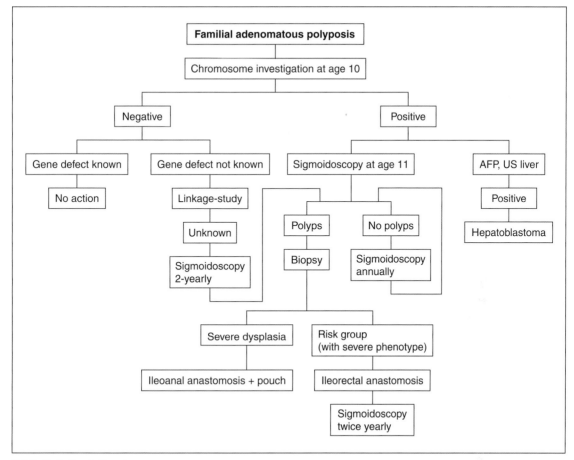

FIGURE 23-3

FOLLOW-UP OF PATIENTS WITH FAMILIAL ADENOMATOUS POLYPOSIS

References

1 Taminiau J. Polyps and tumours of the gastrointestinal tract. In: Buts JP, Sokal EM (eds.), *Management of Digestive and Liver Disorders in Infants and Children*. The Netherlands: Elsevier, 1993, pp. 403–415.

2 Hyer W, Beveridge I, Domizio P, Phillips R. Clinical management and genetics of gastrointestinal polyps in children. *J Pediatr Gastroenterol Nutr* 31:469–479, 2000.

3 Latt TT, Nicholl R, Domizio P, et al. Rectal bleeding and polyps. *Arch Dis Child* 63:144–147, 1993.

4 Verhage J, Mulder CJ, Meyer JW, Reuvers C. Hyperplastic duodenal polyp in a boy. Case report. *J Pediatr Gastroenterol Nutr* 19:326–328, 1994.

5 Corredor J, Wambach J, Barnard J. Gastrointestinal polyps in children: advances in molecular genetics, diagnosis, and management. *J Pediatr* 138(5):621–628, 2001.

6 Waite KA, Eng C. Protean PTEN: form and function. *Am J Hum Genet* 70:829–844, 2002.

7 Schart GM, Becker JHR, Laage NJ. Juvenile gastrointestinal polyposis or the infantile Cronkhite-Canada syndrome. *J Pediatr Surg* 21:953–954, 1986.

8 Mougenot JF, Baldassarre ME, Mashako LM, et al. Recto-colic polyps in the child. Analysis of 183 cases. *Arch Fr Pediatr* 46:245–248, 1989.

9 Woodford-Richens K, Bevan S, Churchman M, et al. Analysis of genetic and phenotypic heterogeneity in juvenile polyposis. *Gut* 46:656–660, 2000.

10 Boardman LA, Thibodeau SN, Schaid DJ, et al. Increased risk for cancer in patients with the Peutz-Jeghers syndrome. *Ann Intern Med* 128:896–899, 1998.

11 McGarrity TJ, Kulin HE, Zaino RJ. Peutz-Jeghers syndrome. *Am J Gastroenterol* 95:596–604, 2000.

12 Nugent KP, Phillips RK, Hodgson SV. Phenotypic expression in familial adenomatous polyposis: partial prediction by mutation analysis. *Gut* 35:1622–1623, 1994.

13 Eccles DM, Lunt PW, Wallis Y, et al. An unusually severe phenotype for FAP. *Arch Dis Child* 77:431–435, 1997.

14 Phillips RKS. FAP: the surgical treatment of the colorectum. *Semin Colon Rectal Surg* 6:33–37, 1995.

15 Burt RW. Colon cancer screening. *Gastroenterology* 119:837–853, 2000.

16 Hamilton SR, Lui B, Parsons RE, et al. The molecular basis of Turcot's syndrome. *N Engl J Med* 332:839–847, 1995.

17 De Rosa M, Fasano C, Panariello L, et al. Evidence for a recessive inheritance of Turcot's syndrome caused by compound heterozygous mutations within the PMS2 gene. *Oncogene* 19:1719–1723, 2000.

18 Menko FH, Sijmons RH. Erfelijke darmkanker. Richtlijnen voor diagnostiek, voorlichting en preventie. Amsterdam: Werkgroep Klinische Oncogenetica, Vereniging Klinische Genetica Nederland, 2001.

24

INTUSSUSCEPTION

Donald Liu

INTRODUCTION

Intussusception is one of the most common causes of intestinal obstruction in infants and young children. It can occur in adults, but it appears primarily in pediatric cases. Intussusception occurs when a portion of the small intestine telescopes into another, causing an invagination and obstruction of the small intestine, venous compression, and bowel wall edema.[1] Approximately 90% of cases of intussusception are ileocolic, but intussusception can also be jejunojejunal, jejunoileal, and duodenojejunal.[2] There is a specific lead point in 2–10% of intussusception cases, but a lead point has an incidence of up to 22% in children over 2 years of age. Recurrent intussusception often indicates the presence of a lead point.

Common lead points include Meckel's diverticulum, polyp, heterotopic pancreatic nodule, enterogenous cyst, adenoma, neurofibroma, hemangioma, or an enlarged hypertrophied ileal lymphoid patch. It has been suggested that adenovirus and other infectious viral agents are associated with intestinal lymphoid hyperplasia and intussusception. Intussusception may also occur following surgery or after abdominal trauma. In the absence of an obvious lead point, however, the disorder remains idiopathic.

The consequences of intussusception can be severe. Portions of the bowel can become ischemic and necrose, leading to bowel perforation and death. Due to these potential complications, it is essential to diagnose intussusception without delay.

EPIDEMIOLOGY

The typical case of intussusception occurs in a male under 10 months of age[1]; 69% of patients are under 1 year and 80% of cases occur in children under 24 months. Incidence has been reported between 1 and 4 per 1000 live births. There is a male-to-female ration of 3:2. There seem to be no trends with respect to race, geographical distribution, or seasonal variation, despite scattered reports suggesting otherwise.

One of the key concerns in the incidence of intussusception is the rate of recurrence. There is a 5–7% recurrence rate in the United States, but this rate is higher in older children. Recurrence usually indicates a lead point; the most common lead point being a Meckel's diverticulum.

DIAGNOSIS

Clinical Symptoms

The "classic triad" of symptoms of intussusception is

- Intermittent abdominal pain
- Vomiting
- Currant jelly stool

This triad, however, occurs in only 10–20% of patients, though the individual symptoms occur with greater frequency.[3] Nonetheless, up to 38% of intussusception cases present without bleeding; up to 24% present without vomiting; 36% without an abdominal mass; and 13% without pain. Abdominal pain can be intermittent when the bowel obstruction is temporarily resolved, but pain is severe enough to cause infants and young children to draw in their legs. Stools take on a red currant jelly appearance as sloughed off mucosa clots and is passed per rectum (this occurs in approximately 60% of cases). Obstruction is often severe enough to cause a palpable abdominal mass, representing the gut proximal to the intussusception. This palpable "sausage-shaped mass" typically appears in the right hypochondrium extending along the line of the transverse colon or to the rectum where it may (on rare occasions) be felt on rectal examination. A history or presence of rectal bleeding also has been found to be an important clinical predictor of intussusception.[1] Given these clinical symptoms, however, it is difficult to distinguish intussusception from other gastrointestinal conditions, and other methods of diagnosis are essential.

Ultrasonography

Ultrasonography classically reveals a "target" or "doughnut" sign in cross-section and a "pseudokidney" sign in longitudinal section. It is useful as a negative indicator, but less useful as a positive indicator of intussusception. It offers the advantage, however, that it is noninvasive and involves no exposure to radiation. The use of ultrasonography to screen cases with atypical presentations for intussusception has been shown to be cost-effective, although an in-depth cost analysis would be required to reach a reliable answer.[3]

Air and Barium Contrast Enemas

Air and barium contrast enemas are considered the gold standard for diagnosis and treatment of intussusception (see section TREATMENT). Air enema can successfully diagnose approximately 95% of cases of intussusception.[4] It involves insufflation of the gut under radiography. The intussusception is revealed on obstruction of this insufflation and, optimally, is reduced. Similarly, barium enema reveals an obstruction of the flow of the enema and, optimally, reduction of the intussusception.

Delay in Diagnosis

A delay in the diagnosis of intussusception can be critical, leading to a high rate (up to 42% according to one study) of complications, including gangrene, ischemia, and perforation. The condition is likely to be fatal after a 2–5-day delay; even if it is not fatal, a delay can result in necrosis of a large portion of the gut and its subsequent loss of viability. Surgical resection is required at this point.

TREATMENT

Nonsurgical Treatment

The main contraindication to hydrostatic reduction is the presence of peritonitis, in which case the patient should have immediate surgery. Mild sedation may be used during the procedure, but anesthesia is usually unnecessary. A surgeon ideally should be in proximity at reduction and if perforation occurs, surgery should follow immediately. Reduction is considered complete when barium is observed as refluxing freely past the point of obstruction or by free passage of air proximally.

The reduction rate of air insufflation is reported as slightly higher than that of barium enema. While both rates have been reported as high as 100% for initial and 95% for recurrent intussusception, these results seem exceptional.[5] Some studies have reported a barium enema reduction rate of 100% if the thickness of the hypoechoic external ring of the "doughnut" was less than or equal to 7.2 mm, a rate of 68.9% if the thickness ranged between 7.5 and 11.2 mm, and the need for surgical resection if the thickness was greater than 11.2 mm.[6] Other studies have suggested that the success rate of hydrostatic

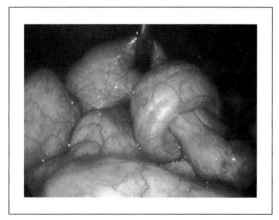

FIGURE 24-1

INTUSSUSCEPTED BOWEL SEGMENT

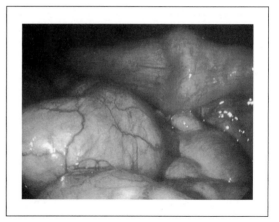

FIGURE 24-2

POSTSURGICAL REDUCTION OF INTUSSUSCEPTION

reduction is 50% if symptoms are present longer than 48 h and 75–80% if reduction is done within the first 48 h of the appearance of symptoms. Nonsurgical treatment, in the absence of contraindicators, however, remains the preferred means of treating intussusception.

Nonsurgical treatment (air and barium enema) has a 5–7% recurrence rate. The overall rate of nonsurgical recurrence has been reported as high as 9%.[5] Recurrence rates with barium enema have been reported as high as 11% and recurrence rates with air enema have been reported as high as 8%.

Surgical Treatment

If enema reduction fails or if small bowel ischemia and necrosis are suspected, it is necessary to reduce the intussusception surgically. Laparotomy or laparoscopy is performed and the intussusception reduced by gentle pressure on the apex of the intussuscepted intestine in the descending or transverse colon (see Fig. 24-2). If a pathologic lead point is recognized, then resection of the involved bowel segment is performed. Resection must also be performed if nonviable intestine is found. Furthermore, if the intussusception cannot be reduced, the involved segment is resected and continuity restored with an anastomosis. Feedings are usually started the day after surgery and rapidly

advance to a regular diet. Antibiotics are commonly discontinued within 48 h, and the child is often discharged shortly thereafter. The recurrence rate after surgical reduction is about 3%. Lead points are most common in children over 2 years of age, and any recurrence is evidence of a lead point.

OUTCOME

Mortality rates due to intussusception have fallen through the twentieth century to less than 1%, as have perforation rates during surgery. The most important concerns are bowel ischemia and the presence of lead points. Bowel ischemia often results from a delay in diagnosis. Recurrence of intussusception indicates the presence of a lead point, especially in older children.

References

1 Kuppermann N, O'Dea T, Pinckney L, et al. Predictors of intussusception in young children. *Arch Pediatr Adolesc Med* 154(3):250–255, 2000.

2 Ko S, Lee T, Ng S, et al. Small bowel intussusception in symptomatic pediatric patients: experiences with

19 surgically proven cases. *World J Surg* 26:438–443, 2002.

3   Harrington L, Connolly B, Hu X, et al. Ultrasono-graphic and clinical predictors of intussusception. *J Pediatr* 132(5):836–839, 1998.

4   Paton Elizabeth A. A 3-month old with blood in the stool: a case scenario. *J Emerg Nurs* 29(1):68–71, 2003.

5   Daneman A, Alton D, Lobo E, et al. Patterns of recurrence of intussusception in children: a 17-year review. *Pediatr Radiol* 28:913–919, 1998.

6   Mirilas P, Koumanidou C, Vakaki M, et al. Sonographic features indicative of hydrostatic reducibility of intestinal intussusception in infancy and early childhood. *Eur Radiol* 11(12):2578–2580, 2001.

25

APPENDICITIS

Mindy B. Statter and Adam Vogel

INTRODUCTION

The term "appendicitis" was coined in 1886 by Harvard pathologist Reginald Fitz, who emphasized in his publication that the disease could be diagnosed before the onset of fatal complications. One year later, T.G. Morton performed the first documented appendectomy for perforated appendicitis. In 1889, the famous "McBurney's Point" was immortalized in surgical literature when Charles McBurney wrote: "I believe that in every case the seat of greatest pain, determined by the pressure of one finger, has been very exactly between an inch and a half and two inches from the anterior spinus process of the ilium on a straight line drawn from that process to the umbilicus."[1] Appendicitis is the most common surgical emergency in children. The diagnosis of appendicitis in children remains challenging because of its varied presentations, delays in seeking medical care, and the difficulties in obtaining an accurate history and physical examination.

INCIDENCE

The diagnosis of appendicitis peaks in the spring. Approximately 1% of all children <15 years of age develop appendicitis, with a peak incidence between 10 and 12 years of age. The incidence of perforation is 20–50%. Appendicitis with perforation is more common in children than adults. This has been shown to be related to delay in presentation to the surgeon rather than specific physiologic differences in children.[2]

ETIOLOGY

In children, obstruction is commonly due to extrinsic compression from lymphoid hyperplasia. The systemic immune response to viral, bacterial, and parasitic infections of the respiratory tract and gut results in hyperplasia of Peyer's patches and immune tissue in the terminal ileum and appendix. Fecaliths, small elements of condensed, hardened stool, can become impacted at the appendiceal orifice resulting in luminal obstruction. Fecaliths are calcified in 10% of patients and visualized on plain abdominal x-rays. Appendiceal carcinoid is the most common neoplasm of the gastrointestinal tract in childhood. The appendix is the most common site for carcinoid tumors. Patients with cystic fibrosis can develop thickened, solid enteric mucus plugs that, like fecaliths, obstruct the appendiceal lumen. Appendiceal disease in cystic fibrosis patients ranges from simple mucous distention to acute appendicitis with perforation. Cystic fibrosis patients with abdominal pain secondary to a noninflamed, distended appendix represent a distinct syndrome cured by appendectomy.[3]

PATHOPHYSIOLOGY

The most important pathologic factor in appendicitis is obstruction of the appendiceal lumen. Luminal obstruction leads to distention as the appendiceal mucosa continues to secrete mucus. This results in increased transmural pressure, impaired venous drainage, and edema with subsequent impaired arterial inflow and local tissue ischemia. This local ischemia and mucosal ulceration enable bacteria to locally invade the appendiceal wall. The combination of bacterial infection and arterial ischemia leads to gangrene and rupture. The process is evidenced by an initial fibropurulent exudate followed by gangrene.[4] The most common organisms involved with perforated appendicitis are gram-negative rods (*E. coli*, *Pseudomonas*, and *Klebsiella*) and anerobes (*Bacteroides*, *Fusobacterium*).[5]

CLINICAL SIGNS AND SYMPTOMS

Appendicitis classically presents with epigastric or periumbilical abdominal pain, anorexia, vomiting, and fever. Embryologically, the appendix develops from the midgut. Intraluminal distention stimulates the visceral afferent nerve fibers of the tenth dermatome which is perceived as dull, achy periumbilical pain. This is often preceded by anorexia and followed by nausea and typically nonbilious emesis.[6]

As the inflammation becomes transmural, the parietal peritoneum becomes irritated, stimulating somatic efferents with localized *right lower quadrant* (RLQ) pain. Rupture can present with an initial relief of pain as the intraluminal obstruction is eliminated before developing more intense RLQ or pelvic pain, or generalized peritonitis. The symptoms of perforated appendicitis include anorexia with vomiting; severe, generalized abdominal pain; fever (>38°C); and diarrhea. Nonverbal children may present with right hip pain mimicking a septic hip. Children <5 years of age, with their sparse omentum, are less capable of "walling off" the perforation and often present with generalized peritonitis.

DIAGNOSIS

The evaluation of right lower quadrant pain and the diagnosis of appendicitis are generally based on the history and physical examination. Although no single aspect of the presentation accurately predicts the presence of the disease, a combination of signs and symptoms may support the diagnosis.[7] The mistakes made in the diagnosis of appendicitis are sometimes due to the failure to realize the variability in the position of the appendix and that appendicitis can mimic many other intraabdominal processes. Table 25-1 lists the differential diagnosis for acute appendicitis.

TABLE 25-1

DIFFERENTIAL DIAGNOSIS OF ACUTE APPENDICITIS

Acute porphyria
Blunt abdominal trauma/rectus sheath hematoma
Cholecystitis, hepatitis, cholangitis
Constipation
Crohn's disease
Duodenal ulcer (with perforation)
Ectopic pregnancy
Gastroenteritis
Hemolytic-uremic syndrome
Henoch-Schonlein purpura
Intussusception
Meckel's diverticulitis
Meconium ileus equivalent
Mesenteric adenitis
Mittleschmerz
Omental torsion and infarction
Ovarian cyst
Ovarian torsion
Pelvic inflammatory disease
Pneumonia
Pyelonephritis
Renal colic 2° renal or ureteral calculi
Sickle cell pain crisis
Small bowel obstruction
Typhlitis in the immunosuppressed patient
Urinary tract infection
Testicular torsion
Torsion of appendix epiplociae

Physical Examination

The physical findings in appendicitis may be quite variable. In general, patients may be irritable or appear sullen. If significant anorexia is present, they may exhibit signs of volume depletion. Early phases of appendicitis may present with a nonspecific, tender abdominal examination. As the parietal peritoneum becomes inflamed, focal right lower quadrant tenderness may develop, with progression to localized peritonitis (tenderness to both palpation and percussion). The localization of pain to the right lower quadrant usually occurs hours after the onset of epigastric or periumbilical pain. With perforation, peritonitis may become diffuse. Appendicitis with a palpable mass is usually a consequence of perforation. The mass may represent either a phlegmon or an abscess. The rectal examination may reveal tenderness in the case of the retrocecal appendix where anterior abdominal wall findings may not be present. In addition, a pelvic abscess may be detected on digital examination.

Laboratory Findings

The laboratory findings should be confirmatory, not diagnostic. A slight-to-moderate elevation in *white blood cell* (WBC) count is commonly seen in acute appendicitis. At least 10% of patients with appendicitis will have a normal WBC and differential.

Perforated appendicitis is almost always associated with a leukocytosis or a predominance of polymorphonuclear cells or significant left shift. A normal WBC count in the setting of localized right lower quadrant pain and tenderness or diffuse peritonitis does not eliminate appendicitis or a surgical abdomen from the differential diagnosis.

A urinalysis is often obtained and can be useful in identifying urinary tract pathology presenting as an acute abdomen. However, in the presence of leukocyte esterase, mild-to-moderate pyuria or hematuria may be seen with appendiceal irritation of the ureter or bladder.[8]

Diagnostic Imaging

The potential consequences of a missed diagnosis of acute appendicitis are serious and include perforation with peritonitis, sepsis, and wound infection. When the history and physical examination are equivocal, radiologic studies are obtained to confirm the diagnosis of appendicitis with the goals of avoiding the consequences of missed diagnosis and negative-finding laparotomies.

Abdominal Radiographs

Radiographic studies are reserved for children with atypical, equivocal, or confusing findings. A calcified fecalith is apparent in 10% of patients. If a fecalith is identified in a child with localized abdominal pain, surgical exploration is indicated. With the finding of small bowel obstruction on abdominal plain film in young children, the differential diagnosis must include perforated appendicitis (see Chap. 7, Fig. 4)

The presence of a fecalith does not absolutely confirm appendicitis as the cause of the patient's illness but supports the diagnosis. *Chest x-ray* (CXR) should be performed to evaluate the lung fields because right lower lobe pneumonia can mimic the abdominal pain of acute appendicitis.[8]

Barium Enema

Barium enema has a limited role in the diagnosis of acute appendicitis. Barium enema should be used in the atypical patient with a protracted acute illness or a history of chronic abdominal pain.[8]

The barium enema findings that suggest appendiceal pathology are nonfilling or incomplete filling of the appendix and extrinsic compression of the cecum. The incomplete filling of the appendix is consistent with the hypothesis that luminal obstruction is an important factor in the pathogenesis of appendicitis.

Ultrasound

Ultrasound has a sensitivity of 75–90% and a specificity of 86–100%, with an overall accuracy of 90–94% for the diagnosis of acute appendicitis.[6]

The advantages of ultrasonography include no radiation exposure, discomfort, or contrast medium. The disadvantages are that it is operator-dependent with regard to the quality and interpretation of the study.

A normal appendix is typically collapsed, compressible, and nonfluid filled, measuring 3–4 mm in cross-sectional diameter. Sonographic characteristics of a fluid-filled, noncompressible lumen, fecalith, periappendiceal fluid, and an appendiceal diameter greater than 6 mm are diagnostic of acute appendicitis. Ultrasound can detect the thickness of all layers of the bowel wall, luminal caliber, and whether the appendix is compressible. An appendix that is >6 mm in diameter or noncompressible is predictive of acute appendicitis, especially when its location corresponds to the point of maximal tenderness. Ultrasound may show matted bowel loops in an inflammatory mass without abscess formation in the right lower quadrant without visualization of the appendix.[8]

Appendicitis may be ruled out if the appendix appears normal; however, if the appendix (normal or diseased) is not seen, physicians are hesitant to make clinical decisions about appendicitis. Other etiologies of RLQ pain may be diagnosed on ultrasound, such as mesenteric lymphadenitis or ovarian pathology.

Computed Tomography

Spiral *computed tomography* (CT) has a sensitivity of 90–100%, a specificity of 91–99%, and an overall accuracy of 94–100%.[6] CT findings consistent with acute appendicitis include visualization of a distended appendix with a diameter >6 mm and/or the appearance of periappendiceal inflammatory changes. CT scans may be useful in atypical patients with undiagnosed abdominal symptoms or in whom satisfactory ultrasound examinations are not possible, e.g., obese children, immunologically suppressed children, or those lacking localizing physical findings. CT scans may also be useful in patients with perforated appendicitis to distinguish phlegmon from abscess and to plan therapeutic interventions, such as percutaneous, transrectal, or transvaginal abscess drainage. A retrospective study reported from Massachusetts General Hospital evaluated whether *focused appendiceal CT with colon contrast* (FACT-CC) increased the accuracy of the preoperative diagnosis acute appendicitis

in children. Preoperative FACT-CC did not increase the accuracy in diagnosing appendicitis when compared with patients diagnosed by history, physical examination, and laboratory studies. The use of CT imaging did not affect the perforation rate in this study; 14.5% in the imaged group versus 13.3% in the nonimaged group. Five patients had preoperative CT scans that were interpreted as negative, but because of high clinical suspicion of appendicitis underwent appendectomy and had appendicitis confirmed at operation and by pathologic examination. The authors concluded that CT scanning may play an important role in the evaluation of patients with an atypical clinical presentation or in older (>11 years) girls.[9]

Partrick et al., in their retrospective study, aimed to determine if the diagnostic accuracy of acute appendicitis in children has improved in concordance with the increased use of CT scanning. Over the 5-year study period, from 1997 to 2001, the use of ultrasound and CT both increased with the proportion of children having CT scan increasing annually. Over this same time interval the number of children proceeding to appendectomy without radiographic evaluation decreased, the rate of perforation remained stable, and the rate of negative appendectomies did not decrease. The authors discuss that the patients receiving CT scans were presumably those with an unclear history, physical examination, or laboratory studies which led clinicians to obtain further diagnostic studies. It may be that this group would have had a greater negative appendectomy rate if no diagnostic study has been obtained. They recommend limiting the use of radiographic studies to children who have been examined and in whom the surgeon cannot conclude that the diagnosis is appendicitis. In light of the recent data concerning the possible harmful sequelae of radiation exposure from pediatric CT scans, the indiscriminate use of CT in the diagnosis of acute appendicitis in children in not warranted.[10]

GUIDELINE TO TREATMENT

The goal of management is to diagnose acute appendicitis before perforation. The risk of perforation within 24 h of the onset of symptoms is <30%. However, after 48 h of onset of symptoms the probability of perforation is >70%. Treatment of choice is early appendectomy. Preoperative resuscitation includes intravenous fluid hydration, nasogastric decompression for protracted emesis and for suspected perforation, and broad-spectrum antibiotic coverage (gram-negative and anaerobic) is indicated. Suggested therapy includes ampicillin, gentamicin, and clindamycin or metronidazole. Exploratory laparotomy and appendectomy is indicated for perforated appendicitis without abscess formation. Postoperatively, antibiotics are continued until fever and leukocytosis have resolved.

Early Appendectomy

Open appendectomy (OA) is performed through a single right lower quadrant abdominal incision. "Muscle-splitting," separation of the muscle fibers parallel to their course rather than division, reduces trauma. After entering the peritoneal cavity, the cecum and then the appendix is delivered into the wound. The appendix is mobilized by dividing and ligating the mesoappendix, the appendiceal blood supply. The base of the appendix may be simply ligated or a pursestring suture may be placed in the cecum adjacent to the base of the appendix, and after the appendix is ligated and amputated, the stump is inverted as the pursestring suture is tied. Cauterization of the residual mucosa of the appendiceal stump prevents formation of a mucocele.

If the appendix is not inflamed, the abdomen should be evaluated for other etiologies of abdominal pain. The terminal ileum should be inspected for "creeping fat," the pathognomonic finding of Crohn's disease; the distal ileum should also be inspected for a Meckel's diverticulum; the ovaries and fallopian tubes should be inspected for gynecologic pathology such as cysts or torsion; the mesentery should be inspected for lymphadenopathy suggestive of mesenteric adenitis.

The operative technique for perforated appendicitis is the same as for acute appendicitis.

Conservative Management and Interval Appendectomy

The standard approach to perforated appendicitis has been limited laparotomy, with drainage of an abscess if present and appendectomy. It has been argued that with this approach, due to the inflammation involving the cecum and surrounding bowel, the procedure can be complicated by greater blood loss, increased risk of bowel injury, and subsequent development of postoperative abdominal and/or pelvic abscesses by entering an established abscess. Alternative approaches depend on whether the mass is a phlegmon or an abscess, as determined by ultrasound or CT. If the mass is determined to be a phlegmon, intravenous antibiotics and volume resuscitation without immediate laparotomy are a safe and effective treatment provided the patient demonstrates clinical improvement, e.g., resolution of fever, leukocytosis, and the abdominal pain. Elective interval appendectomy can be planned 6 weeks later, generally with postoperative hospital stay of 1 day. Laparotomy is indicated if clinical improvement does not occur after 24 h of nonoperative management. If an abscess is identified, after volume resuscitation and intravenous antibiotics, drainage by percutaneous, tranvaginal, or transrectal routes may be performed. With clinical improvement, antibiotic therapy is continued until the patient is afebrile and the leukocytosis and abdominal tenderness have resolved. Elective interval appendectomy can be planned 6 weeks later, generally with postoperative hospital stay of 1 day.

The ability to safely and accurately distinguish perforated from nonperforated acute appendicitis is imperative to the institution of conservative management.[11]

Laparoscopic Appendectomy

Laparoscopic appendectomy (LA) was first described by Semm in the early 1980s.[12] When compared to the traditional open technique, the laparoscopic approach provides visual access to a larger portion of the abdominal cavity allowing evaluation of other etiologies of abdominal pain, superior cosmetic results, and a quicker return to normal activity—this is advantageous to the obese patient.[13] However, in comparing these approaches it is necessary to separate acute and complicated appendicitis. Meguerditchian et al. reviewed 391 cases of pediatric appendectomies performed over a 3-year interval.[14] LA was performed in 126 patients and OA was performed in 262, with 3 conversions to open appendectomy. Perforation was noted in 10.3% of LA cases and in 14.9% of OA cases. Although the LA operative times were slightly longer, the hospitalizations were shorter. The complication rate was not significantly different between the two groups. They noted that their LA patients were older, more frequently female, and that the rate of negative appendectomy was higher with LA (21.4%) than OA (13%) and was not associated with a shortened length of operative procedure or shorter length of hospitalization. The majority of the patients who underwent LA (16/27) and had a negative pathology report presented with either atypical symptoms, pain for >48 h, or inconclusive radiologic findings. These authors concluded that LA is a safe and effective alternative in acute appendicitis.

Horwitz et al. retrospectively reviewed 56 cases of complicated (gangrenous or perforated) appendicitis in children; 27 underwent LA, 22 underwent OA, and there were 7 conversions to open procedures.[15] Complications were more frequent after LA compared to OA (56% vs. 18%). Intraabdominal abscess developed in 13 children; in 2 after OA and in 11 after LA. Based on these findings, the authors suggested that LA should be avoided in children with a preoperative diagnosis of complicated appendicitis because of the increased risk for postoperative intraabdominal abscess and recommend early conversion from LA to OA in children discovered to have complicated appendicits at the time of laparoscopy.

Krisher et al. retrospectively analyzed the records of 453 pediatric patients who were operated on for appendicitis.[16] The surgeon determined the type of appendicitis at the time of operation: acute appendicitis, if the appendix was inflamed without necrotic tissue; gangrenous, if areas of tissue were present without evidence of perforation; perforated, if there was free rupture of intraluminal contents. One-hundred and forty appendectomies were performed laparo-

scopically, 302 were performed using the open technique, and there were 11 conversions from laparoscopic to open procedure. The complication rate for intraabdominal abscess following LA and OA was 6.4 and 3.0%, respectively. The postoperative intraabdominal abscess rate for LA was 2.2% in acute appendicitis, 0% in gangrenous appendicitis, and 24% in perforated appendicitis. The postoperative intraabdominal abscess rate for OA was 2.5% for acute appendicitis, 0% in gangrenous appendicitis, and 4.2% for perforated appendicitis.

McKinlay et al. reviewed retrospectively the charts of 324 children undergoing appendectomy to examine the incidence of intraabdominal abscess.[17] Two-hundred and four were performed laparoscopically, 119 were performed open, and there was 1 conversion from the laparoscopic to the open approach. As in the previous study by Krisher, the distinction between acute, gangrenous, and perforated appendicitis was made clinically based on operative findings. Of the 15 intraabdominal abscesses that occurred, 7 were in the LA group and 8 occurred in the OA group. The incidence of intraabdominal abscess for perforated appendicitis in the LA group was 15% and that for OA was 10%; there was no statistically significant difference.

There is a need for a prospective randomized controlled trial of open versus laparoscopic appendectomy in the pediatric population that specifically addresses perforated appendicitis.

OUTCOMES

There is significant variability in practice patterns and resource usage in the management of acute appendicitis in pediatric hospitals.[18] The median overall negative appendectomy rate was 2.6% (range = 0–17%) and was 2.1% for patients aged 5–17 years. The rate of perforated appendicitis varied markedly and there was no obvious correlation with the patterns of diagnostic testing. The surgical and postoperative management varied widely, with the role of laparoscopy at the time of this study being undefined. The average length of stay was 2 days for acute appendicitis and 6 days for perforated appendicitis.

A standard protocol from Montreal serves as an evidence-based standard-of-care for the management of pediatric appendicitis.[19] The cohort treated under this standard protocol included 648 patients. The negative appendectomy rate was 9.4%. Three-hundred and sixty children (55.6%) had acute appendicitis, 102 (15.7%) had gangrenous appendicitis, and 125 (19.3%) had perforated appendicitis. Hospital stay was 1.39 ± 1.192 days for acute appendicitis, 2.97 ± 1.25 days for gangrenous appendicitis, and 6.31 ± 3.51 days for perforated appendicitis.

COMPLICATIONS

The complication rate is higher in the patient with perforated appendix and ranges from wound infection to intraabdominal abscess and intestinal obstruction.

Wound infection is the most common complication, with a 1–5% incidence in gangrenous or perforated appendicitis. The incidence of intraabdominal infection in patients with perforated appendicitis has been reported at 8%.[19] Small bowel obstruction occurs in 1–2% of patients with perforation, but can complicate the recovery of those patients with acute appendicitis, including those who undergo negative appendectomy.

Due to the proximity of the appendix to the right fallopian tube, one might expect acute or perforated appendicitis to be associated with unilateral tubal infertility. In a relatively recent longitudinal study of women who had prepubertal perforated appendicitis, there was no difference in fertility rates compared to the general population.[20]

Advances in perioperative care and antibiotics have lowered the mortality rate to less than 1%.

MISCELLANEOUS

Asymptomatic Patient with an Incidentally Discovered Fecalith

Data support a role for appendiceal fecaliths (non-calcified and calcified) in the pathogenesis of appendicitis. Appendiceal fecaliths and calculi were found more commonly in patients with acute appendicitis and predispose to appendiceal perforation and

CASE STUDY 25-1

10-Year-Old Female with Perforated Appendicitis

A 10-year-old female presented to the Pediatric Emergency Department with a history of several days (>48 h) of abdominal pain, abdominal distention, anorexia, and fever. Physical examination revealed a child with sick facies, abdominal distention, diffuse tenderness to palpation, and percussion. A CT scan of the abdomen and pelvis demonstrated free peritoneal fluid and fluid collections in the right lower quadrant and pelvis without visualization of the appendix (Fig. 25-1). The CT scan findings were consistent with a diagnosis of perforated appendicitis with phlegmon. The patient was managed conservatively and admitted for IV antibiotic therapy (ampicillin, gentamycin, and metronidazole). The patient's fever resolved. Although her pain localized to the right lower quadrant, her ileus was slow to resolve and she developed diarrhea. A repeat CT scan was obtained after 6 days of antibiotic therapy that demonstrated a large pelvic abscess and a decrease in the amount of free intraperitoneal fluid (Fig. 25-2). The patient was then taken to the operating room for transrectal drainage of the pelvic abscess. She was discharged to home 3 days later afebrile and tolerating a general diet, with resolution of the diarrhea, on a 7-day course of oral antibiotics (Augmentin). She returned 6 weeks later for interval appendectomy under general anesthesia. She was discharged to home the day after her procedure.

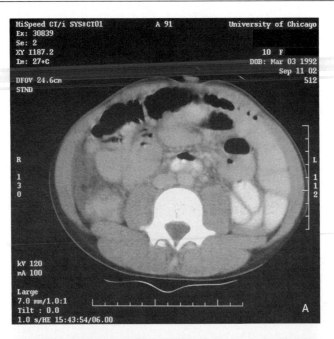

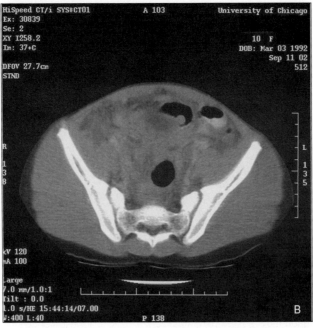

FIGURE 25-1

10-YEAR-OLD FEMALE PRESENTED WITH >48-H HISTORY OF ABDOMINAL PAIN, DISTENTION, ANOREXIA, AND FEVER

(A) CT scan shows free intraperitoneal fluid and (B) fluid collections in the pelvis. These findings were consistent with per-forated appendicitis with plegmon formation.

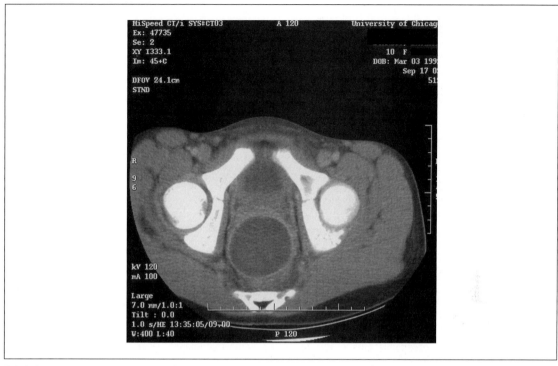

FIGURE 25-2

REPEAT CT SCAN 6 DAYS AFTER ANTIBIOTIC THERAPY DEMONSTRATED A LARGE PELVIC ABSCESS

abscess formation. Appendectomy should be considered in patients in whom an appendiceal calculus is recognized incidentally.[21] Appendectomy is indicated in such a patient if right lower quadrant pain and tenderness develops.

Incidental appendectomy

There remains ongoing debate regarding incidental appendectomy during other abdominal operations. Advocates maintain that the appendix should be removed whenever the exposure allows because the appendix has no function and can cause future morbidity. Incidental appendectomy at the time of abdominal operation for management of solid tumors has been recommended to facilitate the differential diagnosis of right lower quadrant pain and to exclude the diagnosis of acute appendicitis when these patients become neutropenic during subsequent chemotherapy;[22] however, incidental appendectomy may increase operative morbidity.

Reports of reconstructive procedures using the appendix warrant it being left *in situ*. The appendix has been used as a conduit for urinary drainage (Mitrofanoff procedure),[23] a means for delivering antegrade enemas (Malone procedure),[24] and a biliary conduit for biliary atresia, choledochal cyst,[25] and Alagille's syndrome.[26] The appendix should be conserved whenever possible in children with genitourinary anomalies or dysfunctional voiding who may be candidates for urinary reconstruction, congenital biliary anomalies including Alagille's syndrome, spina bifida, chronic constipation, and fecal incontinence.

References

1 Seal A. Appendicitis: a historical review. *Can J Surg* 24:427, 1981.
2 Oldham KT, Colombani PM, Foglia RP. *Surgery of Infants and Children: Scientific Principles and Practice.* Philadelphia, PA: Lippincott-Raven, 1997.

3   Coughlin JP, Gauderer MW, Stern RC, et al. The spectrum of appendiceal disease in cystic fibrosis. *J Pediatr Surg* 25:835, 1990.

4   Schumpelick V, Dreuw B, Ophoff K, et al. Appendix and cecum: embryology, anatomy, and surgical applications. *Surg Clin North Am* 80:295, 2000.

5   Bower RJ, Bell MJ, Ternberg JL. Controversial aspects of appendicitis management in children. *Arch Surg* 116:885, 1981.

6   Silen W. *Cope's Diagnosis of the Acute Abdomen.* New York, NY: Oxford University Press, 1979.

7   Paulson EK, Kalady MF, Pappas TN. Suspected appendicitis. *N Engl J Med* 348:236, 2003.

8   Schwartz MZ, Bulas D. Laboratory evaluation and imaging. *Semin Pediatr Surg* 6:65, 1997.

9   Stephen AE, Segev DL, Ryan DP, et al. The diagnosis of acute appendicitis in a pediatric population: to CT or not to CT. *J Pediatr Surg* 38:367, 2003.

10 Partrick DA, Janik JE, Janik JS, et al. Increased CT scan utilization does not improve diagnostic accuracy of appendicitis in children. *J Pediatr Surg* 38:659, 2003.

11 Weiner DJ, Katz A, Hirschl RB, et al. Interval appendectomy in perforated appendicitis. *Pediatr Surg Int* 10:82, 1995.

12 Semm K. Endoscopic appendectomy. *Endoscopy* 15:59, 1983.

13 Zitsman J. Current concepts in minimal access surgery for children. *Pediatrics* 111:1239, 2003.

14 Meguerditchian AN, Prasil P, Cloutier R, et al. Laparoscopic appendectomy in children: a favorable alternative in simple and complicated appendicitis. *J Pediatr Surg* 37:695, 2002.

15 Horwitz JR, Custer MD, Mehall JR, et al. Should laparoscopic appendectomy be avoided for complicated appendicitis in children? *J Pediatr Surg* 32:1601, 1997.

16 Krisner SL, Browne A, Dibbins A, et al. Intra-abdominal abscess after laparoscopic appendectomy for perforated appendicitis. *Arch Surg* 136:438, 2001.

17 McKinlay R, Neeleman S, Klein R, et al. Intra-abdominal abscess following open and laparoscopic appendectomy in the pediatric population. *Surg Endosc* 17:730, 2003.

18 Newman K, Ponsky T, Kittle K, et al. Appendicitis 2000: variability in practice, outcomes, and resource utilization at thirty pediatric hospitals. *J Pediatr Surg* 38:372, 2003.

19 Emil S, Laberge JM, Mikhail P, et al. Appendicitis in children: A ten-year update of therapeutic recommendations. *J Pediatr Surg* 38:236, 2003.

20 Puri P, McGuinness EPJ, Guiney EJ. Fertility following perforated appendicitis in girls. *J Pediatr Surg* 24:547, 1989.

21 Nitecki S, Karmeli R, Sarr MG. Appendiceal calculi and fecaliths as indications for appendectomy. *Surg Gynecol Obstet* 17:185, 1990.

22 Steinberg R, Freund E, Yaniv I, et al. A plea for incidental appendectomy in pediatric patients with malignancy. *Pediatr Hematol Oncol* 16:431, 1999.

23 Sumfest JM, Burns MW, Mitchell ME. The Mitrofanoff principle in urinary reconstruction. *J Urol* 150:1875, 1993.

24 Griffiths DM, Malone PS. The Malone antegrade continence enema. *J Pediatr Surg* 30:68, 1995.

25 Crombleholme TM, Harrison MR, Langer JC, et al. Biliary appendico-duodenostomy: a non-refluxing conduit for biliary reconstruction. *J Pediatr Surg* 24:665, 1989.

26 Gauderer MW, Boyle JT. Cholecytoappendicostomy in a child with Alagille syndrome. *J Pediatr Surg* 32:166, 1997.

LIVER AND PANCREATIC DISORDERS

26

ACUTE AND RECURRENT PANCREATITIS

Michelle Maria Pietzak, M.D.

INTRODUCTION

Pancreatitis occurs not uncommonly in the pediatric population. However, because its symptoms often mimic more frequently encountered medical conditions, such as acute gastroenteritis, it is often not recognized. The astute physician must have a low threshold to test for the nonspecific symptoms that occur with this inflammatory process. Pancreatitis is an inflammatory process that occurs in the clinical setting of characteristic abdominal and back pain. In the acute state, it should be accompanied by elevations of the pancreatic enzymes—amylase and lipase. The different types of pancreatitis can be classified into acute, chronic, hereditary, hemorrhagic, or necrotic according to the timing of the illness, clinical symptoms, family history, and radiographic findings.

Acute pancreatitis is usually a self-limited process characterized by the classic symptoms of nausea, vomiting, anorexia, epigastric pain, and back pain. Although a child may suffer from repeated bouts of acute pancreatitis, the symptoms and enzyme elevations should completely resolve between attacks. Pancreatic function remains intact and the pancreatic morphology is undisturbed. Acute pancreatitis may lead to chronic pancreatitis if the signs and symptoms of inflammation are

progressive. Chronicity may be accompanied by temporary or permanent loss of both exocrine and endocrine function. The severe pain that accompanies this condition can be debilitating and lead to dependence on narcotics. Within the gland itself, protein plugs may calcify, indicating advanced disease (Fig. 26-1). Patients with hereditary pancreatitis, by definition, will have a family history of the disease. These diseases are autosomal-dominant and affected family members will often present with recurrent bouts of pancreatitis starting in childhood. Hemorrhagic and necrotic pancreatitis are uncommon in the pediatric population, but are a significant cause of morbidity and mortality. A secondary bacterial infection can occur within the gland, leading to bacteremia, shock, and multiorgan system failure.

EPIDEMIOLOGY

Although pancreatitis is seen more often in adults, it is likely underdiagnosed in the pediatric population. Its true identification requires a high index of suspicion on the part of the clinician with a prompt evaluation before its resolution. In the literature, most publications on this disease in childhood are restricted to reports of either an isolated patient or small clusters of patients. Because of this, the true

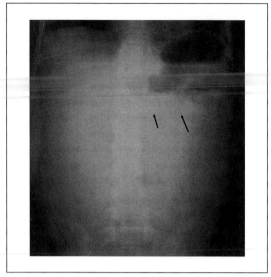

FIGURE 26-1

CALCIFIED PANCREAS SEEN ON KUB
A 6-year-old female presented with a 3-month history of abdominal pain and distention due to severe pancreatitis. KUB revealed ascites and extensive pancreatic calcifications (arrows). Ascitic fluid was markedly hemorrhagic and ERCP was normal. The child was later found to have two different mutations in the CFTR gene.

incidence and prevalence of the disease in this population are unknown. The most common pancreatic disorder in childhood is thought to be acute pancreatitis; the second most common is cystic fibrosis.

ETIOLOGY AND PATHOPHYSIOLOGY

Despite its varied causes, the clinical characteristics of acute pancreatitis follow a similar pattern. Damage occurs to the pancreatic acinar cell by an inciting event, leading to premature activation of the digestive enzymes while still within the cell. This trigger may be infectious, traumatic, metabolic, drug-associated, or related to an underlying anatomic anomaly. An inflammatory response occurs to these damaged cells, activating platelets, and the complement system. Proinflammatory cytokines are released, including nitric oxide, interleukin-1, platelet activating factor, and tumor necrosis factor-alpha.[1] These inflammatory mediators, as well as released additional free radicals and

other vasoactive substances, damage the gland directly, resulting in edema, ischemia, necrosis, and eventual loss of glandular tissue with atrophy. Systemic shock may occur in severe cases, as demonstrated by tachycardia, hypotension, hypoxia, and *adult respiratory distress syndrome* (ARDS).

In contrast to adults, where the majority of cases of pancreatitis are related to either alcohol consumption or gallstone disease, the causes of pediatric pancreatitis are more varied (Table 26-1). In adolescent females, gallstones are a common cause of pancreatitis. In young children, it is more common to have been exposed to an inciting event, such as recent exposure to a medication, infection, or trauma. Recurrent pancreatitis in childhood can be due to hereditary pancreatitis, an anatomic variant of the pancreatic or biliary tree, or an underlying systemic or metabolic disorder. Despite exhaustive investigation, up to 25% of pediatric patients will not have an attributable cause for their pancreatitis.

Anatomic

Congenital defects of the pancreas are rare, but if left uncorrected can lead to chronic pancreatitis. The most common anatomic variant is pancreatic divisum, which occurs when the dorsal and ventral pancreatic ducts fail to fuse during fetal development. This then directs flow primarily to the dorsal duct.[2] While some believe that pancreatic divisum is a variant of normal, and that most people with this anatomy will not experience pancreatitis, others think this variant to be a significant cause of recurrent pancreatitis which requires endoscopic or surgical correction. Any change in anatomy which results in duodenal obstruction, such as strictures, tumors, duplications or diverticula of the duodenum or pancreas, or duodenal hematoma from either accidental or nonaccidental trauma (child abuse) can also lead to pancreatitis.

Traumatic

Trauma is possibly the most common cause of pancreatitis in childhood, and it is likely underestimated in the acute setting. Motor vehicle and bicycle accidents can result in blunt trauma to the pancreas from seat belts and handlebars. Findings

CONDITIONS ASSOCIATED WITH PANCREATITIS IN THE PEDIATRIC POPULATION

Anatomic

Ampullary diverticulum or stenosis

Annular pancreas

Biliary tract malformations

Choledochal cyst or choledochocele

Choledochopancreaticoductal junction anomaly

Cholelithiasis (gallstones)

Common bile duct: absence or anomalous insertion

Duodenal obstruction from diverticulum, hematoma, tumor, or stricture

Duodenal ulcer—perforated

Duplication cyst of the common bile duct, duodenum, gastropancreatic area

Gastric trichobezoar

Pancreatic aplasia, hypoplasia, dysplasia, heterotopy or divisum

Pancreatic duct: absence or anomalous insertion

Pancreatic pseudocyst

Pancreatic tumors

Sclerosing cholangitis

Sphincter of Oddi dysfunction

Hereditary/Metabolic/Systemic

Alpha1-antitrypsin deficiency

Anorexia nervosa/bulimia

Autoimmune disease

Brain tumor

Collagen-vascular disease (dermatomyositis)

Congenital partial lipodystrophy

Cystic fibrosis

Dehydration with hypovolemia and shock

Diabetes mellitus (with or without ketoacidosis)

Glycogen storage disease types Ia and Ib

Hemochromatosis

Hereditary pancreatitis

Hyperalimentation (parenteral nutrition)

Hypercalcemia

Hyperlipidemia types I, IV, and V

Hyperparathyroidism

Hypertriglyceridemia

Hypothermia

Inborn errors of metabolism (cytochrome c oxidase deficiency and organic acidemias, such as homocystinuria, isovaleric acidemia, methylmalonic acidemia, and maple syrup urine disease)

Inflammatory bowel disease (Crohn's disease and ulcerative colitis)

Juvenile tropical pancreatitis

Liver disease (Wilson's disease and Reye's syndrome)

Malnutrition with or without refeeding syndrome

Peritonitis

Renal failure with uremia (hemolytic-uremic syndrome)

Sarcoidosis

Sepsis with shock

Transplantation (bone marrow, heart, kidney, liver, pancreas)

Vascular diseases (Henoch-Schönlein purpura, Kawasaki disease, periarteritis nodosa, systemic lupus erythematosus)

Infectious

Ascaris lumbricoides (duct obstruction)

Campylobacter fetus

Clonorchis sinensis (duct obstruction)

Coxsackie B virus

Cryptosporidium

Cytomegalovirus

Echovirus

Enterovirus

Escherichia coli (verotoxin-producing)

Hepatitis A and B viruses

Human immunodeficiency virus

Influenza A and B viruses

Legionnaire disease

Leptospirosis

Malaria

Measles

Mumps

Mycobacteria

Mycoplasma

Rubella

Rubeola

Toxoplasma

Typhoid fever

Varicella

Yersinia

Traumatic

Blunt injury to the abdomen (motor vehicle and bicycle accidents)

Burns

Contrast from ductal imaging (ERCP and PTC)

Head trauma

Nonaccidental trauma (child abuse)

Radiation to the abdomen

Surgical trauma

Total body cast with immobilization

on physical examination consistent with trauma in the absence of a reliable history should raise the suspicion for child abuse.

Medications

Numerous medications and naturally occurring toxins have been reported as causes of pancreatitis (Table 26-2). Classes of medications most likely to cause pancreatitis include antibiotics, anticonvulsants, antihypertensives, anti-inflammatory, and antineoplastic agents. Most of the drugs mentioned in this chapter have a proposed but unproven pathophysiology, and very few have documented an established causal (as opposed to an associated) relationship to the disease.

Infectious

Worldwide, bacteria, viruses, and parasites account for a significant number of cases of pancreatitis in the pediatric population. For example, the verotoxin-producing strain of *Escherichia coli* associated with *hemolytic uremic syndrome* (HUS) can cause pancreatitis. Varicella and influenza B viruses, associated with Reye's syndrome, have also been implicated in acute pancreatitis of childhood. Parasites common in developing areas, such as *Ascaris* and *Clonorchis*, can migrate into the biliary tree, leading to obstructive jaundice and pancreatitis. Left untreated, this obstruction can lead to severe portal hypertension, liver failure, and death.

The risk for developing acute pancreatitis is higher in children with *acquired immuno deficiency syndrome* (AIDS). One Italian study in symptomatic human immunodeficiency virus (HIV)-infected children demonstrated pancreatic biochemical abnormalities in 15% of patients.[3] At autopsy, children with HIV had frequent pancreatic involvement, defined as edema, inflammation, fibrosis, inspissated material, and enlarged islets of Langerhans.[4] HIV+ patients

TABLE 26-2

DRUGS AND TOXINS ASSOCIATED WITH PANCREATITIS

Antiarrhythmics: procainamide
Antibiotics: erythromycin, isoniazid, metronidazole, nitrofurantoin, paromomycin, penicillin, pentamidine, rifampin, sulfonamides, tetracycline, trimethoprim-sulfamethoxazole
Anticoagulants
Anticonvulsants: carbamazepine, valproic acid
Antihistamines: cyproheptadine, diphenoxylate
Antihypertensives and diuretics: bumetanide, chlorthalidone, clonidine, diazoxide, enalapril, ethacrynic acid, furosemide, methyldopa, thiazides
Anti-inflammatory agents: acetaminophen (when overdosed), corticosteroids, ibuprofen, indomethacin, mesalamine, nonsteroidal anti-inflammatory drugs, piroxicam, salicylates, sulfasalazine, sulindac
Antilipemics: cholestyramine
Antineoplastic agents: asparaginase, azathioprine, cisplatin, cytosine arabinoside, mercaptopurine, cyclophosphamide, methotrexate, vincristine
Antipsychotics: clozapine
Antithyroids: propylthiouracil
Antiviral agents: didanosine (ddI), dideoxycytidine (ddC), lamivudine (3TC), zalcitabine (ddC)
Anxiolytics: meprobamate
Drugs of abuse: alcohol, amphetamines, heroin, narcotics (propoxyphene napsylate), opiates
Histamine2 antagonists: cimetidine, ranitidine
Hormones: corticotropin (ACTH), estrogen, histamine, octreotide
Toxins: boric acid, organophosphates, scorpion venom, spider venom
Vitamins and minerals: calcium, vitamin A (retinoic acid), vitamin D

can develop elevated enzymes due to HIV infection itself, or other coinfections, such as cytomegalovirus (CMV), *Toxoplasma*, *Mycobacterium*, and *Cryptosporidium*. Many of the pharmacologic agents used to inhibit HIV can cause pancreatitis (Table 26-2). In the HIV-infected patient, hyperamylasemia without pancreatitis can occur due to renal failure, AIDS-associated nephropathy, or salivary hyperamylasemia from parotid gland disease. Kaposi's sarcoma and lymphoma can also affect the pancreas, although these are rare in childhood.

Hereditary, Metabolic, and Systemic Diseases

The most common inherited disease of the exocrine pancreas is thought to be cystic fibrosis. This disease, which is autosomal recessive, is caused by mutations in the *cystic fibrosis transmembrane conductance regulator* (CFTR) gene. CFTR is located on the apical membrane of the epithelial cells that line the pancreatic ducts, and it promotes dilution and alkalinization of the secretions as they flow through the ductular network. CF is the only known hereditary disease in which there can be both pancreatitis and pancreatic exocrine insufficiency in the absence of inflammation. Surprisingly, patients with CF and pancreatic insufficiency do not develop acute relapsing pancreatitis, presumably due to loss of functional acinar tissue. Although CF may be one of the more common causes of pancreatitis in childhood, it is believed that only 2% of individuals with CF experience pancreatitis as a result of ductal plugging due to mutant CFTR. Even in the absence of lung disease, there appears to be a strong correlation between specific CFTR mutations and idiopathic and chronic pancreatitis.[5,6] Patients with recurrent pancreatitis without any obvious cause should be screened for CF with a sweat chloride test and CFTR mutational analysis. The role of CFTR in pancreatitis and other diseases of the pancreas is the subject of ongoing research.

The second most common cause of chronic pancreatitis in childhood is believed to be hereditary pancreatitis. The two known types of hereditary pancreatitis are clinically similar, and involve different mutations within the same gene. Both types are autosomal dominant with 80% penetrance.[7] The majority of affected patients report symptoms before the age of 15 years, with some symptomatic even before the age of 5 years. The gene involved is located on chromosome 7q35 and codes for *cationic trypsinogen* (PRSS1). Both mutations result in a form of trypsin that resists degradation by mesotrypsin and enzyme Y, allowing trypsinogen to become activated to trypsin within the pancreas instead of within the duodenum. This leads to uncontrolled activation of other pancreatic enzymes within the acinar cell, resulting in autodigestion and inflammation. The attacks of acute pancreatitis are remarkably only intermittent. It is thought that this uncontrolled activation of other enzymes only occurs when trypsin exceeds the capacity of pancreatic secretory trypsin inhibitor, the "secondary brake" within the pancreatic gland. Identification of those with hereditary pancreatitis is critical, as affected patients are at increased risk for pseudocysts, pancreatic adenocarcinoma, and exocrine and endocrine failure.

Since the discovery that hereditary pancreatitis can be caused by mutations in PRSS1, researchers have been searching for other potential candidate genes that may predispose patients to chronic pancreatitis. Given that the proposed mechanism for pancreatitis with PRSS1 mutations is decreased inactivation, one candidate gene is that which encodes for pancreatic secretory trypsin inhibitor or serine protease inhibitor, *Kazal type I* (SPINK1).[8] SPINK1 mutations have been reported in familial, hereditary, tropical, and idiopathic chronic pancreatitis. Whether or not SPINK1 mutations modify an already underlying genetic disease has yet to be elucidated.

Pancreatitis has been a reported complication in children who have received heart, kidney, liver, pancreas, and bone marrow transplants. Following liver transplantation, it can be life threatening, and is associated with a higher risk for infectious peritonitis and emergency retransplantation. As with autoimmune and collagen-vascular diseases, it is difficult to distinguish between the contributions of medications versus the primary disease process to the development of the pancreatitis.

CLINICAL SIGNS AND SYMPTOMS

The classic signs of acute pancreatitis are nausea, vomiting, anorexia, and abdominal pain. The pain is typically located in the epigastrium, with radiation to the back. However, the pain can also be periumbilical, right upper quadrant, or lower chest. Eating exacerbates the abdominal discomfort and may trigger bilious emesis. The review of systems should inquire about rashes, diarrhea, joint pain, and other signs of vasculitis. A family history of pancreatitis should raise suspicion for hereditary and metabolic diseases.

More common causes of acute abdominal pain in childhood may be differentiated from pancreatitis by a thorough physical examination. Fever, though not always present, is usually low grade. Tachycardia and hypotension may be present early in the course of the illness. Tachypnea with hypoxemia may indicate developing pulmonary edema. In advanced stages of the disease, the child may be icteric and ill appearing, with a distended abdomen and decreased bowel sounds. This may be due to an ileus, ascites, or a mass from a pancreatic phlegmon or pseudocyst. While lying supine, the patient may experience some relief of pain when the knees are drawn up to a flexed trunk. When there has been pancreatic hemorrhage or necrosis, two signs may be present: Grey Turner sign, which is a blue discoloration of the flank; and Cullen's sign, where there is blue discoloration around the pancreas. The child should also be examined for the physical findings of child abuse.

COMPLICATIONS

The complications of pancreatitis can be severe, multisystemic, and life threatening (Table 26-3).

TABLE 26-3

COMPLICATIONS ASSOCIATED WITH PANCREATITIS

Acidosis	Hypoalbuminemia
Adult respiratory distress syndrome	Hypocalcemia
Ascites	Hypotension
Atelectasis	Ileus
Biliary obstruction	Jaundice
Bowel infarction	Mediastinal abscess
Calculi	Pancreatic abscess
Diabetes mellitus	Pancreatic carcinoma
Disseminated intravascular coagulation (DIC)	Pancreatic fibrosis
Duct strictures	Pancreatic necrosis
Electrocardiographic changes	Peptic ulcer
Encephalopathy	Pericardial effusion
Exocrine insufficiency	Phlegmon
Fat emboli	Pleural effusion
Fat necrosis	Pneumonitis
Fistula	Portal vein thrombosis
Gastritis	Pseudocyst
Gastrointestinal fistula	Psychosis
Hemorrhage	Renal failure
Hepatic vein thrombosis	Renal vessel thrombosis
Hepatorenal syndrome	Respiratory failure
Hyperglycemia	Sepsis
Hyperkalemia	Splenic vein varices
Hypertriglyceridemia	Sudden death
	Thrombosis

The major cause of mortality in pediatric patients with acute pancreatitis is infection, which can result in pancreatic abscess, infected pseudocyst, or even necrosis of the gland. Evidence of infection within a defined area can be obtained by a fine-needle aspiration under radiographic guidance using *ultrasound* (US) or *computed tomography* (CT). Gram stain and culture of the aspirate are clinically useful. Often, enteric organisms are recovered, such as *E. coli*, *Klebsiella* species, and other gram-negative rods.[9] In the patient with necrotizing pancreatitis, treatment with an antibiotic which has broad-spectrum activity against both aerobic and anaerobic bacteria is suggested.[10]

Chronic pancreatitis can lead to pancreatic atrophy with exocrine and/or endocrine insufficiency. Severe, prolonged cases may require insulin, pancreatic enzyme replacement, and an elemental or low-fat diet to optimize absorption once enteral feedings are reinitiated.

DIAGNOSIS WITH DIFFERENTIAL

Blood Tests

Routine blood tests can differentiate acute pancreatitis from some of the more common causes of abdominal pain in the pediatric population. A complete blood cell count with differential may reveal leukocytosis with a left shift, or hemoconcentration from dehydration. A routine chemistry panel may reveal hyperglycemia and elevated total bilirubin, *alanine aminotransferase* (ALT), and *aspartate aminotransferase* (AST). Anemia, azotemia, hypoalbuminemia, hypocalcemia, and an elevated lactate dehydrogenase level suggest advanced disease with hemorrhage and pancreatic damage.

The most common laboratory tests used to screen for acute pancreatitis are serum amylase and lipase. Amylase levels begin to rise within 2–12 h and peak at 12–72 h after the initial pancreatic insult.[11] However, an isolated serum amylase level has a relatively low sensitivity (75–92%) and specificity (20–60%).[12] This is because normal amylase levels may be seen with pancreatitis, and hyperamylasemia can result from many diseases that are not of pancreatic origin (Table 26-4). If the amylase level is three to six times above the upper limit of normal for

TABLE 26-4

CONDITIONS OTHER THAN PANCREATITIS ASSOCIATED WITH ELEVATED SERUM AMYLASE

Abdominal aortic aneurysm
Alcoholism
Anorexia nervosa or bulimia
Appendicitis
Biliary tract disease or obstruction
Burns
Cardiopulmonary bypass
Choledocholithiasis
Cirrhosis
Cystic fibrosis
Diabetic ketoacidosis
Drugs
Hepatitis
Heroin addiction
Intestinal infarction, obstruction, or perforation
Lung cancer
Macroamylasemia
Opiates
Ovarian cyst or tumor
Pancreatic duct obstruction or tumor
Parotitis
Peptic ulcer—perforated
Peritonitis
Pneumonia
Prostate tumors
Renal insufficiency
Renal transplant
Ruptured ectopic pregnancy
Salivary duct obstruction
Salpingitis
Trauma (to the head or abdomen)
Viral infections (mumps)

that laboratory, specificity increases for pancreatitis, but at the expense of sensitivity.[12] Serum isoamylase level measurements are more discriminatory, as they differentiate between enzymes of salivary and pancreatic origin. Isoamylase levels should be determined if parotitis from a viral infection is suspected (such as with HIV), in the presence of some cancers, or if ovarian disease is present.

Lipase levels begin to increase 4–8 h after the onset of symptoms, and also peak at about 24 h.[13,14]

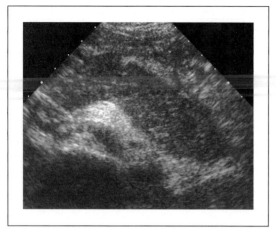

ACUTE PANCREATITIS SEEN ON ABDOMINAL US
A 9-year-old HIV+ female presented with pancreatitis. The head and the body of the pancreas demonstrate decreased echogenicity and are both diffusely enlarged.

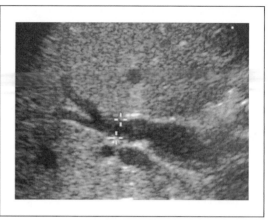

BILIARY DUCTAL DILATATION SEEN ON US
A 7-year-old female presented with chronic pancreatitis. The common bile duct is abnormally dilated, measuring 1.2 cm in diameter. This fusiform enlargement of the common bile duct, proximal to its bifurcation just at the hilus of the liver, is suggestive of a choledochal cyst.

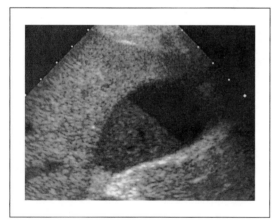

SLUDGE IN THE GALLBLADDER SEEN ON US
Sludge is present in the gallbladder of the same patient as in Fig. 26-2. There is no gallbladder wall thickening or pericholecystic fluid. No calculi were identified; however, they can be obscured by sludge.

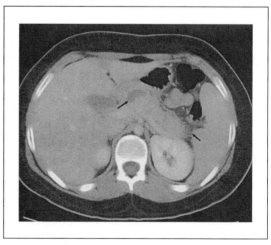

ACUTE PANCREATITIS SEEN ON ABDOMINAL CT
A 4-year-old boy presented with areas of hypodensity within the pancreas, representative of acute pancreatitis. Fluid collections are seen near the pancreatic head and tail (arrows), consistent with inflammatory changes.

However, lipase levels remain elevated for a longer period of time than amylase levels, decreasing over 8–14 days. Serum lipase levels have a reported clinical sensitivity of 86–100% and specificity of 50–99%.[15] If the serum lipase level is greater than three times the upper limit of normal for that laboratory, sensitivity and specificity can be increased to 99–100%.[12] However, significantly elevated lipase, in the presence of normal amylase, has been reported in esophagitis, hypertriglyceridemia, renal insufficiency, acute cholecystitis, and nonpancreatic sources of lipolytic enzymes due to malignant tumors.[16]

Clinical sensitivity for the diagnosis of acute pancreatitis increases to 94% by using serum amylase and lipase level determinations together.[12,16] It is important to note, however, that the degrees of elevation of the amylase and lipase in the plasma in no way reflect the severity of the pancreatic disease process itself. There are serum enzymes more sensitive than amylase which do correlate with disease severity, such as plasma immunoreactive cationic trypsin, pancreatic elastase I, and phospholipase $A_2^{12;}$ however, these tests are not readily available outside of research centers·

Tests of Pancreatic Function

The diagnosis of chronic pancreatitis relies not only on clinical and radiographic findings, but also on tests of pancreatic function.[17] The gold standard for the assessment of pancreatic function involves direct testing for pancreatic insufficiency. This is accomplished via the administration of intravenous secretin or *cholecystokinin* (CCK), and measuring the levels of bicarbonate and pancreatic enzymes from the pancreatic ductal secretions. This requires endoscopic intubation of the duodenum, with accurate placement of a catheter to collect the secretions, under appropriate anesthesia. If performed correctly, the sensitivity and specificity of this procedure for the diagnosis of chronic pancreatitis ranges from 90 to 100%.[18] Because of the challenges in performing and interpreting these examinations, they are usually only available in tertiary centers.

Although not as accurate, noninvasive tests of pancreatic function are more readily available.

Chronic pancreatitis can be demonstrated by decreased enzymes in the blood (amylase, lipase, isoamylase, immunoreactive trypsinogen) or stool (trypsin, pancreatic elastase I), or evidence of malabsorption (increased fecal fat or low serum levels of fat-soluble vitamins). However, because of the generally poor negative predictive value of these tests, chronic pancreatitis cannot be excluded with certainty. False-positive results can be seen with bacterial overgrowth and other mucosal diseases of the small bowel.

Radiographic Studies

A plain abdominal radiograph (KUB: kidney, ureters, and bladder) may demonstrate anomalies in both acute and chronic pancreatitis. Acute pancreatitis may result in an ileus with either a "sentinel" loop of dilated small bowel or colonic distention. Obscured psoas margins and a radiolucent "halo" around the left kidney are also suggestive of pancreatitis. Calcifications can be seen in the area of the pancreatic parenchyma and ductal system with chronic calcific pancreatitis (Fig. 26-1).

Changes in pancreatic size, contour, and texture are best appreciated with an abdominal US.[10] This modality is also excellent at identifying ascites, abscesses, pseudocysts, dilated ducts, and gallstone disease (Figs. 26-2 through 26-4).

An abdominal CT with and without oral and intravenous contrast is useful in imaging the complications of long-standing pancreatitis.[10] CT can provide guidance in the aspiration and drainage of an abscess, phlegmon, or pseudocyst. Prior to any type of surgical intervention, such as necrostomy (surgical debridement for necrosis), CT may be used to further define the peripancreatic anatomy and rule out other complications such as a portal vein thrombosis (Figs. 26-5 through 26-8).

In chronic pancreatitis and recurrent attacks of acute pancreatitis, a more detailed anatomy of the pancreatic and biliary tree is necessary. Cholangiopancreatography may be accomplished by *endoscopic retrograde cholangiopancreatography* (ERCP), *magnetic resonance cholangiopancreatography* (MRCP), or via a direct cholangiogram performed either percutaneously or intraoperatively.

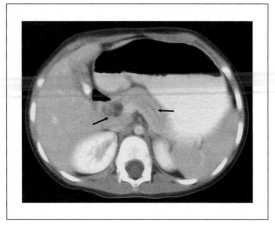

FIGURE 26-6

BILIARY DUCTAL DILATATION DEMONSTRATED ON CT
CT of the abdomen is from the same patient as in Fig. 26-4. The extrahepatic bile duct and pancreatic duct are dilatated (arrows). The pancreas has normal density. Intrahepatic ductal dilatation was seen on other sections. The differential diagnosis of these findings include choledochal cyst, Caroli's disease, and sclerosing cholangitis.

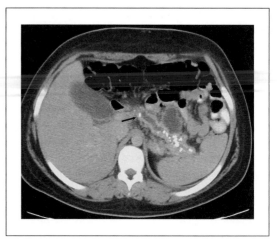

FIGURE 26-7

CALCIFIED CHRONIC PANCREATITIS SEEN ON CT
A 14-year-old obese girl had complained of abdominal pain with nausea and vomiting for several months. She was found to have a hiatal hernia, and underwent laparoscopic fundoplication. Her abdominal pain persisted, and this CT scan was ordered. There is fatty atrophy of the pancreas with multiple punctuate and small calcifications consistent with chronic pancreatitis. The pancreatic duct is dilated, measuring 1.2 cm at the uncinate process. There is a calcification in the duct near the ampulla of Vater (arrow), which appears to be lodged in the common bile duct, causing proximal dilatation. There are several small pseudocysts in the upper abdomen. The largest is in the lesser sac just inferior to the stomach, measuring 3 cm x 4 cm x 3 cm, with inflammation present. This patient remains dependent on parenteral (intravenous) nutrition. Her case emphasizes the need to consider pancreatitis even in older children with the nonspecific complaints of nausea and vomiting.

ERCP is the study of choice to visualize anatomic malformations, such as pancreas divisum or an anomalous pancreaticobiliary duct junction.[2] ERCP may be difficult in very small children due to the large diameter of the endoscope required. ERCP, as opposed to MRCP, has the added benefit of being a therapeutic modality. Sphincterotomy, stent placement, and stone removal can all be performed at the time of the initial diagnostic evaluation. Sphincter of Oddi manometry demonstrating elevated basal pressures consistent with dysfunction is useful, as these patients may benefit from endoscopic sphincterotomy. These procedures should be performed at centers with significant experience in diagnostic and therapeutic ERCP, and in managing severe cases of childhood pancreatitis. A pediatric surgeon should be available at the center, as the complications of ERCP can include duct perforation or worsening of the pancreatitis due to contrast. This may lead to the formation of an abscess, phlegmon, or pseudocyst requiring surgical drainage. However, when performed by experienced endoscopists, therapeutic ERCP in selected pediatric patients has been reported to have a lower rate of complications than in the adult population.[13]

MRCP should be reserved for patients who are too small or too clinically unstable to receive general anesthesia to undergo ERCP. This modality has proven useful in determining the presence of pancreaticobiliary disease, the level of biliary obstruction, and the presence of malignancy or bile duct calculi.[19] The quality of the MRCP images depend on the ability of the patient to remain still (which may require sedation in small children), and if the MRCP equipment and computer programs

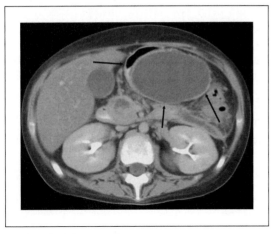

FIGURE   26-8

GIANT PSEUDOCYST SEEN ON CT
An 11-year-old girl presented with chronic pancreatitis undergoing treatment for acute lymphoblastic leukemia. A massive 19 cm × 5.5 cm × 8.5 cm pseudocyst is visualized in the left upper quadrant (arrows). There is also edema and necrosis within the pancreatic tissue, and a smaller pseudocyst within the pancreatic head. Free fluid is present in the abdomen. Stranding within the mesentery of the left upper quadrant is consistent with chronic inflammation. The liver shows fatty infiltration with a normal gallbladder. This pseudocyst remarkably resolved without surgical intervention.

are regularly updated. Interpretation also requires a skilled radiologist familiar with pancreaticobiliary tree anomalies.

If an anatomic variant is suspected and ERCP or MRCP are not possible, the next appropriate step is direct imaging of the pancreaticobiliary system with contrast. This can be performed either percutaneously or intraoperatively. A percutaneous cholangiogram may be performed in the presence of dilated ducts, or through a biliary drain placed postoperatively from pancreatic surgical debridement or orthotopic liver transplant. This type of study requires a skilled interventional radiologist. In the absence of dilated ducts or a biliary drain, transduodenal exploration with intraoperative pancreatography can be performed. Like ERCP, intraoperative imaging can likewise be a therapeutic modality at the time of initial diagnostic evaluation.

If minor or major papillae stenosis is found, surgical sphincteroplasty can be concurrently performed a "sentinel" loop of dilated small bowel.

GUIDELINES FOR TREATMENT AND FOLLOW-UP

The management of acute, uncomplicated pancreatitis in childhood is mainly supportive. The patient should be provided adequate hydration, pain relief, and pancreatic rest.[10] The child should be made *nil per os* in severe cases, which will decrease the cephalic, gastric, and intestinal phases of pancreatic secretion. Continuous or intermittent nasogastric suction may be required in cases with ileus or persistent emesis. If the child is expected to be without enteral feedings for more than 3 days, parenteral nutrition should be initiated to prevent protein catabolism. Recent studies have suggested that nasojejunal feedings with an elemental diet, which bypass the duodenum completely and therefore do not potently stimulate pancreatic secretion, are just as safe as parenteral nutrition in adults with severe to acute pancreatitis. Nasojejunal feeds are also less costly, have less metabolic complications, and may shorten length of stay.[20] Antibiotics are not normally indicated, unless there are signs of sepsis, necrotic pancreatitis, or multiorgan system failure. Histamine (H2) receptor antagonists may help to prevent stress ulceration by reducing duodenal acidification. Current research targeting the inflammatory cascade may also lead to therapies that are beneficial to acute pancreatitis, regardless of the etiology.

Adequate treatment of pain in acute, severe pancreatitis of childhood can be challenging as it may be difficult to relieve a child's pain completely. Opiates have been reported to worsen symptoms by increasing spasm of the sphincter of Oddi. Meperidine is the analgesic of choice of all the pure opiate agonists, because it produces the smallest increase in enterobiliary pressure. We have also used hydromorphone hydrochloride as a continuous infusion in many children with severe, acute pancreatitis, as well as in chronic and complicated pancreatitis, with excellent pain control.

Pancreatic infections may necessitate surgical intervention. However, whether a sterile abscess, pseudocyst or necrosis requires operative management is still controversial.[10] Antibiotics and intensive care usually provide adequate support for the patient who has sterile necrosis. The presence of persistent ileus, bowel perforation, portal vein thrombosis, and multisystem organ failure are "red flags" which indicate urgent surgical intervention. Infected pancreatic necrosis is an absolute surgical indication, requiring necrosectomy, which is thought to stop the progression of the necrotizing process and resultant multiorgan failure. Debridement, rather than total or partial pancreatic resection, is preferred as it preserves exocrine and endocrine function. It may be necessary for the patient to undergo multiple reoperations or continuous lavage with catheters left in the retroperitoneum. Necrosectomy itself may cause further complications such as sepsis; hemorrhage; wound infection; and fistulas of the pancreas, intestine, and biliary system.

SHORT- AND LONG-TERM PROGNOSIS

Most cases of acute pancreatitis in childhood are isolated and uncomplicated, persisting usually for less than a week, and rarely progressing to chronic pancreatitis. The chances of surviving a severe or complicated course of pancreatitis are directly related to the other organ systems involved. Associated complications can affect virtually all organ systems (Table 26-3). The primary morbidity and mortality arise from septic shock, renal failure, respiratory failure, and inflammatory masses of the pancreas.

The *acute physiology and chronic health evaluation* (APACHE-II) and Ranson criteria, that have been developed to predict the outcome from acute pancreatitis in adults, are not as reliable in young children. Pediatric studies have shown a mortality rate of 5–17.5% from an initially mild presentation of acute pancreatitis to upward of 80–100% from hemorrhagic pancreatitis or severe multisystem disorders. After a bout of necrotizing pancreatitis, exocrine and endocrine insufficiency are common.

The degree of dysfunction correlates directly with the extent of parenchymal damage.

For patients with traumatic pancreatitis, in the absence of complete duct transection, nonoperative management is believed to be safe and there are usually no long-term complications.[21] Identification of those with hereditary pancreatitis is critical, as affected family members are at increased risk for pseudocysts, pancreatic adenocarcinomas, and exocrine and endocrine failure.

CONCLUSIONS

The clinician needs to have a high index of suspicion for pancreatitis in the child who presents with the nonspecific but common symptoms of nausea, vomiting, and abdominal pain. A thorough history that emphasizes recent infections, medications, trauma, and any underlying medical condition may clarify the diagnosis. Serum enzyme testing alone (amylase and lipase) for the diagnosis of both acute and chronic pancreatitis may not be adequate, since the clinical specificity remains suboptimal.

Unlike pancreatitis in adults, in which the majority of cases are due to either gallstone disease or alcoholism, this disease in childhood can be from a variety of disparate causes. No identifying factor is present in up to 25% of cases. Common known etiologies include infection, trauma, medications, abnormal anatomy, and hereditary or systemic diseases. A family history of pancreatitis, especially occurring at a young age, should prompt the physician to look for evidence of anatomic abnormalities or inherited biochemical defects.

US remains the initial radiographic study of choice to screen for infection, cholelithiasis, congenital abnormalities, and biliary ductal dilatation. CT is useful in diagnosing and managing the child with a complicated course. If the pancreatitis is chronic or recurrent, further detailed imaging of the biliary system should be performed with ERCP, MRCP, or percutaneous or intraoperative cholangiogram.

Treatment of acute, uncomplicated pancreatitis in the pediatric population is basically supportive, and most children will recover without sequelae. Complications, when they occur, can involve every major organ system and be life threatening. Children with severe or complicated pancreatitis should be managed at a center with expertise in pediatric biliary surgery and nonoperative radiologic and endoscopic interventions.

References

1 Karne S, Gorelick FS. Etiopathogenesis of acute pancreatitis. *Surg Clin North Am* 79:699, 1999.

2 Kamelmaz I, Elitsur Y. Pancreas divisum-the role of ERCP in children. *W V Med J* 95:14, 1999.

3 Carroccio A, Fontana M, Spagnuolo MI, et al. Serum pancreatic enzymes in human immunodeficiency virus-infected children. A collaborative study of the Italian Society of Pediatric Gastroenterology and Hepatology. *Scand J Gastroenterol* 33:998, 1998.

4 Kahn E, Anderson VM, Greco A, et al. Pancreatic disorders in pediatric acquired immune deficiency syndrome. *Hum Pathol* 26:765, 1995.

5 Cohn JA, Friedman KJ, Noone PG, et al. Relation between mutations of the cystic fibrosis gene and idiopathic pancreatitis. *N Engl J Med* 339:653, 1998.

6 Sharer N, Schwarz M, Malone G, et al. Mutations of the cystic fibrosis gene in patients with chronic pancreatitis. *N Engl J Med* 339:645, 1998.

7 Whitcomb DC, Gorry MC, Preston RA, et al. A gene for hereditary pancreatitis maps to chromosome 7q35. *Gastroenterology* 110:1975, 1996.

8 Pfützer RH, Barmada MM, Brunskill APJ, et al. SPINK1/PSTI polymorphisms act as disease modifiers in familial and idiopathic chronic pancreatitis. *Gastroenterology* 119:615, 2000.

9 Luiten EJ, Hop WC, Lange JF, et al. Differential prognosis of gram-negative versus gram-positive infected and sterile pancreatic necrosis: results of a randomized trial in patients with severe, acute pancreatitis treated with adjuvant selective decontamination. *Clin Infect Dis* 25:811, 1997.

10 Banks PA. Practice guidelines in acute pancreatitis. *Am J Gastroenterol* 92:377, 1997.

11 Pieper-Bigelow C, Strocchi A, Levitt MD. Where does serum amylase come from and where does it go? *Gastroenterol Clin North Am* 19:793, 1990.

12 Tietz NW. Support of the diagnosis of pancreatitis by enzyme tests-old problems, new techniques. *Clin Chim Acta* 257:257, 1997.

13 Guelrud M. Endoscopic therapy of pancreatic disease in children. *Gastrointest Endosc Clin North Am* 8:195, 1998.

14 Gwodz GP, Steinberg WM, Werner M, et al. Comparative evaluation of the diagnosis of acute pancreatitis based on serum and urine enzyme assays. *Clin Chim Acta* 187:243, 1990.

15 Agarwal N, Pitchumoni CS, Sivaprasad AV. Evaluating tests for acute pancreatitis. *Am J Gastroenterol* 85:356, 1990.

16 Frank B, Gottlieb K. Amylase normal, lipase elevated: is it pancreatitis? A case series and review of the literature. *Am J Gastroenterol* 94:463, 1999.

17 Clain JE, Pearson RK. Diagnosis of chronic pancreatitis. *Surg Clin North Am* 79:829, 1999.

18 Heiji HA, Obertop H, Schmitz PIM, et al. Evaluation of the secretin-cholecystokinin test for chronic pancreatitis by discriminant analysis. *Scand J Gastroenterol* 21:35, 1986.

19 Hirohashi S, Hirohashi R, Uchida H, et al. Pancreatitis: evaluation with MR cholangiopancreatography in children. *Radiology* 203:411, 1997.

20 Abou-Assi S, Craig K, O'Keefe SJ. Hypocaloric jejunal feeding is better than total parenteral nutrition in acute pancreatitis: Results of a randomized, comparative study. *Am J Gastroenterol* 97:2255, 2002.

21 Holland AJ, Davey RB, Sparnon AL, et al. Traumatic pancreatitis: long-term review of initial non-operative management in children. *Paediatr Child Health* 35:78, 1999.

27

VIRAL HEPATITIS

Lynda Brady

INTRODUCTION

The 1990s were remarkable for the field of viral hepatitis. New viruses were discovered and treatments and vaccines were developed which changed the natural history of viral hepatitis disease. There are six known hepatitis viruses: A, B, C, D, E, and G. The epidemiology, clinical presentation, and treatments of these different forms of infectious hepatitis will be discussed in this chapter. A discussion of hepatitis would not be complete without discussing *fulminant hepatic failure* (FHF) from non-A-G, likely a yet-undiscovered hepatitis virus.

HEPATITIS A

Hepatitis A (HAV) is an RNA picovirus with a single serotype worldwide. HAV causes acute or asymptomatic infection; there is no chronic infection. Immunity conferred from the acute infection is life-long.

Epidemiology

The prevalence of HAV differs throughout the world. It accounts for 20–25% of symptomatic hepatitis worldwide. Endemic areas are found in developing countries that have poor sanitary condi-

tions. These countries have a high incidence of HAV infection in childhood. Infections in these areas are contracted through infected water or food supplies or person-to-person contact. In developed countries, infections usually come in "outbreaks." In these outbreaks, transmission is initially through an infected source then extends through person-to-person contact. It is difficult to stop the spread of the virus since many patients, particularly children, are asymptomatic.

Clinical Presentation

Patients with symptomatic HAV infection characteristically have acute onset of abdominal pain, nausea, vomiting, and fatigue. The presence of jaundice depends on the age of the patients:

- 10% of children under 6 years
- 40–50% of older children (6–14 years)
- 70–80% of older adolescents and adults

The incubation period is 30 days with a range of 15–50 days. The illness is self-limited in the vast majority of cases. Fulminant hepatic failure occurs in 0.1% of patients. Cholestatic hepatitis can develop and take months to resolve and a small number of patients develop relapsing symptoms. Diagnosis is made through detection of anti-HAV IgM (see Fig. 27-1).

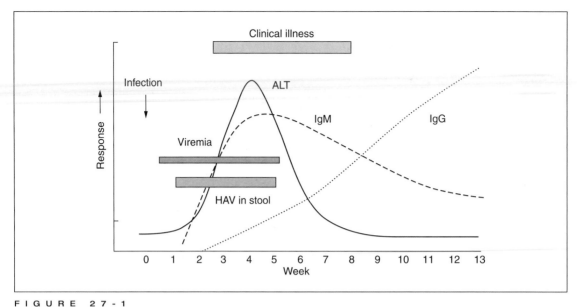

SEROLOGIC CHANGES FOLLOWING HAV INFECTION

Treatment

Hepatitis A infection is usually self-limited with good prognosis for recovery and development of life-long immunity. Treatment during the active infection is supportive. In patients with persistent cholestasis, fat-soluble vitamin supplementation and treatment for pruritis may be necessary. Children with fulminant hepatic failure should undergo liver transplantation.

Prevention

- Hygiene (good hand washing)
- Sanitation (clean water source)
- Hepatitis A vaccine (preexposure)
- Passive immunization (preexposure and postexposure)

The worldwide effort at prevention is aimed at improving sanitation and education about personal hygiene in developing countries. In the United States and developed countries, HAV vaccine has been used in high-risk individuals:

- Travelers to endemic areas
- Lab personnel handling HAV
- Patients with chronic liver disease
- Patients receiving routine clotting factors
- Men who have sex with men
- Illegal drug users
- Institutionalized individuals

Two HAV vaccines were licensed in 1995. The two vaccines are inactivated virus. They are highly immunogenic and efficacious. Approximately 97–100% of children, adolescents, and adults develop protective levels of antibody within 1 month after the first dose of vaccine; essentially 100% develop protective antibody after completing the two-dose series. The vaccines are highly efficacious. In published studies, 94–100% of children were protected against clinical hepatitis A after receiving the equivalent of one dose. In 1996, children in endemic areas in the United States were vaccinated against HAV. In 1999, the program was expanded to include children and adolescents in areas with high rates of infection during a baseline period. The incidence of HAV infection is now the lowest in history.

Passive prophylaxis with HAV immunoglobulin offers 3–6 months of protection. Preexposure prophylaxis can be used for people traveling to endemic areas. Postexposure immunoglobulin is routinely used for household or intimate contacts within 14 days of exposure. In selected situations it will be given in institutions (day care centers) or to those exposed to a common source (infected food). Passive immunization is effective in 80–90% of individuals.

HEPATITIS B

Hepatitis B (HBV) is a double-shelled DNA virus. The virus has several components: the outer surface is the HBV surface antigen (HBsAg), the main component of HBV vaccines that induces the antibody (HBsAb) which confers long-term immunity from disease. Inside the virus are the core antigen (HBcAg) and the e-antigen (HBeAg).

Epidemiology

Hepatitis B poses a huge health burden on the world. Three hundred and fifty million people are infected with HBV. Forty-five percent of the world's population live in areas with a high prevalence of HBV infection (>8% of the population infected). An additional 43% live in areas where the risk is moderate (2–7% of the population infected) and the remaining population live in areas with low risk (<2% of the population infected). In areas with high prevalence, the vast majority of the population acquires the disease through vertical transmission and in early childhood. This modality of transmission carries the highest rates of chronic infection (see Table 27-1). In areas where the risk is

moderate, infections occur throughout all age groups. In countries with low risk of infection, most disease occurs in adults.

Children who develop chronic infection usually are asymptomatic, but they are a source of infection for others and as adults they can develop cirrhosis and *hepatocellular carcinoma* (HCC). This creates a health burden for the country in which they live.

Transmission of Hepatitis B

Concentrations of HBV are high in blood, serum, and wound exudates. Concentrations of the virus are moderately elevated in semen, vaginal secretions, and saliva. Modes of transmission are as follows:

- Perinatal
- Percutaneous/parenteral (IV drugs, tattoo, transfusions, needle sticks)
- Sexual (prostitutes, homosexuals)

Children at risk for acquiring HBV are as follows:

- Children born to HBV-infected mother
- Children from endemic areas
- Close household contacts
- Children attending childcare centers in endemic areas
- Institutional residents and staff
- Adolescents with high-risk behaviors

Clinical Presentation

Acute Infection

The incubation period for HBV infection is 60–90 days (range 45–180). There may be a prodrome illness characterized by malaise, fatigue, low grade fevers, and serum-sickness-like illness. These symptoms will resolve with the onset of jaundice. During acute hepatitis, patients have jaundice, abdominal pain, nausea, vomiting, and fatigue. These symptoms can last several weeks. Acute infection is usually a self-limited illness and requires supportive measures for treatment. Very

TABLE 27-1

RATES OF CHRONIC HBV INFECTION

Age	Rate of Chronic Infection (%)	Acute Symptoms (%)
Birth	80–90	<5
1–4 years	30–50	5–15
Older children and adults	2–10	30–50

TABLE 27-2
SEROLOGIC MARKERS OF HBV INFECTION

HBV Status	HBV DNA	cAb	sAg	sAb	eAg	eAb	ALT/AST
Immunized	Undetected	–	–	+	–	–	Normal
Acute infection	Elevated	IgM	+	–	+[a]	–[a]	Elevated
Resolved infection	Undetected	IgG	–	+	–	+	Normal
Chronic infection	Detected	IgG	+	–	+	–	Elevated
Chronic carrier (replicating)	Detected	IgG	+	–	+	–	Normal
Chronic carrier	Undetected	IgG	+	–	–	+	Normal

[a]There are precore mutant HBV which cannot make e-antigen. The serology will show (–) eAg and (+) eAb. Normally this serologic pattern indicates decreased infectivity, but in precore mutants there is increased infection. In these patients there is a severe form of hepatitis and in pregnant women a likely transmission to the child.

few children have symptomatic infection (see Table 27-1). Acute illness develops into fulminant hepatic failure in only 1% of individuals. Acute hepatitis can progress into a chronic infection; therefore, children with acute HBV infection must be followed until they develop HBsAb.

Chronic Infection

Chronic infection is more common in pediatric patients, where it is usually asymptomatic; anorexia and fatigue, however, can occur. There are three types of chronic infections (see Table 27-2).

- The first is represented by a patient with serologic evidence of HBV infection and chronic liver disease (elevated liver transaminases and histologic evidence of inflammation).
- The second group of patients are chronic carriers with evidence of viral replication but no liver disease. These children are infectious to others and have a small risk for developing liver disease, cirrhosis, and HCC. A large majority of these patients will seroconvert (lose HBV DNA and HBeAg, and develop HBeAb). In children under 5 years old, 3% of infected individuals will seroconvert each year. After age 5 the rate of seroconversion is 5% per year.

- The final group are chronic carriers with no viral replication. These children are not at risk for long-term liver disease.

Diagnosis

Diagnosis of hepatitis B infection is based on evidence of serologic markers, as demonstrated in Table 27-2. Patients with acute infections should be monitored until they develop HBsAb indicating a resolved infection. Patients with chronic disease should undergo liver biopsy to assess the degree of liver inflammation and damage. Chronic carriers do not need to undergo biopsy.

Treatment and Follow-up

Acute HBV has three outcomes and treatment is different for each situation. Treatment for acute hepatitis is supportive. Patients with fulminant hepatic failure will undergo liver transplantation. The final group will go on to develop chronic hepatitis.

The natural history of chronic HBV infection and progression to cirrhosis and HCC is variable. Chronic infection in pediatrics is different than in adults. Adults tend to have higher *alanine aminotransferase* (ALT) levels with a low viral load (HBV DNA), while children have high DNA levels and minimal elevation in ALT. In adults, 15–25% of patients chronically infected will have premature death from liver disease. In pediatric patients <4% developed chronic disease. The majority of patients will seroconvert (lose HBeAg and HBV DNA, and develop HBeAb). Having cirrhosis at diagnosis is a risk factor for poor outcome but even some cirrhotics will seroconvert.

Patients who are chronic carriers should be followed by a physician and have their labs checked yearly. Patients who are chronic carriers with replicating virus need closer follow-up:

Every 6 months:

- Physical examination looking for signs of chronic liver disease and cirrhosis
- Labs: HBsAg, HBsAb, HBeAg, HBeAb, HBV DNA, ALT, AST, α-fetoprotein (screening for HCC)
- Liver ultrasound every year or every other year to screen for HCC

Patients with chronic hepatitis (confirmed by histology) should be treated. The two treatments approved for HBV infection in children are α-interferon (IFN-α_{2b}) and lamivudine.

The aim of treatment for both regimens is viral suppression and remission of liver disease. The end points for treatment success have been loss of DNA, normalization of transaminases, improvement in liver histology, and loss of HBeAg. The limitations of treatment are as follows:

- 50 percent or less respond
- Response not sustained (viral replication occurs again when medication is discontinued)
- Very few patients completely seroconvert (loss HBsAg and develop HBsAb)

Interferon Therapy

Adults treated with interferon, 5–10 million units three times a week, had a 40–50% response rate and it was sustained in 80–90%.

It is clear from the adult trials that the following are predictors of success with interferon therapy:

- Elevated ALT levels
- Low HBV DNA levels
- HBeAg

While the patients less likely to respond are:

- Those with precore mutants
- Those of Chinese ancestry
- Those with normal ALT
- Those with high DNA levels
- Those with decompensated cirrhosis

Children who had factors which predicted success had similar results to adults. The dose of interferon is 6 million units/m^2 given subcutaneously three times per week. Interferon can have significant side effects including fever, malaise, flu-like illness, bone marrow suppression, mood swings, anxiety, and depression.

Lamivudine Therapy

Lamivudine is a nucleoside analog which interferes with HBV reverse transcriptase. Lamivudine use is approved for children and is given as 3 mg/kg (max 100 mg) orally daily for 52 weeks. It is a well-tolerated drug with little side effects. Lamivudine seems to have similar response rates to IFN-α_{2b} therapy. There can be increased response rates with prolonged therapy (>52 weeks). The notable differences between lamivudine and IFN-α_{2b} are as follows:

- Chinese patients have similar response to Whites.
- Response was seen in patients with precore mutants.
- Response was seen in patients with decompensated cirrhosis.

The most concerning side effect of lamivudine is development of YMDD mutations. YMDD is a motif within the DNA polymerase. Mutations develop at increasing rates with prolonged treatment. Patients with mutant can still respond to therapy (DNA suppression, improved liver histology, and transaminases). If a patient has a flare of the disease and worsening liver function with development of mutants, the drug should be discontinued. In patients with mutants who continue to have benefit from the drug, the decision about treatment must be individualized.

Combination therapy with IFN-α_{2b} and lamivudine has not demonstrated any benefit over lamivudine monotherapy. There are ongoing studies looking at other antiviral therapies such as famcyclovir and adefovir.

Patients with chronic liver disease and cirrhosis who do not respond to treatment may go on to develop end-stage liver disease. The rate of recurrent disease after transplantation is high. Untreated recurrent disease is rapidly progressive and destroys the transplanted graft. Treatment with high-dose *HB immunoglobulin* (HBIG) and lamivudine prevent recurrence of HBV after liver transplantation. Studies are ongoing to evaluate the optimal dosing regiments for these drugs.

Prevention

There are limited effective treatments for chronic HBV infection and the complications of the disease can be devastating. Therefore, a major emphasis has been put on prevention. The prevention program for HBV worldwide involved several strategies.

Confer Immunity to those at Risk

- Universal immunization of children beginning at birth
- Children born to HBV-infected mothers were given additional passive immunity with immunoglobulin within 12 h of birth
- Immunize high-risk individuals
  - Health care workers
  - IV drug abusers
  - Homosexuals
  - Prostitutes
- Household/sexual contacts of infected individuals

Interrupt Transmission

- Screening the blood supply and organ donors
- Identifying and educating potential carriers of the disease
  - Counsel on the prevention of transmission to others

- Counsel on the prevention further liver injury (no alcohol)
- Immunize against hepatitis A
- Treating infected individuals

These efforts have dramatically decreased the rate of chronic carriers and the rate of HCC in endemic areas. Similar decreases have been seen in industrialized nations.

HEPATITIS C

Hepatitis C (HCV) is a small RNA virus. The genome consists of a highly conserved 5′ coding region followed by a core and an envelope structural region and five nonstructural regions. There is genetic variability, with several subtypes and distinct geographic distribution. There are six genotypes (1–6) with subtypes designated by letter. In addition, the HCV RNA-dependent polymerase is prone to error. This can lead to viral heterogeneity, known as quasispecies, within the host.

Epidemiology

It is estimated that 170 million people worldwide are chronically infected. Different from HAV or HBV, the prevalence rates worldwide range from 0.3 to 1.5% and industrial countries have high prevalence. In Western Europe and the United States, genotypes 1a, 1b, 2a, 2b, and 3a are represented and type 4 is common in Egypt and the Middle East. The genotypes respond differently to treatment.

Modes of transmission are as follows:

- Intravenous drug use
- Transfusion or transplant prior to 1992
- Occupational exposure
- Birth to infected mother
- Sex with an infected partner
- Multiple sexual partners
- Household contact (very rare)

The vast majority of pediatric patients were infected through transfusion or vertical transmission. The rate of vertical transmission is 5%. In mothers who are coinfected with HIV the rate is 14%.

Clinical Presentation

The average incubation period for hepatitis C is 6–7 weeks. The majority of acute infections are asymptomatic with no acute hepatitis (<20% of infected patients). In adult studies, up to 85% of patients develop chronic HCV infection. Chronic hepatitis from HCV is characterized by fluctuating levels of ALT and occurs in 60–70% of chronically infected individuals. Approximately 20% of these chronically infected patients progress to chronic liver disease and cirrhosis. This is now the most common indication for liver transplant in adult patients. The following are known risk factors for progression of liver disease:

- Alcohol intake
- Age >40 at initial infection
- Coinfection with HIV or HBV

Pediatric patients may have a different disease course than adults. The rate of chronic infection in pediatric patients infected through transfusion may be less than the rates in adults but data are limited. Although pediatric patients have histologic evidence of liver inflammation and fibrosis, there is less progression to clinical chronic liver disease.

Children born to HCV-infected mothers by vaginal delivery or cesarean section have the same rate of infection. HCV has been found in breast milk but there have been no documented cases of infection from breast-feeding. These children have persistent infection with measurable HCV RNA but are clinically asymptomatic and have mild changes on biopsy. In small preliminary studies of patients with perinatally acquired HCV, spontaneous resolution of chronic infection was demonstrated.

Diagnosis

Hepatitis C infection is diagnosed through demonstration of anti-HCV antibody and/or HCV RNA (see Fig. 27-2). The original immunoassay to measure HCV antibody was not sensitive or specific. Prior to the use of second- and third-generation assays, *recombinant immunoblot assays* (RIBA) were used to confirm the diagnosis. Today the third-generation HCV antibody assay is both sensitive and specific and RIBA is no longer necessary for confirmation. The test to confirm HCV infection is a *polymerase chain reaction* (PCR) for HCV RNA. This can also be used to distinguish between active and past infection. This will be positive in actively infected patients and will quantify the viral load. High-risk individuals should be tested. Children born to infected mothers will carry maternal antibodies until 10 months of age and should not be tested for antibody until after age 1 year. If a diagnosis is needed prior to age 1, HCV RNA testing can be done.

Treatment

There have been significant improvements in the treatment of HCV infection in adults over the past 5 years. Early treatment with interferon accomplished sustained viral suppression in less than 20% of patients. The addition of the antiviral drug, ribavirin improved these rates to 50%. The final improvement was the use of pegylated interferon. Pegylated interferon can be given once a week instead of injections three times a week with nonpegylated interferon. This is now the cornerstone of therapy for adults. Treatment is for 24 or 48 weeks depending on the genotype of the virus. An early predictor of success is a decrease in the viral load after 12 weeks of treatment. If this is not seen, treatment can be stopped.

There are no large multicenter trials involving pediatric patients. There are only small uncontrolled trials of interferon treatment in pediatrics, where patients had higher response rates than adults. Currently, trials with pegylated interferon and ribavirin are ongoing. All children with HCV infection and high viral loads should undergo liver biopsy (see Fig. 27-2). Children without hepatitis do not need to be treated. Children with bridging fibrosis or moderate-to-severe hepatitis should be treated with combination therapy. There are no set recommendations about treating pediatric patients with mild hepatitis. There are several factors which may lead to response to treatment:

- Younger age at infection
- Shorter duration of disease

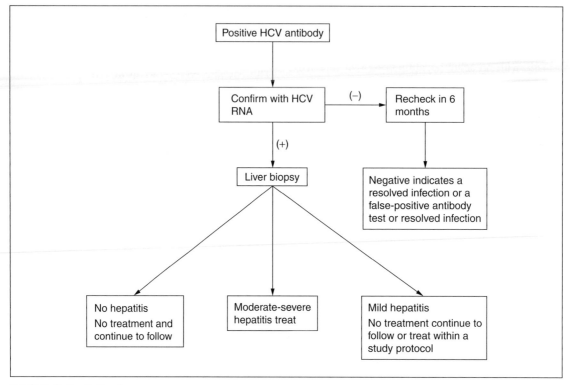

FIGURE 27-2

FOLLOW-UP OF HCV-ANTIBODY POSITIVE PATIENTS

- No alcohol consumption
- Less severe liver disease

These same variables may contribute to the more benign disease which has been documented in pediatric patients. Progression of liver disease in these patients is likely to be very slow and close observation is appropriate. Treatment of these patients should only be done within a study protocol.

Expanding the treatment for hepatitis C has been limited by lack of a small animal model or a cell culture system. The recent development of subgenomic HCV RNA molecules that replicate in transfected cells will allow analysis of the viral life cycle and development of new antiviral therapies. The antiviral therapies may include delivery or expression of antisense RNAs, ribozymes, or dominant negative proteins. In addition, an animal model of transgenic mice with transplanted infected human hepatocytes has been developed. These systems will allow the development of more precise and effective therapies.

Prevention

Prevention of a majority of HCV infections was accomplished by screening blood and blood donors. The rate of new infections in the United States has dropped from 242,000 per year (1985–1989) to 25,000 per year (2001). The majority of infections now come from intravenous drug users and sexual encounters with infected individuals. Current efforts at prevention are as follows:

- Screen and test donors
- Virus inactivation in plasma-derived products
- Safe injections

- Identification and education of high-risk individuals
- Provide HCV-infected individuals:
  - Medical evaluation and treatment
  - Counsel on prevention of further liver damage
  - Counsel on prevention of transmission to others

HEPATITIS D

Hepatitis D (HDV) is a defective single-stranded RNA virus that requires HBV to replicate, therefore, the epidemiology mirrors that of HBV. HDV requires HBV for synthesis of envelope protein composed of HBsAg, which is used to encapsulate the HDV genome.

Epidemiology

Modes of transmission are as follows:

- Percutaneous (IV drug abuse)
- Sexual transmission
- Perinatal (rare)

With these modes of transmission, routine screening for HDV is not necessary in pediatrics. HDV superinfection should be considered in any chronic HBV-infected individual who has decompensation.

Clinical Presentation

There are two types of infection: coinfection and superinfection.

1. Coinfection
   - Acquired at the time of the HBV infection
   - Severe acute disease with a higher rate of fulminant hepatic failure
   - Patients coinfected with HBV-HDV are less likely to develop chronic HBV infection and do not develop chronic HDV
2. Superinfection
   - Acquired in patients chronically infected with HBV

- Likely to develop chronic HDV
- Chronically infected HBV-HDV patients develop chronic liver disease and cirrhosis in 70% versus 15–20% in patients infected with chronic HBV alone

Diagnosis

Diagnosis of HDV infection depends on whether the patient has coinfection or superinfection (see Fig. 27-3). Patients with coinfection will have HDV RNA, IgM anti-HDV, and IgG anti-HDV antibodies in serum during acute infections. Once the infection has resolved there will be no persistent marker demonstrating the patient's previous infection. In patients chronically infected with HBV and superinfected with HDV, several serologic markers appear: HDV RNA, IgM anti-HDV, and IgG anti-HDV antibodies which will persist indefinitely because patients become chronically infected.

Treatment

There is no effective treatment for HDV. The disease will be eradicated once HBV acute and chronic infections are eradicated.

HEPATITIS E

Epidemiology

Hepatitis E (HEV) is a single-stranded RNA virus. Large outbreaks have been reported in Asia, the Middle East, Africa, and Mexico. HEV is transmitted primarily by fecally contaminated drinking water. Although hepatitis E is most commonly recognized to occur in large outbreaks, HEV infection accounts for >50% of acute sporadic hepatitis in both children and adults in high endemic areas. Risk factors for infection among persons with sporadic cases of HEV in endemic areas have not been defined. Unlike hepatitis A virus, which is also transmitted by the fecal-oral route, person-to-person transmission of HEV appears to be uncommon. Virtually all cases of acute HEV in the United

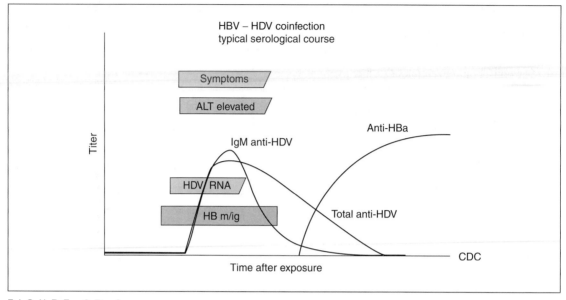

FIGURE 27-3

SEROLOGIC MARKERS OF COINFECTION AND SUPERINFECTION BY HDV

States have been reported among travelers returning from high HEV-endemic areas.

Clinical Presentation

Patients infected with HEV characteristically present with abdominal pain anorexia, dark urine, fever, hepatomegaly, jaundice, malaise, nausea, and vomiting. Other less-common symptoms include arthralgia, diarrhea, pruritus, and urticarial rash. The incubation period following exposure to HEV ranges from 15 to 60 days (mean 40 days). The period of infectivity following acute infection has not been determined but virus excretion in stools has been demonstrated up to 14 days after illness onset. In most hepatitis E outbreaks, the highest rates of clinically evident disease have been in young to middle-age adults. Low rates in young children may be the result of an icteric and/or subclinical HEV infection. No evidence of chronic infection has been detected in long-term follow-up of patients with hepatitis E. The rate of fatality is low except in pregnant women where it is 20–25%. There

have been reported cases of vertical transmission with high perinatal mortality. Diagnosis is made by clinical presentation. Methods to measure IgM and IgG antibodies are available. Measurement of RNA levels is available in research laboratories.

Treatment

Treatment during active infection is supportive. No products are available to prevent hepatitis E. Immunoglobulin prepared from plasma collected in non-HEV-endemic areas is not effective in preventing clinical disease. The efficacy of immunoglobulin prepared from plasma collected in HEV-endemic areas is unknown. There are currently ongoing trials with HEV vaccine.

Prevention

Prevention of HEV relies primarily on the provision of clean water supplies. Hygienic practices that may prevent HEV include avoiding drinking water (and beverages with ice) of unknown purity, uncooked shellfish, and uncooked fruits or vegetables that are not peeled or prepared by the traveler.

HEPATITIS G

Hepatitis G (HGV) was discovered in 1996. It is a single-stranded RNA virus, distantly related to HCV. The virus is transmitted through transfusions. There is a high rate of infection in prostitutes and homosexuals suggesting sexual routes for transmission. Partners of patients have a high rate of infection (42 %) compared to partners of patients with HCV (14%). There is efficient vertical transmission.

There is little evidence that HGV causes any liver disease. It is frequently found coinfected with other viruses but it is also found in normal children.

Diagnosis can be made by PCR for HGV RNA or measurement of antibody to the envelope protein of the virus. Routine testing for this virus is unnecessary.

NON-A-G

The most common cause of fulminant hepatic failure in pediatric patients is viral hepatitis. There are geographic differences in the causes of FHF. Hepatitis A and B are more common in endemic areas. In most series from developed countries, >50% of FHF cases are attributed to non-A-G hepatitis.

Epidemiology

Little is known about the epidemiology of non-A-G. The majority of infected patients present with severe hepatitis or FHF and do not recover from the injury. There is usually no history of transfusion, high-risk behavior in patients, or exposure to others with hepatitis. Details of epidemiology will be limited until a viral agent is identified.

Clinical Presentation

Fulminant hepatic failure is defined as encephalopathy within weeks of the onset of liver disease in a patient with no previously known liver disease. It is rare in pediatrics. The majority of children are pre-

viously healthy children who present with hepatitis. Over days to weeks the child deteriorates with worsening jaundice and signs of encephalopathy. Once this develops, it is easy to recognize that the child is very ill. The work-up for a child with rapid-onset liver disease includes:

- History: rule out previous illnesses, potential exposure to toxins, and family history of FHF
- Physical examination: signs of liver disease, assess degree of encephalopathy
- Laboratory
- Bilirubin, alkaline phosphatase, GGTP, and albumin
- ALT/AST may be elevated or may be decreasing as hepatocytes die
- *Prothrombin time* (PT) to assess for coagulopathy
- Glucose: patients with hepatic necrosis are frequently hypoglycemic
- Blood, urea, and nitrogen (BUN) and creatinine to assess kidney function
- Complete blood count
- Blood cultures if there is suspicion of infection
- Look for causes
  - *Antinuclear antibody* (ANA), antismooth muscle antibody, antiliver kidney microsomal antibody—looking for autoimmune hepatitis
  - Ceruloplasmin-screening for Wilson's disease
  - Hepatitis A, B, and C serology
  - Screen for metabolic disease (tyrosinemia, hereditary fructose intolerance, and fatty acid oxidation defects)
- Ultrasound to look for structural problems (Budd-Chiari syndrome) and malignancy

There is potential for rapid deterioration and patients should be monitored at a transplant center. The complications of FHF include:

- Encephalopathy
- Coagulopathy
- Hypoglycemia
- Renal dysfunction
- Infection

All of these complications are discussed in Chap. 28.

The complication seen more frequently in fulminant hepatic failure compared to chronic liver disease is cerebral edema. Cerebral edema is a major cause of morbidity and mortality in children with FHF. Cerebral edema usually follows stage IV encephalopathy. The pathophysiology is poorly understood. Treatment for cerebral edema is ineffective. Cerebral edema can be anticipated by monitoring cerebral pressures. Cerebral pressure monitors should be placed in all patients with FHF and stage IV encephalopathy. Monitoring intracranial pressure allows for better management and potential prevention of cerebral edema. There are two interventions which are frequently employed in the management of patients: mannitol can be used to treat acute elevations in pressure, while cerebral perfusion pressure can be supported with inotropic agents. Monitoring cerebral perfusion also assists in deciding when a patient is no longer a transplant candidate.

The rate of recovery from FHF varies according to the etiologic agent. Signs of recovery include:

- Improvement in mental status
- Improvement in coagulopathy
- Decreasing ALT/AST if accompanied by stable or improving PT

These signs warrant close monitoring. Continued improvement may indicate there is no need for transplant.

Diagnosis

Known causes of FHF can be diagnosed through the work-up outlined earlier. The known causes of liver disease are discussed in detail in Chap. 28. Non-A-G hepatitis is obviously a diagnosis of exclusion. There have been viruses identified in some cases of non-A-G, but the vast majority of patients do not have serologic or tissue evidence of known viruses.

Treatment

The treatment for FHF is liver transplantation. Patients with non-A-G hepatitis are unlikely to recover from their liver injury and should be transplanted emergently. Posttransplant care is discussed in detail in Chap. 28. Patients with non-A-G have a unique posttransplant complication; they develop aplastic anemia. This can occur in up to 28% of patients. The time course to development of aplastic anemia is variable.

Bibliography

Bortolotti F, Jara P, Crivellaro C, et al. Outcome of chronic hepatitis B in Caucasian children during a 20 year follow-up. *J Hepatol* 29:184–190, 1998.

Centers for Disease Control website. www.cdc.gov HAV and HDV serologic markers obtained from this site.

Davison S. Acute hepatitis and chronic hepatitis. In: Kelly DA (ed.), *Diseases of the Liver and Biliary System in Children*. London: Blackwell Science, 1999, pp. 65–76, 97–123.

Jara P, Bortolotti F. Interferon alpha treatment of chronic hepatitis B in childhood a consensus advisory based on experience in European children. *J Pediatr Gastroenterol Nutr* 29:163–170, 1999.

Jonas MM. Viral hepatitis: from prevention to antivirals. *Clin Liver Dis* 4:849–877, 2000.

Lok A, McMahon B. AASLD guidelines hepatitis B. *Hepatology* 39:1225–1241, 2001.

Pietschann T, Bartenschlager R. Tissue culture and animal models for hepatitis C. *Clin Liver Dis* 7:23–43, 2003.

Vogt M, Lang T, Frosner G, et al. Prevalence and clinical outcome of hepatitis C in children who underwent cardiac surgery prior to implementation of blood donor screening program. *N Engl J Med* 341:866–870, 1999.

Whitington PF, Alonso EM. Fulminant hepatitic failure in children: evidence for an unidentified hepatitis virus. *J Pediatr Gastroenterol Nutr* 33:529–536, 2001.

Yazigi N, Balistreri WF. Acute and chronic hepatitis. In: Suchy F, et al. (eds.), *Liver Disease in Children*. Philadelphia, PA: Lippincott Williams & Wilkins, 2001, pp. 365–429.

CHAPTER

28

LIVER TRANSPLANTATION: INDICATION, MODALITIES, AND MEDICAL FOLLOW-UP

Lynda Brady

INTRODUCTION

Over the past two decades pediatric liver transplantation has become increasingly successful and is now the standard of care for children with end-stage liver disease.

The vast majority of children with pediatric liver disease are managed medically. For a small percentage of patients, however, liver disease progresses and death would be an eventuality without transplantation.

INDICATIONS

Patients are referred for transplantation because of either chronic progressive liver disease or acute liver disease. The vast majority are due to chronic progressive liver disease with biliary atresia accounting for 50% of all pediatric transplants. The diagnostic indications are as follows:

Chronic liver disease

 I. Cholestatic liver disease
   a. Biliary atresia
   b. Neonatal hepatitis

   c. Alagille's syndrome
   d. Persistent familial intrahepatic cholestasis (PFIC)
   e. Nonsyndromic paucity of ducts
 II. Metabolic liver disease
   a. α_1 antityrpsin deficiency
   b. Wilson's disease
   c. Tyrosinemia
   d. Glycogen storage disease type IV
 III. Chronic hepatitis
   a. Viral
   b. Autoimmune
 IV. Other
   a. Cryptogenic cirrhosis

Acute liver failure

 I. Fulminant hepatitis
   a. Viral
   b. Toxins
   c. Autoimmune
 II. Metabolic liver disease
   a. Wilson's disease
   b. Tyrosinemia
   c. Neonatal hemochromatosis
   d. Fatty acid oxidation defects

Others

I. Cystic fibrosis
II. Inherited metabolic disorders
  a. Crigler-Najjar type I
  b. Urea cycle defects
  c. Familial hypercholesterolemia
  d. Primary oxalosis
III. Liver tumors
  a. Hepatoblastoma
  b. Hepatocellular carcinoma

PRETRANSPLANTATION EVALUATION AND MANAGEMENT

Not all children with these diagnoses require liver transplantation. The purpose of the pretransplantation evaluation is to determine which patients would benefit from liver transplantation, when the surgery should be performed, and whether there are contraindications to transplantation.

Evaluation for liver transplantation

I. Nutritional status
II. Assess for hepatic complications
III. Laboratory
  a. Complete blood count
  b. *Alanine aminotransferase* (ALT), *Aspartate aminotransferase* (AST), gamma glutamyl transpeptidase (GGTP), alkaline phosphatase
  c. Bilirubin
  d. Prothrombin time
  e. Electrolytes, blood, urea, and nitrogen (BUN), creatinine
  f. Serology
    • Cytomegalovirus (CMV)
    • Epstein-Barr virus (EBV)
    • Varicella
    • Human immunodeficiency virus (HIV)
    • Hepatitis A, B, and C
IV. Ultrasound liver and spleen for vascular anatomy
V. Cardiac assessment (ECG, Echo, and chest x-ray)
VI. Pulmonary and neurology work-up if indicated

Contraindications for liver transplantation

• Uncontrolled sepsis
• HIV infection
• Unresected extrahepatic malignancy
• Progressive terminal disease (nonhepatic)
• Irreversible neurologic damage

Complications of end stage liver disease

The criteria for listing patients for liver transplantation are based on the degree of hepatic insufficiency and the associated complications:

• Complications of portal hypertension (see Chap. 9)
• Malnutrition
• Coagulopathy
• Encephalopathy
• Spontaneous bacterial peritonitis (SBP)
• Hepatorenal syndrome
• Hepatopulmonary syndrome
• Debilitating pruritus

MALNUTRITION

One of the most commonly encountered complications is malnutrition. Studies have demonstrated that malnourished transplant patients have poorer outcomes than well-nourished patients. Malnutrition in pretransplant patients is multifactorial. Patients may have hepatosplenomegaly and ascites creating mechanical obstruction of the stomach and decreased ability for food intake. Portal hypertension leads to gastropathy with abdominal pain and decrease in food intake as well as malabsorption. Diseased livers are unable to process food and use the calories taken in. Finally, patients with end-stage liver disease have cachexia and decreased appetite. There are several strategies to prevent malnutrition. In infants, a higher calorie dense formula allows the child to receive the same number of calories in a smaller volume. Predigested formulas and formulas with *medium-chain triglycerides* (MCT) as the fat source are more easily absorbed. If a child is unable to take in adequate calories, a nasogastric tube should be placed for supplemental feeds. Children may require a huge number of calories (>150 kcal/kg per day) to overcome the inefficiencies of the intestine and liver. In older children, small frequent meals and additional high calorie liquid supplements should be used. For patients who cannot tolerate oral intake, to maintain growth, *total parenteral nutrition* (TPN) should be considered. TPN is not ideal in this situation. It has complications associated with the central access needed and is not well tolerated by the diseased liver. Most centers consider the need for TPN an indication for transplantation.

The vast majority of pediatric liver transplant patients have cholestatic liver disease. Ursodiol has been shown to improve cholestasis, modulate immune function within the liver, and slow the progression of cholestatic liver disease. It is a benign drug with few side effects and is recommended for all patients with cholestatic liver disease.

In addition to calorie malabsorption, patients develop micronutrient deficiencies. Cholestasis interferes with absorption of fat-soluble vitamins. Vitamin A, D, E, and K must be supplemented to prevent visual problems, rickets neuropathy, and coagulopathy.

COAGULOPATHY

Coagulopathy eventually develops in all patients with end-stage liver disease. The liver produces the majority of clotting factors. Factors II, V, VII, and IX are vitamin-K-dependent; therefore, the first line treatment of coagulopathy is an intramuscular injection of vitamin K. Intramuscular is the ideal route since there may be decreased oral absorption. If the coagulopathy does not respond to the vitamin K, then this indicates the liver is not capable of making adequate clotting factors and is an indication for transplantation. If the coagulopathy does respond to vitamin K, the patients should have vitamin K added to their daily medications or their current dose should be increased. *Fresh frozen plasma* (FFP) and cryoprecipitate are both products which contain clotting factors. Both products have large amounts of sodium and should be used sparingly. Coagulopathic patients undergoing procedures or with evidence of active bleeding should receive

FFP. Those patients with severe coagulopathy should be given FFP to avoid catastrophic bleeding while awaiting liver transplantation.

Patients with cirrhosis and end-stage liver disease often have thrombocytopenia. This can contribute to bleeding. It is unnecessary to give routine infusions of platelets. Platelets should be given prior to invasive procedures if the platelet count is below 50,000 or if there is any evidence of active bleeding.

ENCEPHALOPATHY

Hepatic encephalopathy may be difficult to recognize in children, particularly infants. Early signs are subtle and include irritability, developmental delay, school difficulty, lethargy, and sleep problems. Untreated encephalopathy can progress to decreased consciousness or coma (Table 28-1). The development of hepatic encephalopathy indicates portosystemic shunt and production of toxic metabolites. Encephalopathy is associated with high ammonia levels but there are several theories regarding the pathogenesis.

It is unclear whether ammonia plays a role in the pathogenesis of encephalopathy or is simply a marker. Ammonia is produced from the gut; food proteins are converted to ammonia by colonic bacteria. Even in the absence of protein intake, ammonia can be produced by breakdown of endogenous amino acids. The majority of ammonia is cleared by the liver. This process can be interrupted when the hepatocytes do not function or blood is shunted away from the liver. There is evidence suggesting ammonia plays a role in hepatic encephalopathy; in fact (a) increased protein intake increases the encephalopathy and (b) decreasing ammonia production decreases the encephalopathy. On the other hand, however, ammonia levels do not correlate with the degree of encephalopathy, and in animal models ammonia alone cannot induce hepatic encephalopathy. Other toxins have been proposed as the cause of encephalopathy. Mercaptans and fatty acids are produced by gut bacteria and their levels elevated in patients with encephalopathy. Production of these would be interrupted by the drugs used to decrease ammonia. In the final proposed

TABLE 28-1

STAGES OF HEPATIC ENCEPHALOPATHY

Stage	Clinical Findings	Asterixis	Electroencephalogram (EEG)
I	Personality changes, sleep disturbance, deterioration in intellect	Not present-slight	No changes
II	Disoriented, drowsy, inappropriate behavior	Present	Slowing
III	Sleepy but arousable, delirious, hyperreflexia	Present in cooperative patient	Grossly abnormal slowing
IV	Coma with decorticate or decerebrate posturing	Absent	Depressed amplitudes, delta waves

mechanism of hepatic encephalopathy, *gamma-aminobutyric acid* (GABA) plays a role. GABA is a central nervous system inhibitor. In some animal models increased GABA induces encephalopathy. GABA levels are increased in patients with encephalopathy. Benzodiazepines bind to GABA receptors. In some human studies benzodiazepine antagonist can reverse hepatic encephalopathy. Despite the conflicting data, therapies for hepatic encephalopathy are aimed at reducing ammonia produced in the gut.

Management of mild hepatic encephalopathy is aimed at decreasing ammonia production. Lactulose is an easily tolerated drug and first-line therapy. Lactulose is fermented by the microflora thereby reducing the pH in the colon; as a consequence, the ability to reabsorb ammonia is decreased. Neomycin is used because it changes gut flora decreasing ammonia-producing bacteria. Protein restriction is used in adult patients to treat encephalopathy. Its use is limited in pediatrics because it can contribute to growth failure. Use of sedatives, particularly benzodiazepines, can increase hepatic encephalopathy and should be avoided in patients with end-stage liver disease. Patients who fail a single agent treatment should be given dual therapy for the encephalopathy. Encephalopathy resistant to treatment is an indication for transplantation. Patients who are unable to be transplanted will develop cerebral edema and death will ensue. All symptoms of encephalopathy are reversible prior to the

onset of cerebral edema, but once cerebral edema has occurred, the patient is no longer a transplant candidate.

SPONTANEOUS BACTERIAL PERITONITIS

Spontaneous bacterial peritonitis is a serious complication of ascites in patients with cirrhosis. Diseased livers have decreased immune function, predisposing patients to peritonitis. The clinical presentation is usually abdominal pain and increase in ascites, but they can also present with worsening encephalopathy or shock. Any patient with ascites and abdominal pain or signs of infection should undergo a paracentesis, as the gold standard for diagnosing peritonitis is a positive culture. Laboratory values suggesting the fluid is infected are: *white blood cell* (WBC) >250 and pH <7.2. The majority of patients with peritonitis have bacteria from the *gastrointestinal* (GI) tract: *Escherichia coli, Klebsiella* sp., or *Enterococcus faecalis.* Gram-positive bacteria can also cause SBP; therefore, antibiotic coverage should be broad until a specific microorganism is identified. The mortality from SBP is high and decreases with early diagnosis and treatment. Any patient with high WBC count in the ascitic fluid warrants antibiotic therapy.

Efforts should be made to reduce the volume of ascites:

- Sodium and fluid restriction
- Diuretic use
- When necessary, large volume paracentesis

Recurrence of SBP is common. In patients with large volumes of ascites and recurrent SBP, oral nonabsorbable antibiotics have been shown to decrease the recurrence rates.

HEPATORENAL SYNDROME

Progressive renal insufficiency is common in patients with end-stage liver disease. The pathogenesis is unknown, but the disease is characterized by reduction in cortical blood flow. The clinical presentation is one of rapid renal dysfunction in a patient with cirrhosis. There are no signs or symptoms to predict which patients will develop hepatorenal syndrome. Avoidance of GI bleeding, dehydration, and nephrotoxic drugs are all important. There are other causes for renal insufficiency in patients with end-stage liver disease. Table 28-2 outlines the characteristics which can differentiate hepatorenal syndrome from other causes of renal insufficiency.

The treatment for hepatorenal syndrome is supportive. Initial fluid boluses may help improve renal status. These should be given with care because the course of the disease is progressive and fluid overloading can be detrimental to the patient. Patients can be placed on dialysis to support their renal function. The cure for the syndrome is liver

transplantation, as the renal insufficiency is totally reversible after transplant.

PULMONARY COMPLICATIONS

There are multiple pulmonary complications in children with end-stage liver disease:

- Hepatopulmonary syndrome
- Pulmonary hypertension
- Pleural effusions
- Pneumonia

Hepatopulmonary syndrome is characterized by hypoxia, clubbing, and in severe cases cyanosis. The pathogenesis is multifactorial including intrapulmonary shunting and ventilation-perfusion mismatches. Older children are likely to be asymptomatic except for clubbing. In infants, the combination of hepatopulmonary syndrome and mechanical obstruction from ascites and hepatosplenomegaly may lead to respiratory distress. All children should be screened with oxygen saturation since hepatopulmonary syndrome may make anesthesia more difficult. Symptomatic children may be treated with oxygen and are candidates for immediate transplant. All pulmonary and systemic vascular changes reverse after transplant but recovery may be slow.

DEBILITATING PRURITUS

Cholestasis-associated pruritus can be one of the most severe symptoms for patients. The mechanism is unclear. The treatment for pruritus begins

TABLE 28-2

URINARY FINDING IN PATIENTS WITH LIVER DISEASE

	Prerenal Azotemia	Hepatorenal Syndrome	Acute Tubular Necrosis
Urinary sodium concentration	<10 meq/L	<10 meq/L	>30 meq/L
Urinary osmolality	100 mOsm greater than plasma	100 mOsm greater than plasma	Equal to plasma
Urine/plasma creatinine ratio	>30:1	>30:1	<20:1
Fractional excretion of sodium	<1%	<1%	>2%
Response to volume expansion	Diuresis	No diuresis	No diuresis

with avoidance of anything which starts the patient itching. Use of mild soaps and lotion to avoid dry skin is the first recommendation. Patients should be receiving ursodiol for their cholestasis and pruritus (10 mg/kg per dose three times per day). The next-line drugs are antihistamines, diphenhydramine, and hydroxazine but their use may be limited because of side effects. The last two drugs used in the treatment of pruritus are rifampin and naltraxone (opioid antagonist). Pruritus may be so severe in patients that it warrants immediate liver transplantation. The two diseases which may be an exception to this are Alagille's syndrome and PFIC. Both of these diseases can cause severe pruritus. Biliary diversion has been demonstrated to ameliorate the pruritus particularly in patients with PFIC.

ROUTINE PEDIATRIC CARE

Routine pediatric care is an important part of pretransplantation management. Prior to transplantation it is important for patients to receive all routine immunizations, especially live attenuated viruses [measles, mumps, and rubella (MMR) and Varicella]. Posttransplantation, all immunizations are delayed for at least 6 months until immunosuppression is decreased. There are some studies demonstrating response to live attenuated virus vaccines in posttransplant patients, but the recommendation of the American Academy of Pediatrics is that no immune-compromised patient should receive live vaccines.

Evaluation and treatment of fever is common in pediatric practices. It must be recognized that children with end-stage liver disease are immunocompromised and may have different sources for fever including spontaneous bacterial peritonitis and cholangitis. Children with end-stage liver disease must be evaluated by a physician when they have fever and attempts at determining the source should be made. Any child who appears ill or has significantly abnormal laboratory findings should be hospitalized and observed. Treatment should be directed to the source of the fever. Treatment with antipyretics can be difficult. Acetaminophen is a poor choice for patients with end-stage liver disease.

There is decreased ability to metabolize the drug and the diseased liver is sensitive to the toxic metabolites. Ibuprofen also has side effects which can be detrimental to patients with end-stage liver disease. Patients frequently have splenomegaly and thrombocytopenia. The antiplatelet effects of ibuprofen are undesirable. In addition, patients may already have gastritis that could be aggravated by the drug. Either drug should be used sparingly or not at all.

TRANSPLANT SURGERY

The majority of liver transplants are cadaveric. The graft should have a compatible blood group to the recipient and be an appropriate size. There is no *human leukocyte antigen* (HLA) match required in liver transplantation. There is no absolute age limit for donors, but younger donors are preferred for pediatric patients. Malignancy and bacterial or viral infections are contraindications for organ donation. Over the past decade, the number of pediatric patients and cadaveric donors has been constant; while the number of adults awaiting transplant has increased greatly. This has led to a large organ shortage. In addition, the vast majority of donors are adults while the majority of pediatric patients are <5 years of age. An adult liver cannot fit into the abdomen of a small child. Prior to 1986, a large percentage of pediatric patients died awaiting transplantation.

Beginning in the mid-1980s, several new techniques were developed to expand the donor pool. A rudimentary understanding of liver anatomy is needed to understand these procedures (see Fig. 28-1). The liver has eight anatomical lobes each with a bile duct, hepatic artery, and portal vein segment. This allows a portion of the liver to be separated with an artery, duct, and portal vein attached. The first technique to expand the donor pool for pediatric patients was reducing the size of the graft. Here, the recipient received only a portion of the donor liver. In infants, it is a left lateral segment (segments 2 and 3). The remainder of the liver is discarded. Building on the success of reduced size transplantation, surgeons began splitting a donated

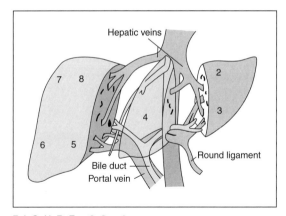

FIGURE 28-1

BASIC ANATOMY OF THE LIVER

organ into two grafts. The left half (segments 2, 3, and 4) or the left lateral segment went to a pediatric patient and the right lobe (segments 5, 6, 7, and 8) went to an adult recipient. In 1989, living-donor liver transplantation was pioneered. Here, the left lobe or the left lateral segment was taken from an adult and given to a child. This technique has now been used to transplant adult patients.

IMMEDIATE POSTOPERATIVE MANAGEMENT

In addition to all the routine care given to a critically ill patient, a liver transplant recipient deserves special consideration (Table 28-3).

Fluid Management

Fluid management can be difficult. Management must take into account fluid losses from abdominal drains. This loss can be significant in patients with severe portal hypertension pretransplantation. In addition, hypovolemia must be avoided. Hypovolemia is a risk factor for clotting the hepatic artery, but too much fluid and a high central venous pressure may lead to venous obstruction and graft congestion.

Infections

Patients who have undergone liver transplantation are vulnerable to multiple infectious complications. Immediate prophylaxis against bacterial, viral, and fungal pathogens is indicated. All patients receive broad-spectrum antibiotic coverage for 48–72 h after transplantation. Since CMV infection can be devastating in the immediate postoperative period and predisposes to chronic rejection and graft loss in the long term-most centers use prophylaxis against CMV. The choice of prophylactic regiments varies center to center. Most centers use intravenous gancyclovir in the immediate postoperative period and then an oral antiviral afterward for a total of 3 months. Oral nystatin is used routinely as antifungal therapy. There are no controlled studies supporting the use of amphotericin or diflucan prophylaxis in pediatric patients. In high-risk patients (those with hepatic necrosis prior to transplant or with possible bowel perforation), systemic antifungals are indicated.

Immunosuppression

While there is significant variability in immunosuppression protocols, all centers initially treat patients with steroids and calcineurin inhibitors (cyclosporine or tacrolimus). It is important to understand the immune system, the mechanism of rejection, and the mechanism of action of these drugs in order to appreciate any center's immunosuppressive regiment (Table 28-4).

Blood group and organ size are the only compatibility needed between donor and recipient. The liver is much less antigenic than other solid organs. Hepatocytes, which make up 80% of the liver mass, have minimal expression of class I HLA antigens. There are *major histocompatibility complex* (MHC) class I and II on bile duct cells and vascular endothelial cells. Sensitization of host T lymphocytes occurs when antigen-presenting cells carry the antigenic markers to the peripheral lymphoid tissue. Circulating lymphocytes are also exposed to foreign antigen within the graft, where Kupffer cells act as antigen-presenting cells. Production of IL-2 and other cytokines are crucial to T-cell proliferation

POSTOPERATIVE MANAGEMENT OF LIVER TRANSPLANT PATIENT

Ventilatory support

Fluid management

Prophylaxis for Infection

Antibiotics: Ampicillin sodium/sulbactam sodium (Unasyn) for GI bacteria and enterococcal prophylaxis

Antiviral: Gancyclovir

Antifungal: Nystatin and systemic antifungals in high risk patients

Cotrimoxazole (PCP prophylaxis)

Antiplatelet Therapy (according to the centers protocol)

Heparin

PGE_1

Aspirin

Dipyridamole

Antacids

Ranitidine

Omeprazole

Immunosuppression

Trough Levels[a]	Cyclosporine (5 mg/kg per dose)[b]	Tacrolimus (0.15 mg/kg per dose)[b]
0–1 month	200–250 ng/L	10–15
1–3 months	200 ng/L	8–12
3–12 months	150–200 ng/L	8–10
>12 months	70–150 ng/L	5–8
	Azathioprine	Prednisone
	Prednisone	

[a]In uncomplicated patients.
[b]Starting dose. Afterward dose is dictated by trough level.

IMMUNOSUPPRESSION DRUGS

	Complications
Steroids	Growth failure, osteoporosis, hypertension, cushingoid features
Cyclosporine	Gingival hyperplasia, hirsutism
Cyclosporine and tacrolimus	Hypertension, renal insufficiency, neurotoxicity, PTLD, hyperlipidemia
Tacrolimus	Diabetes, cardiomyopathy
MMF	GI distress, bone marrow suppression
Azathioprine	GI upset, bone marrow suppression
Rapamycin	Hyperlipidemia, leukopenia, thrombocytopenia
IL-2 receptor antibodies (Basiliximab, Daclizumab)	Unknown secondary to limited use
Thymoglobulin	Significant immunosuppression but infectious and malignant complications in pediatric liver transplant patients are unknown

and activation. These activated T cells "attack" bile duct and vascular endothelial cells, causing rejection. The patient presents with fever, jaundice, and abdominal pain. Laboratory examination demonstrates elevation in bile duct markers (GGTP and alkaline phosphatase). Since hepatocytes are less involved, the transaminases (ALT and AST) are less elevated until rejection is severe or there is compromise of a vessel.

The phases of immunosuppression are: induction, maintenance, and treatment of rejection. During induction very high levels of immunosuppression with glucocorticosteroids and calcineurin inhibitors are maintained. Additional induction agents include

- IL-2 receptor antibodies
- Anti-T-cell antibodies

    Steroids:

- Depress delayed hypersensitivity
- Decreases cytotoxic T-cell proliferation
- Inhibits production of IL-1, IL-2, and γ-interferon
- T-cell sequestration and cytotoxicity
- Decreases local inflammation by depressing neutrophil functions

Calcineurin Inhibitors: Mechanism of Action

Both *cyclosporine* (CSA) and *tacrolimus* (FK) bind to their respective binding protein (CpN, FKBP). These complexes bind to *calcineurin* (CaN) and block the dephosphorylation of *nuclear factor* of *activated T cell* (NF-AT). This prevents NF-AT from translocating to the nucleus where it is required for IL-2 production (see Fig. 28-2).

Additional drugs which can be used for maintenance of immunosuppression include

- Mycophenolate mofetil
- Azathioprine
- Rapamycin

Currently, patients are on at least one immunosuppressant for life. The untoward effects of steroids, especially for pediatric patients, have long

been known. Most centers wean steroids over the first 6–12 months posttransplantation. There are many studies now demonstrating that rapid wean of steroids is safe. There are anecdotal examples of patients who have been weaned totally off immunosuppression. In the only study to attempt weaning patients, only 25% of stable transplant patients could be weaned off immunosuppression. There are no known predictors of which patient will tolerate being off medication. The Holy Grail of transplantation is to be able to induce tolerance and eradicate the need for immunosuppression. This is an area of active investigation.

Once the surgery is successfully completed and the immunosuppressive regiment implemented, the transplant team manages the complications which arise from both. The postoperative period can further be subdivided into problems that may present within the first postoperative week and problems that may develop in the first 3–6 months.

FIRST POSTOPERATIVE WEEK

- Continuation of pretransplantation problems
- Primary graft nonfunction
- Hepatic artery thrombosis
- Hemorrhage
- Bile leak
- Sepsis
- Complications from cyclosporine/tacrolimus
    - Neurologic
    - Renal insufficiency
    - Hypertension
    - Diabetes (tacrolimus)

The problems most easily anticipated are those problems which the child had prior to surgery. Malnutrition, controlled sepsis, respiratory, and renal compromise are all common problems that are seen pretransplantation and will return with the patient from the operating room.

Primary Graft Nonfunction

Primary graft nonfunction is a rare but devastating event. These patients have transaminases over

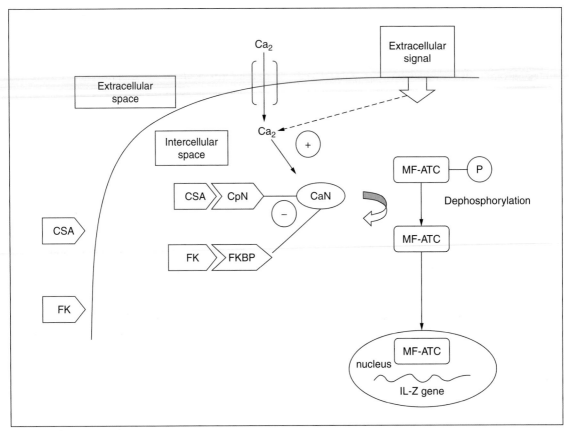

FIGURE 28-2

MECHANISMS OF ACTION OF CYCLOSPORINE AND TACROLIMUS (FK-506)

10,000, severe coagulopathy, encephalopathy, and acidosis. It is unlikely these patients will survive and their demise will be rapid without retransplantation.

Hepatic Artery Thrombosis

Hepatic artery thrombosis has severe consequences in the first postoperative week. The incidence previously was >10% but surgeons have begun using microscopes to complete arterial anastomosis and the incidence has decreased to 4–10%. These patients will appear ill and have acidosis, elevated transaminases, and coagulopathy. Ultrasound of the liver is usually diagnostic. In this immediate postoperative period, the treatment is surgical thrombectomy. Although most centers use some type of anticoagulant to prevent hepatic artery thrombosis, no controlled studies have been done to demonstrate the efficacy of these treatments. Portal vein clots are less likely in the first week but patients with increase in ascites, abdominal drain output, or coagulopathy should undergo ultrasound to examine the portal vein.

Hemorrhage

Patients with severe portal hypertension prior to transplantation are at increased risk of intraabdominal hemorrhage. This is usually obvious with intraabdominal drainage changing from serosanguinous fluid to blood and a decrease in the patient's hemoglobin.

Bile Leak

The drains are also useful to make a diagnosis of a bile leak. The fluid will appear bilious; this can be confirmed by checking the bilirubin level of the fluid. Treatment of a bile leak depends on the source of the leak. Patients with segmental grafts may leak from the cut edge of the graft. Patients with whole grafts are more likely having a breakdown of their biliary anastomosis. This complication may follow a hepatic artery compromise since the artery is the only supply of oxygenated blood to the bile ducts. All patients with a bile leak should undergo a percutaneous cholangiogram to confirm the site of the leak. Anastomotic leaks are repaired in the operating room and cut edge leaks are treated with additional drains.

Infection

Infection and sepsis can accompany any of the technical complications listed earlier. Infections in this early postoperative period can be devastating. There must be close monitoring for signs or symptoms of infection and low threshold for beginning antibiotics and antifungal medication.

Complication from Immunosuppression

The final complications arise from the immunosuppression medications. Renal insufficiency can be seen early-on secondary to the calcineurin inhibitors. This usually occurs if the levels are too high or the patient has other predisposing factors (dehydration, preoperative renal insufficiency, and nephrotoxic drugs).

In addition, these drugs can cause a wide array of neurologic complications. Any child who has seizures, change in mental status, aphasia, or other new-onset neurologic symptoms should be taken off the cyclosporine or tacrolimus. There are characteristic white matter changes seen with calcineurin inhibitors. Most of the neurologic symptoms will resolve once the drug is stopped and are unlikely to recur on a different calcineurin inhibitor.

After the first week posttransplant, the majority of patients have left the intensive care unit and in some instances been discharged from the hospital. Although the patient is doing well, this is still a time for close scrutiny.

THE FIRST 3–6 POSTOPERATIVE MONTHS

- Acute rejection
- Thrombosis/stenosis of vessels
- Bile duct strictures
- Infection
  - Bacterial
  - PCP
  - CMV
  - EBV
- Complications cyclosporine/tacrolimus
  - Neurologic
  - Renal insufficiency
  - Hypertension
  - Diabetes (tacrolimus)
  - Electrolyte abnormalities (Ca^{2+}, HCO_3^-, Mg^{2+})

Acute Rejection

Acute rejection is the most common complication in this time period occurring in up to 60% of patients. Patients may have clinical symptoms of

- Fever
- Abdominal pain
- Jaundice
- Initially maybe asymptomatic

Laboratory values will demonstrate an elevated GGTP, alkaline phosphatase, ALT, and bilirubin. The diagnosis must be confirmed with a liver biopsy. The characteristic histologic features are as follows:

- Portal tract infiltrate
- Endothelialitis
- Bile duct damage

Initial treatment for rejection is a bolus of high dose steroids (10 mg/kg per day for 3 days). The majority of patients respond to this bolus. Patients who do not respond are treated according to their baseline immunosuppression.

Prior to the widespread use of tacrolimus, steroid resistance was treated with a monoclonal antibody, OKT3. Patients who received OKT3 and then tacrolimus had an unacceptable rate of *post-transplant lymphoproliferative disease* (PTLD). This drug is rarely used in pediatric liver transplantation at this time.

Thrombosis and Stenosis of Vessels

Hepatic artery thrombosis outside of the immediate postoperative period can have one of three consequences:

1. Graft loss
2. Chronic bile duct damage from lack of arterial blood leading to retransplantation
3. Development of collaterals and no graft damage

The clinical presentation ranges from a gravely ill patient with hepatic dysfunction to a patient with laboratory evidence of biliary disease or a serendipitous discovery of a clotted artery on ultrasound. Treatment depends on the cause and ranges from retransplantation to simply monitoring the situation (see Fig. 28-3).

Portal vein thrombosis or stenosis presents with signs of portal hypertension (splenomegaly, ascites, and GI bleed). The diagnosis can be made by ultrasound. Most portal vein stenosis can be open by balloon angiography. Patients with recurrent portal vein stenosis can have stents placed with excellent long-term results.

Hepatic vein stenosis can present like a portal vein stenosis. It can be a difficult diagnosis to make on ultrasound and may require angiography to make the diagnosis. Treatment is the same as for portal vein but long-term outcome of stent placement is unknown.

Bile Duct Strictures

Bile duct complications are common and occur in 15% of patients. It is unusual to have bile duct leaks outside the immediate postoperative period but it should be suspected in any patient with signs of peritonitis. The more common biliary problem is bile duct strictures. This is particularly common in reduced-size grafts. Interventional radiologists at most centers can diagnose the problem with percutaneous cholangiogram. Stenotic areas can be ballooned open and recurrent stenosis can be stented.

Infections

Infection is a constant concern and the causative agents change with time. The bacterial sepsis which occurs early on with invasive procedures is less likely outside of the initial postoperative period.

In small children, initial PCP infections may not occur prior to age 5 and many centers continue prophylaxis until that age.

Viral infections are a concern throughout a transplant patient's life. In children who have new-onset GI bleeding, respiratory distress, hepatic dysfunction, or fever of unknown origin, CMV should be considered in the differential diagnosis. CMV culture or quantitative measures in the blood can be used to detect CMV. If invasive disease is suspected, direct examination of the tissue (gut, lung, and liver) may yield the diagnosis. Treatment is intravenous gancyclovir. If the patient has gancyclovir-resistant CMV, foscarnet or cidofovir may be used.

A large percentage of children are EBV seronegative at the time of transplant and will

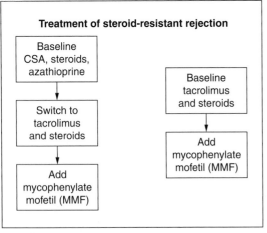

FIGURE 28-3

TREATMENT OF STEROID-RESISTANT LIVER TRANSPLANT REJECTION

undergo a primary EBV infection posttransplant. These are risk factors for the development of PTLD. Pathogenesis of PTLD is linked intimately to EBV. The virus infects and immortalizes human B lymphocytes. EBV is implicated in the pathogenesis of a spectrum of B-cell lymphoproliferative diseases in immunocompromised hosts. Persistence of the EBV genome in transformed B cells occurs following a primary EBV infection. Elimination of these cells is carried out by HLA-restricted, EBV-specific cytotoxic T lymphocytes. These cells are suppressed in transplant patients and allow infected cells to proliferate. According to this paradigm, all PTLDs should represent B-cell proliferations secondary to EBV infection; however, that is not the case. T-cell and natural killer (NK)-cell PTLDs as well as PTLD not associated with EBV also have been reported. A higher proportion of late-developing PTLDs (>2 years posttransplantation) are more likely to be non-B cell or non-EBV related. Patients may present in several clinical pictures: (1) infectious mononucleosis, (2) systemic EBV disease, and (3) lymphoma. Patients are now monitored routinely with quantitative polyermerase chain reaction for EBV DNA. This has allowed for earlier diagnosis and treatment of PTLD. Treatment begins with decrease in immunosuppression and initiation of antiviral therapy. If the disease progresses cessation of calcineurin inhibitors is necessary. There are several additional therapies which may be used: anti-CMV immunoglobulin (Cytogam) or anti-CD20 (anti-B cell) monoclonal antibody (rituximab). If there is lymphoma, surgical resection with the addition of rituximab or appropriate chemotherapy is appropriate. Once the PTLD has resolved, if rejection occurs, calcineurin inhibitors may be reinitiated. Patients must be monitored closely for recurrence of EBV. The improvement in early diagnosis and ability to treat rejection once the PTLD has resolved has greatly improved survival.

Complications from Immunosuppression

Complications from immunosuppression can continue through a transplant patient's life. Hypertension

is common early on when steroid doses are high. The mechanism of action is constriction of medium-sized arterioles in the kidneys. Calcium channel blockers are the first-line drug of choice. If additional agents are needed, β blockers or *angiotensin-converting enzyme* (ACE) inhibitors can be used. Hypertension resolves over the first 3 months in many patients and antihypertensive medications may be discontinued. Patients with persistent hypertension should be treated to avoid long-term renal or cardiovascular problems.

Renal insufficiency progresses over the first year posttransplant. A very small percentage (1–2%) of patients will progress to end-stage kidney disease. It is important to monitor renal function through a transplant patient's life. If there is progression of renal disease, consideration should be given to weaning the calcineurin inhibitors. There has been success weaning calcineurin inhibitors in renal transplant patients to spare renal function.

Long-term survival after pediatric liver transplant is excellent. The *study of pediatric liver transplant* (SPLIT) data demonstrate an 82% 1-year survival and 75% survival at 5 years. The decrease in survival rates from 1 to 5 years is due to continuation of postoperative problems previously described or late complications.

LONG-TERM FOLLOW-UP

- EBV infection
- Graft dysfunction
  - Chronic rejection
  - Recurrent disease
  - *De novo* autoimmune hepatitis
  - Retransplantation
- Growth and development

Infections with EBV occur during this time period and are the same as those described earlier.

Graft Dysfunction

The most common late complication is graft dysfunction. Late acute cellular rejections can occur but usually are associated with decreased immunosuppression. Chronic rejection can occur anytime after transplant. The incidence previously reported was 2–20%. Centers using tacrolimus have seen a decrease in the incidence of chronic rejection. Patients can develop chronic rejection following unresolved acute rejection or can develop independently. These patients present with jaundice accompanied by elevation in GGTP, alkaline phosphatase, and bilirubin. Transaminases may be only mildly elevated. Diagnosis is confirmed on liver biopsy. Histologic features include

- Ductopenia
- Foam cell arteriopathy
- Fibrointimal hyperplasia
- Fibrosis

Treatment includes avoidance of predisposing factors, tacrolimus at higher levels, additional steroids, and mycophenolate mofetil.

Additional graft dysfunction includes recurrence of original disease (autoimmune hepatitis, hepatitis C and B, sclerosing cholangitis) and a newly described *de novo* autoimmune hepatitis following transplantation.

Graft dysfunction or recurrent primary disease may lead to the need for retransplantation. The majority of retransplantations are done in the early postoperative period for primary graft failure or hepatic artery thrombosis. Patient survival after early retransplantation is only slightly lower than that of patients with primary transplantation. Survival is significantly less for patients undergoing late retransplantation. Factors which influence survival after retransplantation include

- The use of reduced size graft
- Age at retransplantation (less than age 3)
- The presence of sepsis or multiorgan failure

Growth and Development

The ultimate goal of liver transplantation is to allow the child long-term survival with good quality of life. Transplant medicine continues to strive for improved survival; however, the excellent results already achieved allow us to begin to concentrate on quality of life issues. Good nutritional

support is crucial for recovery posttransplantation. Despite good nutritional support there is little catch-up growth in the first year posttransplantation. Catch-up growth is seen in the second and third year. Certain children, those with graft dysfunction, retransplants, and those transplanted for fulminant hepatic failure, do not attain normal expected growth. Studies are now underway to assess administration of growth hormone in these children.

Studies regarding quality-of-life issues demonstrate transplant patients return to age-appropriate activities but many experience subtle difficulties. Neuropsychologic testing demonstrates multiple deficits in learning, memory abstract reasoning, and concept formation. The pathogenesis of these difficulties is not completely understood. Neurologic damage from chronic illness may play a role. The contribution of long-term exposure to calcineurin inhibitors, known as neurotoxic drugs, is yet to be discovered. To clarify, these are the important issues for which long-term multicenter trials are needed.

Outcome after Transplant

Although there are many complications encountered after transplant, the overall survival is excellent. The factors which influence outcomes are age at transplant, weight, pretransplantation diagnosis, and the severity of liver disease. The greatest improvement in outcome has been in infants. Technical improvements, improved medical support, and reduced-sized grafts allow these children to be transplanted before they become severely ill. These patients now have survival rates similar to older children and adults.

Bibliography

Cronin DC, Faust TW, Brady L, et al. Modern immunosuppression. *Adv Liver Transplant* 4:619–655, 2000.
Expert reviews in molecular medicine www.ermm.cbcu.cam.ac.uk
Kelly DA, Mayer D. Liver transplantation. In: Kelly, DA (ed.), *Diseases of the Liver and Biliary System*

in Children. London: Blackwell Science, 1999, pp. 293–312.

McDiarmid SV. Liver transplantation: the pediatric challenge. *Clin Liver Dis* 4:879–927, 2000.

Rykman FC, Alonso MH, Bucuvalas JC, et al. In: Suchy F, et al. (eds.). Philadelphia, PA: Lippincott Williams & Wilkins, 2001, pp. 949–970.

Smet F, Sokal EM. Epstein Barr related lymphoproliferative disorders in children after liver transplantation: role of immunity, diagnosis and management. *Pediatr Trans* 6:280–287, 2002.

Whitington PF, Alonso EM, Superina RA, et al. Liver transplantation in children. *J Pediatr Gastroenteral Nutr* 35(Suppl 1):S44–S50, 2002.

29

APPROACH TO THE ASYMPTOMATIC CHILD WITH PROTRACTED HYPERTRANSAMINASEMIA

Pietro Vajro, Nicolina Di Cosmo, and Grazia Capuano

INTRODUCTION

The finding of elevated levels of serum liver enzymes, and specifically of high transaminases, is not an infrequent one. This situation is often a clinical puzzle that should be approached in an orderly and meaningful way. Such problems are discussed in detail in this chapter.

Deeper investigations become necessary after confirmation that the child has persisting hypertransaminasemia which is not due to trivial causes [e.g., self-limiting liver involvement in the course of infections due to minor hepatotropic viruses such as *Epstein-Barr virus* (EBV), *cytomegalovirus* (CMV), or in the course of a treatment with a minimally hepatotoxic drug such as antibiotics].

A correct etiologic diagnosis of a clinically asymptomatic protracted hypertransaminasemia is important because it allows therapeutic intervention, especially for those hepatic diseases which are quickly and silently progressive. Furthermore, it may permit preventive measures of vertical and horizontal transmission to be started for those conditions that are infectious in origin.

SYMPTOMS OR SIGNS LEADING TO FIRST SUSPICION OF HYPERTRANSAMINASEMIA

Clinical Evaluation

Here we are referring to asymptomatic children who discover an unexpected hypertransaminasemia after undergoing a checkup which involves the measurement of serum hepatic enzymes. Clinical signs are therefore usually mild or absent at this time. However, useful and occasionally diagnostic clues are often obtained by careful clinical history and physical examination.

As seen in other parts of this book, clinical evaluation is a very important part of the diagnostic approach. Here we will concentrate on some particular aspects.

The patient's ethnic-geographic origin may give useful information about the etiology: immigrants and internationally adopted children born in endemic areas (e.g., Eastern Europe, Africa, Asia, South America, or Central America) are often affected by chronic viral hepatitis B. Consanguinity or family history of liver disease may suggest a genetic inborn error of metabolism (e.g., α_1 antitrypsin deficiency, cystic fibrosis, Wilson's disease, and hereditary fructose intolerance).

Review of past or recent history may offer immediate useful clues to the underlying disease causing hepatic damage. Inquire about risk factors for viral hepatitis, potential hepatotoxic medications (especially abuse or misuse of acetaminophen or vitamin A), dislike or refusal of sweet foods and fruits ($\rightarrow$ hereditary fructose intolerance), history of recurrent abdominal pain even in the absence of obvious jaundice ($\rightarrow$ choledocal cyst).

Examining the patient, anthropometric measurements are a necessity even in an apparently normal child; borderline short stature may be a clue in the diagnosis of atypical celiac disease or Turner's syndrome-related hypertransaminasemia; obesity may indicate obesity-related liver disease.

PHYSICAL EXAMINATION

Physical examination—in particular abdominal palpation—requires a lot of patience and tact in the pediatric age. Infants often cry and struggle and the consequent abdominal tension makes an adequate examination difficult or impossible. As a result, some pediatric hepatologists prefer to examine an infant in the mother's lap. Older children are more relaxed if they are distracted by friendly conversation during palpation. The liver must be carefully palpated and percussed to assess its span. The normal liver span in children is approximately 5 cm at 1 week, 7–8 cm in boys, and 6–6.5 cm in girls. In general, in infants the lower border of the liver may extend up to 3 cm below the costal margin. In older children, soft liver up to 2 cm below the costal margin is con-

sidered normal. One must keep in mind that in several metabolic liver diseases (e.g., glycogenoses) hepatic consistency may be so soft that even large livers are sometimes difficult to be found under the tips. A hard stony consistency may be found in patients with poorly symptomatic congenital hepatic fibrosis.

The splenic tip may normally be felt during the first 3 months of life. An enlarged spleen along with generalized lymphadenopathy and pharyngitis points to infectious mononucleosis. Splenomegaly may be a sign of a storage disorder or of a previously unrecognized progressive liver disease with cirrhosis and portal hypertension.

Ascites may be present but small amounts of liquid are best assessed by ultrasonography.

Skin manifestations may sometimes offer useful diagnostic clues to the underlying disease causing the hepatic damage. As an example, palmar erythema (blotchy erythema over palmar mounts with central pallor) may be seen in children with silently progressive liver disease as a result of hyperkinetic circulation. A papular dermatitis affecting the extremities (papular acrodermatitis) may be seen in children with hepatitis B. Mild digital clubbing may be a sign of silent underlying cirrhosis or inflammatory bowel disease.

Neurologic abnormalities may be present in postpubertal children with Wilson's disease and ophthalmic assessment may show the presence of the characteristic greenish-orange Kayser-Fleisher ring in the cornea, caused by the deposition of copper. Early stages of copper deposition require, to be properly detected, examination with a slit lamp.

The clinical examination must always be accurate and complete, and focus not only on signs of liver or liver-related disease because poorly symptomatic and protracted hypertransaminasemia in children as in adults could also be due to conditions other than liver disease. This is the case of early presentation of muscular diseases (myopathies) which may produce few clinical symptoms in the pediatric age. It is important to look for the presence of calves' pseudohypertrophy and of the Gower's sign (weakness in leg muscles causes the child to use the hands to climb up the legs in order to assume an upright position from a prone position). These children may suffer from frequent fatigue which could be seen as a clinical sign of liver disease, but instead it represents a problem secondary to the muscular disease.

LABORATORY INVESTIGATION

After evaluation of muscular enzymes, the initial laboratory investigation should include a complete blood count and liver function tests other than transaminases, i.e., *alkaline phosphatase* (ALP), *gamma glutamyl transpeptidase* (GGT), bilirubin fractions, and synthetic liver function (total protein and protein electrophoresis, prothrombin time, glucose, cholesterol, ammonia).

It is important to remember that, in addition to biliary inflammation/obstruction, increased ALP and GGT levels may also reflect osteopenia and enzymatic induction due to anticonvulsant treatments, respectively in children with two common disorders, namely vitamin D rickets and febrile convulsions. As shown in Table 29-1, both enzymes show a significant age dependency. In the pubertal

period, ALP may present a self-limiting, even more striking increase.

Etiology of the Silent Protracted Hypertransaminasemia

After proper clinical examination, and a few laboratory tests including the basic liver function tests and also serum levels of *creatine phosphokinase* (CPK) and *lactate dehydrogenase* (LDH) to rule out muscle and cardiac disease, the following causes of silent liver disease must be considered:

- Viruses (e.g., hepatitis A virus, hepatitis B virus, hepatitis C virus, minor hepatotropic virus. Eventually newly described viruses HGV, TTV, SEN)
- Metabolic disorders (e.g., Wilson's disease, α_1 antitrypsin deficiency, cystic fibrosis, urea cycle disorders, hereditary fructose intolerance)
- Autoimmunity (e.g., autoimmune hepatitis type 1 and 2)
- Gastrointestinal and nutritional diseases (e.g., celiac disease, inflammatory bowel disease, obesity)
- Hepatotoxicity (e.g., acetaminophen, vitamin A)
- Others

TABLE 29-1

AGE DEPENDENCY OF SERUM GGT AND ALP VS. AST AND ALT VALUES (U/L)

	0–1 Month	1–2 Months	2–4 Months	0.4–10 Years	10–15 Years	T assay
GGT	13–147	12–123	8–90	5–32	5–24	37°C
	1–9 Years	10–11 Years	12–13 Years	14–15 Years	16–19 Years	
ALP	145–420	130–560	200–495 m	130–525 m	65–260 m	37°C
			105–420 f	70–230 f	50–130 f	
	0–5 Days	1–9 Years	10–19 Years			
AST	35–140	15–55	5–45			37°C
	0–5 Days	1–9 Years	10–19 Years			
ALT	35–140	15–55	5–45			37°C

Source: Behrman, Kliegman, Jenson. *Nelson Textbook of Pediatrics*, 17th ed. Philadelphia, PA: WB Saunders, 2004.

TABLE 29-2

TABLE 29-2

ASYMPTOMATIC PROLONGED HYPERTRANSAMINASEMIA: INITIAL TESTS

Test	Condition
CPK	Myopathy
ESP : γ globulin	Autoimmune hepatitis
ESP α_1 globulin	α_1 AT deficiency
GGT	Sclerosing cholangitis
HCV-Ab	HCV
HBsAg/Ab HBcAb	HBV
Minor hepatitis viruses	EBV and CMV
Ab Antiendomisium	Atypical celiac disease
Fe/transferrin	Hemocromatosis
Ceruloplasmin	Wilson's disease
Urinary reducing substance	Hereditary fructose intolerance
Ultrasonography	Bright liver → steatosis

TABLE 29-3

ASYMPTOMATIC PROLONGED HYPERTRANSAMINASEMIA: SECOND LEVEL TESTS

Test	Condition
ANA, ASMA, LKM1, LC, ANCA	Autoimmune hepatitis Sclerosing cholangitis
HBV DNA, HCV RNA	HBV and HCV infection
α_1 AT and phenotype	α_1 AT deficiency
Basal and post-penicillamine—urinary copper excretion	Wilson's disease
Sweat test	Cystic fibrosis of pancreas
Molecular test for HFI	Hereditary fructose intolerance
Blood ammonia and amino acids	Urea cycle disorders
Ferritin	Hemocromatosis
Liver biopsy	Histology, EM, Cu, Fe, Enzymes

FIRST AND SECOND LINE DIAGNOSTIC TESTS

Tables 29-2 and 29-3 show, respectively, the first and second line tests that should be obtained to rule out the most common causes of persistent protracted hypertransaminasemia in a child.

It must be stressed that in several liver diseases, isolated hypertransaminasemia may be the only abnormal laboratory parameter for a long period of time. The other laboratory and histopathologic parameters may often also be borderline.

DIAGNOSTIC ALGORITHM

Figure 29-1 shows an algorithm that may be useful for rationally approaching asymptomatic children with protracted hypertransaminasemia of apparent unknown origin. It takes into account a mix of some historic, clinical, laboratory, and instrumental information:

- Exposure to viral hepatitis or hepatotoxic drugs
- Hepatosplenomegaly and overweight
- GGT and immunoglobulin levels
- Hepatic ultrasonography

As shown in the algorithm, history of previous exposure to viral hepatitis and/or particular ethnic origins must point the initial diagnostic approach toward possible viral hepatitis. However, patients with positive markers of viral hepatitis coming from endemic areas may also be affected by other nonviral liver diseases. For this reason, exclusion of progressive and treatable conditions such as *autoimmune hepatitis* (AIH) and Wilson's disease should always remain part of the diagnostic approach.

As shown in the algorithm, the finding of a simultaneous increase of serum GGT values is an important parameter for a correct orientation in the differential diagnosis. In this case, biliary involvement could

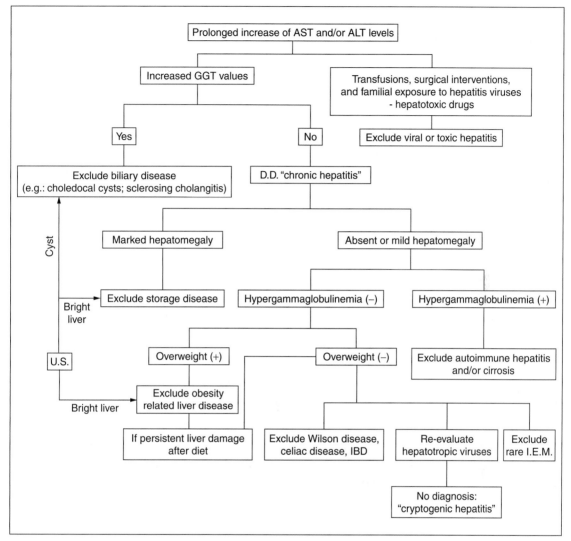

FIGURE 29-1

Approach to a child with prolonged hypertransaminasemia (apply it after exclusion of myopathy and macro-AST as possible causes of increased transaminase levels).

be suspected, even when jaundice is absent. Sclerosing cholangitis is a typical example of such a situation. In these patients liver biopsy (→ bile ducts encircled by inflamed fibrous tissue), *endoscopic retrograde cholangiopanchreatography* (ERCP) or *colangio-magnetic resonance imaging* (MRI) (→ alternance of strictures and dilations of bile duct system), and the finding of an underlying,

sometimes clinically silent, chronic inflammatory bowel disease are important clues for the diagnostic confirmation. It is important to consider that the clinical expression of the inflammatory bowel disease may either precede or follow sclerosing cholangitis. Autoimmunity may coexist [positive antibodies against the cytoplasm of neutrophils, *perinuclear antineutrophilic cytoplasmic antibody* (pANCA) autoantibodies, and peculiar *human leukocyte antigen* (HLA) patterns]. Furthermore, sclerosing cholangitis in childhood may also be associated with systemic diseases, such as histiocytosis X, immune deficiency states, *human immunodeficiency virus* (HIV) infection, neutropenic states, cystic fibrosis, graft versus host disease, chronic pancreatitis, and others.

In the case of normal or slightly elevated GGT values another differential diagnostic pathway must be followed. The clinical examination may already offer assistance. In fact, the finding of marked hepatomegaly which is not explained by severe hepatic disease or hepatitis may suggest the possibility of a silent metabolic storage liver disease. Some metabolic diseases may present only with enlarged liver and minimal liver dysfunction in an otherwise normal child. The softness of the enlarged liver often does not allow correct evaluation of the existing hepatomegaly. Table 29-4 summarizes a selection of the best known causes of marked hepatomegaly in children. Many of them, of course, are not in keeping with the clinical picture of an asymptomatic child with hypertransaminasemia. Some causes may be quickly ruled out after the clinical visit (e.g., developmental delay, coarse facies, and multisystemic involvement).

Other causes of chronic hepatitis enter into the differential diagnosis in the absence of marked hepatomegaly. In this case, it may be important to consider the values of serum gammaglobulins. The presence of hypergammaglobulinemia should lead to the search for an autoimmune hepatitis, which must be confirmed by testing non-organ-specific autoantibodies (antinuclear, ANA and/or antismooth muscle, SMA in AIH type 1, antiliver and kidney microsomes, LKM and/or antiliver cytosol, LC in AIH type 2) and by evaluating the liver histology (presence of portal tract inflammation and piecemeal necrosis). As autoimmune hepatitis quickly progresses to cirrhosis in the pediatric age and in still asymptomatic individuals, a rapid work-up is mandatory before starting appropriate immunosuppressive treatment.

Ultrasonographic examination is an important step of the diagnostic pathway of cryptogenic hypertransaminasemia in children since it may

show a fatty liver. Steatosis may be the expression of a primary metabolic liver disease (as in the case of several inborn errors of metabolism) or it may be obesity-related (*nonalcoholic steatohepatitis*, NASH, or *nonalcoholic fatty liver disease*, NAFLD). The patient's obesity may have been overlooked or not seriously considered by most of these young patients and their doctors. Measuring weight and height, weight/height ratio, and ponderal excess should therefore be mandatory in every child with protracted hypertransaminasemia of unknown origin because correct dietary measures may revert to normal—both obesity-related ultrasonographic and laboratory abnormalities, thus halting the vicious circuit of the etiology tracing.

In obese children who still present hypertransaminasemia despite weight loss and in those who are not able to comply with slimming diets, other causes of liver disease must be ruled out. Wilson's disease (carrier rate 1:90) is of particular importance in the pediatric age because it may have no clinical peculiarities and the signs are often difficult to distinguish from those of other silent chronic liver diseases. Neurologic and psychiatric symptoms are absent in the pediatric age. Due to the progressive nature of the disease (→ liver cirrhosis) it is of crucial importance to perform several tests (serum ceruloplasmin and copper levels, basal and postpenicillamine urinary copper excretion, hepatic copper levels, molecular test for the Wilson's disease gene) to rule out doubts regarding the diagnosis. Similarly, hepatic presentation of atypical celiac disease may be very difficult to recognize unless systematic screening is performed. These patients generally are identified at an older age than is typical with celiac disease, have minor and nonspecific histologic hepatic abnormalities which revert to normal after starting a gluten-free diet, unless an autoimmune disorder has been triggered. In this case, liver disease is unresponsive to diet and needs immunosuppressive treatment.

In the case where *aspartate-aminotransferase* (AST) is the only elevated enzyme, one should look at the possibility of several diseases affecting extrahepatic or extramuscular organs which also produce AST (pancreas, kidney, central nervous system, hemolytic diseases) or to pharmacologic

SELECTED CAUSES OF MARKED HEPATOMEGALY IN CHILDREN

Mechanism	Condition	Selected Helpful Diagnostic Criteria
Inflammation	Viral hepatitis	Viral markers
	Autoimmune hepatitis (often)	AutoAbs
	Systemic disease. Juvenile rheumatoid arthritis	
Fibrosis	Congenital hepatic fibrosis	Ultrasonography, liver biopsy
Venous congestion	Decreased cardiac function	Ultrasonography
	Abnormal suprahepatic vs. Budd-Chiari	
Storage of metabolic substances	Obesity, malnutrition, diabetes mellitus	Hepatic fat → ultrasonographic bright liver; histologic steatosis
	Galactosemia, hereditary fructose intolerance	Urine reducing substances. Enzyme assays, molecular tests. Coagulopathy
	Fatty acids oxidation defects	Minor viral illness → severe ALT increase; hypoglycemia; abnormal urine organic acid profile
	Oxidative phosphorylation defects	Lactic acidosis; neurologic/muscular disease. Liver failure
	Reye's syndrome	Minor viral illness → hypoglycemia; vomiting. CPK increase. Liver failure. Cerebral edema at CT scan
	Lysosomal enzyme acid lipase deficiency: cholesterol ester storage disease, Wolman's disease	Asymptomatic, neurologic deterioration, GI symptoms, x-rays calcifications of adrenals
	Glycogen storage diseases	Type I: Hypoglycemia, hyperlipidemia, hyperuricaemia, increased lactic acid, acidosis. Short stature.
		Type III: Milder than I. Type VI and IX: sometimes only hepatomegaly
	Mucopolysaccharidoses (+ splenomegaly)	Coarse facies. Bone x-rays. Eye visit. Urine MPS increased
	Abetalipoproteinemia	Acantocytosis; very low serum levels of cholesterol and triglycerides.
		Ataxia; retinitis pigmentosa
	Nieman Pick disease (+ splenomegaly)	Lipid laden foam cells bone marrow and affected tissue. CNS involvement
	Gaucher (+ splenomegaly)	Gaucher's cells in bone marrow or affected tissue
	α_1 antitrypsin deficiency	Abnormal α_1 AT molecules along the ER Serum electrophoresis
	Congenital defects of the glicosylation (CDG)	Multisystemic involvement Isoelectric focusing of serum transferrin
	Copper storage: Wilson's disease	See text
Neoplastic disease	Primary tumors: hepatoblastoma, hemangioendothelioma, teratomas, embryonal rhabdomyosarcoma of the biliary tree	CT scan. Liver biopsy. αFP. Urinary vanilmandelic acid excretion
	Tumors secondarily infiltrating the liver: neuroblastoma, Wilm's tumor, lymphoma	

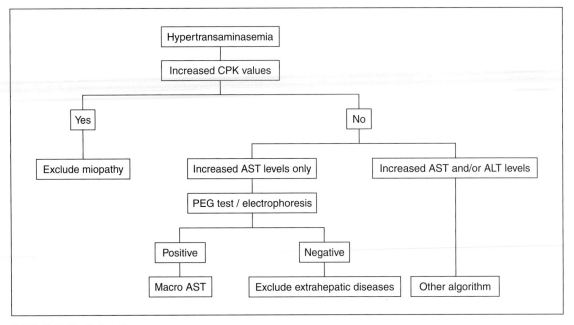

FIGURE 29-2

Approach to a child with prolonged hypertransaminasemia when serum CPK is elevated or when serum AST is the only elevated transaminase.

interferences like antibiotic treatment with macrolids. Another possible cause of the increase in the isolated AST is the reduced renal clearance of a high molecular weight complex (normal AST + IgG) the so-called macro-AST (Fig. 29-2). It is not certain whether this is truly a rare condition or whether the apparent rarity is a consequence of missed diagnoses due to poor knowledge of this abnormality by doctors and biochemical pathologists. Figure 29-3 shows the two tests which are necessary for making a diagnosis.

Unfortunately, despite the accuracy of the work-up, no etiologic diagnosis is possible in a considerable percentage of children with asymptomatic protracted hypertransaminasemia (approximately 10–20% of cases). In this case, the patient must be told that other tests may become available in the near future which could help to identify the cause and possibly a treatment of hypertransaminasemia. The histologic correlate of cryptogenetic hypertransaminasemia is generally either a nonspecific reactive hepatitis or a liver steatosis, the latter

suggesting an unknown metabolic abnormality. Some of these patients may sometimes present spontaneous remission. Liver transplantation remains an option in the case of progressive downhill disease.

LIVER BIOPSY IN SPECIFIC DISEASES

In asymptomatic children with protracted hypertransaminasemia of unknown cause, a diagnostic needle liver biopsy should be performed after at least 6 months of disease duration, unless some laboratory signs of AIH or of Wilson's disease are present. In this situation, liver biopsy is necessary to confirm the diagnosis and should be performed as soon as possible before further progression of the hepatic damage.

Liver biopsy is important for histologic confirmatory diagnosis for every form of chronic hepatitis and for its grading and staging before starting a treatment (e.g., interferon and steroids). In AIH,

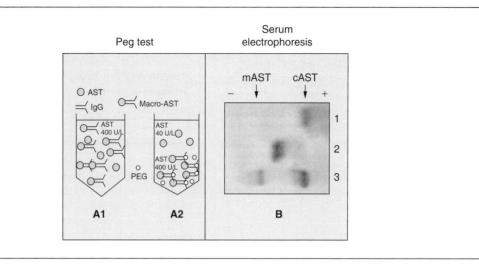

FIGURE 29-3

Panels A1 and A2 shows the polyethylene glycol (PEG) precipitation test in a patient with macro-AST. After native serum (panel A1) is added with PEG and has undergone centrifugation, the enzyme activity is markedly decreased in the supranatant, the highest activity being found in the pellet (panel A2).

Panel B shows the corresponding serum electrophoresis on cellulose acetate: the migration pattern of macro-AST is characterized by a position intermediate between the mitochondrial (mAST) and cytoplasmic (cAST) isoenzymes. Lane 1 refers to a normal individual; lane 2 to a patient with macro-AST; lane 3 to a patient with viral hepatitis.

complete long-term normalization of liver inflammation after treatment is also necessary for deciding on the opportunity of discontinuing treatment without the risk of a relapse.

Pending definite single valid and noninvasive criteria for diagnosis of Wilson's disease, liver biopsy is very often crucial. In fact, in addition to revealing steatosis ± inflammation, it may also show ultrastructural abnormalities of mitochondrial cristae which help to confirm the diagnosis in early phases of the disease. Most importantly, it also allows the measurement of hepatic copper (>250 μg/dry weight is diagnostic) which may also be monitored for tailoring the correct chelating treatment during follow-up.

Liver biopsy may help in the diagnosis of sclerosing cholangitis (see previous sections).

The need for liver biopsy in the diagnostic work-up of obesity-related liver disease in the pediatric age is still a controversial subject.

THERAPY

A detailed approach to therapy is beyond the scope of this chapter. Here we should remember that the treatment of asymptomatic children with hypertransaminasemia obviously depends on its cause and it may include the following:

- Interferon (HBV and HCV hepatitides) and lamivudine (HBV hepatitis) in hepatic viral diseases. Unfortunately therapeutic trials in the pediatric age have shown the same limited efficacy or complications (e.g., YMDD mutants after lamivudine) as were reported in the adult population
- Dietary treatment in metabolic disorders: fructose-free diet in hereditary fructose intolerance, frequent meals in glycogenosis, and weight loss in obesity-related liver disease

- Chelation and/or interference with absorption of toxic metals (e.g., penicillamine or trentine or zinc in Wilson's disease)
- Steroids ± azathioprine or cyclosporine in autoimmune disorders
- Ursodeoxycholic acid in sclerosing cholangitis, cystic fibrosis-related liver disease, and sometimes as an *ex adjuvantibus* treatment in some cryptogenetic liver diseases
- Avoidance of offending toxic food or drugs (e.g., gluten-free diet in celiac disease; interruption of treatment with a putatively toxic drug)

PROGNOSIS

Prognosis depends on etiology of hypertransaminasemia and on whether a valid treatment exists. Most untreated cases with chronic viral hepatitis B lose markers of active viral replication (negativization of HBeAg and HBV DNA) before reaching adulthood. Patients treated with the existing antiviral drugs may present acceleration in serum conversion in approximately one-third to one-half of cases.

It must be stressed that the prognosis of autoimmune hepatitis and of Wilson's disease mostly depends on the speed of diagnosis and on correct specific therapy before cirrhosis is established.

FOLLOW-UP

A close follow-up is advised to rule out the possibility of progression of the liver disease (e.g., monitoring of synthetic functions of the liver and ultrasonographic or endoscopic search of signs of portal hypertension; monitoring of αFP as a marker of neoplastic evolution and delta agent superinfection in chronic hepatitis B) and of response to treatment (e.g., monitoring of liver function tests (LFTs), viral loads, autoantibodies titers, urinary copper, antibodies antiendomisium and antitransglutaminase values, weight loss, and ultrasonographic bright liver).

SOME EXAMPLES REGARDING PREVENTION OF HYPERTRANSAMINASEMIA

Prevention of hepatitis B is now done through vaccination programs. Hepatitis B immune globulin administration within 4–6 h of birth followed by the hepatitis B vaccine can prevent the disease in infants born to mothers who are positive for hepatitis B surface antigen.

The incidence of hepatitis C may be reduced through correct screening of blood and blood products. Breast-feeding is not a risk factor for HCV transmission from mother to infant and should not be discouraged.

Obesity-related liver disease has unfortunately become an overwhelming entity also in the pediatric age in spite of affordable prevention through correct dietary habits and weight loss programs.

Decreased use, abuse, or misuse of drugs might reduce the incidence of hepatotoxicity.

Genetic counseling is important for liver disease due to inborn errors of metabolism.

Bibliography

D'Agata ID, Balistreri WF. Evaluation of liver disease in the pediatric patient. *Pediatr Rev* 20:376–390, 1999.

Limdi JK, Hyde GM. Evaluation of abnormal liver function tests. *Postgrad Med J* 79:307–312, 2003.

McDiarmid SV. The liver and metabolic diseases of childhood. *Liver Transpl Surg* 4(5 Suppl 1):S34–S50, 1998.

Mieli-Vergani G, Vergani D. Immunological liver diseases in children. *Semin Liver Dis* 18:271–279, 1998.

O'Connor JA. Acute and chronic viral hepatitis. *Adolesc Med* 11:279–292, 2000.

Pratt DS, Kaplan MM. Evaluation of abnormal liver-enzyme results in asymptomatic patients. *N Engl J Med* 342:1266–1271, 2000.

Wolf AD, Lavine JE. Hepatomegaly in neonates and children. *Pediatr Rev* 21:303–310, 2000.

IV

PHARMACOTHERAPY AND NUTRITION

C H A P T E R

30

COMMONLY EMPLOYED DRUGS: DOSAGE RECOMMENDATIONS AND SIDE EFFECTS

Zahangir Khaled

Pediatric pharmacology is complex. Several factors must be considered before prescribing a pediatric medication. These include (a) patient's weight, (b) drug absorption and distribution, (c) side effects, (d) drug interaction, (e) growth and development, (f) nutritional requirements, and (g) family dynamics and schooling. This chapter is designed to provide students in clinical training, house staff, and practicing physicians a clear and concise concept of the medication commonly used in different gastrointestinal (GI) disorders. All information about the drugs has been collected from North American Society for Pediatric Gastroenterology, Hepatology, and Nutrition (NASPGHAN) drug formulary, Physicians Desk Reference (PDR), assorted Pediatric Gastrointestinal books, and from other latest available sources.

Drugs	Formulation	Dosing	Side Effects	Mechanism of Action	Comments
Acetylcysteine (Mucomyst)	Solution: 100, 200, mg/mL	Acetaminophen poisoning: loading dose 140 mg/kg, then 70 mg/kg q 4 h × 17 doses PO or NG is preferred. IV only indicated in PO or NG intolerance, GI bleeding or obstruction, toxicity	*Common*: Nausea, vomiting, diarrhea, and headache *Less common*: Tinnitus, urticaria, flushing, angioedema, tachycardia, bronchospasm, and renal stone formation	It is a reducing agent with antioxidant and mucolytic activity. It prevents liver damage by regenerating liver stores of glutathione	Most effective when administered within the first 8 h of ingestion. Adequate hydration is necessary to prevent crystallization in renal tubules

Drugs	Formulation	Dosing	Side Effects	Mechanism of Action	Comments
		from maternal over-dose in neonate Meconium ileus: 5–10 mL/kg of 10% solution per rectum via soft rubber catheter			
Acyclovir (Zovirax)	Suspension: 200 mg/ 5 mL Tablet: 400 and 800 mg Capsule: 200 mg Injection: 50 mg/mL	Mucocutaneous HSV: 750 mg/m² per day or 15 mg/kg per day IV, tid × 5–7 days. Or 1200 mg per day (max 80 mg/kg per day) PO, tid × 7–10 days HSV prophylaxis: 750 mg/m² per day IV, tid or 600–1000 mg per day PO, qid during risk period CMV prophylaxis: 1500 mg/m² per day IV, tid or 800–3200 mg per day PO, qid during risk period (max 80 mg/kg per day)	*Common*: General feeling of bodily discomfort, nausea, vomiting, diarrhea, phlebitis, elevation of blood urea nitrogen (BUN) and creatinine *Less common*: Agitation, rash, elevation of transaminases, anemia, neutropenia, thrombocytopenia, thrombocytosis, leukocytosis, neutrophilia, hematuria, dizziness, skin peeling, seizures, coma, and swollen face and throat	It is a synthetic purine nucleoside analogue. It stops replication of herpes viral DNA by competitive inhibition of viral DNA polymerase	Oral absorption is unpredictable. IV infusion must be accompanied by adequate hydration
Albumin, human (Albuminar, Albutein, Buminate, Plasbumin)	5 and 25% solution	Hypoproteinemia: 0.5–1 g/kg per dose IV over 1/2 h to 2 h, repeat 1–2 days prn Hypovolemia: 0.5–1 g/kg per dose IV rapid infusion, repeat prn	*Common*: Fluid overload *Less common*: Hypersensitivity reaction and hypernatremia	Plasma volume expander	Contraindicated in severe anemia and CHF. Use 5% solution in premature infants, 25% increase the risk of intraventricular hemorrhage (IVH)
Aluminum hydroxide (Amphojel, Dialume, Nephrox, Alu-Tab)	Suspension: 320 mg/ 5 mL, 450 mg/ 5 mL, 600 mg/ 5 mL, and 675 mg/ 5 mL	Peptic ulcer: 320–960 mg per dose q 3-6 h or 1 and 3 h after meals and at bedtime GI bleeding prophylaxis: Infants: 120–320 mg per dose q 1-2 h	Constipation, decreased intestinal motility, hypophosphatemia	Neutralize gastric acid and reduce pepsin activity	Rarely use for GI bleeding prophylaxis. Interferes with the absorption of iron, isoniazid (INH), digoxin, indomethacin, and tetracyclines

Drugs	Formulation	Dosing	Side Effects	Mechanism of Action	Comments
	Tab: 300, 500, and 600 mg	Children: 320–960 mg per dose q 1-2 h			
Aluminum hydroxide with mag- nesium hydroxide (Maalox, Mylanta)	Cap: 400, 475, and 500 mg Suspension: Maalox: 225 mg aluminum hydroxide (AlOH) + 200 mg magne- sium hydrox- ide (MgOH)/ 5 mL Mylanta: 200 mg AlOH + 200 mg MgOH + 20 mg Simethicone (antiflatulent)/ 5 mL Chewable tabs: 200 mg 200 mg AlOH + 200 mg MgOH	Peptic ulcer: Children: 5–15 mL per dose q 3-6 h GI bleeding prophylaxis: Neonates: 1 mL/kg per dose q 4 h prn Infant: 2–5 mL per dose q 1-2 h Children: 5–15 mL q 1-2 h	Diarrhea, constipation, and hypokalemia	Neutralize gastric acid and reduce pepsin activity	Rarely use for GI bleeding prophylaxis. Interferes with the absorption of iron, INH, digoxin, indomethacin, and tetracyclines
Amitriptyline (Elavil, Emitrip, Endep, Enovil)	Tab: 10, 25, 50, 75, 100, and 150 mg	Recurrent abdominal pain (low dose): 0.2–0.4 mg/kg per day or 10–50 mg per day at bedtime For depression dose starts with 1–1.5 mg/kg per day	*Common*: Dry mouth, constipation, urinary hesitancy, blurred vision, sleepiness, drowsiness, confu- sion, orthostatic hypotension, arrhythmias, and weight gain *Less common*: Seizure, tremor, insomnia, aggrava- tion of psychosis, and sexual disturbances	Increases cen- tral nervous system (CNS) concentration of serotonin and norepi- nephrine by inhibiting reuptake	Abrupt discontin- uation may cause with- drawal syn- drome. Do not use in patients with seizure, cardiac dis- order, narrow angle glaucoma, receiving or received mono- amine oxidase (MAO) inhibitors in last 2 weeks
Amoxicillin (Amoxil, Trimox, Polymox)	Suspension: 125, 200, 250 and 400 mg/5 mL	Infection: 25–50 mg/kg per day PO, tid	*Common*: Nausea, vomiting, loose stool or diarrhea, and skin rashes	Inhibits bacter- ial cell wall mucopeptide biosynthesis	Better absorbed from the gut than ampicillin

Drugs	Formulation	Dosing	Side Effects	Mechanism of Action	Comments
	Tabs: 500 and 875 mg Chewable tabs: 125, 200, 250, and 400 mg Caps: 250 and 500 mg	SBE prophylaxis: 50 mg/kg PO 1 h before procedure	*Less common:* Abdominal discomfort, anaphylaxis, serum sickness type reactions, pseudomembranous colitis, interstitial nephritis, eosinophilia, and hemolytic anemia		
Amoxicillin-clavulanic acid (Augmentin)	Suspension: 125, 200, 250, and 400 mg amox/ 5 mL ES: 600 mg amox/5 mL Tabs: 250, 500, and 875 mg Chewable tabs: 125, 250, 200, and 400 mg amox (dose based on amoxicillin)	Infection: <3 months: 30 mg/kg per day PO, bid >3 months: 20–40 mg/kg per day PO, bid-tid	*Common:* Nausea, vomiting, loose stool or diarrhea, and skin rashes *Less common:* Abdominal discomfort, anaphylaxis, serum sickness type reactions, pseudomembranous colitis, interstitial nephritis, eosinophilia, and hemolytic anemia	Amoxicillin: Inhibits bacterial cell wall mucopeptide biosynthesis Clavulanic acid: Protects hydrolyzable amoxicillin from inactivation by beta lactamase enzymes	Effective against *Staphylococcus aureus, Streptococcus, Haemophilus influenzae, Moraxella catarrhalis, Escherichia coli, Klebsiella,* and *Bacteroides fragilis*
Ampicillin	Suspension: 125, 250, and 500 mg/5 mL Caps: 250 and 500 mg Injection: 125, 250, and 500 mg; 1, 2, and 10 g	Endocarditis prophylaxis in high risk patient: 50 mg/kg (max 2 g) IV/IM, 30 min before procedure. Then 25 mg/kg (max 1 g) PO/IV/ IM 6 h later	*Common:* Nausea, vomiting, loose stool or diarrhea, and skin rashes *Less common:* Abdominal discomfort, anaphylaxis, serum sickness type reactions, pseudomembranous colitis, interstitial nephritis, eosinophilia, and hemolytic anemia	Inhibits bacterial cell wall mucopeptide biosynthesis	
Ampicillin/ sulbactum (Unasyn)	Injection: 1.5 and 3 g (amp: sulbac = 2:1)	Infection: 100–200 mg/kg per day	*Common:* Diarrhea, thrombophlebitis, and rash	Ampicillin: Inhibits bacterial cell wall	Effective against *S. aureus, Streptococcus,*

Drugs	Formulation	Dosing	Side Effects	Mechanism of Action	Comments
		(max 8 g per day) IV/IM, qid (dose based on ampicillin)	*Less common:* Anaphylactic reaction, nausea, vomiting, itching, candidiasis, fatigue, malaise, headache, chest pain, flatulence, abdominal distension, pseudomembranous colitis, glossitis, urine retention, dysuria, edema, facial swelling, erythema, chills, tightness in throat, substernal pain, epistaxis, and mucosal bleeding	mucopeptide biosynthesis Sulbactum: Extends spectrum by inhibiting beta lactamase	*H. influenza,* *M. catarrhalis,* *E. coli, Klebsiella,* and *B. fragilis.* Lower dose in patient with renal impairment
Amphotericin B (Fungizone, Amphocin)	Suspension: 100 mg/mL Injection: 50 mg vials	Systemic fungal infection: Test dose: 0.1 mg/kg per dose (max 1 mg) IV Initial dose: 0.25 mg/kg per day IV, qd Maintenance: 0.25–1 mg/kg per day IV, qd	*Common:* Chills, fever, nausea, vomiting, diarrhea, renal failure, hypokalemia, hypertension, leukopenia, thrombocytopenia, and abdominal or chest pain *Less common:* Liver failure, hypomagnesemia, infection, coagulation defect, seizure, joint pain, and transient vertigo	Acts by binding to sterols in fungal cell wall	Monitor: CBC, BUN, creatinine, serum potassium, AST, and ALT. Use 0.1 mg/mL for peripheral and 0.2 mg/mL for central line (dilute in D_5W)
Azathioprine (Imuran)	Suspension: 2 and 50 mg/mL Tab: 50 mg Injection: 5 mg/mL (100 mg in 20 mL vial)	Inflammatory bowel disease: 2–2.5 mg/kg per day PO/IV, qd	*Common:* Elevated liver enzymes, leukopenia, infections, nausea, and pancreatitis *Less common:* Vomiting, diarrhea, anorexia, stomach pain, skin rash, stomatitis,	Inhibit synthesis of DNA, RNA, and proteins. Antagonize purine metabolism	Metabolized to 6-MP and ultimately to 6-TG and 6-MMP. Metabolism rate may vary depending on thiopurine methyl transferase activity

Drugs	Formulation	Dosing	Side Effects	Mechanism of Action	Comments
			bone marrow suppression, and hyperuricemia Chronic use may increase the risk of lymphoma and skin cancer		Monitor: CBC, ALT, BUN, and creatinine Therapeutic 6-TG level: > 235 pmol/8 × 10^8 RBC Allopurinol and probenecid increase drug level
Baclofen (Lioresal)	Tab: 10 and 20 mg Suspension: 5 and 10 mg/mL Injection: 0.5 and 2 mg/mL	Investigational drug for GERD. In pediatric population 2.5 mg PO, qd was found effective	*Common:* Drowsiness, hypotonia, dizziness, paresthesia, nausea, vomiting, headache, and hypotension *Less common:* Fever, dyspnea, rash, urinary frequency, and hallucination	Centrally acting skeletal muscle relaxant. Exert its effects by stimulation of the $GABA_B$ receptor	
Bethanechol chloride (Urecholine)	Suspension: 1 mg/mL Tab: 5, 10, 25, and 50 mg Injection: 5 mg/mL	Prokinetic: 0.1–0.2 mg/kg per dose PO, tid-qid	Nausea, belching, abdominal cramps or discomfort, diarrhea, excessive salivation, urinary urgency, headache, flushing, sweating, bronchial constriction, lacrimation, and miosis	Parasympathomimetic agent. It stimulates gastric motility	The injection is for subcutaneous use only
Bisacodyl (Dulcolax, Bisco-lax, Carter's little pills, Fleet Laxative)	Tab: 5 mg Enema: 10 mg/30 mL Powder: 1.5 mg with tannic acid 2.5 g/pack Suppository, rectal: 5 and 10 mg	Constipation: Rectal suppository: <2 years: 5 mg qd 2–11 years: 5–10 mg qd >11 years: 10 mg qd Oral: 3–12: 0.3 mg/kg per day (max 10 mg per day) >12 years: 5–15 mg per day	*Common:* Nausea, vomiting, abdominal cramps, rectal irritation. *Less common:* Chronic use may result laxative dependence	Diphenylmethane derivatives. It decreases water absorption from the lumen and stimulates intestinal secretion (stimulant laxative)	Laxative effect is seen in 6–12 h. It is reabsorbed via enterohepatic circulation and has increased risk of abuse or overdose

Drugs	Formulation	Dosing	Side Effects	Mechanism of Action	Comments
Bismuth subsalicylate (Pepto-Bismol)	Liquid: 262 mg/ 15 mL, 524 mg/ 15 mL Chewable tabs: 262 mg Cap: 262 mg	Diarrhea: 100 mg/ kg per day divided in 5 doses × 5 days *H. pylori* gastritis: dose not well established in children	*Common*: GI upset, darkening of tongue, and black stool *Less common*: Decrease platelet aggregation	Possible mechanisms: (a) normalizing fluid movement via an antisecretory mechanism, (b) binding bacterial toxins, and (c) antimicrobial activity	Not recommended in children with flu-like symptoms, chicken pox, and severe renal failure
Calcium carbonate (Tums, Oscal, Rolaids)	Elemental calcium in parenthesis Tums: 500 mg (200 mg) Tums EX: 750 mg (300 mg) Oscal: 1250 mg (500 mg) Caltrate: 1500 mg (600 mg) Rolaids: 500 mg (200 mg) and 1000 mg (400 mg)	Recommended dietary allowance (RDA) of elemental calcium in mg: 0–6 months: 210 6–12 months: 270 1–3 years: 500 4–8 years: 800 9–18 years: 1300	*Common*: Constipation *Less common*: Hypercalcemia, hypophosphatemia, hypomagnesemia, nausea, and headache	Replete the body content of calcium	May decrease absorption of tetracycline and iron
Carnitine (Levocarnitine, Carnitor, VitaCarn)	Solution: 100 mg/mL Tab: 330 mg Cap: 250 mg Injection: 200 mg/mL	Carnitine deficiency: Neonate: 10–20 mg/kg per day IV or in TPN Infant and children: 50–100 mg/kg per day (max 3 g) PO, bid-tid Carnitine deficient dialysis patient: 10–20 mg/kg IV after each dialysis in addition to usual dose	Nausea, vomiting, abdominal cramps, diarrhea, body odor (dose related), dizziness, seizures, paresthesia, hypertension, hypercalcemia, and muscle weakness	It is a carrier molecule in the transport of long-chain fatty acids across the inner mitochondrial membrane. Carnitine can promote the excretion of excess organic or fatty acids in patients with defects in fatty acid metabolism and/or specific organic acidopathies that bioaccumulate acyl-CoA esters	

Drugs	Formulation	Dosing	Side Effects	Mechanism of Action	Comments
Cefazolin (Ancef, Kefzol, Zolicef)	Injection: 0.25, 0.5, 1, 5, 10, and 20 g	Infection: 50–100 mg/kg per day (max 6 g), IV or IM, tid-qid Endocarditis pro-phylaxis in peni-cillin allergic children: 25 mg/kg (max 1 g), IV or IM 30 min prior to procedure	Most common is hypersensitivity reactions. Others are similar to penicillin. 5–10% of penicillin sen-sitive persons are also hyper-sensitive to cephalosporins	Inhibits bacterial cell wall mucopeptide biosynthesis	First generation cephalosporins. Effective against S. aureus, Streptococcus, E. coli, Proteus, and Klebsiella. May cause false positive urine reducing substance
Ceftazidime (Fortaz, Tazimide, Tazicef, Ceptaz)	Injection: 0.5, 1, 2, 6, and 10 g	Pseudomonas infection: 90–150 mg/kg per day (max 6 g per day) IV/IM, tid	Common: Phlebitis, hyper-sensitivity reac-tion, diarrhea, nausea, vomit-ing, abdominal pain, elevation of liver enzymes, and eosinophilia Less common: Headache, dizzi-ness, paresthesia, pseudomembra-nous colitis, and aplastic anemia	Semisynthetic, broad-spectrum, beta-lactam antibi-otic. It inhibits the enzymes responsible for cell wall synthesis	Third generation cephalosporins. Effective against gram-positive and gram-negative organisms including Pseudomonas. Can cause false-positive test for urinary glucose and positive Coombs test without hemolysis
Ceftriaxone (Rocephin)	Injection: 0.25, 0.5, 1, 2, and 10 g	Infection: 50–75 mg/kg per day (max 4 g), IV/IM, qd-bid	Reversible cholestasis, sludging in gall bladder, and jaundice Others are same as ampicillin	Inhibits bacterial cell wall muco-peptide biosyn-thesis. It has a high degree of stability in the presence of beta lactamase, both penicilli-nases and cephalospori-nases, of gram-negative and gram-positive bacteria	Third generation cephalosporins. Effective against gram-positive and gram-negative organisms. 5–10% of peni-cillin sensitive persons are also hypersen-sitive to cephalosporins

Drugs	Formulation	Dosing	Side Effects	Mechanism of Action	Comments
Cephalexin (Keflex, C-Lexin)	Drop: 100 mg/mL Suspension: 125 and 250 mg/ 5 mL Tab: 250, 500, and 1000 mg Cap: 250 and 500 mg	Infection: 25–100 mg/kg per day (max 4 g per day) PO, qid	Most common is hypersensitivity reactions. Others are similar to penicillin. 5–10% of penicillin sensitive persons are also hypersensitive to cephalosporins	Inhibits bacterial cell wall mucopeptide biosynthesis	First generation cephalosporins. Effective against *S. aureus, Streptococcus, E. coli, Proteus,* and *Klebsiella.* Give 2 h before or 1 h after meal
Chloral hydrate (Noctec)	Syrup: 250 and 500 mg/5 mL Cap: 250 and 500 mg Suppository: 324, 500, and 648 mg	Sedation for procedures: 25–100 mg/kg per dose PO or PR (max 1 g in infant and 2 g in children)	Paradoxical excitement, hypotension, respiratory depression	It is a sedative-hypnotic	Rapid onset and short duration of action. Contraindicated in gastritis
Cholestyra-mine (Questran, Questran Light, Prevalite)	Anhydrous resin per pack: Questran: 4 g/9 g packet Questran light: 4 g/5 g pack Prevalite: 4 g/5.5 g pack	Nonspecific diarrhea: Dose based on anhydrous resin: 250–500 mg/kg per day PO, bid-tid	*Common:* Constipation, abdominal distension, vomiting, and fat soluble vitamin deficiency. *Less common:* Hypochloremic metabolic acidosis and rash.	Nonabsorbable anion exchange resin. It binds with bile acids and thereby increases fecal excretion	Other oral medicine should be given 1 h before or 4 h after administration of cholestyramine. Contraindicated in biliary atresia and Roux-en Y portoenterostomy
Cimetidine (Tagamet)	Syrup: 300 mg/ 5 mL Tab: 100, 200, 300, 400, and 800 mg Injection: 150 mg/mL	GERD, erosive esophagitis, and peptic ulcer: Neonate: 5–20 mg/ kg per day PO/IV/ IM, bid-qid Infant: 10–20 mg/ kg per day PO/IV/ IM, bid-qid Children: 20–40 mg/kg per day, PO/IV/IM, qid	*Common:* Headache, diarrhea, dizziness, gynecomastia, disorientation, and confusion *Less common:* Nausea, vomiting, rash, neutropenia, agranulocytosis, thrombocytopenia, hypotension, elevated liver enzymes, bradycardia, arthralgia, and myalgia	Competitive inhibitor of H2 receptor. It blocks the histamine-mediated acid secretion from parietal cells	It increases the level of phenytoin, lidocaine, diazepam, and theophylline and decreases absorption of iron, ketoconazole, and tetracyclines

Drugs	Formulation	Dosing	Side Effects	Mechanism of Action	Comments
Ciprofloxacin (Cipro)	Injection: 10 mg/mL Tab: 100, 250, 500, and 750 mg Suspension: 250 and 500 mg/5 mL	Inflammatory bowel disease: 20–30 mg/kg per day (max 1.5 g), PO bid. Or 10–20 mg/kg per day (max 800 mg) IV, bid	*Common*: Nausea, diarrhea, vomiting, abdominal pain or discomfort, headache, restlessness, and rash *Less common*: Foot pain, dizziness, drowsiness, anorexia, seizure, oral candidiasis, *C. difficile* colitis, chest pain, renal failure, pruritus, and epistaxis	Block bacterial DNA synthesis by inhibiting topoisomerase II and IV	May increase level of theophylline, warfarin, and cyclosporine
Cisapride (Propulsid)	Suspension: 1 mg/mL Tab: 10 and 20 mg	Prokinetic: 0.1–0.3 mg/kg per dose (max 10 mg per dose) PO, tid-qid	*Common*: Headache, diarrhea, abdominal pain, constipation, dyspepsia, flatulence, rhinitis, dizziness, vomiting, and dry mouth *Less common*: Palpitation, chest pain, fatigue, back pain, dehydration, and myalgia Rare but serious: QT prolongation, cardiac arrhythmias, in some cases resulting in death	Promotes gastric motility by enhancing the release of acetylcholine at the myenteric plexus	Concurrent use of the following drugs increase serum cisapride level: ketoconazole, itraconazole, miconazole, fluconazole, erythromycin, clarithromycin, nefazodone, indinavir, and ritonavir. Avoid concurrent use of drugs known to prolong QT interval: Tricyclic antidepressants, quinidine, and procainamide
Cromolyn sodium (Gastrocrom)	Cap: 100 mg Oral concentrate: 100 mg/ 5 mL	Food allergy: Less than 2 years: 20 mg/kg per day PO, qid	*Common*: Headache and diarrhea	Stabilizes mast cells, thereby inhibiting the release of	

Drugs	Formulation	Dosing	Side Effects	Mechanism of Action	Comments
		>2 years: 100 mg (max 1.6 g per day) PO, qid	*Less common:* Abdominal pain, dysphagia, pruritus, rash, urticaria, arthralgia, angioedema, tachycardia, paresthesia, abnormal liver function test (LFT), tinnitus, and systemic lupus erythematosus (SLE)-like syndrome	histamine and leukotrienes (SRS-A)	
Cyclosporine (Neoral, Sandimmune)	Solution: 100 mg/mL Caps: 25, 50, and 100 mg Injection: 50 mg/mL	Immunosuppression: 5–10 mg/kg per day PO, bid (titrate to desired serum trough levels) Inflammatory bowel disease: 5–7.5 mg/kg per day	*Common:* Nausea, vomiting, leukopenia, hyperkalemia, hyperuricemia, nephrotoxicity, paresthesia, hypertrichosis, tremor, hypertension, hirsutism, gingival hypertrophy, and hepatotoxicity *Less common:* Leg cramps, headache, acne, seizure, leukopenia, hematuria, chest pain, mouth sore, joint pain, pancreatitis, swallowing difficulties, weight loss, weakness, opportunistic infection, and lymphoproliferative disease	Inside the T cell it binds to a protein called cyclophilin A and inhibits calcium-dependent activation of the cell	Monitor: CBC, BUN, creatinine, uric acid, potassium level 2 weekly × 3 months and then monthly Erythromycin, ketoconazole, fluconazole, and verapamil may increase drug level. Carbamazepine, rifampin, phenobarbital, and phenytoin may decrease drug level Vaccination may be less effective. Avoid live attenuated vaccines Neoral cannot be used interchangeably with Sandimmune, as the absorption is different
Cyproheptadine (Periactin)	Syrup: 2 mg/ 5 mL Tab: 4 mg	Appetite stimulant: 2 mg PO, QHS, increases every 2–3 weeks (max 8 mg per day)	*Common:* Sedation, dry mouth, thickened bronchial secretions,	Antihistaminic and antiserotonergic agent	Contraindicated in neonates, asthma, glaucoma,

Drugs	Formulation	Dosing	Side Effects	Mechanism of Action	Comments
		Allergic conditions: <2 years: 0.25 mg/kg per day PO, bid-tid 2–6 years: 2 mg PO, bid-tid (max 12 mg per day) 7–14 years: 4 mg PO, bid-tid (max 16 mg per day)	bronchospasm, urinary retention, and blurred vision. *Less common:* Hemolytic anemia, thrombocytopenia, jaundice, photosensitivity, hypotension, and fatigue		GI or GU obstruction, and concomitant use of MAO inhibitors
Deferoxamine Mesylate (Desferal Mesylate)	Injection: 500 mg	Acute iron poisoning: 15 mg/kg per hour IV or 50 mg/kg per dose IM Q 6 h (max 6 g per day) Chronic iron overload: 15 mg/kg per hour IV for 8–12 h	Flushing, erythema, urticaria, hypotension, tachycardia, nausea, vomiting, diarrhea, leg cramps, fever, dizziness, hearing loss, dyspnea, and dysuria	Chelating agent. It binds to iron and promotes excretion	Consider supplementing vitamin C. It increases availability of iron for chelation <10 years: 50 mg daily >10 years: 100 mg daily
Diphenhydramine	Syrup: 12.5 mg/5 mL Liq: 6.5 mg/5 mL Elixir: 12.5 mg/5 mL Tab: 25 and 50 mg Chewable tabs: 12.5 mg Injection: 10 and 50 mg/mL	Allergic rash or urticaria: 5 mg/kg per day PO/IM/IV (max 300 mg per day), q 6 h For anaphylaxis: 1–2 mg/kg slow IV	*Common:* Sedation *Less common:* Paradoxical excitation, convulsion, and postural hypotension	Competitively blocks histamine at H1 receptor	Contraindicated in acute asthma, GI or urinary obstruction
Docusate sodium (Colace)	Syrup: 16.7 and 20 mg/5 mL Solution: 10 and 50 mg/mL Tab: 100 mg Cap: 50, 100, 240, and 250 mg	Constipation: Infants: 5 mg/kg per day, qd-qid <3 years: 10–40 mg per day, qd-qid 3–6 years: 20–60 mg per day, qd-qid 6–12 years: 40–150 mg per day, qd-qid >12 years: 50–500 mg per day, qd-qid	Abdominal cramping, nausea, and rash	Surface-active agent helps to keep stools soft for easy passage	Not habit forming. Oral solution can be given with formula, milk, or fruit juice

Drugs	Formulation	Dosing	Side Effects	Mechanism of Action	Comments
Erythromycin (Erythrocin, Pediamycin)	Drop: 100 mg/ 2.5 mL Suspension: 200, 400 mg/5 mL Ethyl succinate: Tab: 400 mg Chewable tabs: 200 mg Estolate: Tab: 500 mg Cap: 125 and 250 mg Chewable tabs: 125 and 250 mg Suspension: 125 and 250 mg/5 mL Drop: 100 mg/mL Gluceptate: Injection: 1000 mg	Prokinetic: 3 mg/kg per dose IV, tid Adult PO dose 250 mg tid. PO dose for pediatric patient is not established	*Common*: Nausea, vomiting, abdominal pain, diarrhea, and anorexia *Less common*: Cholestatic hepatitis, cardiac arrythmias, vertigo, seizure, and pseudomembranous colitis	Inhibits protein synthesis by binding to 50S ribosomal subunit	Good for short-term use. Do not use for more than 3 weeks
Esomeprazole (Nexium)	Cap: 20 and 40 mg	GERD, erosive esophagitis, gastric and duodenal ulcer: Adult dose 20 or 40 mg qd Pediatric dose not available	*Common*: Headache, diarrhea, nausea, abdominal pain, flatulence, constipation, and dry mouth *Less common*: Back and chest pain, tinnitus, dyspepsia, elevation of transaminases, dysphagia, asthma aggravation, coughing, pharyngitis, rhinitis, sinusitis, and rash	Suppresses gastric acid secretion by inhibition of the H^+/K^+-ATPase in the gastric parietal cell	Unable to take capsule: Open capsule, mix the pellets with applesauce and then swallow immediately. Do not chew or crush the pellets. The pellet and applesauce mixture should not be stored for future use
Famotidine (Pepcid)	Liq: 40 mg/5 mL Tab: 10, 20, and 40 mg Chewable tabs: 10 mg Injection: 10 mg/mL	GERD, gastric, and duodenal ulcer: Infants and children: 1–2 mg/kg per day (max 40 mg per day) PO/IV, qd-bid	*Common*: Headache, dizziness, constipation, and diarrhea *Less common*: Nausea, vomiting, abdominal discomfort,	Competitive inhibitor of H2 receptor. It blocks the histamine-mediated acid secretion from parietal cell	

Drugs	Formulation	Dosing	Side Effects	Mechanism of Action	Comments
			thrombocytope-nia, increased liver number, rash, pruritus, bronchospasm, and anaphylaxis		
Fentanyl (Sublimaze, Duragesic)	Injection: 50 ug/mL	Sedation for procedure: 1–3 µg/kg per dose IV over 3–5 min, repeat 30–60 min prn	*Common:* Respiratory depression, apnea, bradycar-dia, respiratory arrest, hyperten-sion, hypoten-sion, dizziness, and drowsiness *Less common:* Blurred vision, nausea, vomiting, diaphoresis, rigidity, pruritus, constipation, miosis urticaria, laryngospasm, and anaphylaxis	Narcotic analgesic	Less emetic than either morphine or meperidine
Ferric gluconate (Ferrlecit)	Injection: 12.5 mg elemental iron/mL	Iron deficiency anemia: No published data is available. Some children centers use the following protocol: >40 kg: 62.5 mg IV × 10 doses 20–40: 31.2 mg × 10 doses <20 kg: 15.6 mg IV × 10 doses	*Common:* Injection site reaction, hypotension, hypertension, headache, dizzi-ness, nausea, vomiting, diar-rhea, dyspnea, cough, chest pain, leg cramps, and pruritus. *Less common:* Hypersensitivity reaction and anaphylaxis	Replete the body content of iron	Contraindicated if there is any evidence of iron overload
Iron dextran (InfeD)	Injection: 50 mg elemental iron/mL	Iron deficiency anemia: dose calculation: Dextran in mL = 0.0476 × wt in kg ×	Anaphylaxis, hypotension, rash, myalgia, arthral-gia, fever, and skin discoloration.	Replete the body content of iron	Administer test dose: Infant: 12.5 mg Children: 25 mg, IM or IV and

Drugs	Formulation	Dosing	Side Effects	Mechanism of Action	Comments
		(desired Hb – measured Hb) + 1 mL/5 kg body weight (up to max of 14 mL) Max daily dose (IV/IM): <5 kg: 25 mg 5–10 kg: 50 mg >10 kg: 100 mg			wait for an hour before starting the dose. Maximum rate of IV infusion: 50 mg/min
Ferrous sulfate (Fer-in-sol, Feosol)	Elemental iron: 20% Drop: 75 mg/0.6 mL (15 mg Fe); 125 mg/mL (25 mg Fe) Syrup: 90 mg Fe/ 5 mL (18 mg Fe) Elixir: 220 mg/ 5 mL (44 mg Fe) Tab: 195 mg (39 mg), 300 mg (60 mg), and 324 mg (65 mg)	Iron deficiency anemia: 3–6 mg elemental iron/kg per day, qd-bid Prophylaxis: 1–2 mg elemental iron/kg per day, qd-bid	*Common*: Nausea, epigastric discomfort, abdominal pain, constipation, and black stool *Less common*: Diarrhea and discoloration of teeth (by liquid prep)	Replete the body content of iron	Give with or after meal. Consider adding vitamin C to enhance absorption (200 mg/30 mg of iron)
Ferrous gluconate	Elemental iron: 12% Elixir: 300 mg/ 5 mL (34 mg Fe) Tab: 240 mg (27 mg Fe), 300 mg (34 mg Fe), 320 mg (37 mg Fe), and 325 mg (38 mg Fe)	Iron deficiency anemia: 3–6 mg elemental iron/kg per day, qd-bid Prophylaxis: 1–2 mg elemental iron/kg per day, qd-bid	*Common*: Nausea, epigastric discomfort, abdominal pain, constipation, and black stool *Less common*: Diarrhea and discoloration of teeth (by liquid prep)	Replete the body content of iron	Give with or after meal. Consider adding vitamin C to enhance absorption (200 mg/30 mg of iron)
Fluconazole (Diflucan)	Suspension: 10 and 40 mg/mL Tab: 50, 100, 150, and 200 mg Injection: 2 mg/mL	*Candida* or *Cryptococcus* infection: Neonate: 6–12 mg/ kg IV/PO Children: 10 mg/kg (max 400 mg) IV/PO Maintenance: 3–6 mg/kg per day	*Common*: Headache, nausea, abdominal pain, dyspepsia, dizziness, vomiting, diarrhea, and skin rash *Less common*: Hepatitis,	It is a highly selective inhibitor of fungal cytochrome P450 sterol C-14 alpha-demethylation	May cause cardiac arrythmias when used with cisapride, terfenadine, and astemizole

Drugs	Formulation	Dosing	Side Effects	Mechanism of Action	Comments
		IV/PO, qd × 20 days	cholestasis, fulminating hepatic failure, seizure, anaphylaxis, leucopenia, and hypokalemia		
Flucytosin (Ancobon, 5-FC, 5-Fluorocytosine)	Liq: 10 mg/mL Cap: 250 and 500 mg	*Candida* or *Cryptococcus* infection: Neonates: 80–160 mg/kg per day PO, qid Children: 50–150 mg/kg per day PO, qid	*Common*: Nausea, vomiting, abdominal pain, diarrhea, mylosuppression, nephrotoxicity, aspasate aminotransferase (AST), and alanine aminotransferase (ALT) elevation. *Less common*: Rash, ataxia, hearing loss, headache, paresthesia, parkinsonism, peripheral neuropathy, and weakness	Two mechanisms: (a) Competitive inhibition of purine and pyrimidine uptake and thus inhibits fungal DNA synthesis (b) One of its metabolic products, 5-fluorouracil interferes with RNA processing and function	Monitor: CBC, LFT, and renal function Use with caution in patients with impaired renal function Normal peak level: 40–60 mg/L
Flumazenil (Romazicon)	Injection: 0.1 mg/mL	Reversal of benzodiazepine sedation: 0.01 mg/kg (max 0.2 mg) IV, followed by 0.005–0.01 mg/kg per dose IV every min, total cumulative dose of 1 mg. Repeat in 20 min, max of 3 mg in 1 h	*Common*: Injection site pain, nausea, vomiting, dizziness, increased sweating, flushing, headache, blurred vision, and agitation *Less common*: Hiccup, seizures, arrhythmias, bradycardia, shivering, and dysphonia	It antagonizes the actions of benzodiazepine on the CNS	
Fluticanose propionate (Flonase, Flovent)	Aerosol inhaler (MDI): 44, 110, and 220 µg/ actuation Dry powder inhaler (DPI): 50, 100, and 250 µg per dose	Eosinophilic esophagitis: 2 sprays in mouth and then swallow bid-tid	*Common*: Pharyngitis, laryngitis, dysphonia, oropharyngeal candidiasis *Less common*: Cushingoid features,	It is a synthetic glucocorticoid with potent anti-inflammatory activity	Rinse mouth after each use

Drugs	Formulation	Dosing	Side Effects	Mechanism of Action	Comments
		poor growth in children and adolescents, hyperglycemia, osteoporosis, and weight gain			
Folic acid (Folvite)	Solution: 1 mg/mL Tab: 0.4, 0.8, and 1 mg Injection: 5 mg/mL	Folic acid deficiency: Initial dose: <1 year: 15 µg/kg per dose (max 50 µg per day) PO/IV/IM/SC, qd-tid 1–10 years: 1 mg per dose PO/IM/IV/SC, qd-tid >10 years: 1–3 mg per dose PO/IM/IV/SC, qd-tid Maintenance: <1 year: 30–45 µg/kg per day PO, qd 1–10 years: 0.1–0.4 mg per day PO, qd >10 years: 0.5 mg per day PO, qd	None known. May mask hematologic effects of vitamin B$_{12}$	Replete the body content of folic acid	RDA: Up to 1 year: 25–35 µg 1–10 years: 50–100 µg >10 years: 125–200 µg
Foscarnet (Foscavir)	Injection: 24 mg/mL	Acyclovir resistant herpes simplex: 40 mg/kg per dose tid × 3 weeks or until lesions heal	*Common*: Fever, nausea, diarrhea, vomiting, headache, anemia, bone marrow suppression, nephrotoxicity, seizures, and electrolyte abnormalities (hypocalcemia, hypophosphatemia, hyperphosphatemia, hypomagnesemia, and hypokalemia) *Less common*: Peripheral neuropathy, hallucinations,	It inhibits replication of cytomegalovirus and herpes simplex virus types 1 and 2	Stop if Cr ≥ 2.9 mg/dL

Drugs	Formulation	Dosing	Side Effects	Mechanism of Action	Comments
			elevation of AST and ALT, hypertension, coughing, dyspnea, pruritus, and skin rash		
Furazolidone (Furoxone)	Suspension: 3.3 mg/mL Tab: 100 mg	Protozoal diarrhea: 1 month and older: 5–8.8 mg/kg per day (max 400 mg per day) PO, qid	*Common*: Hypotension, urticaria, fever, and arthralgia *Less common*: Nausea, vomiting, headache, drowsiness, dizziness, urine discoloration, and mild reversible intravascular hemolysis	Act by inhibiting several enzyme systems	May cause hemolytic anemia in infants <1 month old due to immature enzyme system It does not significantly alter the normal bowel flora May exhibit a disulfiram-like reaction to alcohol
Furosemide (Lasix, Furomide)	Solution: 8 and 10 mg/mL Tab: 20, 40, and 80 mg Injection: 10 mg/mL	Edema and hypertension: 1–2 mg/kg per dose (max 6 mg/kg per dose) PO or IV, bid	*Common*: Hypokalemia, dehydration, hyperuricemia, increased urine calcium excretion, dizziness, vertigo, hyponatremia, hypomagnesemia, photosensitivity, ototoxicity, and nephrocalcinosis *Less common*: Cholestatic jaundice, hysersensitivity reaction, aplastic anemia, rash, and pruritus	Loop diuretics. It inhibits active NaCl reabsorption in the thick ascending limb of the loop of Henle	Chance of ototoxicity increase when used with aminoglycosides
Gancyclovir (Cytovene)	Cap: 250 and 500 mg Injection: 500 mg	CMV infection: 3 months and older: induction: 10 mg/kg per day IV, bid × 2–3 weeks	*Common*: Neutropenia, thrombocytopenia, anemia, elevation of creatinine,	It is a deoxyguanosine analog that inhibits replication of CMV	Intestinal absorption is poor. IV route is preferred

Drugs	Formulation	Dosing	Side Effects	Mechanism of Action	Comments
		Maintenance: 5 mg/kg per day IV, qd, 5 days per week CMV prevention in transplant recipient: induction same as above but duration 1–2 weeks, followed by maintenance at same dose	catheter infection, and retinal detachment *Less common*: Pneumonia, paresthesia, confusion, elevation of AST and ALT, weight loss, alopecia, and dry skin		IM and SC injections are contraindicated because of high pH of the solution
Gentamicin (Garamycin)	Injection: 10 and 40 mg/mL	Endocarditis prophylaxis (in high risk): 1.5 mg/kg (max 120 mg) IM/IV 30–60 min before procedure with ampicillin or vancomycin For infection: 6–7.5 mg/kg per day IM/IV, tid	*Common*: Nephrotoxicity and ototoxicity *Less common*: Neuromuscular blocked, respiratory depression, visual disturbances, rash, generalized burning, itching, leukopenia, eosinophilia, and AST and ALT elevation	It binds to 30S ribosomal subunit, prevents the formation of initiation complex, which is necessary for bacterial cell wall synthesis	Therapeutic peak level 6–10 mg/L and trough level <2 mg/L
Glucagon	Injection: 1 and 10 mg/vial	Hypoglycemia: 0.03–0.1 mg/kg per dose (max 1 mg), repeat in 20 min if needed GI procedure (decreased motility): Pediatric dose not available	*Common*: Nausea, vomiting, hypoglycemia, respiratory distress, and inhibition of GI motility *Less common*: Urticaria and hypersensitivity reaction	It induces liver glycogen breakdown, releasing glucose from the liver	Blood glucose concentration rises within 10 min of injection and maximal concentrations are attained at approximately a half hour after injection
Glycerin (Fleet Babylax)	Supp: Infant, adult Rectal solution: 4 mL/application	*Constipation*: Neonate: 0.5 mL/kg per dose PR, qd-bid <6 years: 2–5 mL solution or 1 supp PR qd-bid	Rectal irritation, abdominal pain, bloating, and dizziness	Osmotic laxative	Best effect when supp retained for 15 min or longer

Drugs	Formulation	Dosing	Side Effects	Mechanism of Action	Comments
		>6 years: 5–15 mL solution as an enema or 1 adult supp PR, qd-bid			
Granisetron (Kytril)	Tab: 1 mg Injection: 1 mg/mL	Chemotherapy-induced nausea and vomiting: 2 years and older: 10–20 µg/kg per dose IV, 15–60 min before chemotherapy, followed by 2–3 prn doses in 24 hr. Or a single dose of 40 µg/kg IV, 15–60 min before chemotherapy	*Common*: Headache, asthenia, somnolence, diarrhea, constipation, elevation of AST and ALT, hypertension, fever, and taste disorder *Less common*: Agitation, bradycardia, skin rash, and hypersensitivity reaction	It is a selective 5-hydroxytryptamine 3 (5-HT$_3$) receptor antagonist with little or no affinity for other serotonin receptors. It prevents 5-HT$_3$ receptor-mediated activation of vagal nerve	
Hydrocortisone enema (Cortenema)	100 mg/ 60 mL	Proctitis, distal, and left-sided colitis: one application 1–2 times a day for 2–3 weeks	Similar to prednisolone	Potent anti-inflammatory activity. It inhibits NFKβ and decreases release of proinflammatory cytokines IL-1 and IL-2	Rectally administered aminosalicylates are superior to hydrocortisone enemas
Infliximab (Remicaide)	Injection: 100 mg/20 mL	Inflammatory bowel disease: 5 mg/kg per dose (max 10 mg/kg per dose) IV infused over 2–3 h (0, 2, and 6 weeks, and then every 8 weeks)	*Common*: Anaphylaxis, fever, rash, headache, sore throat, dyspnea, chest pain, hypotension, nausea, dysphagia, diarrhea, and serum sickness (3–12 days later) *Less common*: Myalgias, polyarthralgias, hand and facial edema, lupus-like syndrome, and lymphoma	Anti-TNF-α antibody. It binds to both soluble and transmembrane forms of TNF-α. It is a chimeric IgG1 × monoclonal antibody, composed of human constant and murine variable regions	Purified protein derivative (PPD) must be done before infusion. Contraindicated in tuberculosis, systemic fungal infection, and hypersensitivity to murine proteins

Drugs	Formulation	Dosing	Side Effects	Mechanism of Action	Comments
Interferon alpha 2b (Intron A)	3, 5, 18, and 50 million units/mL	Chronic hepatitis B and C: 3 million units/M^2 SC/IM three times a week (TIW) for 1st week, followed by 6 million unit/M^2 TIW × 16–24 weeks (may extend for 18–24 months based on clinical response)	*Common*: Flu-like symptoms (fever, headache, chills, and myalgia), neutropenia, thrombocytopenia, epistaxis, hypertension, edema, anorexia, and urinary tract infection (UTI) *Less common*: Depression, goiter, neurotoxicity, virilism, rhinorrhea, and increased saliva	Inhibits virus replication in virus-infected cells. Enhances phagocytic activity of macrophages and augments specific cytotoxic activity of lymphocytes for target cells	Stop treatment if no clinical response in 24 weeks
Iodoquinol (Yodoxin)	Tab: 210 and 650 mg	Intestinal amebiasis: 30–40 mg/kg per day (max 2 g per day) PO, tid × 20 days	*Common*: Nausea, vomiting, abdominal cramps, diarrhea, pruritus ani, headache, vertigo, and skin eruptions *Less common*: Agitation, thyroid enlargement, optic neuritis, and peripheral neuropathy	Mechanism of action is unknown	Contains 64% organically bound iodine. Contraindicated in hepatic damage Long-term use may cause optic neuritis, optic atrophy, and peripheral neuropathy
Lactulose (Kristalose, Cephulac)	Syrup: 10 g/15 mL	Constipation: 1 mL/kg (max 60 mL) PO, qd-bid Hepatic encephalopathy: Infant: 2.5–10 mL per day PO, tid-qid Children: 40–90 mL per day PO, tid-qid (adjust dose to produce 2–3 soft stools a day)	Flatulence, cramping, nausea, vomiting, and diarrhea	Nonabsorbable sugar. Increase osmotic pressure	Contraindicated in galactosemia. Monitor: Serum ammonia and electrolyte level in encephalopathic patient

Drugs	Formulation	Dosing	Side Effects	Mechanism of Action	Comments
Lamivudine (Epivir)	Solution: 5 and 10 mg/mL Tab: 100, 150, and 300 mg	Hepatitis B infection: 3 mg/kg per day (max 100 mg per day) PO, qd	*Common:* Headache, fatigue, nausea and vomiting, diarrhea, anorexia, abdominal pain, dyspepsia, pancreatitis, neutropenia, elevated liver enzymes, insomnia, peripheral neuropathy, cough, and myalgia *Less common* but serious: Lactic acidosis and severe hepatomegaly with steatosis	Nucleoside analogue. It inhibits reverse transcriptase (RT) and also acts as a DNA chain terminator	Monitor: CBC, LFT, amylase, lipase, and serum HBV DNA Posttreatment exacerbations of hepatitis B, and emergence of viral mutants associated with reduced drug susceptibility and diminished treatment response may occur
Lansoprazole (Prevacid)	Cap: 15 and 30 mg For oral suspension: 15 and 30 mg pack	GERD, erosive esophagitis, and peptic ulcer: 1–2 mg/kg per day PO (max 30 mg per day), qd-bid Zollinger-Ellison syndrome: adult dose, 60 mg daily. Pediatric dose not available	*Common:* Headache, constipation, diarrhea, abdominal pain, and nausea *Less common:* Back and chest pain, tinnitus, dyspepsia, elevation of transaminases, dysphagia, asthma aggravation, coughing, pharyngitis, rhinitis, sinusitis, and rash	Suppresses gastric acid secretion by inhibition of the H^+-/K^+-ATPase in the gastric parietal cell	Oral suspension: Add the granules in 10 mL of water, stir well, and drink immediately. Do not crush or chew the granules
Loperamide (Imodium)	Solution: 0.2 mg/mL Tab: 2 mg Cap: 2 mg	Acute diarrhea (initial dose with in 24 h of symptoms): 2–6 years: 1 mg PO, tid 6–8 years: 2 mg PO, bid	Nausea, vomiting, constipation, sedation, cramps, dry mouth, and rash	Acts by slowing intestinal motility and by affecting water and electrolyte movement through the bowel	Discontinue if no clinical improvement in 2 days

Drugs	Formulation	Dosing	Side Effects	Mechanism of Action	Comments
		> 8 years: 2 mg PO tid Chronic diarrhea: 0.08–0.24 mg/kg per day (max 2 mg per day) PO, bid-tid			
Magnesium citrate (Evac-Q-Mag)	5 mL = 3.9–4.7 meq Mg	Constipation: <6 years: 2–4 mL/kg per day PO, qd-bid 6–12 years: 100–150 mL per day PO, qd-bid >12 years: 150–300 mL per day PO, qd-bid	*Common:* Hypermagnesemia, muscle weakness, and hypotension *Less common:* Respiratory depression	Poorly absorbed ions that retain water in lumen by osmosis and causes reflex increase in peristalsis	Decrease absorption of H2 antago-nist, pheny-toin, iron salt, and steroid
Magnesium hydroxide (Milk of Magnesia)	Liq: 390, 400, and 800 mg/ 5 mL Suspension: 2.5 g/30 mL	Antacid: 2.5–5 mL per dose, PO, qd-qid Laxative: 1–2 mL/ kg per dose (max 60 mL per dose) PO, qd-qid	*Common:* Hypermagnesemia, muscle weakness, and hypotension *Less common:* Respiratory depression	Poorly absorbed ions that retain water in lumen by osmosis and causes reflex increase in peristalsis	Decrease absorption of H_2 antago-nist, pheny-toin, iron salt, and steroid
Megestrol (Megace)	Suspension: 40 mg/mL Tabs: 20 and 40 mg	Appetite stimulant: Children: 10 mg/kg per day (max 800 mg per day) PO, bid	*Common:* Headache, flatu-lence, decreased glucose tolerance, and throm-bophlebitis *Less common:* Constipation, dry mouth, palpitation, dyspnea, oral moniliasis, alope-cia, UTI, gyneco-mastia, and seizure	The precise mechanism is unknown	Safety and effectiveness in pediatric patients have not been established
Meperidine (Demerol)	Syrup: 10 mg/ mL Tabs: 50 and 100 mg Injection: 10, 25, 50, 75, and 100 mg/mL	Analgesia: Children: 1–1.5 mg/kg per dose PO/IV/IM/SC q 3-4 h prn	*Common:* Lightheadedness, dizziness, drowsi-ness, sedation, nausea, vomiting, and sweating, res-piratory depression,	Narcotic analgesic. Binds to opiate receptors in CNS	Onset of action: PO 10–15 min IV 5 min Use lower dose in renal impairment

Drugs	Formulation	Dosing	Side Effects	Mechanism of Action	Comments
			hypotension, and bradycardia *Less common*: Hallucination, paradoxical excitation, constipation, pruritus, urinary retention, seizures, and physical and psychologic dependence		
6-Mercap-topurine (Purinethol)	Tabs: 50 mg	Inflammatory bowel disease: 1.5 mg/kg per day PO, qd	*Common*: Elevated liver enzymes, leukopenia, infections, nausea, and pancreatitis *Less common*: Vomiting, diarrhea, anorexia, stomach pain, skin rash, stomatitis, bone marrow suppression, and hyperuricemia Chronic use may increase the risk of lymphoma and skin cancer	Inhibits synthesis of DNA, RNA, and proteins. Antagonize purine metabolism	Metabolized to 6-TG and 6-MMP. Metabolism rate may vary depending on thiopurine methyl transferase activity Monitor: CBC, ALT, BUN, and creatinine Therapeutic 6-TG level: >235 pmol/ 8×10^8 RBC Allopurinol and probenecid increase drug level
Mesalamine (Asacol, Pentasa, Claversal, Salofalk Rowasa, Canasa)	Asacol: 400 mg enteric-coated tablet Pentasa: 250 mg control release cap Claversal: 500 mg tab Salofalk: 250 mg tab Rowasa: rectal enema 4 g/60 mL	Inflammatory bowel disease: Active disease: 50–100 mg/kg per day (max 4 g per day) PO, bid-tid Maintenance: 50 mg/kg per day (max 3 g per day) PO, bid-tid For distal ulcerative colitis, proctosigmoiditis or	*Common*: Diarrhea, headache, nausea, abdominal pain, dyspepsia, vomiting, and rash *Less common*: Abdominal distension, anorexia, mouth ulcer, GI bleeding, pancreatitis, liver enzyme elevation, pruritus, photosensitivity,	5-Aminosalicylic acid (5-ASA) is the active ingredient. It inhibits leukotriene biosynthesis	Capsules may be opened for administration Tablets must be swallowed whole Pentasa releases throughout the small intestine and colon

Drugs	Formulation	Dosing	Side Effects	Mechanism of Action	Comments
	Canasa: 500 mg rectal suppositories	proctitis: Rowasa enema 2 g daily preferably at bedtime. Or Canasa 500 mg supp. bid-tid	myalgia, arthralgia, acne, and alopecia		Asacol releases in distal ileum and right colon
Methotrexate	Tabs: 2.5 mg Injection: 25 and 50 mg/mL	Inflammatory bowel disease: 15–25 mg or 15 mg/M^2 IM/SC q weekly. Low dose therapy PO not preferred	*Common*: Ulcerative stomatitis, leukopenia, nausea, abdominal distress, malaise, undue fatigue, chills and fever, dizziness, hepatotoxicity, and decreased resistance to infection *Less common*: Vomiting, diarrhea, nephropathy, alopecia, photosensitivity, urticaria, skin pigmentation, and seizure	Inhibits the conversion of folic acid to tetrahydrofolate, an important step for the synthesis of DNA	May cause fetal death or congenital anomalies. Not recommended for women of childbearing potential. Pregnancy should be avoided if either partner is receiving methotrexate
Methylcellulose (Citrucel)	Powder: orange flavor regular or sugar free 2 g/packet Tab: 500 mg	Constipation: Children 6–12 years: 1/2 pack (1 g) in 8 oz of cold water 1–2 times per day	Diarrhea	Bulk forming agent. It increases luminal mass, which stimulates peristalsis	Contraindicated in fecal impaction and swallowing difficulty
Methylprednisone (Solu-Medrol)	Tabs: 2, 4, 8, 16, 24, and 32 mg Injection: 40, 125, 500, 1000, and 2000 mg Depo-Medrol: 20, 40, and 80 mg/mL	Inflammatory bowel disease: 1–2 mg/kg per day (max 60 mg per day) PO/IV, qd-bid	*Common*: Acne, moon face, hirsutism, cutaneous striae, peptic ulcer disease, mood swing, hyperglycemia, and hypertension *Less common*: Headache, pseudotumor cerebri,	Multifactorial: (a) Decreased release of inflammatory cytokines IL-1 and IL-2 (b) Decreased capillary permeability, impaired chemotaxis, and stabilize	Never stop abruptly. Do not use if fungal infection present Consider calcium and vitamin D supplementation in patient

Drugs	Formulation	Dosing	Side Effects	Mechanism of Action	Comments
			psychosis, proximal myopathy, hyperpigmentation, GI bleeding, renal calculi, and aseptic necrosis of femoral head *Long-term use*: Growth retardation, osteoporosis, and posterior subcapsular cataract	lysosomal membranes (c) Enhance sodium and water absorption	on long-term steroid
Metoclopromide (Reglan, Clopra, Maxolon)	Syrup: 1 mg/mL Tab: 5 and 10 mg Injection: 5 mg/mL	Prokinetic: 0.1–0.2 mg/kg per dose (max 15 mg per day) PO/IM/IV, qid Post-op nausea and vomiting: 0.1–0.2 mg/kg per dose PO/IM/IV, qid Chemotherapy-induced emesis: 1–2 mg/kg per dose PO/IM/IV, q 2-6 h	*Common*: Restlessness, drowsiness, fatigue, lassitude, insomnia, headache, confusion, and dizziness *Less common*: Extrapyramidal reactions including tardive dyskinesia, Parkinson-like symptoms and motor restlessness, galactorrhea, gynecomastia, nausea, diarrhea, and leucopenia	It is a cholinergic stimulant, dopamine receptor antagonist. It increases the amplitude and duration of contraction in the esophagus, stomach and duodenum by releasing acetylcholine	Major disadvantage is its side effects compared to its beneficial effects
Metronidazole (Flagyl, Metro)	Suspension: 50 and 100 mg/mL Tab: 250 and 500 mg Cap: 375 mg Injection: 5 mg/mL	Anaerobic infection: 30 mg/kg per day (max 4 g per day) PO/IV, q 6 h Giardiasis: 15 mg/kg per day PO, tid × 7–10 days *Clostridium difficile* infection: 20–30 mg/kg per day PO, tid × 10–14 days Amebiasis: 35–50 mg/kg per day PO, tid × 10 days	*Common*: Nausea, headache, dry mouth, and metallic taste *Less common*: vomiting, diarrhea, insomnia, urticaria, dizziness, stomatitis, urethral burning, pancreatitis, and peripheral neuropathy	Cut the supply of reducing equivalents. May also inhibit DNA synthesis and alter DNA repair	Disulfuram reaction if patient takes alcohol IV: Slow infusion over 1 h

Drugs	Formulation	Dosing	Side Effects	Mechanism of Action	Comments
		Crohn's disease: 10–20 mg/kg per day PO, tid			
Midazolam (Versed)	Syrup: 2 mg/mL Oral solution: 2.5 and 3 mg/mL Injection: 1 and 5 mg/mL	Sedation for procedure: 6 months–5 years: 0.05–0.1 mg/kg per dose IV over 2–3 min. May repeat prn 2–3 min intervals, max dose 6 mg 6–12 years: 0.025–0.05 mg/kg per dose, repeat prn in 2–3 min intervals, max 10 mg >12 years: 0.5–2 mg per dose over 2 min, repeat prn in 2–3 min intervals, max 10 mg	*Common*: Respiratory depression, nausea, vomiting, hypotension, and hiccups *Less common*: Paradoxical excitement and amnesia	Facilitate γ-aminobutyric acid (GABA) mediated inhibition of neuronal activity	May use IV prep for oral administration. Flumazenil can be used to reverse its effect
Mineral oil (Kondremul, Fleet mineral oil enema)	Fleet mineral oil enema 118 mL/ bottle	Constipation: PO: 1–3 mL/kg per day divided qd-tid Rectal: 2–12 years: ½ bottle (59 mL) qd > 12 years: 1 bottle (118 mL) qd	*Common*: Nausea, vomiting, diarrhea, and abdominal cramps *Less common* but serious: Lipid pneumonitis	Coats fecal contents and thereby inhibits absorption of water	Use with caution in babies and young children for risk of aspiration May interfere absorption of fat-soluble vitamins
Misoprostol (Cytotec)	Tabs: 100 and 200 μg	NSAID ulcer prevention: Adult: 100–200 ug PO, qid Pediatric dose not available	*Common*: Nausea, flatulence, headache, dyspepsia, vomiting, and constipation *Less common*: Abdominal pain, vaginal bleeding, menstrual irregularities, rash, and drowsiness	Synthetic prostaglandin E_1 analog. Inhibits gastric acid secretion and protects mucosa	Should be taken for the duration of NSAID therapy. Use with caution in adolescent female. It may cause abortion, premature birth, or birth defects
Mycophenolate mofetil (Cellcept)	Cap: 250 mg Tab: 500 mg	Immunosuppression: 600 mg/m² per day (max 2 g per day)	*Common*: Nausea, GI bleeding, abdominal pain,	It blocks the *de novo* synthesis of guanosine	Patient should avoid exposure to UV light by

Drugs	Formulation	Dosing	Side Effects	Mechanism of Action	Comments
	Suspension: 200 mg/mL	PO, bid. Or 30 mg/kg per day PO, bid	fever, infection, sepsis, diarrhea, vomiting, pharyngitis, respiratory tract infection, hypertension, anemia, constipation, neutropenia, and bone marrow suppression *Less common*: Insomnia, hepatitis, pancreatitis, back pain, hyperglycemia, and possible development of lymphoma	nucleotide by inhibiting inosine monophosphate dehydrogenase (IMPDH). T and B lymphocytes are critically dependent for their proliferation on *de novo* synthesis	wearing protective clothing or using a sunscreen cream
Naloxone (Narcan)	Injection: 0.02, 0.4, and 1 mg/mL	Opiate intoxication: <20 kg: 0.1 mg/kg per dose IV/IM/SC/ETT, repeat prn 2–3 min >20 kg: 2 mg per dose, repeat prn 2–3 min, max 10 mg	*Common*: Nausea, vomiting, sweating, tachycardia, increased blood pressure, and tremulousness *Less common*: Seizures, ventricular tachycardia and fibrillation, pulmonary edema, cardiac arrest, and even death	Opioid antagonist	May precipitate acute opiate withdrawal syndrome
Nystatin (Mycostatin)	Suspension: 100,000 U/mL Tab: 500,000 U	Oral candidiasis: 4–6 mL swish and swallow qid × 2–3 weeks	It is well tolerated even on prolonged administration. May cause diarrhea	Acts by binding to sterols in fungal cell wall. It is both fungistatic and fungicidal	
Octreotide (Sandostatin)	Injection: 50, 100, 200, 500, and 1000 µg/mL	GI bleeding: 1 µg/kg IV bolus, then 1 µg/kg per hour continuous infusion Secretory diarrhea: 1–10 µg/kg per day, divided bid, IV/SC (max 1500 µg per day)	*Common*: Headache, dizziness, diarrhea, nausea, abdominal discomfort, flatulence, hypo or hyperglycemia, bradycardia, constipation, flushing, edema, pruritus, and UTI	Somatostatin analog. Decreases splanchnic blood flow, and inhibits release of serotonin, gastrin, vasoactive intestinal peptide, secretin, motilin,	Long-term use may cause growth hormone suppression

Drugs	Formulation	Dosing	Side Effects	Mechanism of Action	Comments
			Less common: Hepatitis, pancreatitis, arthritis, chest pain, tachycardia, biliary sludge, gall bladder polyp, syncope, seizure, hearing loss, and hematuria	and pancreatic polypeptide. Also inhibits growth hormone, glucagon, and insulin secretion.	
Olsalazine (Dipentum)	Cap: 250 mg	IBD: Weight base children dose is not available. Adult dose: 1 g per day PO, bid	*Common*: Diarrhea, abdominal cramps, nausea, dyspepsia, headache, and arthralgia *Less common*: Anorexia, vomiting, stomtitis, fatigue, depression, rash, increased URI, pancreatitis, neutropenia, and hepatitis	Its metabolites 5-ASA inhibits leukotriene biosynthesis	Used in patients who are intolerant of sulfasalazine Contraindicated in salicylate hypersensitivity
Omeprazole (Prilosec)	Suspension: 2 mg/mL Cap: 10 and 20 mg	GERD, erosive esophagitis, duodenal, and gastric ulcer: 0.5–1.5 mg/kg per day (max 20 mg) PO, qd-bid Zollinzer-Ellison syndrome: requires higher dose	*Common*: Headache, diarrhea, abdominal pain, nausea, rash, and constipation *Less common*: Vitamin B_{12} deficiency, hypertension, pancreatitis, esophageal candidiasis, gastric fundic gland polyps, weight gain, dry skin, and pruritus	Suppresses gastric acid secretion by inhibition of the H^+/K^+-ATPase in the gastric parietal cell	Recipe for making oral suspension: Open one 20 mg capsule and mix with 10 mL of sodium bicarbonate injection (1 meq/mL). Stable for 2 weeks at room temperature
Ondansetron (Zofran)	Solution: 0.8 mg/mL Tab: 4, 8, and 24 mg Orally disintegrated tablets (ODT): 4 and 8 mg Injection: 2 mg/mL	Chemotherapy-induced nausea and emesis: 0.15 mg/kg per dose IV. Or 4–11 years: 4 mg PO >12 years: 8 mg PO 30 min before, 4 and 8 h after	*Common*: Headache, fatigue, constipation, diarrhea, rash, elevation of AST and ALT *Less common*: Bronchospasm, hiccups, tachycardia, chest pain, anaphylaxis, hypokalemia,	$5-HT_3$ receptor antagonist. Activation of this receptor in the CNS and GI tract is a key component in triggering vomiting	

Drugs	Formulation	Dosing	Side Effects	Mechanism of Action	Comments
		chemotherapy followed by q 4 h prn	seizure, and dystonic reaction		
Pancreatic enzyme supplement (Pancrease, Ultrase, Creon, Viokase, Cotazym)	Enteric-coated microspheres and microtablets	Exocrine pancreatic insufficiency: Infants: 2000–4000 units lipase per 120 mL formula or per breast-feeding 1–4 years: 1000 units lipase/kg per meal >4 years: 500 units lipase/kg per meal (max 16,000 units/meal) Take one-half of the meal doses with snacks	*Common*: Abdominal cramps, diarrhea, greasy stools, flatulence, and allergic reactions *Less common*: Colonic stricture (with higher dose >6000 units/kg per meal) and GI bleeding	Hydrolyzes fats into fatty acids and glycerol, split protein into amino acids, and converts carbohydrates to dextrins and short chain sugars	Do not chew microspheres and microtablets. Concurrent use of H2 receptor antagonist or proton-pump inhibitor (PPI) may enhance enzyme activity
Penicillamine (Cuprimine, Depen)	Suspension: 50 mg/mL Tab: 250 mg Cap: 125 and 250 mg	Wilson's disease: <6 months: 250 mg PO, qd 6 months–12 years: 250 mg PO, bid-tid >12 years: 250 mg PO, qid	*Common*: Anorexia, epigastric pain, nausea, vomiting, oral ulceration, pruritus, rash, diminish or total loss of taste perception, leukopenia, thrombocytopenia, and proteinuria *Less common*: Aplastic anemia, hemolytic anemia, nephritic syndrome, glomerulonephritis, peripheral neuropathy, optic neuritis, and myasthenia gravis	Chelating agent	Monitor: CBC, UA Consider adding pyridoxine 25–50 mg per day
Phenobarbital	Elixir: 3 and 4 mg/mL Tab: 8, 15, 16, 30, 32, 60, 65, and 100 mg	For HIDA scan: 5 mg/kg per day PO, bid × 5 days For cholestatic jaundice: 3–10 mg/kg per day PO, bid	*Common*: Sedation, rash, and hypotension *Less common*: Arrhythmias, respiratory depression,	Induces hepatic microsomal enzymes and increases bile acid independent bile flow	Expected serum level in cholestasis 10–20 µg/mL. For cholestasis it

Drugs	Formulation	Dosing	Side Effects	Mechanism of Action	Comments
	Cap: 16 mg Injection: 30, 60, 65, and 130 mg/mL		megaloblastic anemia, and elevation of liver enzymes		is a less preferred agent
Piperacillin/ tazobactum (Zosyn)	Injection: 2, 3, and 4 g (piperacilline to tazobactam ratio 8:1)	Infection: Doses based on piperacilline <6 months: 150–300 mg/kg per day IV, tid-qid 6 months and older: 300–400 mg/kg per day (max 18 g per day) IV, tid-qid	*Common*: Diarrhea, sedation, nausea, vomiting, dyspepsia, constipation, headache, insomnia, rash, pruritus, fever, agitation, moniliasis, hypertension, dizziness, abdominal pain, chest pain, edema, and rhinitis *Less common*: Anaphylaxis, pseudomembranous colitis, vertigo, convulsion, tinnitus, photophobia, flushing, cholestatic jaundice, and Stevens-Johnson syndrome	Piperacillin inhibits bacterial cell wall synthesis. Tazobactum, a beta lactamase inhibitor increases the spectrum of piperacilline activity	Effective against *S. aureus*, *H. influenzae*, *Enterobacter*, *Serratia*, *E. coli*, *P. aeruginosa*, *Bacteroides*, and *Acinetobacter*. Associated with an increased incidence of fever and rash in cystic fibrosis patients
Polyethylene glycol electrolyte solution (Golytely, Nulytely, Colyte)	Golytely powder: polyethylene glycol-3350 236 g, Na sulfate 22.74 g, Na bicarbonate 6.74 g, NaCl 5.86 g, KCl 2.97 g. After dissolving in 4 L of water (isosmotic solution with salty taste) the solution contains	Bowel preparation for colonoscopy or disimpaction of stool in constipation: 25–50 mL/kg per hour until rectal effluent is clear	*Common*: Nausea, abdominal fullness, and bloating *Less common*: Abdominal cramps, vomiting, urticaria, and dyspnea with pulmonary edema	Acts by inducing osmotic diarrhea	Patient should be NPO 3–4 h before administration

Drugs	Formulation	Dosing	Side Effects	Mechanism of Action	Comments
	PEG-3350 17.6 mmol/L, sodium 125 mmol/L, sulfate 40 mmol/L, chloride 35 mmol/L, bicarbonate 20 mmol/L, and potassium 10 mmol/L Nulytely: contains 420 g polyethylene glycol-3350, 5.72 g sodium bicarbonate, 11.2 g sodium chloride, 1.48 g potassium chloride. When dissolved in water to a volume of 4 L, it is an isoosmotic solution having a pleasant mineral water taste				
Polyethylene glycol 3350 powder (Miralax)	Powder: 17 g per capsule	Constipation: 0.8 g/kg per day PO, qd (mix in water or juice 2 g/oz)	*Common*: Nausea, abdominal bloating, and flatulence *Less common*: Abdominal cramps and urticaria	Acts by inducing osmotic diarrhea	It has no taste
Prednisolone Prelone, Pediapred, Delta-Cortef)	Syrup: Pediapred 1 mg/mL, Prelone 3 mg/mL Tab: 5 mg	Inflammatory bowel disease: 1–2 mg/kg per day (max 60 mg per day) PO, qd-bid	*Common*: Acne, cushingoid face, hirsutism, cutaneous striae, hypertension, hyperglycemia, and peptic ulcer *Less common*: Mood changes, GI bleeding, seizures, increased intracranial	Glucocorticoid with potent anti-inflammatory activity. It inhibits NFKβ and decreases release of proinflammatory cytokines IL-1 and IL-2	Immunization should not be undertaken in patients who are on high dose corticosteroids. Consider calcium and vitamin D

Drugs	Formulation	Dosing	Side Effects	Mechanism of Action	Comments
			pressure, proximal myopathy, aseptic necrosis of femoral head, and renal calculi *Long-term use:* Impairment of linear growth, bone resorption, and posterior subcapsular cataract		supplementation in patients who are on long-term steroid therapy
Prednisone	Syrup: 1 mg/mL Tab: 1, 2.5, 5, 10, 20, and 50 mg	Inflammatory bowel disease: 1–2 mg/kg per day (max 60 mg per day) PO, qd-bid	*Common:* Acne, cushingoid face, hirsutism, cutaneous striae, hypertension, hyperglycemia, and peptic ulcer *Less common:* Mood changes, GI bleeding, seizures, increased intracranial pressure, proximal myopathy, aseptic necrosis of femoral head, and renal calculi *Long-term use:* Impairment of linear growth, bone resorption, and posterior subcapsular cataract	Glucocorticoid with potent anti-inflammatory activity. It inhibits NFKβ and decreases release of proinflammatory cytokines IL-1 and IL-2	Immunization should not be undertaken in patients who are on high dose corticosteroids. Consider calcium and vitamin D supplementation in patients who are on long-term steroid therapy
Prochlorperazine (Compazine)	Syrup: 1 mg/mL Tab: 5, 10, and 25 mg Slow release cap: 10, 15, and 30 mg Suspension: 2.5, 5, and 25 mg Injection: 5 mg/mL	Antiemetic: 2 years and older: 0.4 mg/kg per day PO/PR, tid-qid. Or 0.1–0.15 mg/kg per dose (max 40 mg per day) IM, tid-qid	*Common:* Sedation, dry mouth and blurred vision *Less common:* Nausea, vomiting, excitation, convulsions, postural hypotension, photosensitivity, dystonic reaction, tardive dyskinesia, and neuroleptic	Competitive inhibitor of H1 receptor	Decrease seizure threshold. Use with cautious in patients with known seizure disorder

Drugs	Formulation	Dosing	Side Effects	Mechanism of Action	Comments
			malignant syndrome		
Promethazine (Phenargon, Provigan)	Syrup: 6.25 and 25 mg/ 5 mL Tab: 12.5, 25, and 50 mg Sup: 12.5, 25, and 50 mg Injection: 25 and 50 mg/ mL	Antihistaminic: 0.1 mg/kg per dose PO, q 6 h prn Nausea and vomiting 0.25–1 mg/kg per dose PO/IM/IV, q 4-6 h prn Motion sickness: 0.5 mg/kg per dose, 30–60 min before departure followed by q 12 h prn	*Common*: Sedation, dry mouth, and blurred vision *Less common*: Nausea, vomiting, excitation, convulsions, postural hypotension, photosensitivity, dystonic reaction, and neuroleptic malignant syndrome	Competitive inhibitor of H1 receptor	Decrease seizure threshold. Use with cautious in patients with known seizure disorder.
Propranolol (Inderal)	Suspension: 1 mg/mL Solution: 4, 8, and 80 mg/mL Tab: 10, 20, 40, 60, 80, and 90 mg Extended release cap: 60, 80, 120, and 160 mg Injection: 1 mg/mL	Portal hypertension prophylaxis: 0.6–0.8 mg/kg per day PO, bid-qid	*Common*: Exacerbation of asthma and bradycardia *Less common*: Nausea, vomiting, abdominal cramp, constipation, insomnia, thrombocytopenic purpura, SLE, and ischemic colitis	Decrease splanchnic and portal perfusion by blocking the β_2 receptor in the splanchnic bed	Use nonselective agent
Ranitidine (Zantac)	Syrup: 15 mg/mL Tab: 75, 150, and 300 mg	GERD, erosive esophagitis, and peptic ulcer disease: 5–10 mg/kg per day PO, bid-tid	*Common*: Headaches, dizziness, diarrhea, constipation, fatigue, irritability, rash, thrombocytopenia, and elevation of AST and ALT *Less common*: Arrythmias, leukopenia, pancreatitis, rash, and bronchospasm	Competitive inhibitor of H2 receptor. It blocks the histamine mediated acid secretion from parietal cell	Patients with impaired renal function require dose adjustment

Drugs	Formulation	Dosing	Side Effects	Mechanism of Action	Comments
Rifampin (Rifadin, Rimactane)	Suspension: 10 and 15 mg/mL Cap: 150 and 300 mg Injection: 600 mg	Pruritus due to cholestasis: 10–20 mg/kg per day PO/IV, bid	*Common*: Nausea, vomiting, heartburn, headache, jaundice, and discoloration of skin and body secretions *Less common*: Ataxia, bone marrow suppression, rash, myalgia, hemolytic anemia, and pseudomembranous colitis	Precise mechanism is unknown. Possible mechanisms: (a) Enhances hepatic microsomal enzyme activities (b) Inhibits bile acid uptake into the hepatocytes (c) Facilitates metabolism and urinary excretion of bile acids	To reduce GI side effect recommends taking with food
Senna (Senokot)	Syrup: 43.6 mg/ mL Granules: 326 mg/tsp Tab: 187, 217, 374, and 600 mg Supp: 652 mg	Constipation: 0–1 year: 1.25–2.5 mL PO, HS (max 5 mL per day) 1–5 years: 2.5–5 mL PO, HS (max 10 mL per day) 5–15 years: 5–10 mL PO, HS (max 20 mL per day) 15 years and older: 2–4 tabs PO, HS	Nausea, vomiting, abdominal cramps, urine discoloration, and electrolyte and fluid imbalance	It decreases water absorption from the lumen and stimulates intestinal secretion (stimulant laxative)	Active metabolites may stimulate Auerbach's plexus
Simethicone (Mylicon, Phazyme, Mylanta Gas, Gas-X)	Drop: 40 mg/ 0.6 mL Chewable tab: 40, 80, and 125 mg Tab: 60 and 95 mg Cap: 125 mg	Antiflatulent: <2 years: 20 mg PO, qid 2–12 years: 40 mg PO, qid >12 years: 40–125 PO, qid (max 500 mg per day)	None known. Considered safe	In the stomach and intestines it alters the surface tension of gas bubbles enables them to coalesce, thereby freeing and eliminating the gas more easily by belching or passing flatus	Avoid carbonated beverage
Sodium phosphate/ bisphonate (Fleet, Fleet Phospho-Soda)	Fleet enema, pediatric size 67.5 mL (6 g Na phosphate + 16 g Na	Constipation: 1–12 years: 1 pediatric enema PR, may repeat if needed >12 years: 1 adult	Hypocalcemia, hyperphosphatemia, hypernatremia, hypotension, dehydration, and acidosis	Retain water in the lumen by osmosis and causes a reflex increase in peristalsis	Onset of action 5–15 min after rectal and 3– 6 h after

Drugs	Formulation	Dosing	Side Effects	Mechanism of Action	Comments
	biphosphate/ 100 mL) Adult enema: 133 mL, twice the pediatric size Fleet Phospho-Soda: 30, 45, 90, and 237 mL (18 g Na phosphate + 48 g Na biphosphate/ 100 mL)	enema (133 mL) PR, may repeat if needed Phospho-Soda: 5–9 years: 5 mL PO × 1 10–12 years: 10 mL PO × 1 > 12 years: 20–30 mL PO × 1			oral administration
Spironolactone (Aldactone)	Suspension: 1, 2, and 5 mg/mL Tab: 25, 50, and 100 mg	Edema: 1–3.3 mg/kg per day (max 200 mg per day) PO, bid	*Common:* Hyperkalemia, hyponatremia, hyperchloremic metabolic acidosis, and gynecomastia *Less common:* Nausea, vomiting, and rash	It inhibits the action of aldosterone by competitively binding to the cytoplasomic receptor	Contraindicated in renal insufficiency. Use with caution in presence of liver disease
Sucralfate (Carafate)	Suspension: 100 mg/mL Tab: 1 g	GERD, erosive esophagitis, and peptic ulcer disease: 40–80 mg/kg per day (max 4 g per day) PO, qid	*Common:* Constipation *Less common:* Dry mouth, nausea, vomiting, flatulence, gastric discomfort, pruritus, rash, dizziness, insomnia, vertigo, headache, and back pain	It forms an ulcer-adherent complex that covers the ulcer site and protects it against further attack by acid, pepsin, and bile salts	May decrease absorption of fat-soluble vitamins, phenytoin, ketoconazole, and digoxin
Sacoridase (Sucraid)	8500 IU sacrosi-dase/mL	Congenital sucrase-isomaltase deficiency (CSID): 1–2 mL (8500–17,000 IU) PO with each meal or snack diluted with 2–4 oz of water, milk, or infant formula	*Common:* Abdominal pain, vomiting, nausea, diarrhea, and constipation *Less common:* Insomnia, headache, nervousness, and dehydration	Replacement of the enzyme	Do not reconstitute in juice. It may decrease enzyme activity

Drugs	Formulation	Dosing	Side Effects	Mechanism of Action	Comments
Sulfasalazine (Azulfidine)	Tab: 500 mg	Inflammatory bowel disease: Active disease: 50–75 mg/kg per day (max 4 g) PO, tid-qid Maintenance: 50 mg/kg per day (max 3 g) PO, tid-qid	*Common*: Anorexia, headache, nausea, vomiting, dyspepsia, and reversible oligospermia (in one-third of the patients) *Less common*: Pruritus, urticaria, fever, hemolytic anemia (Heinz bodies), agranulocytosis, cyanosis, pancreatitis, hepatitis, bloody diarrhea, hypersensitivity skin rash, fibrosing alveolitis, and alopecia	Its metabolites 5-ASA inhibits leukotriene biosynthesis	Contraindicated in hypersensitivity to sulfasalazine, its metabolites, sulfonamides or salicylates, intestinal or urinary obstruction, and porphyria Monitor: CBC and renal function
Tacrolimus (Prograf)	Suspension: 0.5 mg/mL Caps: 1 and 5 mg Injection: 5 mg/mL	Liver transplant: 0.15–0.3 mg/kg per day divided bid, titrate dose to therapeutic levels IV: continuous infusion 0.05–0.1 mg/kg per day (rarely use) IBD: same dose as above	*Common*: Anorexia, nausea, diarrhea, vomiting, constipation, headache tremor, insomnia, hypertension, hyperglycemia, hypokalemia, hyperkalemia, hypomagnesemia, anemia, abdominal pain, back pain, fever, nephrotoxicity, hepatotoxicity, pruritus, and rash. *Less common*: Myalgia, seizure, cardiomyopathy, opportunistic	Macrolide antibiotic. It binds to FK binding protein in the lymphocyte and inhibits the calcium-dependent pathway of lymphocyte activation (on a weight basis it is 10–100 times more potent immunosuppressor than cyclosporine)	Avoid using simultaneously with cyclosporine Monitor: Serum potassium level Therapeutic trough level: 10–19 ng/mL Blood level may decrease by phenobarbital, phenytoin, carbamazepine, and rifampin Blood level may increase by calcium

Drugs	Formulation	Dosing	Side Effects	Mechanism of Action	Comments
			infection, and lymphoprolifera-tive disorder		channel block-ers, antifungal imidazole group, macrolide antibiotics, cimetidine, cyclosporine, methylpred-nisolone, and grapefruit juice
Thalidomide	Cap: Thalomid 50 mg	Inflammatory bowel disease: Adult: 100–300 mg per day PO, qd, preferably at bed-time. Dose for pediatric patients is not available	*Common*: Teratogenicity, drowsiness, somnolence, rash, peripheral neuropathy, dizziness, orthostatic hypotension, and neutropenia *Less common*: Dry mouth, thrombocytope-nia, hyper-glycemia, hyperkalemia, hypocalcemia, leg cramps, arthritis, and hepatospleno-megaly	It is an inhibitor of TNF-α	Contraception must be used for at least 4 weeks before and for 4 weeks follow-ing discontin-uation of thalidomide therapy. Thalidomide is present in the semen. Males receiving thalidomide must com-pletely abstain from hetero-sexual contact or always use a latex condom during sex
Ursodeoxy-cholic acid (Actigal)	Suspension: 60 mg/mL Cap: 300 mg	Cholestatic jaundice: 10–30 mg/kg per day PO, bid Cystic fibrosis (to improve fatty acid metabolism): 15–30 mg/kg per day PO, qd-tid	*Common*: Diarrhea, dys-pepsia, vomiting, arthritis, pharyn-gitis, back pain, and dizziness *Less common*: Constipation, headache, and alopecia	Hepatoprotective agent. Possible mechanisms: (a) enhance hepatocyte excretion of toxic bile acids in bile, (b) improve bile flow,	It is the major bile acid of black bear. Normally present only small quanti-ties in human

Drugs	Formulation	Dosing	Side Effects	Mechanism of Action	Comments
				(c) stabilize hepatocyte membrane, and (d) protect hepatocyte mitochondria from permeability transition	
Vancomycin (Vancocin)	Solution: 1 and 10 g powder. Reconstitute to 500 mg/6 mL (83.33 mg/mL) Cap: 125 and 250 mg Injection: 500 mg; 1, 2, 5, and 10 g	*C. difficile* colitis: 20–40 mg/kg per day PO, qid × 7–10 days Endocarditis prophylaxis in penicillin allergic patient: 20 mg/kg (max 1 g) IV over 1–2 h plus gentamicin 1.5 mg/kg (max 120 mg) IM/IV completed 30 min before the procedure	*Common:* Nephrotoxicity, ototoxicity, and neutropenia *Less common:* Red man syndrome, anaphylaxis, drug fever, chills, nausea, eosinophilia, rashes, Stevens-Johnson syndrome, toxic epidermal necrolysis, and rare cases of vasculitis	Inhibits cell wall biosynthesis. In addition, it also alters bacterial cell membrane permeability and RNA synthesis	For *C. difficile* infection vancomycin should always be given orally
Vasopressin (Pitressin)	Injection: 20 U/mL	GI bleeding: start at 0.002–0.005 U/kg per min, then increase dose as needed up to 0.01 U/kg per min	*Common:* Tremor, sweating, vertigo, nausea, vomiting, abdominal discomfort, hypertension, and bradycardia *Less common:* Bronchoconstriction, anaphylaxis, and water intoxication	It causes contraction of smooth muscles of the vascular bed	Antidiuretic hormone analog. Taper dose before discontinuation
Vitamin A (Aquasol A)	Drop: 5000 IU/ 0.1 mL Tab: 5000 IU Cap: 10,000, 25,000, and 50,000 IU	Cholestasis: 5000–25,000 IU PO, qd Cystic fibrosis: 5000 IU PO, qd	Hepatotoxicity, rash, headache, pseudotumor cerebri, papilledema, hypercalcemia, and irritability	Replete the body content of vitamin A	RDA: Up to 1 year: 1250 IU 1–3 years: 1333 IU 4–6 years: 1667 IU

Drugs	Formulation	Dosing	Side Effects	Mechanism of Action	Comments
	Injection: 50,000 IU/mL				7–10 years: 2333 IU 11–18 years: 2667–3333 IU
Vitamin A, D, E, and K	Drops and chewable tablets	Cystic fibrosis: 0–1 year: 1 mL PO, qd 1–2 years: 2 mL PO, qd 2–12 years: 1 tablet PO, qd >12 years: 2 tablets PO, qd	Most common is nausea	Replete the body content of vitamin A, D, E, and K	1 mL of drop contains: A—3170 IU D—400 IU E—40 IU K—100 μg Each chewable tablet contains: A—9000 IU D—400 IU E—150 IU K150 μg
Vitamin D 1,25-OH (Rocaltrol)	Cap: 0.25 and 0.5 μg Injection: 1 μg/mL	Cholestasis: 0.05–0.3 μg/kg per day PO, qd	Hypercalcemia, nephrocalcinosis, and constipation	Replete the body content of vitamin D	RDA: Preterm: 400–800 IU <1 year: 300 IU 1 year and older: 400 IU
Vitamin D 25-OH (Calderol)	Cap: 20 and 50 μg	Cholestasis: 3–5 μg/kg per day PO, qd	Hypercalcemia, nephrocalcinosis, and constipation	Replete the body content of vitamin D	RDA: Preterm: 400–800 IU <1 year: 300 IU 1 year and older: 400 IU
Vitamin D₂ Ergocalciferol (Drisdol)	Drops: 8000 IU/mL Tab: 50,000 IU Injection: 500,000 IU/mL	Cholestasis: 5000–8000 IU PO, qd Cystic fibrosis: 400 IU PO qd	Hypercalcemia, nephrocalcinosis, and constipation	Replete the body content of vitamin D	RDA: Preterm: 400–800 IU <1 year: 300 IU 1 year and older: 400 IU
Vitamin E (Aquasol E, Liqui-E)	Aquasol E: 50 IU/mL Liqui-E: 25 IU/mL	Cholestasis: Liqui-E: 15–25 IU/kg per day PO, qd	Headache, diarrhea, rash, decreased serum thyroxine and triiodothyronine	Replete the body content of vitamin E	RDA: 3–10 IU per day. Liqui-E better absorbed than Aquasol E

Drugs	Formulation	Dosing	Side Effects	Mechanism of Action	Comments
		Aquasol E: 50–400 IU/kg per day PO, qd Cystic fibrosis: Aquasol E: 25– 400 IU PO, qd	level, and blurred vision		
Vitamin K (Mephyton)	Tab: 5 mg Injection: 10 mg/mL	Cholestasis: 2.5–5 mg PO/IM/ SC/IV qd-twice per week Vitamin K deficiency: 1–2 mg IM/SC/IV Liver failure: 1 mg per year of age (max 10 mg) IM/SC/IV Cystic fibrosis: <1 year on no antibiotic: 2–5 mg PO per week <1 year on antibiotic: 2–5 mg PO, twice per week >1 year on antibiotic or associated liver disease: 2–5 mg PO, twice per week	Transient flushing, dizziness, rapid and weak pulse, sweating, and dyspnea Rare but serious: Anaphylactoid reaction	Replete the body content of vitamin K	RDA: Up to 1 year: 5 µg 1–6 years: 10–20 µg 7–10 years: 30 µg 11 years and older: 45– 65 µg
Zinc sulfate	Liq (acetate): 5 and 10 mg elemental Zn/mL Tab and cap: 23% elemental Zn as sulfate Tab: 66 mg (15 mg elemental Zn), 110 mg (25 mg elemental Zn). Cap: 110 mg (25 mg elemental Zn), 220 mg (50 mg elemental Zn) Injection: 1 and 5 mg elemental Zn/mL	Zinc deficiency: Children: 1 mg/kg per day elemental zinc PO, bid-tid. Supplement in TPN (IV): Premature infants: 400 µg/kg per day <3 months: 300 µg/ kg per day >3 months to 5 years: 100 µg/kg per day (max 5 mg per day) >5 years: 2–5 mg per day	Common: Nausea, vomiting, leukopenia, and diaphoresis Less common: Tachycardia, hypotension, gastric ulcer, and jaundice	Replete the body content of zinc	Administer with food to reduce GI side effect

Bibliography

Gunn VL, Nechyba C (eds). *The Harriet Lane Handbook*, 16th ed. Philadelphia, PA: Mosby, 2002.

Katzung BG (ed.). *Basic and Clinical Pharmacology*, 7th ed. New York, NY: McGraw-Hill, 2002.

North American Society for Pediatric Gastroenterology, Hepatology, and Nutrition (NASPGHAN). *Drug Formulary*.

Physicians Desk Reference (PDR), 57th ed. New Jersey, NJ: Medical Economic Company, 2003.

Walker WA, Durie PR, Hamilton JR, Walker-Smith JA, Watkins JB (eds.). *Pediatric Gastrointestinal Disease*, 3rd ed. Ontario, ON: BC Decker, 2000.

Web site for updated drug information: PDR.net and MEDLINEplus drug information.

Wyllie R, Hyams J (eds.). *Pediatric Gastrointestinal Disease*, 2nd ed. Philadelphia, PA: WB Saunders, 1999.

31

MEDICAL NUTRITION THERAPY IN THE PEDIATRIC PATIENT

Melanie R. Silverman, Angela Dye,
and JoAnn Kaiser Froehlke

INTRODUCTION

This chapter provides an overview of pediatric nutrition, covering four subject areas: general pediatric nutrition, disease-specific diets, tube-feeding, and parenteral nutrition. While the authors of this chapter have attempted to give ample nutrition information, this does not replace the need for consultation with a pediatric registered dietitian. Dietitians are considered foremost experts in food and nutrition, able to recommend appropriate diets, tube-feeding formulas, and parenteral nutrition regimens necessary to achieve maximum growth potential. In hospital settings there should be dietitians available for consult, otherwise contact the American Dietetic Association (www.eatright.org).

THE PEDIATRIC PATIENT'S RELATIONSHIP TO FOOD

Food plays an important role in the growth and development of a child. The macronutrients (carbohydrate, protein, and fat) provide energy for the formation of cells and the synthesis of enzymes, hormones, and transport molecules. The micronutrients (vitamins, minerals, and trace elements (TE)) function as cofactors and coenzymes in metabolic reactions.[1] In addition, food has an important emotional significance for children. For example, food is often the central focus of holidays, birthdays, weekends, and family vacations. When certain foods must be eliminated due to a disease process, families face emotional challenges. Parents often feel isolated preparing special formulas or foods. Older pediatric patients may feel frustrated and sad, not able to eat the same foods as their friends. Physicians and other members of the medical team need to be sensitive to these emotions. Understanding the everyday challenges, while providing sound nutritional advice, will help families better confront the nutritional and medical challenges ahead.

THE GROWING CHILD'S NUTRITIONAL NEEDS

Nutrient Requirements

The Food and Nutrition Board of the National Research Council published the first edition of the recommended dietary allowances (RDAs) in 1941, outlining the essential nutrients needed for most healthy populations. Since 1941, the levels have been revised several times to include new scientific knowledge.[2] Recently, dietary reference intakes (DRIs) were developed, specifically targeted to prevent nutritional deficiencies, reduce the risk of chronic diseases, promote optimal health, and prevent toxicities.[3] The DRIs consist of four reference values, including the RDAs:

- *Adequate intakes (AI).* The daily nutrients recommended based on observed or experimentally determined approximations of intake by groups of healthy people.
- *Estimated average requirements (EAR).* The daily intake value that is estimated to meet the requirement defined by a specified indicator of adequacy in 50% of an age- and gender-specified group.
- *Recommended dietary allowances.* The average daily dietary intake levels that are sufficient to meet the nutritional needs of 97–98% of healthy people in a group.
- *Tolerable upper intake levels (UL).* The highest levels of daily nutrients that would not be hazardous to health. As intake increases above this level, the risk of adverse effects increases.

When estimating the calorie and protein needs of a healthy child, the RDAs are a good starting point as listed below:[3]

Age of Pediatric Patient	Calories Per Kilogram Body Weight	Protein Grams per Kilogram Body weight
Birth to 6 months	108	2.2
6–12 months	98	1.6
1–3 years	102	1.2
4–6 years	90	1.1
7–10 years	70	1.0
Females: 11–14 years	47	1.0
Females: 15–18 years	40	0.8
Males: 11–14 years	55	1.0
Males: 15–18 years	45	0.9

Fluid

Fluid estimations for infants and children are based on their body water content and the limited capacity of their kidneys to handle high solute loads. In general, fluid is lost through the gastrointestinal (GI) tract, kidneys, lungs, and skin. The Holliday-Segar and body surface area methods are two equations used to estimate fluid maintenance for children.

1. Holliday-Segar method[4]
   - 1st 10 kg body weight: 100 mL/kg
   - 2nd 10 kg body weight: 1000 mL + 50 mL/kg >10 kg
   - Each additional kg: 1500 mL + 20 mL/kg >20 kg
2. Body surface area method[5]
   - 1500 mL/m^2 24 h

The amount of fluid lost increases when there is an increase in respiratory rate or fever. Increases can also be attributed to a hot or dry environment, injuries to the skin or tissue, diarrhea, vomiting, ketoacidosis, and hyperosmolar nonketotic dehydration.

Nutritional Aspects in Different Ages and Stages of Childhood

Each age group has unique growth patterns and exhibits different feeding characteristics. Patients can be categorized into four stages with respect to age: infancy (birth to 2 years old), preschool years (2–6 years old), middle childhood (7–10 years old), and adolescence (11–18 years old).[5]

Premature Infants

Premature infants are initially classified according to birth weight.

- Low birth weight (LBW): less than 2500 g
- Very low birth weight (VLBW): less than 1500 g
- Extremely low birth weight (ELBW): less than 1000 g

Physical parameters such as weight, length, and head circumference are then plotted on intrauterine growth curves. Two of the most common curves are the Denver Growth Chart reported by Lubchenco and group and the Babson/Benda Intrauterine and Postnatal Growth Chart. Both have their limits, but are among the most useful charts available.[6]

Once premature infants are assessed on growth curves, they are designated as small for gestational age (SGA) or less than the 10th percentile; appropriate for gestational age (AGA) or between the 10th percentile and 90th percentile; or large for gestational age (LGA) or greater than the 90th percentile.[6] Premature infants are expected to gain an average of 14.9 g/kg per day or 25.2 g per day until they reach full-term.

Feeding Issues

Premature infants have the highest calorie and protein needs per kilogram. Recommended enteral nutrient intakes for premature, low birth weight infants are 105–130 calories per kilogram (cal/kg) and 3–4 grams of protein per kilogram (g/kg). Values should be adjusted depending on the patient's medical condition and size.[7]

Human milk is strongly encouraged for the premature infant, but premature formulas are also available. The feeding route depends on the premature infant's gestational age. Coordinated suck and swallow mechanisms are not developed until 32–34 weeks gestation; therefore, tube-feeding is often necessary.[8] While enteral nutrition is the preferred feeding route for these patients, feeding intolerance, especially in very small infants, is common.

Infancy: Birth to 2 Years of Age

An infant's weight, length, head circumference, and weight-to-height ratio can be plotted on sex-specific growth charts published by The National Center for Health Statistics (NCHS) www.cdc.gov/growthcharts. The percentile distributions represent a cross-section of children in the United States. Healthy children should follow a predictable path of growth along these curves.[4]

Infants will lose weight after birth, but should regain the weight in 8–10 days. Healthy infants are expected to double their weight in 6 months and triple it in a year.

Feeding Issues

The infant's primary nutritional source should be breast milk for the first 6 months of life. When breast milk is not used, infant formula is available.

Introduction of solid foods, beginning with iron-fortified rice cereal, occurs at 5–6 months. Feeding progression must be balanced with nutrient needs and physical readiness (Table 31-1).[5]

At 1 year of age, children will show preferences in foods. Parents or caregivers are responsible for what, when, and where a child eats; the child is responsible for determining how much and whether he or she will eat. Children are excellent regulators of their appetite, so force-feeding is never recommended.

Preschool Years: 2–6 Years of Age

Beginning at age 2, the body mass index (BMI) or the Quetelet index of a child can be plotted on growth curves in addition to weight, height, and weight-for-height (www.cdc.gov/growthcharts). BMI is calculated by dividing weight in kilograms by height in meters squared [wt (kg)/ht^2 (m^2)]. BMI is a simple method for obesity screening, but reviewing other parameters is helpful in evaluating a pediatric patient's adiposity.[3]

Feeding Issues

Children at this age will begin to exert more independence in their eating and developing habits that could put them at risk for obesity later in life. Healthy food options must be made available.

Portion sizes are difficult to estimate for preschool children. A long-standing rule of thumb is to offer one tablespoon of each food group for every year of age with more provided according to appetite. Because of the relatively small gastric size, snacks are important and should be planned accordingly. In total, a child may need to eat four to six times per day.

Excessive juice intake has been shown to lead to failure to thrive (FTT) and chronic diarrhea; it should be limited. In addition, parents and/or caregivers need to be aware of foods that are potential choking hazards at this age, such as hot dogs, grapes, raw vegetables, popcorn, peanut butter, nuts, and hard candy.[9]

Middle Childhood: 7–10 Years of Age

Physicians continue to plot children on curves to track growth (www.cdc.gov/growthcharts). Children's bodies prepare for the changes that will occur during adolescence.[5]

TABLE 31-1

INTRODUCTION OF SOLID FOODS

Food Groups	Birth to 4 Months	4–5 Months	5–7 Months	7–9 Months	9–12 Months
Breastmilk	On demand	On demand	On demand	On demand	On demand
Iron-fortified infant formula (oz)	1st month = 20–26 2nd month = 24–31 3rd month = 26–35 4th month = 30–39	5th month = 32–38	6th month = 30–36 7th month = 28–34	8th month = 26–32 9th month = 26–30	10th month = 24–28 12th month = 22–26
Iron–fortified dry infant cereal		1/4 to 1/3 cup rice cereal once or twice a day (use breast milk or formula to mix with cereal)[a]	1/4 to 1/3 cup cereal twice daily (delay use of barley, oats, and wheat until 6 months old)	1/3 to 1/2 cup cereal once per day	1/2 to 3/4 cup cereal once per day
Vegetables			2–6 tbsp well cooked, plain mashed vegetables once or twice per day	3–8 tbsp well cooked, mashed vegetables twice per day	1/4 to 1/3 cup well cooked, mashed or chopped vegetables twice per day
Fruits			2–6 tbsp plain, strained fruits or 1/4 cup mashed banana once or twice per day	3–8 tbsp soft, mashed fruit twice per day	1/4 to 1/3 cup chopped, soft fruits twice per day
Meats and protein foods				1/4 to 1/3 cup strained meat or poultry, 1/8 cooked egg yolk, cooked mashed dried beans or tofu	1/8 to 1/4 cup small tender pieces of meat, poultry, cottage cheese, egg yolk, yogurt, cooked dried beans or tofu
Juice, unsweetened				1–2 oz from a cup	2–4 oz from a cup
Crackers or bread				2–4 saltine squares	2–4 saltines or 1/2 slice bread, 1/4 cup rice or pasta twice per day

[a]Cereal can be delayed until 6 months if desired. Breast milk or formula provides adequate nutrition.

Source: Permission for use granted by NCES, Inc., 1904 East 123rd Street, Olathe, Kansas 66061 (800)445-5653 www.ncescatalog.com.

Feeding Issues

Children exert more independence at this age and may begin to prepare their own food. Family meals may become infrequent as activities increase outside of the home. Skipping breakfast is common, though undesirable since missing meals can later lead to overeating. Parents and/or caregivers should pay close attention to provide healthy food, snack options, and structured mealtimes as much as possible.[9]

Adolescence: 11–18 Years of Age

The adolescent population experiences dynamic physical and emotional changes. During this stage of development, patients often become overly sensitive to their bodies. The risk for unsafe dieting and use of diet products is high, resulting in the susceptibility to eating disorders. Eating disorders are complex issues with medical, social, cultural, and nutritional issues. Physicians should be aware of how to identify these issues and refer a patient to a trained professional for assistance.[9] The American Academy of Pediatrics (AAP) published a recent policy statement on identifying and treating eating disorders (www.aap.org/policy/020003.html).

Feeding Issues

Appetite, age, gender, and activity level should guide adolescent food intake. Unfortunately, these patients often develop irregular eating patterns, spending more time socializing away from home, and eating inexpensive fast food. Encouraging patients to limit their consumption and choose healthier menu items is the appropriate recommendation.[9]

FEEDING THE GROWING CHILD

Breast Milk and Breast-feeding

Breast milk is the optimal nutritional source for growth and development of an infant. In 1997, the AAP updated its breast-feeding policy statement due to the considerable advancements in scientific knowledge. There is strong evidence that human milk decreases the incidence and/or severity of diarrhea, respiratory infections, otitis media, bacteremia, bacterial meningitis, botulism, urinary tract infections, and necrotizing enterocolitis. There is also some evidence, though not as strong, that breast-feeding may have a protective effect against sudden infant death syndrome, insulin-dependent diabetes mellitus, Crohn's disease, ulcerative colitis, allergic diseases, and other chronic digestive diseases. Rarely is breast-feeding contra-indicated due to a disease state or medication in a mother or infant. The International Lactation Consultants Association (ILCA) at http://www.ilca.org can answer questions about breast-feeding. The complete policy statement from the AAP is located online at www.aap.org/policy/re9729.html.

Formula Feeding

When a mother chooses not to breast-feed or cannot for medical reasons, infant formulas are available. It should be noted that nutrients are absorbed and used more efficiently in breast milk than formula. Consequently, formulas are higher in protein, vitamins, and minerals to ensure adequate nutrient intake.[10]

The AAP recommends that infants start cow's milk at 1 year, though many parents begin feeding cow's milk prior to that time. One of the negative consequences of starting cow's milk too early is the risk of iron deficiency anemia. Special toddler formulas were developed for older infants and younger children to reduce the problems associated with early cow milk introduction. These formulas comply with the Infant Formula Act of 1980, mandating certain levels of nutrients. Physicians should encourage those parents providing cow's milk early to use one of the toddler formulas instead.[10]

Fatty Acids in Formula

Recently, there has been much research and debate about the inclusion of long-chain polyunsaturated fatty acids (LCPUFAs), docosahexaenoic acid (DHA), and arachidonic acid (ARA) in infant formulas. Breast milk naturally contains these important fatty acids and breast-fed infants have higher levels of these fatty acids in their blood and tissues. Some studies have suggested that these additives may have important roles in cognitive development, visual acuity, and growth.[11] Several formula companies have begun to fortify formulas with DHA and ARA, hoping to achieve an infant formula closer to the composition of breast milk. At this time, the AAP has not issued an official position statement on the addition of fatty acids to infant formulas; clearly further research is needed.

Formula Categories

Some of the commonly used pediatric formulas in the United States are listed in Table 31-2. While the authors have attempted to provide a comprehensive listing of formulas, it may not be complete as formula manufacturers are constantly reformulating and improving products. For the most updated nutritional information, contact the manufacturers directly. The contact information is available in the bibliography section. Detailed information about each formula category is listed in Table 31-2.

Premature Infant Formulas

- *Human milk fortifiers.* This is a powder added to premature infants fed breast milk. Fortification is necessary because of the increased needs in calories, protein, vitamins, and minerals that human milk cannot solely supply to the very low birth weight infant.
- *Premature formulas.* Formulas contain higher calorie, protein, and mineral concentrations to compensate for prematurity.[12]
- *Transition formulas.* These formulas have more calories, protein, vitamins, and minerals than term formulas for ex-premature infants. The recommended use is throughout the first year of corrected gestational age.

Cow Milk Based Infant Formulas

- *Term infant formulas—Cow milk based.* The formulas contain lactose, intact protein, and a low-to-moderate osmolality. Formulas with lower electrolytes or added rice starch for reflux are included in this group.[12]
- *Lactose free formulas.* These formulas are available for infants with lactase deficiency.

- *Modified fat formulas.* Formulas contain 60–86% of fat as medium chain triglycerides (MCT) and are useful in the management of steatorrhea, chylous ascites, or chylothorax.

Soy Formulas for Infants and Children Over 1 Year

Soy and lactose free formulas. These formulas contain intact protein, low-to-moderate osmolality, and are used for primary or secondary lactase deficiency or galactosemia.[12,13] Soy or lactose free formulas are not recommended for infants with suspected or proven cow's milk protein allergy. It is well known that up to 50% of the infants allergic to milk protein will develop allergy to soy protein when switched to soy formulas.

Semielemental Formulas for Infants and Children Over 1 Year

Formulas are lactose free with partially hydrolyzed protein, partial medium chain triglycerides, and a low-to-moderate osmolality. Formulas are recommended for steatorrhea, intestinal resection, cystic fibrosis, chronic liver disease, inflammatory bowel disease (IBD), diarrhea, cow's milk allergy, and soy protein allergy.

Elemental Formulas for Infants and Children over 1 Year

Formulas are lactose free, low in fat, and have a high osmolality. Protein is provided in the free amino acid form and is useful in feeding patients intolerant to the semielemental formulas.[12]

Formulas for Children 1–10 Years of Age

Formulas are approximately 30 calories per ounce (100 cals/100 mL) with a high renal solute load, a low-to-moderate osmolality, and some can contain fiber.

Modular Components

The components provide individual carbohydrate, protein, and fat components that can be added to formulas or food.[4]

T A B L E   3 1 - 2

INFANT AND PEDIATRIC FORMULAS

Cow, Soy, Rice and Lactaid Milks

Milk	Cals (100 kcal)	Vol/oz (mL)	Kcal/oz (30 mL)	Carb. Source	Carb (g)	Protein Source	Protein (g)	Fat Source	Fat (g)	A (IU)	D (IU)	E (IU)	K (µg)	Thiamin (µg)	Riboflavin (µg)	B6 (µg)	B12 (µg)	Niacin (µg)	Folate (µg)	Pantothenic Acid (µg)	Biotin (µg)	C (mg)	Choline (mg)	Inositol (mg)	Ca mg (meq)	P (mg)	Mg (mg)	Fe (mg)	Zn (mg)	Mn (µg)	Cu (µg)	I (µg)	Se (µg)	Na mg (meq)	K mg (meq)	Cl mg (meq)	Renal Solute Load mOsm	Osmol mOsm/kg water	Lactose Free?	Gluten Free?	Milk Protein Free?	Fiber (gms)
Whole milk	100	159	20	Lactose	7.7	Cow milk (casein predominant)	5.39	Butterfat	5.48	207	67	0.1	6	62	266	69	0.59	138	8	515	5.1	2	33	7	195 (9.7)	152	21.3	0.08	0.6	4	21	7	n/a	80 (3.5)	249 (6.4)	164 (4.6)	50.1	285	No	Yes	No	-
2% milk	100	194	15	Lactose	9.6	Cow milk (casein predominant)	6.70	Butterfat	3.80	410	82	0.1	4	78	330	86	0.7	172	10	640	n/a	2	n/a	n/a	244 (12.2)	190	28	0.1	0.8	5	27	9	n/a	100 (4.3)	308 (7.9)	204 (5.8)	62.3	n/a	No	Yes	No	-
1% milk	100	234	11	Lactose	12	Cow milk (casein predominant)	7.80	Butterfat	2.34	n/a	95	n/a	n/a	94	400	101	0.9	210	12	772	n/a	2.4	n/a	n/a	299 (15)	226	33	0.12	0.9	7.8	23	n/a	5.2	121 (5.3)	374 (9.5)	n/a	n/a	n/a	No	Yes	No	-
Skim milk	100	272	10	Lactose	13.8	Cow milk (casein predominant)	10.50	Butterfat	0.54	562	111	n/a	n/a	100	390	109	1.1	245	13.9	916	n/a	2.8	n/a	n/a	335 (17)	281	31	0.11	1.1	9.1	27	n/a	5.8	144 (6.3)	462 (12)	n/a	n/a	n/a	No	Yes	No	-
Soy milk	100	300	10	Soybeans, rice syrup	5.54	Soybeans	8.40	Soybeans	5.80	98	n/a	n/a	n/a	490	210	130	0	450	6.1	150	n/a	0	n/a	n/a	12 (0.6)	150	58	1.8	0.7	520	370	n/a	3.9	37 (1.6)	43 (1.1)	n/a	n/a	n/a	Yes	Yes	Yes	4 g/100 kcal
Rice milk[a]	100	200	15	brown rice	2.1	(minimal)	0.83	Expeller pressed high oleic Safflower oil	1.70	n/a	n/a	n/a	n/a	n/a	n/a	n/a	n/a	n/a	n/a	n/a	n/a	n/a	n/a	n/a	75 (3.3)	n/a	n/a	n/a	n/a	n/a	n/a	n/a	n/a	n/a	n/a	n/a	n/a	n/a	Yes	No	Yes	-
Enriched rice milk[a]	100	200	16	brown rice	21	(minimal)	0.83	Expeller pressed high oleic Safflower oil	1.70	385	n/a	0.92	n/a	n/a	n/a	n/a	1.1	n/a	n/a	n/a	n/a	n/a	n/a	n/a	231 (12)	n/a	n/a	n/a	n/a	n/a	n/a	n/a	n/a	n/a	n/a	n/a	n/a	n/a	Yes	No	Yes	-
Lactaid milk 2%	130	240	16	Lactase enzymes added	12	Cow milk (casein predominant)	8.00	Butterfat	5.00	n/a	n/a	n/a	n/a	n/a	n/a	n/a	1.1	n/a	n/a	n/a	n/a	n/a	n/a	n/a	n/a	n/a	n/a	n/a	n/a	n/a	n/a	n/a	n/a	n/a	n/a	n/a	n/a	n/a	Yes	Yes	No	-

Human Milk and Human Milk Fortifiers for Premature Infants

	Cals 100 kcal	Vol (mL)/oz	Kcal/oz (30 mL)	Carb. Source	Carb (g)	Protein Source	Protein (g)	Fat Source	Fat (g)	A (IU)	D (IU)	E (IU)	K	Thiamin (µg)	Riboflavin (µg)	B6 (µg)	B12 (µg)	Niacin (µg)	Folate (µg)	Pantothenic Acid (µg)	Biotin (µg)	C (mg)	Choline (mg)	Inositol (mg)	Ca mg (meq)	P (mg)	Mg (mg)	Fe (mg)	Zn (mg)	Mn (µg)	Cu (µg)	I (µg)	Se (µg)	Na mg (meq)	K mg (meq)	Cl mg (meq)	Renal Solute Load mOsm	Osmolality mOsm/kg water	Lactose Free?	Gluten Free?	Milk Protein Free?	Fiber (gms)
Human milk (Term)	100	147	20	Lactose	10.6	Human milk (whey predominant)	1.54	Human milk	5.74	331	3	0.6	0.3	30	n/a	n/a	0.07	221	7	265	0.6	6	14	22	41 (2.2)	21	5.1	0.04	0.18	0.51	1	37	16	26 (1.0)	78 (1.9)	62 (1.8)	14.4	286	No	Yes	No	-
Human milk (Preterm)	100	149	24	Lactose	9.9	Human milk (whey predominant)	2.10	Human milk	5.80	581	3	1.6	0.3	72	22	n/a	0.07	224	5	269	0.6	16	14	22	37 (1.8)	19	4.6	0.18	0.51	1	96	16	2.2	37 (1.6)	85 (2.2)	82 (2.3)	18.7	290	No	Yes	No	-
Similac human milk fortifier (Ross) powder[c]	14	per 4 pkts or 3.6 gms	–	Lactose, corn syrup solids	1.8 per 4 pkts	Nonfat milk & whey protein concentrate	1.0 per 4 pkts	Medium chain triglycerides	0.36 per 4 pkts	620	120	3.2	8	233	417	211	0.64	3570	23	1500	26	25	2.9	3.9	117 (5.8)	67	7	0.4	1	7	170	n/a	0.5	15 (0.65)	63 (1.6)	38 (1.1)	11.2	385	No	Yes	No	-
Similac natural care advance (Ross) RTF	100	124	~24	Corn syrup solids & lactose	10.6	Nonfat milk & whey protein concentrate	2.71	50% MCTs, 30% Soy, 18.3% Coconut oils (0.25% DHA, 0.40% ARA)	5.43	1250	150	4.0	12	250	620	250	0.55	5000	37	1900	37	37	10	5.5	210 (10.5)	116	12	1.44	0.72	10	250	6	1.8	43 (1.9)	129 (3.3)	81 (2.3)	26.7	280	No	Yes	No	-
Enfamil human milk fortifier (Mead Johnson) powder[c]	14	per 4 pkts	–	Corn syrup solids & lactose	<0.40 per 4 pkts	Milk protein isolate, whey protein isolate hydrosylate	1.1 per 4 pkts	70% MCT, 30% Soy oils	1.0 per 4 pkts	950	150	4.6	4.4	150	220	115	0.18	3000	25	730	2.7	12	n/a	n/a	90 (4.5)	50	n/a	1.44	0.72	10	44	10	n/a	16 (0.70)	29 (0.74)	13 (0.37)	9.7	35 mOsm/kg for 4 pkts to 100 mL breastmilk	No	Yes	Yes	-

[a] Manufactured with barley enzyme. May contain a residual amount of barley protein from processing.

[b] Varies with maternal diet stage of lactation and among mothers.

[c] 1 packet to 50 cc of breastmilk adds 2 calories more per ounce. 1 packet to 25 cc of breast milk adds 4 calories more per ounce.

T A B L E   3 1 - 2

INFANT AND PEDIATRIC FORMULAS (CONTINUED)

Premature Infant Formulas for Hospital Use/Premature Discharge Formulas

	Vol. (mL) per 100 Cals	Kcal/oz (30 kcal mL)	Carbohydrate (g) Source	gms	Protein (g) Source	gms	Fat (g) Source	gms	Vitamins (IU) A	D	E	K	Vitamins (µg) Thia-min	Ribo-flavin	B6	B12	Nia-cin	Fo-late	Panto-thenic Acid	Bio-tin	Vitamins (mg) C	Cho-line	Ino-sitol	Minerals (mg) Ca (meq)	P	Mg	Fe	Minerals (µg) Zn	Mn	Cu	I	Se	Minerals (mg) Na (meq)	K (meq)	Cl (meq)	Other Characteristics Renal Solute Load mOsm	Osmol-ality, mOsm/kg water	Lactose Free?	Gluten Free?	Milk Protein Free?	Fiber (gms)
Similac special care advance 20 with iron (Ross) RTF	148	20	Corn syrup solids & lactose	10.6	Nonfat milk & whey protein concentrate	2.71	50% MCT, 30% Soy & 18.3% Coconut oils (0.25% DHA, 0.40% ARA)	5.43	1250	150	4	12	250	620	250	0.55	5000	37	1900	37	37	10	5.5	180 (9.0)	100	12	1.8 (low iron: 0.37)	1.5	12	250	6	1.8	43 (1.9)	129 (3.3)	81 (2.3)	26.2	235	No	Yes	No	-
Similac special care advance 24 with iron (Ross) RTF	124	24	Corn syrup solids & lactose	10.6	Nonfat milk & whey protein concentrate	2.71	50% MCT, 30% Soy & 18.3% Coconut oils (0.25% DHA, 0.40% ARA)	5.43	1250	150	4	12	250	620	250	0.55	5000	37	1900	37	37	10	5.5	180 (9.0)	100	12	1.8 (low iron: 0.37)	1.5	12	250	6	1.8	43 (1.9)	129 (3.3)	81 (2.3)	26.2	280	No	Yes	No	-
Enfamil premature lipil 20 with iron (Mead Johnson) RTF	148	20	Corn syrup solids & lactose	11.0	Whey protein concentrate & nonfat milk	3.00	40% MCT, 30% Soy & 27% high oleic vegetable oils (3% ARA & DHA)	5.1	1250	240	6.3	8	200	300	150	0.25	4000	40	1200	4	20	20	44	165 (8.3)	83	9	1.8 (low iron: 0.5)	1.5	6.3	120	25	2.8	58 (2.5)	98 (2.5)	90 (2.5)	27	240	No	Yes	No	-
Enfamil premature lipil 24 with iron (Mead Johnson) RTF	123	24	Corn syrup solids & lactose	11.0	Whey protein concentrate & nonfat milk	3.00	40% MCT, 30% Soy & 27% high oleic vegetable oils (3% ARA & DHA)	5.1	1250	240	6.3	8	200	300	150	0.25	4000	40	1200	4	20	20	44	165 (8.3)	83	9	1.8 (low iron: 0.5)	1.5	6.3	120	25	2.8	58 (2.5)	98 (2.5)	90 (2.5)	27	300	No	Yes	No	-
Similac neosure advance (Ross) RTF	134	22	Maltodextrin & lactose	10.3	Nonfat milk & whey protein concentrate	2.60	44.7% Soy, 29% Coconut oil 24.9% MCT oil (0.15% DHA, 40% ARA)	5.50	460	70	3.6	11	220	150	100	0.4	1950	25	800	9	15	16	6	105 (5.2)	62	9	1.8	1.2	10	120	15	2.3	33 (1.4)	142 (3.6)	75 (2.1)	27	250	No	Yes	No	-
Enfamil enfacare lipil (Mead Johnson) powder	135	22	Corn syrup solids & lactose	10.4	Whey protein concentrate & nonfat milk	2.80	34% High oleic vegetable, 29% Soy, 20% MCT & 14% Coconut oils, (3% ARA & DHA)	5.3	450	80	4	8	200	200	100	0.3	2000	26	850	6	16	24	30	120 (6.0)	66	8	1.8	1.25	15	120	21	2.8	35 (1.6)	105 (2.7)	78 (2.2)	24	260	No	Yes	No	-

TABLE 31-2

INFANT AND PEDIATRIC FORMULAS (CONTINUED)

Cow Milk-Based Formula

	Cals	Vol (mL)/100 kcal	Kcal/oz (30 mL)	Carbohydrate (g) gms	Carbohydrate Source	Protein (g) gms	Protein Source	Fat (g) gms	Fat Source	A (IU)	D	E	K	Thiamin	Riboflavin	B6	B12	Niacin	Folate	Pantothenic Acid	Biotin	C	Choline (mg)	Inositol	Ca (meq)	P	Mg	Fe	Zn	Mn	Cu	I	Se	Na (meq)	K (meq)	Cl (meq)	Renal Solute Load (mOsm)	Osmolality (mOsm/kg water)	Lactose Free?	Gluten Free?	Milk Protein Free?	Fiber (gms)
Similac advance (Ross) RTF[d]	100	148	20	10.8	Lactose	2.07	Nonfat milk & whey protein concentrate	5.40	40% High-oleic Safflower, 30% Soy, 29% Coconut oils (0.15%, 0.40% ARA).	300	60	1.5	8	100	150	60	0.25	1050	15	450	4.4	9	16	4.7	78 (3.9)	42	6	1.8	0.75	5	90	6	1.8	24 (1.0)	105 (2.7)	65 (1.8)	18.7	300	No	Yes	No	--
Similac lactose free advance (Ross) powder	100	148	20	10.7	Maltodextrin & sucrose	2.14	Milk protein isolate	5.40	40% High-oleic Safflower, 30% Soy, 29% Coconut oils (0.15%, 0.40% ARA).	300	60	3	8	100	150	60	0.25	1050	15	450	4.4	9	16	4.3	84 (4.2)	56	6	1.8	0.75	5	90	9	1.8	30 (1.3)	107 (2.7)	65 (1.8)	19.9	200	Yes	No	No	--
Similac pm 60/40 (Ross) powder[d]	100	148	20	10.2	Lactose	2.22	Whey protein concentrate & sodium caseinate	5.59	50% Corn, 38% Coconut & 12% Soy oils	300	60	2.5	8	100	150	60	0.25	1050	15	450	4.5	9	12	24	56 (2.8)	28	6	0.7	0.75	5	90	6	1.9	24 (1.0)	80 (2.2)	59 (1.7)	18.3	280	No	Yes	No	--
Similac 2 (for 9–24 months of age) (Ross) powder	100	148	20	10.6	Lactose	2.07	Nonfat milk & whey protein concentrate	5.49	40% High-oleic Safflower, 30% Coconut & 20% Soy oils	300	60	3	8	100	150	60	0.25	1050	15	450	4.4	9	16	4.7	118 (5.9)	64	6	1.8	0.75	5	90	6	1.8	24 (1.0)	105 (2.7)	65 (1.8)	19.5	300	No	Yes	No	--
Enfamil lipil with iron (Mead Johnson) RTF[d]	100	148	20	10.9	Lactose	2.10	Reduced mineral whey & nonfat milk	5.3	44% Palm oleic, 19.5% Soy, 19.5% Coconut 14.5% high oleic Sunflower oils (2.5% ARA & DHA)	300	60	2	8	80	140	60	0.3	1000	16	500	3	12	12	6	78 (3.9)	53	8	1.8 (low iron : 0.7)	1	15	75	10	2.8	27 (1.2)	108 (2.8)	63 (1.8)	19.2	260	No	Yes	No	--
Enfamil lacto free lipil (Mead Johnson) powder	100	148	20	10.9	Corn syrup solids	2.10	Milk protein isolate	5.3	44% Palm oleic, 19.5% Coconut, 14.5% high oleic Sunflower oils (2.5% ARA & DHA)	300	60	2	8	80	140	60	0.3	1000	16	500	3	12	12	6	82 (4.1)	55	8	1.8	1	15	75	15	2.8	30 (1.3)	110 (2.8)	67 (1.9)	20	200	Yes	Yes	No	--
Enfamil ar lipil (Mead Johnson) powder	100	148	20	11.0	Lactose, pregelatinized rice starch, maltodextrin	2.50	Nonfat milk	5.1	44% Palm oleic, 19.5% Soy, 19.5% Coconut, 14.5% high oleic Sunflower oils (2.5% ARA & DHA)	300	60	2	8	80	140	60	0.3	1000	16	500	3	12	12	6	78 (3.9)	53	8	1.8	1	15	75	10	2.8	40 (1.7)	108 (2.8)	75 (2.1)	22	230	No	Yes	No	--
Parent's choice lipids (Wyeth) powder[d]	100	148	20	10.6	Lactose	2.20	Whey & casein	5.3	36% Palm, 21% Coconut, 21% oleic, 21% Soy, 1% lecithin	300	60	1.4	8	100	150	62.5	0.2	750	7.5	315	2.2	8.5	15	4.1	63 (3.2)	42	7	1.2	0.8	15	70	9	2.1	22 (0.95)	83 (2.1)	55.5 (1.5)	19.8	280	No	Yes	No	--
Parent's Choice 2 with iron (>4 months old) (Wyeth) powder	100	148	20	10.1	Lactose	2.60	Whey & casein	5.4	34.6% Palm, 20.2% Soybean oil, 20.2% oleic, 2.5% lecithin, (0.75% ARA, 0.5% DHA)	368	65	2	9.9	147	221	88	0.29	1021	15	441	2.9	13.2	14.7	4	120 (6)	84	9.9	1.8	0.885	5.9	85	10	n/a	32 (1.4)	124 (3.2)	81 (2.3)	17.5	280	Yes	No	No	--
Good start supreme (Nestle) powder[d]	100	150	20	11.2	Lactose, corn maltodextrin	2.20	100% Partially hydrolyzed whey protein	5.1	46% Palm olein, 25% Soy oil, 21% Coconut oil, 6% high oleic Safflower (0.32% DHA 0.64% ARA)	300	60	2	8	100	140	75	0.33	1050	15	450	4.4	9	12	6	64 (3.2)	36	7	1.5	0.8	7	80	12	1.16	27 (1.2)	108 (2.8)	65 (1.4)	13.5	265	No	Yes	No	--
Good start essentials (Nestle) powder	100	150	20	11.2	Lactose, corn syrup	2.20	Whey & casein	5.1	47% Palm olein, 26% Soy oil, 21% Coconut oil, 6% high oleic Safflower	300	60	2	8	80	140	65	0.25	1000	15	450	3	9	12	6	75 (3.8)	42	7	1.5	0.8	7	80	10	1.16	24 (1.1)	105 (2.7)	63 (1.4)	12.6	299	No	Yes	No	--
Good start 2 essentials (>4 months old) (Nestle) powder	100	150	20	13.2	Corn maltodextrin, corn syrup	2.60	Whey & casein	4.1	47% Palm olein, 21% Coconut oil, 6% high oleic Safflower	250	60	2	8	80	140	65	0.25	1000	15	480	3	9	12	5	120 (6)	80	8	1.8	0.8	7	85	10	1.16	39 (1.7)	135 (3.5)	90 (2)	12.1	326	No	Yes	No	--
Portagen (Mead Johnson) powder	100	100	30	11.0	Corn syrup solids	3.40	Sodium caseinate	4.6	87% MCT oil & Corn oil	750	75	3	15	150	180	200	0.6	2000	15	1000	7.5	7.8	12.5	4.5	90 (4.5)	68	20	1.8	0.9	12	150	7	n/a	53 (2.3)	120 (3.1)	83 (2.4)	30	350	Yes	Yes	No	--

[d]Formulas available without DHA/ARA.

TABLE 31-2

INFANT AND PEDIATRIC FORMULAS (CONTINUED)

Soy Formulas for Infants and Children Over 1 Year

	Cals	Vol (mL) per 100 kcal	Kcal/oz (30 mL)	Carbohydrate (g) gms	Carbohydrate Source	Protein (g) gms	Protein Source	Fat (g) gms	Fat Source	A	D	E	K	Thia-min	Ribo-flavin	B6	B12	Nia-cin	Fol-ate	Panto-thenic Acid	Bio-tin	C	Cho-line	Ino-sitol	Ca (meq)	P	Mg	Fe	Zn	Mn	Cu	I	Se	Na (meq)	K (meq)	Cl (meq)	Renal Solute Load, mOsm	Osmolality, mOsm/kg water	Lactose Free?	Gluten Free?	Milk Protein Free?	Fiber Free? (gms)
Similac isomil advance (Ross) RTF[a]	100	148	20	10.3	Corn syrup & sucrose	2.45	Soy protein isolate & L-methionine	5.46	40% High oleic, 30% Saffflower, 29% Soy & Coconut oils (0.15% DHA, 0.40% ARA)	300	60	1.5	11	60	90	60	0.45	1350	15	750	4.5	9	12	5	105 (5.2)	75	7.5	1.8	0.75	25	75	15	1.8	44 (1.9)	108 (2.8)	62 (1.7)	22.8	200	Yes	Yes	Yes	–
Similac isomil 2 (for 9–24 months of age) (Ross) powder	100	148	20	10.3	Corn syrup solids & sucrose	2.45	Soy protein isolate & L-methionine	5.46	40% High-oleic Safflower, 30% Coconut & 30% Soy oils	300	60	1.5	11	60	90	60	0.45	1350	15	750	4.5	9	12	5	135 (6.7)	90	7.5	1.8	0.75	25	75	15	1.8	44 (1.9)	108 (2.8)	62 (1.7)	23.3	200	Yes	Yes	Yes	–
Similac isomil DF (Ross) RTF	100	148	20	10.1	Corn syrup & sucrose	2.66	Soy protein isolate & L-methionine	5.46	60% Soy & 40% Coconut oils	300	60	1.5	11	60	90	60	0.45	1350	15	750	4.5	9	12	5	105 (5.2)	75	7.5	1.8	0.75	25	75	15	1.8	44 (1.9)	108 (2.8)	62 (1.7)	24	240	Yes	Yes	Yes	0.9 g/100 kcal
Enfamil prosobee lipil (Mead Johnson) powder[a]	100	148	20	10.6	Corn syrup solids	2.50	Soy protein isolate	5.3	44% Palm olein, 19.5% Soy, 19.5% Coconut,14.5% high oleic Sunflower oils (2.5% ARA & DHA)	300	60	2	8	80	90	60	0.3	1000	16	500	3	12	12	6	105 (5.2)	83	11	1.8	1.2	25	75	15	2.8	36 (1.6)	120 (3.1)	80 (2.2)	24	200	Yes	Yes	Yes	–
Enfamil nextstep prosobee lipil (Mead Johnson) powder 1–3 yers	100	150	20	11.8	Corn syrup solids & sucrose	3.30	Soy protein isolate	4.4	44% Palm olein, 19% Soy, 19% Coconut, & 15% high oleic Safflower oils (3% ARA/DHA)	300	60	2	8	80	90	60	0.3	1000	16	500	3	12	12	17	115 (2.8)	90	8	1.8	1.2	25	75	15	2.8	45 (2.0)	150 (3.8)	100 (2.8)	30	260	Yes	Yes	Yes	–
Ross carbohydrate free (Ross) liquid Concentrate	100	148	20		Selected by Physician	2.96	Soy protein isolate & L-methionine	5.33	40% High-oleic Safflower, 30% Coconut & 30% Soy oils	300	60	1.5	11	60	90	60	0.45	1350	15	750	4.5	9	12	5	105 (5.2)	75	7.5	1.8	0.75	25	75	15	2.1	44 (1.9)	108 (2.8)	62 (1.7)	25.8	168	Yes	Yes	Yes	–
Parent's choice soy (Wyeth) powder	100	148	20	10.2	Corn syrup solids & sucrose	2.70	Soy protein isolate	5.3	36% Palm, 21% Coconut, 6% high oleic Safflower	300	60	1.4	8.3	100	150	62.5	0.3	750	7.5	450	5.5	8.3	12.8	15	90 (4.5)	63	10	1.8	0.8	30	70	9	2.1	30 (1.3)	105 (2.7)	56 (1.6)	23.3	220	Yes	Yes	Yes	–
Good start essentials soy (Nestle) powder	100	150	20	11.1	Corn maltodextrin & sucrose	2.80	100% Soy	5.1	47% Palm olein, 26% Soy, 21% Coconut, 6% high oleic Safflower oil	300	60	3	8	60	94	60	0.3	1300	16	470	5	12	12	5	105 (5.2)	63	11	1.8	0.9	34	120	15	2.0	36 (1.6)	116 (3.0)	71 (2.0)	16.4	200	Yes	Yes	Yes	–
Good start 2 essentials soy (Nestle) powder	100	150	20	12.0	Corn maltodextrin & sucrose	4.40	100% Soy	4.4	47% Palm olein, 26% Soy, 21% Coconut, 6% high oleic Safflower oil	310	60	2.4	7.8	90	94	86	0.31	1200	16	470	7.8	16	12	18	135 (6.7)	90	13	1.8	1.2	37	120	12	2	42 (1.8)	118 (3.0)	79 (2.2)	26	200	Yes	Yes	Yes	–

[a]Formula available without DHA/ARA.

INFANT AND PEDIATRIC FORMULAS (CONTINUED)

Semi-elemental Formulas for Infants and Children Over 1 Year

	Cals per 100 kcal	Vol (mL) per 100 kcal	Kcal/oz (30 mL)	Carbohydrate (g) Source	gms	Protein (g) Source	gms	Fat (g) Source	gms	Vit A (IU)	Vit D (IU)	Vit E (IU)	Vit K	Thiamin	Riboflavin	B6	B12	Niacin	Folacin	Pantothenic Acid	Biotin	C	Choline	Inositol	Ca (meq)	P	Mg	Fe	Zn	Mn	Cu	Se	I	Na (meq)	K (meq)	Cl (meq)	Renal Solute Load mOsm	Osmolality mOsm/kg water	Lactose Free?	Gluten Free?	Milk Protein Free?	Fiber (gms)
Semilac alimentum advance (Ross) powder	100	148	20	Sucrose, modified tapioca starch	10.2	Casein hydrolysate, L-cystine, L-tyrosine, L-tryptophan	2.75	38% Safflower, 33% MCT, 28% Soy oil (0.15% ARA, 0.40% DHA)	5.54	300	45	3	15	60	90	60	0.45	1350	15	750	4.5	9	8	5	105 (5.2)	75	7.5	1.8	0.75	8	75	15	1.8	44 (1.9)	118 (3.0)	80 (2.3)	25.3	370	Yes	Yes	Yes	–
Enfamil nutramigen lipil (Mead-Johnson) powder	100	148	20	Corn syrup solids, modified corn starch	11.0	Casein hydrolysate, L-cystine, L-tyrosine, L-tryptophan	2.80	44% Palm olein, 19.5% Soy, 19.5% Coconut, 14.5% high oleic	5	300	50	2	8	80	90	60	0.3	1000	16	500	3	12	12	17	94 (4.7)	63	11	1.8	1	25	75	15	2.8	47 (2.0)	110 (2.8)	86 (2.4)	25	320	Yes	Yes	Yes	–
Enfamil pregestimil (Mead Johnson) powder	100	148	20	Corn syrup solids, modified corn starch	10.2	Casein hydrolysate, L-cystine, L-tyrosine, L-tryptophan	2.80	55% MCT, 25% Soy, 10% corn, 10% high oleic Safflower oils	5.6	380	50	3.8	12	80	90	60	0.3	1000	16	500	3	12	12	17	115 (5.8)	75	11	1.8	1	25	75	15	2.8	47 (2.0)	110 (2.8)	86 (2.4)	16.9	320	Yes	Yes	No	–
Pepdite one + (SHS) powder	100	100	30	Corn syrup solids	10.6	Hydrolyzed protein, free amino acids	3.10	35% MCT oil & 65% canola & hybrid Safflower oils	5.00	243	32	1.6	2.7	100	100	100	0.2	1200	30	400	2	9.3	37.5	22	113 (5.7)	94	18	1.4	1.4	200	110	9.6	3	41 (1.8)	136 (3.5)	63 (1.75)	28	430–440	Yes	Yes	Yes	–
Compleat pediatric (Novartis) RTF	100	100	30	hydrolyzed cornstarch, apple juice, vegetables, fruits	13	Beef, caseinates	3.80	32% High oleic Sunflower, 28% Soybean, 18% MCT oils, 12% beef fat, 10% mono & diglycerides	3.90	330	48	2.2	3.8	260	200	250	0.56	1600	35	960	30.4	9.6	28	7.6	100 (5.0)	100	19	1.3	1.2	220	120	14	5.2	68 (3.0)	150 (3.8)	72 (2.0)	23.2	380	Yes	Yes	No	4.4 g/Liter
Peptamen junior (Nestle) powder	100	100	30	Malto- dextrin & sucrose	13.6	Hydrolyzed whey protein	3.00	60% MCT 40% LCT (Soybean, Canola Soy, residual milk fat)	3.84	150	40	1.5	4	60	80	80	0.15	600	22	300	1.5	8	25	n/a	92 (4.6)	61	12	1	1	160	80	8	2.4	66 (2.9)	135 (3.5)	81 (2.2)	20.5	260–320	Yes	Yes	No	–

INFANT AND PEDIATRIC FORMULAS (CONTINUED)

Elemental Formulas for Infants and Children Over 1 Year

Formula	Cals	Vol. (mL) per 100 kcal	Kcal per oz (30 mL)	CHO gms	CHO Source	Protein gms	Protein Source	Fat gms	Fat Source	A (IU)	D (IU)	E (IU)	K (IU)	Thiamin (µg)	Riboflavin (µg)	B6 (µg)	B12 (µg)	Niacin (µg)	Folate (µg)	Pantothenic Acid (µg)	Biotin (µg)	C (mg)	Choline (mg)	Inositol (mg)	Ca (mg/meq)	P (mg)	Mg (mg)	Fe (mg)	Zn (mg)	Mn (µg)	Cu (µg)	I (µg)	Se (µg)	Na (mg/meq)	K (mg/meq)	Cl (mg/meq)	Renal Solute Load, mOsm	Osmolality, mOsm/kg water	Lactose Free?	Gluten Free?	Milk Protein Free?	Fiber (gms)
Vivonex pediatric (Novartis) powder	100	125	24	16.2	Maltodextrin & modified corn starch	3.00	Free amino acids	3.00	68% MCT 32% Soybean oil	312	63	3.75	5	188	225	250	0.38	2500	25	625	12.5	12.5	25	7.5	121 (6.1)	100	25	1.25	1.5	250	150	15	3.75	50 (2.2)	150 (3.8)	125 (3.6)	17	360	Yes	Yes	Yes	-
Neocate (SHS) powder	100	150	20	11.7	Corn syrup solids	3.10	L-amino acids	4.50	5% MCT & 95% LCT	409	87	1.14	8.79	92.6	137.8	123.5	0.17	1544	10.2	620	3.1	9.26	13.1	23.3	124 (6.2)	93.1	12.4	1.85	1.66	90	124	15.4	3.73	37.3 (1.6)	155.1 (4.0)	77.2 (2.1)	13	375	Yes	Yes	Yes	-
Neocate junior (SHS) powder	100	100	30	10.4	Corn syrup solids	3.00	L-amino acids	5.00	65% LCT & 35% MCT	243	32.3	1.7	2.7	100	100	100	0.2	1200	30	390	2	9.3	37.6	22	113 (5.7)	94	18	1.4	1.4	200	110	9.6	3	41 (1.8)	137 (3.5)	63 (1.75)	35	607	Yes	Yes	Yes	-
Pediatric E028 (SHS) RTF	100	100	30	14.6	Corn syrup solids & sucrose	2.50	L-amino acids	3.50	35% MCT 65% LCT (Canola & Safflower)	117	31	0.82	1.5	60	70	80	0.07	900	6	240	2	3.1	18.3	1.8	62 (3.1)	62	9	0.77	0.77	100	100	6	1.54	20 (0.9)	93 (2.3)	35 (0.97)	14	820	Yes	Yes	Yes	-
Elecare (Ross) powder	100	100	30	10.7	Corn syrup solids	3.01	L-amino acids	4.76	39% High-oleic Safflower, 33% MCTs & 28% Soy oils (39-33-28)	273	42	2.1	6	210	105	101	0.42	1680	30	421	4.2	9	8	5.1	108 (5.4)	81	8	1.8	1.1	105	126	7	2.3	45 (2.0)	151 (3.8)	60 (1.7)	27.3	551	Yes	Yes	Yes	-
Neocate one plus (SHS) powder	100	100	30	14.6	Corn syrup solids	2.50	L-amino acids	3.50	35% MCT & 65% LCT (Canola & Safflower)	117	31	0.82	1.5	60	70	80	0.07	900	6	240	2	3.1	18.3	1.8	62 (3.1)	62	9	0.77	0.77	100	100	6	1.54	20 (0.9)	93 (2.3)	35 (0.97)	14	610	Yes	Yes	Yes	-

Formulas for Children 1–10 Years

Formula	Cals	Vol. (mL) per 100 kcal	Kcal per oz (30 mL)	CHO gms	CHO Source	Protein gms	Protein Source	Fat gms	Fat Source	A (IU)	D (IU)	E (IU)	K (IU)	Thiamin (µg)	Riboflavin (µg)	B6 (µg)	B12 (µg)	Niacin (µg)	Folate (µg)	Pantothenic Acid (µg)	Biotin (µg)	C (mg)	Choline (mg)	Inositol (mg)	Ca (mg/meq)	P (mg)	Mg (mg)	Fe (mg)	Zn (mg)	Mn (µg)	Cu (µg)	I (µg)	Se (µg)	Na (mg/meq)	K (mg/meq)	Cl (mg/meq)	Renal Solute Load, mOsm	Osmolality, mOsm/kg water	Lactose Free?	Gluten Free?	Milk Protein Free?	Fiber (gms)
Pediasure enteral (Ross) RTF†	100	100	30	11.4	Sucrose & maltodextrin	3.00	Sodium caseinate & whey protein concentrate	4.98	50% High-oleic Safflower, 30% Soy & 2% MCTs	257	51	2.3	4	270	211	262	0.6	1688	37	1013	32	10	30	8	97 (4.8)	80	19.8	1.4	1.8	101	101	10	2.3	38 (1.7)	131 (3.3)	101 (2.9)	27.6	345–520	Yes	Yes	No	-
Pediasure with fiber (Ross) RTF	100	100	30	11.3	Sucrose & maltodextrin	3.00	Sodium caseinate & whey protein concentrate	4.98	50% High-oleic Safflower, 30% Soy & 2% MCTs	257	51	2.3	4	270	211	262	0.6	1688	37	1013	32	10	30	8	97 (4.8)	80	19.8	1.4	1.8	101	101	10	2.3	38 (1.7)	131 (3.3)	101 (2.9)	27.6	335–345	Yes	Yes	No	0.5 g/100 kcal
Kindercal oral/tube feeding (Mead Johnson) RTF	100	94	32	12.7	Maltodextrin & sugar	2.82	Milk protein concentrate	4.14	40% Canola, 28% high oleic Safflower, 20% MCT, 12% Corn oil	394	50	3.5	3	160	197	197	0.55	1974	15	1231	15	24	25	8	95 (4.8)	80	19.7	1	1.2	197	122	12	3	34 (1.5)	123 (3.2)	70 (1.9)	27.6	345–520 (flavor dependent)	Yes	Yes	No	0.63-g/L
Nutren junior (Nestle) RTF	100	100	30	12.8	Maltodextrin & sucrose		Milk & whey protein	4.20	Soybean, 25% MCT, Canola, Soy lecithin	240	56	2.8	3	240	200	240	0.6	2000	40	1000	30	10	30	8	100 (5.0)	80	20	1.4	1.5	150	100	12	3	46 (2.0)	132 (3.5)	108 (3)	20.4	350	Yes	Yes	No	-
Carnation follow-Up formula (Nestle) powder	100	150	30	13.2	Corn syrup solids, lactose, corn???	2.60	Nonfat milk	4.10	47% palm oleic, 26% Soy, 21% Coconut, 6% high oleic Safflower oil	250	60	2	8.1	80	96	66	0.32	1280	16	1480	2	8	12	18	120 (6.0)	80	8.4	1.8	0.63	7	76	12	3	39 (1.7)	135 (3.6)	90 (2.5)	18	326	No	Yes	No	-
Resource just for kids (Novartis) w/wo fiber RTF	100	100	30	11	Hydrolyzed corn starch & sucrose	3.00	Sodium & calcium caseinate & whey protein concentrate	5.00	42% High oleic Sunflower, 38% Soybean, 20% MCT oil	240	33	2.3	4	120	150	160	0.24	1700	37	1000	15	10	40	8	114 (5.7)	80	20	1.4	1.2	200	100	12	4	59 (2.6)	114 (2.9)	510 (14)	19	390	Yes	Yes	No	1.4 g/8 ounces
Next Step (1–3 years of age) (Mead Johnson) powder	100	100	30	11.1	Lactose & corn syrup solids	2.60	Nonfat milk	5.00	45% Palm olein, 20% soy, 20% Coconut, & 15% high oleic Sunflower oils	300	60	2	8	100	150	100	0.25	1050	15	450	4.4	9	16	4.7	120 (6.0)	84	8	1.8	0.9	7	90	8	2.8	41 (1.8)	130 (3.4)	86 (2.4)	25	260	No	Yes	No	-

†Pediasure enteral formula contains less sucrose and is lower in osmolality than flavored Pediasure. Enteral Vanilla 335 mOsm/kg vs. Vanilla flavor 430 mOsm/kg.

INFANT AND PEDIATRIC FORMULAS (CONTINUED)

Modulars

	Calories	Carbohydrate (g)		Protein (g)		Fat (g)	
		Source	gms	Source	gms	Source	gms
Carbohydrate Modulars							
Polycose (Ross) *powder*	8 kcal/1 tsp or 23 kcal/1 TBSP	Glucose polymers	25 g per 100 kcal	--	--	--	--
Polycose (Ross) *Liquid*	2 kcal/1mL or 60 kcal/1 ounce	Glucose polymers	25 g per 100 kcal	--	--	--	--
Moducal (Mead Johnson) *powder*	3.8 kcal/g or 8 g/TBSP	Maltodextrin	95 g/100 g	--	--	--	--
Duocal (SHS) *powder*	492 kcal/100 gms	Hydrolyzed corn starch	72.7 kcal/100 gms	--	--	Corn, Coconut & MCT oil	22.3 g/100 g
Protein Modulars							
Casec (Mead Johnson) *powder*	3.8 kcal/g 17 kcal/TBSP	Lactose	0.4 g/100 g	100% Calcium caseinate	90 g/100 g	Milk protein & Soy lecithin	2 g/100 g
Promod (Ross) *powder*	28 kcal/1 scoop	--	--	Whey protein concentrate & Soy lecithin	5 g/1 scoop or 6.6 gms	--	--
Fat Modulars							
Vegetable Oil *liquid*	40 kcal/1 tsp	--	--	--	--	Corn oil	4.54 g/1 tsp
Microlipid (Mead Johnson) liquid	6.75 kcal/1 TBSP or 15 mL	--	--	--	--	Safflower oil & polyglycarol esters of fatty acids	11.1 g/100 kcal
MCT oil (Mead Johnson) *liquid*	115 kcal/1 TBSP	--	--	--	--	Fractionated Coconut oil	28.00

TABLE 31-3

FORMULA MIXING INSTRUCTIONS

Powder Formulas

Caloric Density Calorie per Ounce (cal/oz)[a]	Water (oz)	Unpacked Level Scoop (Powdered Formula)	Approximate Yield (Fluid Ounces)
20 (standard mixture)	2	1	2
22	3.5	2	4
24	5	3	6
27	4.25	3	5

Caloric Density Calorie per Ounce (cal/oz)[b]	Water (oz)	Unpacked Level Scoop (Powdered Formula)	Approximate Yield (Fluid Ounces)
20	4.5	2	5
22 (standard mixture)	2	1	2
24	5.5	3	6.5
27	8	5	9

Caloric Density Calorie per Ounce (cal/oz)[c]	Water (oz)	Packed Level Scoop (Powdered Formula)	Approximate Yield (Fluid Ounces)
20	2	1	2.25
22	3.5	2	4
24	8	5	9.25
27	7	5	8.25
30 (standard mixture)	5	4	6

Caloric Density Calorie per Ounce (cal/oz)[d]	Water Milliliter (oz)	Powder	Approximate Yield Milliliter (oz)
20 (standard mixture)	59 (2)	1 scoop	65 (2.2)
24	48 (1.6)	1 scoop	54 (1.8)
27	42 (1.4)	1 scoop	48 (1.6)
30	38 (1.3)	1 scoop	44 (1.5)

Concentrated Liquid Formulas

Caloric Density Calorie per Ounce (cal/oz)[e]	Water (oz)	Liquid Concentrate (Ounces)	Approximate Yield (Fluid Ounces)
20 (standard mixture)	1	1	2
22	2.5	3	5.5
24	2	3	5
27	1	2	3

TABLE 31-3

FORMULA MIXING INSTRUCTIONS (*CONTINUED*)

Caloric Density Calorie per Ounce (cal/oz)[f]	Water (oz)	Liquid Concentrate (oz)	Approximate Yield (Fluid Ounces)
20 (standard mixture)	13	13	26
22	11	13	24
24	9	13	22
27	6	13	19
Caloric Density Calorie per Ounce (cal/oz)[g]	Water (oz)	Liquid Concentrate (oz)	Approximate Yield (Fluid Ounces)
20 (standard mixture)	13	13	26
24	9	13	22
27	6	13	19
30	4.5	13	17.5

[a]To prepare Similac with iron, Similac low iron, Similac advance, Similac 2, Similac lactose free, Similac isomil, Similac isomil advance, Similac isomil 2, Similac PM 60/40, and Similac alimentum powder.

[b]To prepare Similac neosure advance powder.

[c]To prepare Elecare powder make certain to use a packed level scoop of powder.

[d]To prepare Enfamil Lipil with iron, Enfamil low iron, Enfamil with iron, Enfamil A.R., LactoFree Lipil, Nutramigen, ProSobee, ProSobee Lipil, next step toddler formula, next step soy toddler formula, and Pregestimil. Note: Enfamil A.R. should not be diluted to caloric concentrations higher than 24 cal/oz because of increased viscosity. Nutramigen and Pregestimil powders should be packed, level scoops. All other formulas use unpacked, level scoops.

[e]To prepare Similac with iron, Similac low iron, Similac advance, Similac lactose free, Similac isomil.

[f]Shows the quantity of water to mix with one 13 fluid ounce can of liquid concentrate.

[g]Enfamil Lipil with iron, Enfamil low iron, Enfamil with iron, LactoFree Lipil, Nutramigen, ProSobee, ProSobee Lipil.

Source: Used with permission of Ross Products Division, Abbott Laboratories Inc., Columbus, OH 43215. From Pediatric Nutritionals Product Guide, Ross Products Division, Abbott Laboratories Inc. Courtesy of Mead Johnson Nutritionals, Evansville, Indiana.

Formula Mixing

Infant formulas are available in powder, liquid concentrate, and ready-to-feed liquid forms; powder is the least expensive and ready-to-feed is the most expensive. The liquid concentrate and powdered formulas require water for preparation. Infant formulas are available in 20 calories per ounce (20 cal/oz) or 67 cal/100 mL. When a child needs an increase in calories or a volume restriction, formula can be mixed to as high as 30 cal/oz or 100 cal/100 mL. Increasing the caloric density changes the renal solute load and osmolality, which in turn may affect the hydration status and tolerance of the formula. Symptoms of intolerance include vomiting, diarrhea, delayed gastric emptying, and—in enterally fed infants—increased gastric residuals and abdominal distention.

Formulas can be concentrated in two ways: (1) less water can be added to powdered or liquid concentrate forms or (2) modulars in the form of carbohydrates, protein, or fat can be added. Table 31-3 lists examples of recipes for some common formulas. Contact the formula manufacturer directly if mixing instructions for a particular formula are not listed.

Introduction of Solid Foods in Normal Infants (see also Table 31-1)

Infants have an extrusion reflex that enables them to swallow only liquids. By 4–5 months of age, an infant's extrusion reflex has disappeared, allowing a child to swallow safely. The first food introduced is iron-fortified rice cereal on a small spoon. Pureed single vegetables and then fruits, one at a time, are good choices after rice cereal. Initial refusal of new foods and flavors is common; food should be reintroduced several times before ruling out a child's acceptance of the food. If an infant is introduced to food or a drink before they are physiologically ready there is an increased risk of digestive problems and food allergies. Signs of intolerance or allergy can include rashes, vomiting, diarrhea, irritability, or wheezing.[4]

THE NUTRITIONAL ASSESSMENT

A thorough nutritional assessment requires a review of four parameters: anthropometric, biochemical, clinical, and dietary. Pediatricians should be proficient in gathering nutrition assessment parameters to customize medical care.[4]

Anthropometric Data

Anthropometric data include body weight, recumbent length/height, and head circumference. Body weight is a routine measure that can provide insight to the nutritional health of a patient. Length is an indicator of linear growth with respect to bone growth. Serial length measurements may provide insight about whether short stature is due to genetics or some other etiology. Head circumference, as previously discussed, is used to measure brain growth. If a patient is severely malnourished and has a slow growing head, this may be a sign of immature brain development.

Biochemical Data

The biochemical assessment can be divided into the following categories:[3]

- Visceral protein status
- Somatic protein status
- Hematology
- Immunology

Micronutrient deficiencies could also be assessed by checking serum concentrations, but results are often inaccurate and will vary depending on a patient's medical condition.[1]

Visceral Protein Status

Albumin is the most commonly used laboratory value for visceral protein analysis because it is the most abundant protein in blood and the test is relatively inexpensive. The value is affected by critical illness and has a long half-life. Albumin is a negative acute phase reactant, meaning it will fall due to decreased hepatic synthesis or fluid shifts.

Prealbumin, retinol binding protein, and transferrin levels may be better indicators of visceral protein status because of their shorter half-lives, 2–3 days, 12 h, and 8–9 days, respectively. These visceral proteins are catabolized early in starvation or injury, making these measurements good markers for energy reserves; however, there are disadvantages to these lab values. Similar to albumin, prealbumin and retinol binding protein measures are negative acute-phase reactants. Transferrin can be affected by hepatic failure, nephrotic syndrome, iron deficiency, and neoplasia.

Somatic Protein Status

Somatic protein status is an assessment of lean body mass. One method to evaluate lean body mass is to use upper arm and skin fold measurements: triceps skin fold (TSF), mid-arm circumference (MAC), and mid-arm muscle circumference (MAMC). Measurements are performed and compared to published standards to evaluate body composition.

Hematology

The complete blood count is valuable in detecting anemia that can be due to chronic diseases or deficiencies in iron, vitamin B_{12}, or folate. It should be noted that iron deficiency anemia is the most common pediatric problem in the United States.[3]

Immunology

Protein-energy malnutrition and subclinical deficiencies of nutrients can affect the immune response and increase the risk for infection. Total lymphocyte count (TLC) can serve as a measure of a patient's immune function. The value can be derived from white blood cell (WBC) counts as follows:

$$WBC/mm^3 \times lymphocytes = TLC/mm^3$$

In the immunologic assessment, values less than 1500 are associated with nutritional depletion. In infants less than 3 months, values less than 2500 may be abnormal.[3] In addition, delayed or an absent response of cutaneous anergy is often found in moderate-to-severe malnutrition; however, the relationship is nonspecific.[1]

Clinical Elements

All physicians should perform a clinical examination to assess the nutritional status of a patient. The hair, face, eyes, mouth, tongue, gums, skin, nails, glands, musculoskeletal and neurologic system can provide clues to a possible nutrient deficiency. Specifically, look for rashes or dermatitis, nail or hair changes, pale or dry mucous membranes, decreased skin turgor, red or bleeding gums, dental caries, missing or broken teeth, subnormal body temperature, and pulse or blood pressure.[4]

Dietary Assessment

Perhaps the most important component of the nutritional assessment is the dietary assessment. A physician can perform a brief dietary intake evaluation asking parents or caregivers for information on a child's daily diet. Socioeconomic, religious, and ethnic factors should be considered when discussing the types of food a patient consumes. Questions related to the following information are a good guide to elicit necessary information about a child's diet:

- Frequency, amount, and type of feedings
- Use of oral supplements such as milk, juices, water
- Vitamin, mineral, and herbal usage
- Introduction of solid foods for infants
- Allergies or intolerances
- Aversions or preferences
- Chewing or swallowing difficulties

MALNUTRITION AND FAILURE TO THRIVE

Throughout childhood, healthy pediatric patients should gain steady weight and plot appropriately on growth curves. Lack of weight gain or weight loss is

cause for concern in a child and should be promptly addressed. However, it is necessary to evaluate a trend of growth rather than one isolated point on a growth curve. Plotting the child's weight versus height ratio on the chart provides valuable information. A child whose weight is below the fifth percentile, but whose weight/height ratio is within normal limits is likely to have a height gain problem rather than a primary nutritional deficiency. Weight-for-height is in addition a measure used to identify thin, tall children who are at nutritional risk and would be missed if relied on weight/age charts alone.

A weight decrease of more than two major percentiles (e.g., falling, in time, from the 75th to the 25th percentile) is considered evidence of growth failure. The following points are some of the criteria used to identify growth failure:

1. Growth below a specified percentile on growth charts: weight-for-age plotting less than the fifth percentile in the absence of developmental delay or weight-for-height plotting less than the fifth percentile.
2. Poor growth velocity: decreased growth velocity where weight falls more than two major percentiles over 3–6 months or decrease of more than two standard deviations over a 3–6-month period.

Failure to Thrive

On the spectrum of growth failure is the diagnosis of failure to thrive. FTT is a complex diagnosis that involves a multitude of factors including the health of the child as well as family, economic, and psychosocial conditions. Historically, failure to thrive was classified as either organic or nonorganic. Organic failure to thrive was identified as malnutrition related to a medical condition causing inadequate intake, absorption, or usage of nutrients. Nonorganic failure to thrive was related to social or behavioral dysfunction leading to inadequate nutrition.

Classification of Malnutrition

If a patient meets the criteria for failure to thrive, the degree of growth failure must be assessed with the use of equations before making nutrition recommendations and deciding if a patient needs hospitalization. The Waterlow classification is used to assess the degree of malnutrition from acute malnutrition (wasting) to chronic malnutrition (stunted growth). NCHS growth charts (www.cdc.gov/ growthcharts) are used to obtain percentiles for the following formulas:

Acute nutritional status

$$= \frac{\text{actual weight} \times 100}{\text{50th percentile weight/height}}$$

Chronic nutritional status

$$= \frac{\text{actual weight} \times 100}{\text{50th percentile height/age}}$$

Nutritional Status	Acute	Chronic
Stage 0 (normal)	Greater than 90%	Greater than 95%
Stage 1 (mild)	81–90%	90–95%
Stage 2 (moderate)	70–80%	85–89%
Stage 3 (severe)	Less than 70%	Less than 85%

If there are recent weight changes in a patient, they may be due to acute issues. A good rule of thumb to evaluate a significant weight change is >2% weight loss in 1 week, 5% weight loss in 1 month, 7.5% weight loss in 3 months, and 10% weight loss in 6 months. The following formulas evaluate body weight fluctuations:

% ideal body weight (IBW)

$$= \frac{\text{actual weight}}{\text{IBW at 50th percentile for age}} \times 100$$

$$\% \text{ usual body weight} = \frac{\text{actual weight}}{\text{usual weight}} \times 100$$

$$\% \text{ weight change} = \frac{\text{actual} - \text{usual weight}}{\text{usual weight}} \times 100$$

Calculating Higher Nutrient Needs

If a patient is diagnosed with failure to thrive, the goal is to promote catch-up growth and correct nutrient deficiencies. Catch-up growth is achieved by providing calories and protein in excess of the RDAs. Severely malnourished children have needed up to 150–240 cal/kg and 3.1–4.4 g/kg of protein for catch-up growth. Guidelines for estimating catch-up growth are as follows:[4,12]

1. Plot the child's height and weight on the NCHS growth chart
2. Determine the child's recommended calories for age (RDA)
3. Determine the ideal weight (50th percentile) for the child's height
4. Multiply the RDA calories by the ideal body weight for height (kg)
5. Divide this value by the child's actual weight

Catch-up Growth Requirements

1. Calories:

$$\frac{\text{RDA calories for age} \times \text{ideal weight for height (kg)}}{\text{actual weight}}$$

2. Protein:

$$\frac{\text{RDA for protein age} \times \text{ideal weight for height (kg)}}{\text{actual weight}}$$

Gastrointestinal Diseases and Failure to Thrive

A gastrointestinal disease is a common cause for FTT, but other medical conditions should be evaluated too. Table 31-4 reports some GI causes of FTT, which should be assessed when evaluating a child with FTT. If a patient is referred to a gastroenterologist for failure to thrive, diet therapy or other sources of nutritional support may become necessary.

MEDICAL NUTRITION THERAPY FOR GI DISORDERS

A number of gastrointestinal disorders require specific medical nutrition therapy. Recommendations are different from the nutrition regimens previously

TABLE 31-4

GASTROINTESTINAL SIGNS AND SYMPTOMS ASSOCIATED WITH INADEQUATE INTAKE OR EXCESSIVE LOSSES

Finding	Diagnostic Considerations
Inadequate Intake	
Pain (esophageal, abdominal)	Gastroesophageal reflux
	Hiatal hernia
	Milk-protein intolerance
	Lactose intolerance
	Overfeeding
	Acute gastroenteritis
	Inflammatory bowel disease
	Inflammation or obstruction of biliary tract
	Pancreatitis
	Intermittent volvulus
	Intussusception
Swallowing difficulties (dysphagia)	Tracheo-esophageal fistula
	Mass or tumor
	Atresia or stenosis
	Stricture, web, ring
	Neuromuscular dysfunction
	Viral or fungal mucosal infection
Poor appetite	Excessive gastric acidity
	Dysmotility
	Zinc deficiency
	Dehydration or inadequate caloric intake
	Constipation
Excessive Losses	
Regurgitation/spitting up	Gastroesophageal reflux
	Esophageal disorders
Vomiting—nonbilious emesis	Gastric outlet obstruction
	Protein hypersensitivity
	Gastroenteritis
	Pancreatitis
	Hepatitis
	Cholecystitis
	Appendicitis
Vomiting—bilious emesis	Volvulus
	Adhesions
	Intussusception
	Intestinal malformation

TABLE 31-4

GASTROINTESTINAL SIGNS AND SYMPTOMS ASSOCIATED WITH INADEQUATE INTAKE OR EXCESSIVE LOSSES (*CONTINUED*)

Finding	Diagnostic Considerations
Excessive Losses (Continued)	
Diarrhea and malabsorption	Milk-protein hypersensitivity
	Carbohydrate malabsorption
	Cystic fibrosis
	Celiac disease
	Inflammatory bowel disease

Source: Used with permission from Krebs NF. Gastrointestinal problems and disorders. In: Kessler DB, Dawson P (eds.), *Failure to Thrive and Pediatric Undernutrition*. Baltimore, MD: Paul H. Brookes, 1999, pp. 215–225.

described for normal pediatric patients and often include conventional medical therapy. The reader should obviously refer to the specific chapter in this book for a strictly medical approach to these disorders. This section of the chapter will only serve as a guideline to assist in the nutritional management of patients with the following conditions:

- Gastroesophageal reflux disease (GERD)
- Diarrhea
- Constipation
- Short bowel syndrome (SBS)
- Chronic liver disease
- Food allergy
- Irritable bowel disease
- Celiac disease (CD)
- Pancreatitis
- Lactose intolerance (LI)
- Irritable bowel syndrome

Gastroesophageal Reflux Disease

Infants

A common first-line therapy for gastroesophageal reflux disease in infants is using feed-thickeners. From a nutritional standpoint, thickened feedings increase the carbohydrate content of the diet, diluting the overall nutrient density of the formula or breast milk. Although there is no evidence from randomized, controlled trials to support the efficacy of the treatment,[13] there is some evidence suggesting that thickened feedings may indeed decrease the number of episodes of vomiting in infants with GERD. Therefore, up to 1 oz of rice cereal can be added per 2 oz of formula or breast milk.

Further dietary instruction for GERD includes careful infant feeding and burping, as well as preventing overfeeding. Larger feedings can increase gastric pressure and cause reflux; therefore, smaller, frequent feedings are recommended. To reduce reflux symptoms, infants should be kept in an upright position following feeding and avoid postprandial diaper changes. In addition, wearing loose clothing may help to minimize intraabdominal pressure, thereby reducing symptoms.[4]

Most cases of GERD resolve spontaneously in healthy infants. Infants with medical problems, such as cystic fibrosis, bronchopulmonary dysplasia, heart disease, and cerebral palsy, may develop pathologic GERD, leading to multiple episodes of emesis, feeding problems, and failure to thrive. Transpyloric, continuous tube feedings can be effective in correcting GERD-related emesis and FTT in infants.

Toddlers and Children

Toddlers and children experiencing GERD may show improvement if food is avoided 1–2 h prior to naps and bedtime. Certain foods should not be unnecessarily restricted, as food irritants vary from child to child. In general, foods that decrease lower esophageal sphincter (LES) pressure (chocolate, peppermint, and fatty foods) and esophageal irritants (citrus and tomato) can exacerbate GERD symptoms. If citrus and tomato are eliminated due to symptoms, alternate dietary sources of vitamin C should be offered.

The evaluation of nutrient intake of patients with GERD is difficult because of frequent reflux episodes. Use pediatric growth curves (www.cdc.gov/growthcharts) and follow growth parameters closely to help determine the adequacy of the diet.

Diarrhea

Excess consumption of high-sorbitol juices, such as apple or pear juice, is a common cause of diarrhea in young children. A thorough diet history is necessary before initiating therapy. No specific dietary changes (e.g., lactose-free milk and use of soy formulas) are recommended for infants and children with acute diarrhea. The old theories of bowel rest or diet restriction are no longer common practice (see Chap. 3). Unrestricted, age-appropriate diets do not worsen mild diarrhea and may actually lower stool output compared with oral replacement therapy (ORT) or intravenous fluids alone. Restricting the diet in an attempt to reduce diarrhea symptoms can contribute to malnutrition.[14,15]

For an infant or child with persistent diarrhea who cannot or will not ingest an adequate diet, tube-feeding is an option, provided that the child has some gastrointestinal absorptive capacity. In cases of persistent postenteritis diarrhea, infants may develop cow's milk protein allergy, which is best treated with the use of an oral or tube-fed protein hydrolysate formula.[15] Parenteral nutrition is used if the gastrointestinal tract is not a viable option for feeding; however, this feeding route can cause gut atrophy and promote bacterial translocation.[16]

Vitamin and Mineral Supplementation

Multivitamin and mineral supplements are given to most children with persistent diarrhea because micronutrients, such as folic acid, thiamin, vitamin B_{12}, vitamin K, vitamin A, iron, copper, calcium, magnesium, zinc, phosphorous, and selenium are often malabsorbed. Zinc deficiency in malnourished children with diarrhea, particularly for children in underdeveloped countries, is an issue.

Studies have found that zinc supplementation for children and infants with zinc deficiency significantly decreases the duration and amount of diarrhea, while improving nutritional status.[15]

Constipation

The Role of Fiber

Rarely, in clinical practice, can constipation be solely attributed to inadequate oral intake of fiber. However, nutrition therapy focusing on appropriate fiber and fluid intake is beneficial. When initiating a high-fiber diet, stress the gradual introduction of more fiber, as rapid introduction can cause abdominal gas, bloating, and pain.

High-fiber diets usually are not necessary for infants less than 12 months. Contrary to a widely held belief, the iron contained in infant formula has not been shown to cause constipation in infants. Nevertheless, if parents choose a low-iron formula, iron supplementation will become necessary at 4–6 months when iron stores deplete.

Calculation of Fiber Requirements

The fiber recommendation for children over 4 years old is 0.5 g of fiber/kg body weight. The recommended grams of fiber per day can also be calculated by taking the child's age and adding 5. For example, a 5-year-old child would have a goal of 10 g of fiber per day. Foods that are naturally high in fiber include fruits, vegetables, whole grains, bran, legumes, nuts, and seeds. Generally, children should have approximately 24–32 oz of fluid per day depending on age. In addition six to eight servings of fruits and vegetables each day is recommended with serving sizes varying according to the child's age. High-fiber diets are generally adequate in vitamins and minerals, as long as a variety of foods are selected.

Short Bowel Syndrome

Initial Nutritional Management

Total parenteral nutrition (TPN), or intravenous nutrition, should be started as soon as possible for a new patient with short bowel syndrome, customizing calories and protein for age. Replacement fluids may be needed to replace gastrointestinal losses and to facilitate fluid and electrolyte management. This solution should replicate the electrolyte composition of lost fluids.[17] Gastric contents approximately contain:

- Na: 140 meq/L
- K: 15 meq/L
- Cl: 155 meq/L

Additional sodium and zinc may be necessary to compensate for losses once the patient begins to have ostomy output or bowel movements.

Ileostomy output approximately contains:

- Na: 80–140 meq/L
- K: 15 meq/L
- HCO_3: 40 meq/L
- Cl: 115 meq/L
- Zn: 12 mg/L

While long-term parenteral nutrition is essential for some children with SBS, it is crucial to initiate enteral feedings soon because luminal nutrients promote intestinal adaptation. See Chap. 6 for a more complete presentation.

Enteral Nutrition

There is controversy about the optimal formula for infants and toddlers with SBS. If available, human milk is the optimal source of nutrition because it contains factors that stimulate mucosal hyperplasia and the activity of brush-border enzymes. Protein hydrolysate formulas or amino acid-based formulas are often used in infants with SBS. These formulas may reduce the risk of food allergy, which can develop during therapy for SBS. Older infants and toddlers may benefit from a fiber-containing enteral tube-feeding.

Fats

Enteral fats seem to be the most significant macronutrients for gastrointestinal adaptation. In animal models, long chain fats appear to be more effective than medium chain triglycerides in inducing this adaptation. Although MCTs might be absorbed slightly better, their lower caloric density

(7.0 kcal/g vs. 9.0 kcal/g) and higher osmotic load make them less desirable.

Carbohydrates

Carbohydrate excesses are problematic for the child with SBS. Infants, in particular, suffer from osmotic diarrhea when given large carbohydrate loads. While short chain fatty acids (SCFA) can be absorbed well and provide an important calorie source in the older child, this is not the case with infants and small children. Infants have such a rapid transit that the SCFA are produced in much lower quantities.

Oral Feedings

Careful attention is given to oral motor stimulation in the infant who is unable to eat by mouth. While continuous enteral feedings will remain the primary route of nutrition, an oral stimulation program will develop feeding skills, crucial in preventing oral aversion later in life. It can take months to years to wean a patient to exclusive oral nutrition. If possible, solid foods should be introduced at developmentally appropriate ages. There is a tremendous amount of variation in specific food tolerances, so foods should be introduced slowly, allowing 3 days to pass before trying any new foods. In general, meats might be better tolerated than a high-carbohydrate food like rice cereal because they are higher in protein and fat. Fruit juice should be avoided as it causes osmotic diarrhea. Lactose can be introduced later in the course of therapy.

Vitamin and Mineral Supplementation

Vitamin and mineral supplementation including iron, folate, and magnesium supplements is needed for the child with SBS who is completely weaned from TPN. Intramuscular vitamin B_{12} may be required in a dose of 1 mg every 3 months. Calcium and vitamin D absorption and bone density should be carefully monitored.

Chronic Liver Disease

Children with chronic liver disease often exhibit protein-energy malnutrition and growth failure secondary to fat malabsorption, poor oral intake, altered nutrient metabolism, and impaired liver synthetic function. Nutritional goals for this patient population include preventing protein-energy malnutrition and treating any nutritional deficits.[4] In addition, goals should optimize nutritional status before and after transplantation to precipitate a better outcome.[18]

The nutrition assessment is difficult in infants and children with chronic liver disease. Weight is confounded by fluid if ascites is present, and serum protein synthesis is depressed secondary to decreased liver synthetic function. Traditional markers of nutritional status, described earlier in this chapter, such as weight-for-height, weight-for-age, serum albumin, and serum prealbumin are no longer valid. In this case, skin fold thickness and mid-arm circumference measurements may be better nutritional markers.

Energy Requirements

Energy needs vary depending on the type of liver disease present. For infants and children with extrahepatic biliary atresia, the most common form of chronic liver disease, a 30% increase in resting metabolic rate has been reported.[19] Infants and children with end-stage liver disease may require 130–150% of the RDA for energy. Energy requirements in older children and adolescents with chronic liver disease have not been studied. Continuous tube feedings are often required to meet the high nutritional requirements. If feasible, small amounts of oral feeds should be encouraged so feeding skills do not regress after transplantation.

Protein Requirements

Protein requirements vary depending on the stage and severity of liver disease. To start, the recommended dietary allowance for protein is recommended to prevent malnutrition and wasting. Optimal protein needs in this patient population are closer to 2.0–3.0 g/kg per day. Low protein diets are not recommended unless there is clinical evidence of protein intolerance, such as elevated plasma ammonia or hepatic coma.[4]

Carbohydrate Requirements

Patients with chronic liver disease are at risk for hypoglycemia secondary to decreased glycogen synthesis, impaired gluconeogenesis, and increased insulin levels. Due to these metabolic derangements, carbohydrates are an important energy source. Glucose polymers can be added to food or enteral feedings to help meet high caloric needs and prevent hypoglycemia. Small, frequent meals may also help to maintain euglycemia and meet nutritional needs.

Fat Requirements

Fat malabsorption is not present in all types of chronic liver disease; however, it does occur in conditions such as cholestatic liver diseases where there is decreased bile acid secretion into the intestinal tract. Medium chain triglycerides do not require bile acids and can be used to replace up to 75% of fat calories. MCTs can be added to the child's diet either by using one of several commercial infant and pediatric formulas that contain 40–85% of fat calories as MCT, or by adding them to milk or food. Older children may be able to use MCT oil in cooking or add a water-miscible form to drinks. In all cases, MCTs should be introduced slowly to avoid gastrointestinal symptoms. Care should be taken to prevent essential fatty acid deficiency by providing at least 3–4% of daily calories as linoleic and linolenic acid or 10% of total energy intake as long chain fat.

Vitamin and Mineral Supplementation

Malabsorption of fat-soluble vitamins can result in severe deficiencies, such as hyperkeratosis and xeropthalmia (vitamin A), rickets (vitamin D), neurologic abnormalities (vitamin E), and hemorrhagic disease (vitamin K). Supplementation with water-soluble forms of the vitamins is necessary in the presence of severe fat malabsorption. Suggested doses are as follows:

- Vitamin A : 5000–15,000 IU per day
- Vitamin D (25-hydroxycholecalciferol): 5–7 µg/kg per day

- Vitamin E: 100–500 mg per day
- Vitamin K: 1–10 mg per day

Serum levels should be checked every 3 months to avoid toxicity.

Calcium requirements may be higher in the patient with chronic liver disease secondary to malabsorption and poor vitamin D status. When cholestasis or bone disease is present, 25–100 mg/kg per day of elemental calcium and 25–50 mg/kg of phosphorous may be required to correct bone abnormalities. Iron, zinc, magnesium, and water-soluble vitamins may also require supplementation.

Liver Transplantation

Following liver transplantation, TPN is indicated until the gastrointestinal tract can be used. Tube feedings may become necessary until nutritional needs can be met orally. Oral aversion and developmental delay may be problematic in this patient population because of prolonged use of nutrition support prior to transplant. Occupational or speech pathologists should be consulted to assist with a treatment plan for these problems.

Ultimately, the patient should be transitioned to an age-appropriate, regular diet. Multivitamins may be needed in the posttransplant period. Additionally, magnesium and sodium bicarbonate may be required as some immunosuppressive medications waste these minerals.

Food Allergy

The overall goal of nutrition therapy for pediatric patients with food allergy is to avoid life-threatening reactions, while promoting growth and development. Simply providing a list of foods to avoid is not as helpful. After the diagnosis of food allergy has been made, a dietitian should provide the nutritional therapy. Therapy involves eliminating the identified food allergen(s) from the diet. Patients and caregivers must be educated on common food allergens, such as the milk, eggs, soy, wheat, and nuts hidden in foods. For example, processed meats, with the exception of kosher products, usually contain milk as filler and pose a problem to patients allergic to milk.

Elimination of the Allergen

While eliminating one food allergen may be relatively easy, eliminating two or more allergens is more challenging, increasing the likelihood of nutritional inadequacy. Vitamin and mineral supplements will become necessary to meet the RDAs, if requirements cannot be met with food. For example, a milk-free diet is deficient in calcium, protein, riboflavin, and vitamins A and D, unless sufficient substitutions are made. Nondairy creamers and rice milk are poor substitutes, as they do not contain high-quality protein and calcium. A diet that restricts milk, eggs, meats, and fish is protein-deficient and requires supplementation. Grain-free diets, particularly when multiple grains are restricted, are deficient in B vitamins, iron, calories, and carbohydrates. Diets that eliminate citrus are deficient in vitamin C and folic acid and require supplementation.

Feeding the Allergic Patient

Breast milk is the optimal source of nutrition for infants, some infants may develop symptoms of food allergy while breast-fed (see the specific chapter). In this instance, maternal restriction of cow's milk, soy, egg, fish, peanuts, and tree nuts may be helpful. If this does not improve symptoms or if the diet restrictions become too difficult for the mother to adhere to, hypoallergenic infant formulas based on protein (extensive) hydrolysates should be used as a breast-feeding alternative.[20] Hypoallergenic formulas include Alimentum (Ross Laboratories, Columbus, OH), Pregestimil (Mead Johnson, Evansville, IN), and Nutramigen (Mead Johnson, Evansville, IN). These formulas are preferred over soy-based products, as approximately 25–60% of infants with food-induced proctocolitis and enterocolitis have parallel reactions with soy. Rarely (about 5% of allergic babies), these reactions can also occur with both whey and casein hydrolysate formulas. In this instance, or in the presence of multiple, severe food hypersensitivity, true elemental diets, i.e., amino acid-based formulas, are required to decrease symptoms while meeting nutritional needs. Elemental formulas, such as Neocate, Neocate One Plus, and E028 (Scientific Hospital Supplies,

Gaithersburg, MD), as well as Vivonex Pediatric (Sandoz, Minneapolis, MN) can be used in these challenging situations (refer to Table 31-2 for detailed macro- and micronutrient values on the formulas).

Patient Resources

Educating patients and families about manufacturer ingredient changes and product recalls is essential in the ongoing management of food allergy. The Food Allergy and Anaphylaxis Network (FAAN) has many helpful resources. Their contact information is available in the resource section.

Inflammatory Bowel Diseases

The objectives of nutrition therapy in inflammatory bowel disease are to control symptoms, maintain electrolyte balance, prevent growth retardation and nutritional deficiencies, and allow for temporary remission of IBD. Chronic malnutrition appears to be the primary cause of growth impairment that is common in children with IBD. Self-limited intake, in an attempt to reduce symptoms of cramping and diarrhea, is the major cause of malnutrition in this group of patients; a careful diet history, with attention to symptoms, is imperative.

Energy Needs

As many children with IBD may require catch-up growth, 140–150% of the RDA for both calories and protein may be needed. Because these needs are difficult to meet by oral intake alone, nutrition support may be warranted. Some studies have demonstrated increased growth rates with parenteral nutrition support and others have achieved similar beneficial results with enteral nutrition support. As parenteral nutrition is associated with greater complications and cost, enteral nutrition should be used as the primary feeding route for the nutrition support of children with IBD.

Low Residue Diets and Lactose Use

Controlled studies have not supported the use of a low-residue diet. However, such a diet should be used in the management of IBD, when there is a history of stricture or when the colon is extensively involved. Patients do not need to restrict lactose, as lactase deficiency and lactose intolerance are no more common in this patient population than what is seen in an age- and ethnically-matched control population. Moreover, as no therapeutic diet offers long-term benefit, an unrestricted, healthful diet should be encouraged in the absence of active disease.

Vitamin and Mineral Supplementation

If malabsorption is present, which is more common in Crohn's disease than ulcerative colitis, vitamins and minerals need to be supplemented. Fat-soluble vitamins, A, D, E, and K, are required for the patient with fat malabsorption, and therapeutic doses of iron, calcium, magnesium, zinc, vitamin B_{12}, and folic acid may also be required.

Celiac Disease

Celiac disease is unique in that it is one gastrointestinal disorder that is solely managed by lifelong, strict adherence to a diet: the gluten-free diet.

Gluten is a protein consisting of gliadin and glutenin. Prolamines are the water-insoluble fraction of gluten. The prolamines that are toxic in CD are gliadin in wheat, hordein in barley, and secalin in rye. Avenin, the prolamine in oats, was for a long time included in the toxic group; strong scientific evidence that supports that consuming oats is safe for both adults and children with CD. Although oats have been proven to be absolutely safe for children and adults with CD, many support groups and professional medical associations do not freely advocate their use because uncontaminated oats may be difficult to find due to concerns on possible manufacturing contamination.

The Gluten-free Diet

Foods, supplements, and medications containing wheat, barely, rye, and their derivatives need to be avoided. This can be quite daunting, as gluten is present in so many processed foods, and food labeling is often ambiguous. The gluten-free diet can be nutritionally complete, as long as a variety of foods are chosen. One exception may be a risk of inadequate dietary thiamin, riboflavin, and niacin, as many gluten-free products are not enriched with these vitamins.

If malabsorption is present, patients may need extensive supplementation to correct nutritional deficiencies. Iron, folate, B_{12}, calcium, fat-soluble vitamins, and zinc may all be required. While lactose intolerance can coexist with CD, it is usually temporary and lactase activity rebounds with villous regeneration. Lactose is restricted only if symptoms are present (see Chap. 18).

Pancreatitis

Acute

The nutritional goal for the child with pancreatitis is to prevent malnutrition and growth failure, while providing an adequate diet that does not exacerbate symptoms. For a child with a complex, lengthy course of acute pancreatitis, oral feeding may not be possible for several weeks. In these circumstances, to prevent nutritional deficits that can develop quickly, TPN should be started. There are no evidence-based guidelines for managing the refeeding phase in children with acute pancreatitis. Relying on serum levels of amylase and lipase is not a valid parameter. It is generally accepted to try clear liquids when the ileus has resolved and the patient feels hungry.

Chronic

Chronic pancreatitis places a child at greater risk of malnutrition and subsequent growth failure because of recurrent pain, poor oral intake, and steatorrhea. The use of oral nutritional supplements, enteral feeding, or TPN is indicated to prevent or correct malnutrition in the child with chronic pancreatitis. In general, fat should not be restricted in order to control symptoms. Rather, adequate dietary fat should be encouraged, with the use of pancreatic enzymes, if required.

Lactose Intolerance

Lactose intolerance is the term used to describe the adverse clinical effect of lactose ingestion in individuals who have either congenital lactase deficiency or late-onset (also called "adult-type") lactase deficiency. Congenital lactase deficiency is extremely rare and presents in neonatal mage with profuse osmotic type diarrhea at first feedings (see Chap. 3). This exceptionally rare condition clearly requires strict adherence to a lactose-free diet. Patients with late-onset lactose intolerance, the most common form, typically tolerate a low lactose regimen.

Several lactose-free infant formulas are available for infants with LI as shown in Table 31-2. Older children should eliminate milk and dairy products from their diets. In this instance, the risk for nutritional deficiencies is similar to that of children following a milk-free diet (see section FOOD ALLERGY).

Tolerance to lactose-containing foods varies amongst patients. Most patients can handle the small amounts of lactose in foods such as yogurt with active cultures or aged cheeses. Commercially available lactose-free products and lactase enzyme drops and tablets are also used in the management of LI.

Irritable Bowel Syndrome

It is generally accepted (see Chap. 6) that dietary manipulation and drug therapy can help to relieve symptoms in this poorly understood disorder. To promote bowel regularity, a regular diet with adequate fiber is recommended.[4] If painful gas is problematic, patients should avoid gum chewing, rapid eating, excess amounts of carbonated beverages, legumes, cruciferous vegetables, and fructose or sorbitol-containing foods.

TUBE-FEEDING

Indications

When a pediatric patient cannot ingest, digest, or absorb an adequate amount of macro- and micronutrients through oral diets, tube feedings become necessary. Patients can rely on a tube-feeding regimen as their sole source of nutrition or partial supplementation. Tube-feeding regimens can be creatively scheduled to maximize calories and protein and minimize time on a feeding pump.

There are several medical conditions that necessitate the use of tube feeding. Functional indications include

- Neurologic disorders
- Neuromuscular diseases
- Prematurity
- Genetic and metabolic conditions
  Structural indications include
- Tracheoesphageal fistula
- Esophageal atresia
- Cleft palate

Obstruction indications consist of cancer of the head/neck, as well as intubation. Injury indications include trauma or sepsis and surgery.

Feeding Routes

A tube-feeding enterostomy can be placed at a variety of sites along the gastrointestinal tract. Two factors to consider when determining what type of tube and which feeding route is best is the risk of aspiration and the duration planned for the feeding. When there is an aspiration risk, such as patients with an impaired gag reflex, delayed gastric emptying, frequent vomiting, or severe gastroesophageal reflux, feeding into the small bowel is the preferred choice since there is a reduced risk of aspiration beyond the pylorus. With respect to duration, feeding tubes through the nose, whether gastric or enteric, should be in place for a few weeks. If tube-feeding will last longer than about 4–6 weeks, the patient should be considered for a more permanent enterostomy for feeding.

Formula Selection

Formula selection is dependent on several factors: nutritional and fluid requirements, age, activity level, medical condition, gastrointestinal function, route of delivery, osmolality, renal solute load, caloric density, viscosity, cost, food intolerance, allergy, and family lifestyle and schedule.

Methods of Delivery

The two most common methods of enteral nutrition delivery are continuous and intermittent feeding. The choice depends on the route of administration and the ability of a patient to take nutrition by mouth.

Continuous feeds infuse at constant rate from several hours per day to a full 24 h. These feedings are recommended for patients at risk for refeeding syndrome, fed postpylorically, or when the intestinal mucosa is extensively damaged by disease or surgery. Continuous feeds can run overnight for those patients taking minimal oral intake during the day.

Intermittent bolus feeding mimics mealtimes during the day and requires minimal equipment. Feedings are administered by gravity over 15–30 min on a schedule of about every 2–4 h. This method of delivery is best for the ambulatory patient, allowing freedom away from pump.

The Use of Breast Milk in Tube Feedings

The intermittent or bolus feeding schedule is the preferred method of tube feeding delivery of human milk. When breast milk is delivered at a continuous rate, fat in the milk separates and collects in the infusion system: 20% of calories can be lost. When residual milk is flushed, a large fat bolus will be delivered to the patient and patients with impaired gastrointestinal tracts may not tolerate this bolus.

Initiation and Advancement of Tube Feedings

The modalities of initiating and advancing tube feedings vary from institution to institution. In general, continuous drip feedings should begin at 1–2 mL/kg per hour and advance 0.5–1.0 mL/kg per hour every 8–24 h until feeding reaches nutritional goal. Intermittent feedings begin at 25% of volume goal on the first day, dividing the formula equally over 5 to 8 feedings. Increase volume by 25% per day as tolerated. Intermittent feedings should be administered by gravity for 15–30 min.

Evaluation and Monitoring of Tube Feedings

A patient's tolerance to a tube-feeding regimen requires close evaluation and monitoring. Presence or absence of diarrhea, vomiting, and abdominal distention are gastrointestinal parameters to check frequently, especially with a new tube feeding regimen. Electrolytes, fluid status, and renal function should be routinely monitored. The mechanical intricacies, such as tube position and site care, cannot be ignored. Growth parameters such as height, weight, and head circumference should be monitored to assess the effectiveness of the regimen.

There is controversy about holding tube feedings for residuals in the stomach, especially for the critically ill. A single high residual of >1.5–2 times the hourly rate of infusion should not require feedings to stop. Physicians and the medical team should review medications and the medical condition of the patient as a contributing factor in a high residual. Treatment can involve decreasing the rate by half for a few hours or placing the tube in the transpyloric position.

Complications of Tube Feedings

Tube feeding complications are classified as mechanical, metabolic/nutritional, gastrointestinal, and developmental problems. The composition of the formula, patient's clinical condition, and mechanical administration of tube-feeding should guide any changes made to a tube-feeding or schedule if a patient has any of the listed complications below:

- *Mechanical*: Complications are related to size, position of tube, and the flow of formula through a tube-feeding. The tube may be uncomfortable for patient due to its size and may need to be switched for a smaller tube. In addition, the tube can become occluded from medications. Routine flushing after medication administration can help prevent any occlusions.
- *Metabolic/nutritional*: The most common complication is over- or underhydration. This condition is more common with renal, cardiac, or hepatic diseases. Other complications include hypoglycemia, electrolyte imbalances, inadequate weight gain, and vitamin, mineral, or trace element deficiencies. Routine

monitoring of lab values, I/Os, and clinical status is imperative when addressing these issues.
- *Developmental*: If patients have feeding tube access for long periods of time, they may not learn to take nutrition by mouth and miss important developmental skills in feeding. Pediatric speech pathologists or occupational therapists should work closely with patients to preserve oral function.
- *Gastrointestinal*: These complications include nausea, vomiting, diarrhea, constipation, and fat malabsorption. Physicians should evaluate whether complications stem from formula intolerance, a mechanical cause, or some other factor such as medications. Sometimes the smell of a tube-feeding formula will make patients nauseous.

Transition to Oral Feeds

The transition to oral feedings requires a thorough evaluation of the nutritional status of the patient. Criteria include

- Resolution of the initial reason a tube-feeding was started
- Quality of oral and motor skills
- Speech and swallow pathologist documenting adequate and safe swallowing mechanisms
- Evaluation of social situation and caretaker readiness

The transition is completed slowly. Patients receiving continuous tube-feeding should move toward bolus or nocturnal feedings while oral feedings are evaluated during daytime hours. Tube-feeding should be decreased in 25% increments to carefully evaluate the patient's ability to consume adequate calories by mouth. Once a patient is taking 75% of estimated calories, a tube-feeding can be discontinued.

TOTAL PARENTERAL NUTRITION

Parenteral nutrition or intravenous nutrition becomes necessary for patients who cannot meet their requirements through the enteral route by either oral intake or the previously described tube feedings. Parenteral nutrition does not enter the lymphatic system or portal circulation, but circulates in a form used by cells for energy production, maintenance, and growth of tissues. Nutrients routinely included in parenteral nutrition solutions are glucose, amino acids, fat emulsion or lipid, vitamins, minerals, and trace elements. Individual institutions should have policies on the administration of medications included in a parenteral nutrition regimen.

Clinical Indications

Neonates

Parenteral nutrition support should begin if the neonate will have little to no enteral feeding for at least 3 days. Recent data for the very low birth weight (<1500 g) infant indicates that parenteral nutrition should be initiated within 24 h of birth. Some institutions provide standard intravenous solutions of amino acids, dextrose, and electrolytes as the patient's first fluids and begin lipids within 24 h. Premature infants are at greater risk for nutritional deficiencies because of their higher metabolic rate, lower body stores of nutrients, and immature digestive and absorptive capacity. In addition, premature infants are at risk for developing necrotizing enterocolitis, affecting the ability to tolerate enteral feedings.

Pediatric Patients

In the older child, parenteral nutrition should be initiated if the patient will have little to no oral or enteral intake for 5–7 days. Indications for parenteral nutrition in the pediatric patient include, but are not limited to, gastrointestinal dysfunction due to congenital or acquired anomalies (e.g., short gut syndrome), inflammatory bowel disease, hepatic failure, pancreatitis, severe pulmonary disease, respiratory failure, and hypercatabolic states such as burn injury, trauma, cancer, and chylothorax.

Vascular Access

Vascular access depends on the age of the patient coupled with the medical condition. The common

term used for parenteral nutrition by central access is total parenteral nutrition. Central access is recommended if parenteral nutrition is needed for more than 7 days and nutrient needs are high. Peripheral access, known as peripheral parenteral nutrition (PPN), is most often used as a nutritional source for less than 7–14 days or if central line access is not available. The peripheral route is not ideal for fluid restricted infants and small children. These patients require solutions with dextrose greater than 12.5% and amino acids in concentrations that would increase the osmolality of the solution and place the patients at risk for phlebitis and skin sloughing.

Nutritional Components of Parenteral Nutrition

Two guides were developed at the University of Chicago to calculate parenteral nutrition for neonatal and pediatric patients. Methods by other institutions may vary. While reading the text, refer to Table 31-5 for the neonatal population and Table 31-6 for the pediatric population.

Fluids

Fluid management requires balancing estimated needs with the dynamic changes in clinical status. For example, a sick newborn may only need 40–80 cc/kg for the first day of life and move toward 100–150 cc/kg by 1 week of life. In contrast, if the patient has minimal to no urine output, fluid needs may be only 45 cc/kg. In conditions of extreme fluid needs, such as diabetes insipidus, requirements may be as high as 400 cc/100 kcal.

When an arterial line is needed for blood gas monitoring, the equivalent fluid and sodium provided by the arterial line are subtracted from the fluid and sodium in the parenteral nutrition solution. In addition, fluid needed for medications, such as dopamine and midazolam, must be considered in the total fluid requirements

Calories

Calorie requirements are influenced by many of the same factors that affect fluid status. Parenteral requirements for energy are lower than enteral

TABLE 31-5

NEONATAL PARENTERAL NUTRITION GUIDE

1. Determine calculation weight: Use birthweight until reachieved; actual weight thereafter
2. Determine fluids allowance for TPN: Total fluids = dextrose and protein (HAL) + intralipid/fat (IL)
3. Sources of calories:
    a. Fat (IL): Start at 1.0 g/kg using 20% IL; advance 0.5 g/kg every other day to IL goal of 2.5–3.0 g/kg. Check triglyceride weekly. Do not advance if TG >150 mg/dL; do not exceed 1.0 g/kg if on phototherapy for first week of life (especially for patients <30 weeks)

    To determine cc/h: (1.0 g/kg × wt (kg) × 100 cc/20 g)/24 h. For example: 20% IL = 20 g/100 cc

    b. Carbohydrate (dextrose): Start at 6-8 mg/kg per min; advance daily by 0.5–1.0 mg/kg per min; usually do not exceed 10–12 mg/kg per min, especially if patient is NPO. Check blood sugars daily. Do not exceed 12.5% in a PIV and usually 20–25% in central line

    To determine mg/kg per min = ((dextrose/6) × infusion rate)/weight

    c. Protein (amino acids): TrophAmine; start at 1.5 g/kg and advance daily by 0.5 g/kg per day to goal of 2.5–3.5 g/kg; provide 3.5 g/kg for preterms <1200g. Add cysteine (40 mg/g of TrophAmine in dextrose/protein bag). Limit TrophAmine in renal/liver failure. Limit amino acids to 2.0% with peripheral IV/peripheral PCVC
4. Determining calorie (kcal) content: Caloric goals: 90–100 kcal/kg per day
    a. Dextrose: % dextrose = g dextrose/100cc; therefore kcal from dextrose = (g dextrose/100 cc) × (vol. in cc dextrose/protein (HAL) received) × 3.4 kcal/g dextrose. For example: 150 cc of 12.5%: ((12.5 g/100 cc) × 150cc) × 3.4 kcal/g = 63.8 kcal
    b. Intralipid: 2 kcal/cc for 20% IL
    c. Protein: Consider protein as a source for maintenance and growth of protein stores/muscle; 4 kcal/g
5. Calcium: 300–600 mg/kg Ca gluconate; start at low end and increase as needed; limit to 200–300 mg/kg in a peripheral line
6. Phosphorus: Start at 0.7 mmol/kg in most cases; advance to 1–2 mmol/kg; write as meq of cation (1.5 meq K Phos provides 1 mmol Phos; 1.3 meq Na Phos provides 1 mmol Phos). Restrict in renal failure
7. Magnesium: 0.1–0.5 meq/kg. Restrict in renal failure, may not need Mg in the first few days of life if serum level is high due to maternal $MgSO_4$; requirements may increase with Amphotericin
8. Electrolytes:
    a. Sodium: 2–4 meq/kg; may not need first few days of life; greater than normal requirements may indicate greater than normal losses (note: arterial line fluid contains Na: 0.45NS = 77 meq/L; 0.9NS = 154 meq/L)
    b. Potassium: 2–3 meq/kg; may not need first few days of life; greater than normal requirements may indicate greater losses; furosemide, chlorothiazides, Amphotericin increase losses; spironolactone decreases losses; restrict in renal failure
    c. Acetate/chloride: % of each anion used depends on acid/base balance or acetate can be used as a source of base in acidotic patient
9. Vitamins: MVI-Pediatric: 2 cc/kg up to 5 cc; no need for extra phytonadione
10. Trace elements: Not needed in short term (1–2 weeks) TPN; Dose Peds TraceLyphomed for premature/full-term infants: 0.2 cc/kg; decrease to 0.1 cc/kg or withhold in cholestasis; decrease to 0.1 cc/kg if urine output inadequate
11. Zinc: Premature: 0.4 mg/kg; full term: 0.3 mg/kg with no TE; decrease to 0.3 g/kg and 0.2 mg/kg with TE
12. Selenium: Not needed for short term TPN; dose at 2 μg/kg to max of 30 μg per day
13. Heparin: 1 U/cc for central lines, but not for peripheral lines

TABLE 31-5

NEONATAL PARENTERAL NUTRITION GUIDE (*CONTINUED*)

14. Peripheral TPN: Do not exceed 800 mOsm/L. Dextrose and protein contribute the majority of mOsm
15. Calcium/phosphorus precipitation: The Pediatric Nutrition Support Service uses precipitation curves to determine Ca/Phos limits

Routine monitoring

I/Os, blood and urine glucose (q day), basic metabolic panel, Ca, Mg, P (q day until stable then 2–3 times/week). Hepatic panel, GGTP, triglyceride level (baseline then 1 time/week). Weights, head circumference (q day to QOD). Length (q 1–2 weeks). Follow neonatal normal laboratory values for respective institutions

Source: For use at the University of Chicago Children's Hospital under the guidance of the Pediatric Nutrition Support Service, Department of Pharmaceutical Services, University of Chicago Hospitals: JoAnn Kaiser Froehlke, R.D; Ellen Newton, R.N (revised 8/03).

TABLE 31-6

PEDIATRIC PARENTERAL NUTRITION GUIDE

1. Determine calculation weight: Use birthweight until reachieved; actual weight thereafter
2. Determine fluids allowance for TPN: Total fluids = dextrose and protein (HAL) + intralipid/fat (IL)
3. Sources of calories:
   a. Fat (IL): Start at 1.0 g/kg using 20% IL; advance 0.5 g/kg every day to achieve caloric goals. Check triglyceride weekly. Do not advance if TG > 200 mg/dL

      To determine cc/hr: (1.0 g/kg × wt (kg) × 100 cc/20 g)/24 h. For example: 20% IL = 20 g/100 cc

   b. Carbohydrate (dextrose): Start at 4–6 mg/kg per min and advance daily by 1.0–1.5 mg/kg per min; usually do not exceed 10 (>12 years) or 10–12 (<12 years) mg/kg per min, especially if patient is NPO. Cycled TPN (see no. 16) may go above limits since TPN infuses over shorter time and faster rate. Check blood sugars daily. Do not exceed 10% in a peripheral IV and usually 20–25% in central line; central PICC lines are confirmed by x-ray as central line; peripheral PICC can go to 12.5% dextrose

      To determine mg/kg per min = (% dextrose × infusion rate)/(6 × weight)

   c. Protein (amino acids): Using TrophAmine for infants/children <2 years and Travesol for >2 years; start at 1.0 g/kg and advance daily by 0.5 g/kg per day to protein goal (1.0–2.5 g/kg depending on age and diagnosis); use cysteine at a dose of 40 mg/g of TrophAmine. Limit protein in renal/liver failure usually to 1.0 g/kg
4. Determining calorie (kcal) content: Individualized based on recommended dietary allowances (see section RDA)
5. Calcium: 50–100 mg Ca gluconate/kg (lower doses for older children/adolescence; usually a max of 4.0 g Ca gluconate/bag for teenagers and young adults)
6. Phosphorus: Usually start at 0.3–1.0 mmol/kg; start at lower dose; write as meq of cation. (1.5 meq K Phos provides 1 mmol Phos; 1.3 meq Na Phos provides 1 mmol Phos). Restrict in renal failure
7. Magnesium: 0.2–0.5 meq/kg. Restrict in renal failure; requirements may increase with Amphotericin
8. Electrolyte requirements
   a. Sodium: 2–4 meq/kg; need for greater than normal requirements may indicate greater than normal losses (e.g., gastrointestinal, urine, or chest tube losses)
   b. Potassium: 2–3 meq/kg; restrict in renal failure; requirements may increase with furosemide, chlorothiazide, Amphotericin; decrease with spironolactone
   c. Acetate/chloride: % of each anion used depends on acid/base balance

(Continued)

TABLE 31-6

PEDIATRIC PARENTERAL NUTRITION GUIDE (*CONTINUED*)

9. Vitamins: <11 years: use MVI-Pediatric: 2 cc/kg up to 5 cc; ≥11 years: use MVI-12: 10 cc per day + phytonadione 1 mg per day (do not need additional phytonadione when using Infuvite)

10. Trace elements <11 years: PedsTE: 0.2 cc/kg; ≥11 years: MTE-4: 1 cc per day; withhold in cholestasis; decrease if urine output inadequate

11. Zinc: May be needed if patient has ostomy output or diarrhea

12. Selenium: 2 μg/kg to max of 30 μg per day

13. Heparin: Not used for central line unless infusion rate is slow (<10 cc/h). PCVCs require heparin at 1 U/cc

14. Peripheral TPN: Do not exceed 800 mOsm/L. Dextrose and protein contribute the majority of mOsm

15. Calcium/phosphorus precipitation: The Pediatric Nutrition Support Service uses precipitation curves to determine Ca/Phos limits

16. Cycling: Determine no. of hours in cycle (example: 24 → 20 → 16 →12). Divide volume of HAL by 1 h less than desired (e.g., if 20-h cycle, divide by 19 = rate for 18 h then divide rate in half to give the rate for the 1st hour and the 20th hour)

Routine monitoring

I/Os and blood glucose (1–2 times per week while advancing; then as needed if low/high blood sugars or on steroids). Hepatic profile, GGTP and triglyceride level (baseline then 1 times per week). Basic metabolic panel, Ca, Mg, P (q day until stable, then 2–3 times per week). Weight (every other day). Head circumference (if less than 3 years q 2 weeks). Length/height (weekly to monthly if followed outpatient). Follow pediatric normal laboratory values for respective institutions

Source: For use at the University of Chicago Children's Hospital under the guidance of the Pediatric Nutrition Support Service, Department of Pharmaceutical Services, University of Chicago Hospitals: JoAnn Kaiser Froehlke, R.D.; Ellen Newton, R.N.

requirements because calories are not needed for the digestion and absorption of nutrients. Clinicians often use the recommended dietary intakes as a starting place for energy requirements.[2] The calories provided can be modified based on an individual's clinical status. Specially designed ventilators or metabolic carts can be used in selected circumstances to determine resting energy expenditure using indirect calorimetry.

Fat

Fat, or lipid, is necessary for proper development of the retinas, brain, cell structure and function, and is a source of the essential fatty acids linolenic and linoleic acids. At least 4% of total calories must be provided in the form of lipid to prevent essential fatty acid deficiency.

Lipids should comprise 30–50% of calories. The goal for fat infusion on a kilogram (kg) basis varies depending on the patient's caloric needs and clinical status. Dosing of lipids in the preterm and very sick infant must be done carefully as the activity of the lipoprotein lipase, hepatic function, and supply of carnitine may be low or not fully developed. High doses of lipid may adversely affect the pulmonary and immune systems and solutions with more than 60% of calories as lipid may cause ketonemia. In any infant or child, stress can also contribute to the body's inability to metabolize lipid in an efficient manner. Therefore, serum triglyceride should be measured approximately once a week as part of a liver panel and levels should not exceed 150–200 mg/dL. Twenty percent lipid emulsions appear to be better tolerated than 10% lipid emulsions, especially in preterm infants, due to the relatively lower phospholipid/triglyceride weight ratio.

Carbohydrates

Dextrose is the major source of nonprotein calories in parenteral nutrition. It provides 3.4 cal/g and is dosed in terms of an infusion rate (mg/kg per min). An equation to determine mg/kg per min is shown in the parenteral nutrition guides.

Osmolarity

Dextrose and amino acids contribute to the osmolarity of the parenteral nutrition solution. Therefore, care must be given to the amount of dextrose and amino acid relative to fluid, as well as the type of access available for the solution.

At the University of Chicago, the dextrose and amino acid components are limited to a maximum of 800 mOsm/L for a peripheral line. To determine the contribution of mOsm from the dextrose and amino acids, each percent of dextrose contributes 50 mOsm/L, while each percent of amino acids contributes 100 mOsm/L.

Example. The dextrose in a 12.5% solution will contribute 625 mOsm/L.

$$12.5\% \times 50 \text{ mOsm/L} = 625 \text{ mOsm/L}$$

The protein in a 2.5% amino acid will contribute 250 mOsm/L.

$$2.5\% \times 100 \text{ mOsm/L} = 250 \text{ mOsm/L}$$

If combined, the two nutrients would contribute 875 mOsm/L. In peripheral parenteral nutrition, this would be excessive in osmolarity. To decrease the mOsm, fluid allowed for the TPN would need to be increased or the amount of dextrose or amino acids decreased.

Protein

Amino acids are needed for synthesis and maintenance of somatic and visceral proteins, enzymes, neurotransmitters, hormones, bile salts, and immunoglobulins. Commercial amino acid solutions provide 4 kcal/g and 0.16 g nitrogen per gram.

Specific amino acid requirements vary based on medical conditions, including prematurity. TrophAmine, the pediatric crystalline amino acid product, is used in the neonatal population because it mimics the plasma amino acid profile of the breast-fed infant and contains the essential amino acids taurine and tyrosine. Cysteine may become conditionally essential, but is added separately to parenteral solutions because of its unstable properties. For adequate nitrogen accretion, appropriate amounts of nonprotein calories are needed. For the preterm infant, approximately 70 nonprotein calories will achieve this goal. In the older child and adolescent, positive nitrogen balance is achieved with a nonprotein calorie (NPC) to nitrogen (N) ratio of 150–300:1.

Electrolytes

Electrolytes move from one space to another by concentration gradient, bulk flow, and active transport. Sodium, chloride, and bicarbonate are the predominant electrolytes in the extracellular space. Potassium and magnesium are the predominant electrolytes in the intracellular space. Certain types of stress, disease states, and medications can affect their distribution. Managing TPN electrolytes and intravenous fluids can be challenging and each electrolyte should be evaluated often and adjusted according to the medical course of a patient.

Calcium and Phosphorus

Adequate calcium and phosphorus are essential in bone mineralization. This is especially true for the premature infant, as 80% of calcium and phosphorus is accrued in bones during the last trimester. In TPN regimens, calcium and phosphorus amounts are limited because they can combine to form calcium phosphate that would precipitate. Conditions that increase the chances of the two combining in a solution include restricted volume, limited amino acids and dextrose, warm temperature of the TPN bag, exclusion of cysteine, and overdosing of calcium and phosphorus beyond recommendations. For optimal mineral retention and mineral homeostasis, a ratio by weight of calcium to phosphorus of 1.3–1.7:1 is recommended.

Trace Elements

Trace elements are substances that are found in the human body at concentrations less than 0.01% and function as cofactors in many enzymatic reactions. The essential trace elements include chromium, molybdenum, manganese, iron, cobalt, copper, selenium, and zinc. Deficiencies can occur, especially in the long-term TPN patient. Trace elements are not needed in short-term TPN usage. In patients with cholestasis, the dose of trace elements is either eliminated or reduced because of the risk of copper and manganese toxicity.

Iron

Iron is rarely added to parenteral nutrition solutions due to possible allergic reactions and the risk of iron overload. In preterm infants, frequent blood draws and low initial stores can cause iron deficiency. Blood transfusions can become a frequent source of iron during the critical periods. Once a preterm infant is being fed enterally and iron indices indicate that the patient is producing red blood cells, enteral iron supplementation can be added to the regimen. In children and adolescents on TPN, iron dextran is sometimes added to those patients with gastrointestinal blood loss.

Vitamins

The American Medical Association and the American Society of Clinical Nutrition recommend a separate parenteral vitamin solutions for infants and children less than 11 years of age and for older children and adults. Optimally, a specific preparation for preterm infants needs to be developed to provide doses appropriate to their needs. The present dose of 2 cc/kg up to 5cc per day may provide excess of some water-soluble vitamins and an inadequate amount of vitamin A.

Administration Considerations

Once the patient begins to feed, a sliding scale can be used to administer the combination of parenteral and enteral feeds. If a patient is eating, calorie counts can be evaluated to assist in the TPN weaning process. Fluid from tube feeds is subtracted from the total fluid allotted to the TPN. In the beginning of the wean, the parenteral nutrition prescription is still written as if the patient is not fed enterally in case the tolerance is an issue. As the patient tolerates more oral feeding or tube feeding, TPN can be weaned.

Example. If the infant weighs 1.5 kg and the fluid order for the TPN and feeds together equals 150 cc/kg, but the feeding order is 3 cc of breast milk (BM) every 3 h or 24 cc of BM per day, then:

150 cc/kg × 1.5 kg
    = 225 cc total volume per day or 9.4 cc/h
      (for 24 h)

225 cc − 24 cc of BM per day
    = 201 cc per day (volume remaining for TPN)
      or 8.4 cc/h

Cycling Parenteral Nutrition

In critically ill patients, the TPN is administered over 24 h because of the potential for metabolic and electrolyte abnormalities. Once a patient is more stable, the time needed to administer the TPN can be slowly shortened. This most often is applicable to children greater than 2 years of age and adolescents. In most cases, the TPN is tapered down by 1–4 h per day; the rate of TPN at the beginning and end of the cycle is half of the full rate.

TPN is often cycled at less than a 24-h rate because of medication incompatibility and insufficient access. Amphotericin B, acyclovir, metronadizole, and fentanyl cannot be administered in the same line as TPN. For example, if there is only one line available to infuse TPN and amphotericin then the TPN is stopped for 4 h to allow for the administration of the amphotericin. Each institution should have a different list of medications for which this is applicable.

Patient Monitoring and Complications

Patients receiving parenteral nutrition solutions need routine monitoring in the following areas:[7]

- Growth indicators such as weight, head circumference (for children less than 3 years old), and length or height should be measured daily to weekly to assess the nutrition provided.
- Gastrointestinal tolerance of any enteral nutrition or readiness for enteral nutrition can

be evaluated daily by monitoring abdominal girth, gastric residuals, episodes of emesis, and stool frequency and consistency.

- Electrolytes, minerals, blood counts should be measured initially and then weekly. Vitamins, trace elements, and other iron indices should be measured as needed.
- Fluid balance should be monitored daily to determine if fluids provided need modification.
- Daily blood glucose and weekly triglyceride levels monitor metabolic tolerance. Many of the metabolic complications are caused by either an under- or overdosed nutrient. A patient can exhibit signs of hyperglycemia on a glucose infusion rate that he or she has tolerated the previous week. To manage this patient, not only will the dextrose in the TPN need to be decreased, but the access site must be carefully examined for signs of infection. Another metabolic complication of parenteral nutrition is TPN-related cholestasis, commonly seen in infants receiving TPN for more than 2 weeks. Factors involved in the etiology of cholestasis include sepsis, lack of enteral feeding, and gastrointestinal complications that required surgery.
- Mechanical complications are associated with the catheter at the time of insertion and problems that may occur after insertion. Patients are at risk for pneumothorax during insertion of a central line. If heparin is not added to a central line, or a line is kinked, occlusion can occur. Phlebitis can occur if the concentration of dextrose, amino acids, or calcium is too high.
- Psychosocial complications often occur in the older child and adolescent receiving TPN. The patient may feel isolated because the joy and social aspect of eating and drinking with family and friends is not possible. In addition, the illness that necessitates parenteral nutrition includes frequent visits to the hospital or clinic, causing stress on the patient and family. A good support system in and out of the hospital is an important aspect of patient care.

Total Nutrient Admixtures

Total nutrient admixtures (TNAs) are parenteral nutrition solutions that contain all three macronutrients in one bag. The biggest advantage of using TNAs is convenience, which is significant in home administered TPN. When TNAs are used, it is important to examine the bag for any abnormalities, adhere to allowable hang times, and store the solution properly until use. The risk for physical changes in the solutions can occur, placing a patient at risk. For example, it is difficult to detect calcium and phosphorus precipitation due to the whitish color of the solution. In addition, if an excess cation is added to a TNA, phase separation can occur resulting in a layer of free oil. This separation may go undetected at first, but over time, a layer of yellow-brown oil droplets forms. It should also be noted that intravenous iron cannot be added to a TNA.

Home Parenteral Nutrition

Stable patients can receive parenteral nutrition at home if they are not able to meet enteral requirements. Indications for home parenteral nutrition (HPN) include short gut syndrome, intestinal pseudoobstruction, inflammatory bowel disease, acute pancreatitis, prolonged postoperative ileus, preparation for organ transplant, and cancer. A cycled TPN regimen is preferred to give more independence to a patient. The medical team should work with the home TPN patient to advance enteral feeds and eventually discontinue the use of the TPN.

The Role of the Home Care Company

Medical and educational support for the home parenteral nutrition patient is often a hospital-based team of physicians, nurses, social workers, dietitians, and pharmacists. TPN home care is costly, but is less than if the patient remained in the hospital for care. Nurses will visit homes and intervene if problems arise. Risk of septic complications is less at home because the patient is no longer exposed to sick patients in the hospital. The rate of at-home sepsis is also related to the ability of the patient or family member to take care of the catheter required for the parenteral nutrition and any medications.

References

1 Loughrey CM, Duggan C. Assessment of nutrition status: the role of the laboratory. In: Soldin SJ, Rifai N, Hicks JM (eds.), *Biochemical Basis of Pediatric Disease*. Washington DC: AACC Press, 1998, pp. 571–597.
2 National Research Council. Recommended Dietary Allowances, 10th ed. Washington, DC: National Academy Press, 1989.
3 Bessler S. Nutritional assessment. In: Samour PQ, Helm KK, Lang CE (eds.), *Handbook of Pediatric Nutrition*, 2nd ed. Maryland, MD: Aspen Publishers, 1999, pp. 17–42.
4 Williams CP. *Pediatric Manual of Clinical Dietetics*. Chicago, IL: The American Dietetic Association, 1998.
5 Chumlea WC, Guo SS. Physical growth and development. In: Samour PQ, Helm KK, Lang CE (eds.), *Handbook of Pediatric Nutrition*, 2nd ed. Maryland, MD: Aspen Publishers, 1999, pp. 3–15.
6 Anderson DM. Nutritional implications of premature birth, birth weight, and gestational age classification. In: Groh-Wargo S, Thompson M, Cox JH (eds.), *Nutritional Care for High-Risk Newborns*, 3rd ed. Chicago, IL: Precept Press, 2000, pp. pp. 4–5.
7 Groh-Wargo S. Recommended enteral nutrient intakes. In: Groh-Wargo S, Thompson M, Cox JH (eds.), *Nutritional Care for High-Risk Newborns*, 3rd ed. Chicago, IL: Precept Press, 2000, pp. 231–263.
8 Wessel JJ. Feeding methodologies. In: Groh-Wargo S, Thompson M, Cox JH (eds.), *Nutritional Care for High-Risk Newborns*, 3rd ed. Chicago, IL: Precept Press, 2000, pp. 321–339.
9 Lucas B. Normal nutrition from infancy through adolescence. In: Samour PQ, Helm KK, Lang CE (eds.), *Handbook of Pediatric Nutrition*, 2nd ed. Maryland, MD: Aspen Publishers, 1999, pp. 99–120.
10 Hansen JW, Boettcher JA. Human milk substitutes. In: Tsang RC, Zlotkin SH, Nichols BL, et al. (eds.), *Nutrition During Infancy*. Cincinnati, OH: Digital Educational Publishing, 1997, pp. 441–446.
11 Auestad N, Halter R, Hall RT, et al. Growth and development in term infants fed long-chain polyunsaturated fatty acids: a double-masked, randomized, parallel, prospective, multivariate study. *Pediatrics* 108:2, 2001.
12 Nevino-Folino N, Miller M. Enteral nutrition. In: Samour PQ, Helm KK, Lang CE (eds.), *Handbook of Pediatric Nutrition*, 2nd ed. Maryland, MD: Aspen Publishers, 1999, pp. 513–549.
13 Huang R-C, Forbes DA, Davies MW. Feed thickener for newborn infants with gastro-esophageal reflux. Cochrane Database Syst Rev (3):CD003211, 2002.
14 Baker SS, Davis AM. Hypocaloric oral therapy during an episode of diarrhea and vomiting can lead to severe malnutrition. *J Pediatr Gastroenterol Nutr* 27:1–5, 1998.
15 Guandalini S, Dincer AP. Nutritional management in diarrhoeal disease. *Baillieres Clin Gastroenterol* 12(4):697–717, 1998.
16 Hadfield RJ, Sinclair DG, Houldsworth PE, et al. Effects of enteral and parenteral nutrition on gut mucosa permeability in critically ill. *Am J Respir Crit Care Med* 23:1055–1060, 1995.
17 Warner BW, Vanderhoof JA, Reyes JD. What's new in the management of short gut syndrome in children. *J Am Coll Surg* 190(6):725–736, 2000.
18 Shepard RW, Chin SE, Cleghorn GJ, et al. Malnutrition in children with chronic liver disease accepted for liver transplantation: clinical profile and effect in outcome. *J Pediatr Child Health* 27:295–299, 1991.
19 Pierro A, Koletzko B, Carnielli V, et al. Resting energy expenditure is increased in infants and children with extrahepatic biliary atresia. *J Peditr Surg* 24:534–538, 1989.
20 American Academy of Pediatrics, Committee on Nutrition: Hypoallergenic infant formulas. *Pediatrics* 106(2):346–349, 2000.

Bibliography

Support Groups/Research Organizations

American Dietetic Association, 120 South Riverside Plaza, Suite 2000, Chicago, IL 60606-6995, 800-877-1600, www.eatright.org.
American Society for Parenteral and Enteral Nutrition, 8630 Fenton Street, Suite 412, Silver Spring, MD 20910, 800-727-4567, www.nutritioncare.org.
Celiac Disease Foundation, 13251 Ventura Blvd, Suite 1, Studio City, CA 91604-1838, 818-990-2354, www.celiac.org.

Crohn's & Colitis Foundation of America, Inc, 386 Park Avenue South, 17th Floor, New York, NY 10016-8804, 800-932-2423 or 212-685-3440, www.ccfa.org.

IBS Self Help Group, 3332 Yonge Street, PO Box 94074, Toronto, Ontario, Canada M4N 3RI, www.ibsgroup.org.

International Lactation Consultant Association, 1500 Sunday Drive, Suite 102, Raleigh, North Carolina, 27607, 919-861-5577, www.ilca.org.

Mead Johnson Nutritionals, 2400 West Lloyd Expressway, Evansville, Indiana 47721, 812-429-6399, www.mediajohnson.com.

National Digestive Diseases Information Clearinghouse (NDDIC), National Institute of Diabetes and Digestive and Kidney Diseases (NIDDK), National Institutes of Health (NIH), 2 Information Way, Bethesda, MD 20892-3570, 800-891-5389 or 301-654-3810, Email: nddic@info.niddk.nih.gov, Website: http://www.niddk.nih.gov.

Nestle Infant Nutrition, P.O. Box AW, Wilkes-Barre, Pennsylvania 18703, 800-628-2229, www.verybestbaby.com.

North American Society for Pediatric Gastroenterology, Hematology & Nutrition, 1501 Bethlehem Pike, P.O. Box 6, Flourtown, PA 19031, 215-233-0808, www.naspghan.org.

Novartis Nutrition, Consumer & Product Support, 445 State Street, Fremont, MI 49412, 800-333-3785, www.novartisnutrition.com.

Pediatric Crohn's & Colitis Association, Inc., P.O. Box 188, Newton, MA 02168, 617-489-5854, http://pcca.hypermart.net.

R.O.C.K. (Raising Our Celiac Kids), 3527 Fortuna Ranch Road, Encinitas, CA 92924, 858-395-5421, www.celiackids.com.

Ross Products Division, Abbott Laboratories, Inc., Columbus, Ohio 43215-1724 USA, 800-227-5767, www.rosspediatrics.com.

SHS North America, 9900 Belward Campus Dr., Suite 100, Rockville, MD 20850 800-365-7354, www.shsna.com.

The Celiac Sprue Association/USA, Inc., P.O. Box 31700, Omaha, NE 68131-0070, 402-558-0600, www.csaceliacs.org.

The Food Allergy and Anaphylaxis Network (FAAN), 10400 Eaton Place, Suite 107, Fairfax, VA 22030, www.foodallergy.org.

The Gluten Intolerance Group, 15110 10th Ave S.W., Suite A, Seattle, WA 98166-1820, 206-246-6652, www.gluten.net.

The Oley Foundation, 214 Hun Memorial, A-28, Albany Medical Center, Albany, NY 12208-3478, 800-776-6539, www.c4isr.com/oley.

Wyeth Nutrition, 170 Radnor-Chester Road, St. Davids, Pennsylvania 19087, 610-902-1200, www.wyethnutritionals.com.

INDEX

Page numbers followed by italic *f* or *t* indicate figures or tables, respectively.